PSYCHOLOGY OF TERRORISM

Psychology of Terrorism

EDITED BY

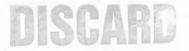

Bruce Bongar
Lisa M. Brown
Larry E. Beutler
James N. Breckenridge
Philip G. Zimbardo

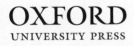

OXFORD

UNIVERSITY PRESS

2007

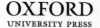

OXFORD
UNIVERSITY PRESS

Oxford University Press, Inc., publishes works that further
Oxford University's objective of excellence
in research, scholarship, and education.

Oxford   New York
Auckland   Cape Town   Dar es Salaam   Hong Kong   Karachi
Kuala Lumpur   Madrid   Melbourne   Mexico City   Nairobi
New Delhi   Shanghai   Taipei   Toronto

With offices in
Argentina   Austria   Brazil   Chile   Czech Republic   France   Greece
Guatemala   Hungary   Italy   Japan   Poland   Portugal   Singapore
South Korea   Switzerland   Thailand   Turkey   Ukraine   Vietnam

Library of Congress Cataloging-in-Publicaton Data
Psychology of terrorism / edited by Bruce Bongar . . . [et al.].
   p.   cm.
Includes bibliographical references.
ISBN–13 978–0–19–517249–2
ISBN 0–19–517249–3
1. Terrorism—Psychological aspects.   2. Disasters—Psychological aspects.
3. Victims of terrorism—Mental health.   I. Bongar, Bruce Michael.
[DNLM: 1. Terrorism—psychology.   2. Stress, Psychological —therapy.
3. Survivors— psychology.   WA 295 P9743 2006]

RC569.5.T47P83 2006
363.32019—dc22   2005034001

9 8 7 6 5 4 3 2 1
Printed in the United States of America
on acid-free paper

This book is dedicated to all those who fight terrorism, to all those who strive to prevent terrorism, and to all those whose lives have been irreparably scarred by terrorism.

Foreword

How do I answer the preschooler who asks, "Why does that man want to kill us?" during a nightly news broadcast. Why do wealthy suburbanites beg their primary care physicians to write prescriptions for Cipro (ciprofloxacin) when no outbreak of anthrax has ever occurred within hundreds of miles? How do we provide explanations of dispositional perceived risk, negativity bias, attributional error, and social amplification to the nightly news reporter who wants psychological sound bites? Not long ago few of us would have dreamed that we would face such questions.

What happens to people, both as individuals and members of social groups, when we suddenly find ourselves forced to question our fundamental assumptions about our basic safety, security, and well-being? What happens when that challenge appears suddenly in the form of massive destruction and loss of life from unanticipated sources and directions, accompanied by continuing threats from others we do not know and whose motives we cannot comprehend? Today, we know the answer: anxiety, fear, dread, and terror.

Terrorism in human history dates back at least to biblical times, although September 11, 2001, brought the full psychological and societal impact of massively destructive terrorist acts into sharp

emotional focus for Western society. During the following years we have had to confront the horror of significant civilian casualties, live with uncertainty and fear compounded by stumbling and intrusive efforts by government to protect us, all the while attempting to comprehend the willingness of other people from different cultures to gladly die in an effort to kill as many of us as possible.

As behavioral scientists and mental health practitioners, the years since 9/11 have forced us to contemplate a range questions long overlooked by many of our colleagues. Should we regard those who organize and perpetrate acts of terror as criminals or revolutionaries; antisocial personalities or religious ideologues; psychopaths or self-sacrificing advocates of radical social change; or all of the above? What treatment strategies will prove most effective for helping people who experience post traumatic stress, chronic reactive anxiety, burnout, and related physical symptoms? Does the development of a complex fluctuating color coded threat level system, and announcement that future attacks will almost certainly occur. facilitate or hinder coping? Do existing treatment models actually work or must we abandon conventional ideas for new intervention paradigms? What can we do to promote resilience in coping with uncertain risk, chronic threat of future attacks, and inconsistent messages from government authorities? Traditional education and training of mental health professionals and behaviorally scientists has done little to prepare us for addressing these critical questions.

Bongar and his talented colleagues offer us significant assistance in overcoming the gaps in our training. They have compiled a broad and deep array of exceptionally useful information aimed at helping readers both to understand the psychology of the terrorist and the best scientifically grounded remedies for the terrorized. These experts from academic, medical, military, and clinical settings cover the full range of theoretical, clinical, social psychological, work site, developmental, and historical contexts. The authors also look well beyond the scope of 9/11, addressing a wide range of historical events, as well as domestic terrorism such as the threats posed by the "Unabomber," Oklahoma City Bombing, and postal anthrax incidents.

As we prepare ourselves and our students to serve the contemporary needs of society, the contents of this volume provide an incredibly valuable and vital resource. The work of these contributors will enable our profession to more readily step forward and engage in research and clinical endeavors aimed at reducing both terrorist threats and the accompanying psychological consequences. Although I rue the need for this excellent resource, I remain grateful for it.

Gerald P. Koocher
Boston
March 23, 2006

Acknowledgments

I, along with millions of others who watched the events of September 11, 2001, unfold, felt the immediate shocking impact of the terrorist attacks—all the more so as my son frequently traveled on that fateful flight from Boston to San Francisco and could have easily been on the plane that terrible day. As a clinical psychologist, I immediately volunteered my services to the American Red Cross (ARC). While awaiting an assignment to go to Manhattan, I completed the required ARC Disaster Mental Health Level 1 training to work at a disaster site. As both a scientist and a practitioner, I was astonished to learn that scientifically validated methods were not being used for training, and the need to provide responders, victims proximally and remotely affected with the best possible psychological tools to deal with this horror became evident and provided a challenge for me.

While awaiting any available opening for an ARC assignment to go back to New York City, I took it upon myself immediately to go to New York, and without identifying myself in any way, informally assessed the situation as best I could. An insight soon emerged. These people had attacked not just the United States of America, but my Dad's "home." For my father, Moses Bongar, was a "true New Yorker" (and though he traveled far and wide,

New York City was always there in his soul). Before my trip, I was honored to be invited as a specialist in clinical emergencies and crises to come to Washington, D.C. to discuss disaster mental health and its role with regard to 9/11 with Dr. Bernadine Healy, the head of the American Red Cross. After spending several days in New York City, and being astonished at the incredible resilience of this remarkable city and its people, I was able to meet at some length with Dr. Healey and her senior aid at ARC headquarters. In this meeting, I emphasized the critical role of the American Psychological Association, through its Disaster Response Network (DRN), and the efforts of Dr. Russell Newman and senior DRN staff who served as vital resources that stood ready to work closely with the ARC and its then head of disaster mental health, Dr. John Clizbe.

Most importantly, I had a remarkable evening with the individual whom I consider to be the foremost authority on suicide terror in the world, Professor Ariel Merari. It was through this meeting at the Willard Hotel that I realized how little I and other interested mental health professionals really knew about terrorism and what this heinous attack America would entail in the years to come. That evening with Ariel changed my life. For Professor

Merari shared with me his vast experience and that of his Israeli colleagues who have waged battle against this ghastly sort of event since the founding of the State of Israel. He quickly convinced me that America would soon find itself deluged with a panoply of so-called terrorism experts—all of whom would be more than willing to provide their learned opinions (often for a substantial fee). Unfortunately, as I had already learned decades ago, one good scientific study is worth a thousand "learned opinions." Thus, Professor Merari inspired me to coordinate the first ever American-based international conference on the psychology of terrorism. Science, rather than "opinion," would be the heart and soul of this endeavor. I would also be remiss in not mentioning another remarkable, accomplished Merari, Professor Dalia Merari, whose sage counsel helped me focus on what would be of most interest and value in the applied sphere.

My colleagues at the first North Atlantic Treaty Organization conference on the prevention of suicide terror, organized by Professors Ariel Merari and Scott Atran, and held in Lisbon in 2004 were ever in my mind as we headed for the finish line. In particular, I wish to acknowledge Dr. Simon Wesley and Professor Atran for their generous efforts to educate me on the nuances and vital dimensions of both basic and applied science after such evil events. London and Madrid proved their prescience. At the NATO conference I also learned how science and its cutting edge applications can be best mobilized through teamwork and discussion. At several dinners, I was fortunate enough to be educated in the complexities of how science can impact assessment, risk management and intervention by a wise and wonderful colleague, Major General Issac Ben-Israel.

It is crucial to note that neither the initial conference in Palo Alto on the psychology of terrorism nor this book could ever have come to fruition without the faith and support of a truly remarkable woman, Joan Bossert of Oxford University Press (OUP). For it was Joan and the other leaders at OUP who, without missing a beat, immediately recognized that such a conference was not only timely, but represented a sea change in how psychological science and its application would be the key to understanding the role that psychology would play in making a difference in how we assess, manage, treat, and prevent the inevitable psychological trauma that is inherent in any human-created mass casualty event.

Thanks to Joan and to her dedicated colleagues and staff at OUP for guidance and assistance in preparing this massive missive. It is essential to acknowledge the magnificent role that OUP's Joseph Zito, Jennifer Rappaport, Mallory Jensen, and Anne Enenbach played in making this book a reality.

I would be remiss in not acknowledging the critical additional financial support for the conference that was solicited by President Allen Calvin of the Pacific Graduate School of Psychology and, in particular, wish to thank Racky Newman and her foundation and Rabbi Stephen Pearce of Temple Emanu-El for support of this event.

This book also owes a great debt to the input and wise counsel of Col. Larry James of the United States Army; an equal debt is owed to Captain Elizabeth Holmes of the United States Naval Academy (and to my colleagues Brad Johnson and Rocky Lall). I would also like to thank and acknowledge Dr. Patrick DeLeon for his sage counsel. I also wish to thank my colleagues Drs. Paul Stockton, Phillip Zimbardo, Larry Beutler, and James Breckenridge for their dedicated work in crafting a marvelous course on the psychology of terrorism at the United States Naval Postgraduate School (NPS) in Monterey, California. Professors often dream of having a class of students so dedicated, so wise, and most importantly, so motivated to learn that teaching is not a mere pleasure, but a life-changing event. The first class in the NPS Master's degree program in Homeland Security humbled all five of us with their amazing range of intellect, experience and talents (both individually and collectively). You know who you are and I, for one, will be forever grateful for the experience of being your student and your professor.

Any book of this magnitude rises or falls on the perseverance, resiliency and good spirits of one's senior support staff. Laura Pratchett, my graduate student assistant from my PGSP-STANFORD doctor of psychology program, functioned at the level of a junior colleague rather than a beginning graduate student (here her training in Scotland as a solicitor brought a laser beam focus to this old professor's tome). My former graduate students Drs. Glenn Sullivan and Eric Crawford also insured that the conference from which this work sprung was run like a Swiss watch (a Rolex for that matter). I also want to acknowledge that Dr. Sullivan will carry the torch on my own work on suicide terror long after I have sailed off to retirement. I am also indebted to my personal assistant, Briana Breen, for her perseverance, resiliency and consistent good spirits in getting this book completed through her role as a senior coordinator. Briana tirelessly endured "herding cats"—especially yours truly.

From a personal standpoint, I also wish to acknowledge the incredible support of Professor Larry Beutler, my beloved colleague and writing partner of so many years—Larry was always there and his gimlet editorial eye suffuses many of the chapters herein. Blanche Dubois in the Tennessee Williams masterpiece, *A Street Car Named Desire*, once remarked that "I have always depended on the kindness of strangers." More than 20 years ago, Professor Phillip Zimbardo, already a legend as teacher of psychology, most generously recommended to his publisher that a young colleague be asked to review a critical chapter or two in his classic introductory text. That young professor Bongar (now grown a bit long in the tooth) hopes that 20 years from now, if he is lucky, he will have the energy, intellectual mastery and drive that Phil continues to demonstrate to the world. Professors lucky enough to have many years of mentoring doctoral students know that if one is extremely lucky, one has a few super stars, destined early on to surpass their professor's own research and scientific accomplishments. It is clear that my colleague and former doctoral student Dr. Lisa Brown is already on such a trajectory and her enormous efforts, along with those of my colleagues Larry, Phil, and Jim are ever present in this work.

Psychologists who wish to understand the psychology of terrorism can learn much from our sibling social sciences, in particular from the discipline of anthropology. My life-long friend, mother of our son Brandon, and my former wife, the noted cultural anthropologist Professor Debbora Battaglia, who for almost 13 years honored me by allowing me to accompany her on many of her professional journeys. For most of my adult life, I have not been a deeply religious person, but I continue to thank God every day that our son was not on that plane.

Most of all, this book is dedicated to my son, Brandon Fortune Bongar—for so many years you

have been my hero. The reader may wonder about such an odd place to tell his son this—for both father and son are old-fashioned guys who are easily embarrassed about telling each other how much they love one another. Parents in all cultures know that the greatest pride is the pride one takes in the accomplishments of one's children.

I am always indebted to my family and thank my Mom, my amazingly gifted and talented sister Hallie, her husband James White and my Native American nephew and nieces, my wonderfully entrepreneurial brother Andrew, his wife Kim and the boys, and my intrepid sister Debbie and her children in Israel.

I would also like to thank specifically for their unflagging support for the National Center on Disaster Psychology and Terrorism, our distinguished chair of psychiatry, Alan Schatzberg, Dean Pizzo of Stanford Medical School, the chair of our joint doctor of psychology program, Bruce Arnow, Javaid Sheikh of VAPAHCS, and last but never least our visionary, President Allen Calvin of the Pacific Graduate School. I would also like to thank my friends and colleagues Eric Harris and Susan Brooks, Wendy and Sy Packman, Ben Patty and Bennie, Linda Crothers and Dani, my fellow "Lotus Eaters" David Clark, Andrew Slaby, and Terry Maltsberger, Art and Barbara Frankel, David and Marilyn Rigler, Don Bersoff, Kirk Hubbard, Bruce and Diane Ogilvie, and Kevin Murphy. In addition, since 1978, I have been honored beyond measure to have as my esteemed friend and colleague, the current president of the American Psychological Association, Dean Gerald Koocher.

Randy Travis, a famous American country-western balladeer, once sang the lyrics "your heroes will help you find good in yourself, your friends won't desert you for somebody else." Thank you RAH, IF, CSF, ACD, WS, SF, CR, WBG, HW, AM PL, BCO, DR, MHE, DR, LGP, CR, JKG, JR, WSC and JPJ, LV, CP, JP, GN, and SW.

For over twenty five years I have been privileged to be a scientific fellow among a remarkable band of brothers and sisters, The Explorers Club, who have "pushed the limits for more than a century"—thank you for allowing this "shrink" to learn that "home is where when you go there, they have to take you in."

While my colleagues Lisa, Larry, Phil, and Jim kindly and generously put their names and considerable skills into this volume, as a bluewater sailor with thousands of miles under my keel, I know that to escape chaos, in the end someone must take full responsibility as the "skipper" for all that is contained herein. I fully accept such responsibility, and I trust that the readers of this book will soon realize that all chapter authors involved in this project strove at every juncture to provide the intended audience with the most accurate, useful and scientifically sound chapters possible. In particular I am indebted to Professors Tony Taylor and Douglas Paton of New Zealand for inviting me to give a plenary address on the psychology of terrorism to the New Zealand Psychological Society—the best (and most honestly critical audience) I have ever addressed. I am honored to have had the chance to work with every contributor to this volume and hope that each reader will find that the assembled chapters meet both their professional and personal needs.

Finally, to the sunshine of my life: John, Gordo, Frank, Las Vegas Larry, M, Jeff, Joel, Sarah, Robyn The Wonder Dog, to Donna Olsen Satterfield, my former internship supervisor who for 30 years has been my best friend, and last but never least, first among equals, to My Funny Valentine, Cookie (who taught me the real meaning of true love that lasts forever—it was always you from the start).

Contents

Contributors

Editors

Bruce Bongar is Calvin Professor of Psychology at the Pacific Graduate School of Psychology and Consulting Professor of Psychiatry and Behavioral Sciences at Stanford University School of Medicine. He founded and is the executive director of the National Center on Disaster Psychology and Terrorism. Along with Larry Beutler, the Director of the Palo Alto Medical Reserve Corps (MRC) of the Office of the Surgeon General of the United States, Professor Bongar recently volunteered his services and has joined the senior staff of the San Mateo County Coastside Medical Reserve Corp (MRC). Professor Bongar, along with his close colleague Professor Ariel Merari, of Tel Aviv University, will be undertaking an international collaborative study to attempt to scientifically understand and prevent acts of suicide terror such as those that occurred on 9/11 and the bombings in London and Madrid—a study that grew out of the first NATO conference on the prevention of suicide terrorism—organized by Merari and Scott Atran. Dr. Bongar is an authority on suicide and life threatening behaviors and on clinical and legal standards of care. He founded the Oxford University Press Clinical Psychology Series and is the winner of both the Shneidman award for early career achievement and Dubin award for lifetime career achievement in the scientific understanding of suicide from the American Association of Suicidology, and is past president of Section VII, Clinical Emergencies and Crises, of the Division of Clinical Psychology (Division 12) of the American Psychological Association. Professor Bongar is a fellow of the American Psychological Association, the Academy of Psychosomatic Medicine, and the American Psychological Society. A practicing clinical psychologist and psychotherapist for almost 30 years, Dr. Bongar is a licensed psychologist, a chartered clinical psychologist of the British Psychological Society, and a Diplomate of the American Board of Professional Psychology.

Lisa M. Brown is an Assistant Professor in the Department of Aging and Mental Health, Florida Mental Health Institute, and the Department of Psychiatry and Behavioral Medicine, University of South Florida. Brown is interested in how adults cope with adverse personal or societal life events. Her research on mental health and disasters has evolved from her longstanding interest in the effects of adverse events and pathological conditions on the mental and physical health of older adults. Brown and her colleague John A. Schinka have recently completed a longitudinal study that examines the effects of the 2004 and 2005 hurricanes on a cohort of elderly Floridians. She is currently evaluating the effectiveness of a mental health intervention that was developed to reduce hurricane related distress and put into practice statewide after the 2004 hurricane season. Along with Kathryn Hyer, Brown is examining the response and recovery of long-term care facilities during disasters and working to develop policy and best practices to protect institutionalized adults.

Larry E. Beutler is the William McInnes Distinguished Professor of Psychology at Pacific Graduate School of Psychology (PGSP), and is a Consulting Professor of Psychiatry and Behavioral Sciences at Stanford University School of Medicine. He is also a Visiting Professor of Homeland Security and Defense at the Naval Post-Graduate School in Monterey and the former Chair of the Ph.D. Program and Director of Clinical Training at Pacific Graduate School of Psychology. Beutler has published over 20 scholarly books and 350 scientific articles and papers on psychological assessment, training, and treatment. He is a Past President of the Society for Clinical Psychology (Division 12, APA), the Division of Psychotherapy (APA), and the International Society for Psychotherapy Research.

James N. Breckenridge is the Associate Director of the Stanford Center for Interdisciplinary Policy, Research, and Education on Terrorism. He retired recently from his positions as Chief of the Psychology Services at the Veterans Affairs Palo Alto Health Care System. Breckenridge is also Professor of Psychology at the Pacific Graduate School of Psychology, and Director of Training of the PGSP-STANFORD Psy.D. Consortium, and Consulting Professor of Psychiatry and Behavioral Sciences at Stanford University School of Medicine. He teaches graduate courses in the psychology of terrorism at the Center for Homeland Defense and Security at the Naval Post-Graduate School, where he is a Distinguished Senior Fellow. Breckenridge is also a Fellow of the American Psychological Association and is chair-elect of the Veterans Af-

fairs section of Division 18 (Public Service). He recently received the Division's National Outstanding Researcher Award for his work in health economics, risk adjustment, and other statistical modeling approaches to healthcare utilization. The Department of Veterans Affairs Under Secretary for Health recognized Dr. Breckenridge in 2005 for his Robert Wood Johnson funded research on national patterns of intensive care and palliative care alternatives.

Philip G. Zimbardo is internationally recognized as the "voice and face of contemporary psychology" through his widely seen PBS-TV series, *Discovering Psychology*, his media appearances, best-selling trade books on shyness, and his classic research, the Stanford Prison Experiment. Zimbardo has been a Stanford University professor since 1968, having taught previously at Yale, NYU, and Columbia University. He is now an Emeritus Professor but is still teaching more new and intense undergraduate courses. He has been given numerous awards and honors as an educator, researcher, writer, and service to the profession. Most recently he was awarded the 2005 Havel Foundation Prize from the Czech Republic for his lifetime of research on the human condition. Among his more than 350 professional publications and 50 books is the oldest current textbook in psychology, *Psychology and Life*, going into its 18th edition. His current research interests are in the domain of experimental social psychology with a scattered emphasis on everything and anything interesting to study from time perspective to political psychology. Zimbardo is currently enmeshed in his major opus, Zimbardo is past President of the Western Psychological Association (twice), President of the American Psychological Association, the elected Chair of the Council of Scientific Society Presidents (CSSP) representing 63 scientific, math and technical associations (with 1.5 million members), and is now Chair of the Western Psychological Foundation and President of the Philip Zimbardo Foundation that collects funds for college scholarships and computers for children in his ancestral Sicilian village town of Cammarata. Zimbardo is also the director of a new terrorism center sponsored jointly by Stanford and the Naval Postgraduate School, The Interdisciplinary Center for Policy, Education, and Research on Terrorism (CIPERT).

Contributors

Col. L. Morgan Banks, PhD
Psychological Applications Directorate, Ft. Bragg, NC

Larry E. Beutler, PhD, ABPP
Naval Postgraduate School, Monterey, CA
National Center on the Psychology of Terrorism

Bruce Bongar, PhD, ABPP, FAPM
Pacific Graduate School of Psychology, Palo Alto, CA
Department of Psychiatry and Behavioral Sciences,
 Stanford University School of Medicine,
 Stanford, CA *and*
National Center on the Psychology of Terrorism

Susan Brandon, PhD
Department of Psychology, Yale University, New
 Haven, CT

James N. Breckenridge, PhD
Naval Postgraduate School, Monterey, CA

Lisa M. Brown, PhD
Aging and Mental Health Department,
 Louis de la Parte Florida Mental Health
 Institute, University of South Florida,
 Tampa, FL *and*
National Center on the Psychology of Terrorism

Richard Bryant, PhD
Department of Psychology, University of New
 South Wales, Sydney, Australia

Lisa D. Butler, PhD
Department of Psychiatry and Behavioral Sciences,
 Stanford University School of Medicine,
 Stanford, CA

David Chiriboga, PhD
Aging and Mental Health Department, Louis de
 la Parte Florida Mental Health Institute,
 University of South Florida, Tampa, FL

John A. Clizbe, PhD
American Red Cross, Washington, DC

Donna Cohen, PhD
Aging and Mental Health Department, Louis de
 la Parte Florida Mental Health Institute,
 University of South Florida, Tampa, FL

Dennis D. Embry, PhD
PAXIS Institute, Tucson, AZ

**Brian W. Flynn, EdD, RADM, U.S. Public
Health Services, Ret.**
Center for the Study of Traumatic Stress,
 Uniformed Services University of the Health
 Sciences, Bethesda, MD

Zeno Franco
Pacific Graduate School of Psychology,
 Palo Alto, CA

Scott Gerwehr
Defense Group Inc., Center for Intelligence
 Research and Analysis, Santa Monica, CA

Richard Gist, PhD
Department of Psychology, University of Missouri–
 Kansas City, Kansas City, MO
Principal Assistant to the Director, Kansas City Fire
 Department, Kansas City, MO

Susan Hamilton, PhD
American Red Cross, Washington, DC

Jennifer Housley
Pacific Graduate School of Psychology,
 Palo Alto, CA

Kirk M. Hubbard, PhD
Operational Assessment Division, Central Intelligence Agency, Washington, DC

Larry James, PhD
Department of Psychology, Tripler Army Medical
 Center, Honolulu, HI *and*
National Center on the Psychology of Terrorism

John Kalafat, PhD
Graduate School of Applied and Professional
 Psychology, Rutgers University, Piscataway, NJ

Timothy A. Kelly, PhD
Fuller Graduate School of Psychology, Pasadena,
 California

Gregory A. Leskin, PhD
National Center for Post-Traumatic Stress Dis-
 order, VA
Palo Alto Healthcare System, Palo Alto, CA

Joy Kohlmaier, PhD
Louis de la Parte Florida Mental Health
 Institute, University of South Florida,
 Tampa, FL

Brett T. Litz, PhD
National Center for Post-Traumatic Stress
 Disorder, Behavioral Science Division,
 Boston, MA

Shira Maguen, PhD
Post-Traumatic Stress Disorder Program, San
 Francisco Veterans Administration Medical
 Center, San Francisco, CA

Charles R. Marmar, MD
San Francisco Department of Veterans Affairs
 Medical Center, San Francisco, CA

Clark McCauley, PhD
Psychology Department, Bryn Mawr College, Bryn Mawr, PA

Rose McDermott, PhD
Political Science Department, University of California, Santa Barbara, CA

Ariel Merari, PhD
Psychology Department, Tel Aviv University, Tel Aviv, Israel *and*
National Center on the Psychology of Terrorism

Fathali M. Moghaddam, PhD
Psychology Department, Georgetown University, Washington, DC

Leslie Morland, PsyD
National Center for Post-Traumatic Stress Disorder, Veterans Affairs Pacific Island Healthcare System, Honolulu, HI

Douglas Paton PhD, CPsychol
School of Psychology, University of Tasmania, Launceston, Tasmania, Australia *and*
National Center on the Psychology of Terrorism

Joseph W. Pfeifer
Fire Department of New York, NY

Laura Pratchett, LLB (Hons)
Pacific Graduate School of Psychology–Stanford PsyD Consortium, Palo Alto, CA

Dori Reissman, MD
Centers for Disease Control and Prevention, Atlanta, GA

Stephan G. Reissman, PhD, CEM
Centers for Disease Control and Prevention, Atlanta, GA

Gil Reyes, PhD
School of Psychology, Fielding Graduate University, Santa Barbara, CA

Josef I. Ruzek, PhD
National Center for Post-Traumatic Stress Disorder, VA Palo Alto Health Care System, Palo Alto, CA

Joel Shurkin
National Center on the Psychology of Terrorism Baltimore, MD

Andrew Silke, PhD
School of Law, University of East London, Stratford, London, England

Nicci Spinazzola, EdS, LMFT, LPC
Richard Hall Community Mental Health Center, Somerville, NJ

Glenn R. Sullivan, PhD
Pacific Graduate School of Psychology, Palo Alto, CA *and*
National Center on the Psychology of Terrorism

A. J. W. Taylor
School of Psychology, Victoria University of Wellington, Wellington, NZ

Maureen Underwood, LCSW
Morristown, NJ

John M. Violanti, PhD
School of Public Health and Health Professions, Social and Preventative Medicines, State University of New York–Buffalo, Buffalo, NY

Rachel Yehuda, PhD
Psychiatry Department, Mount Sinai School of Medicine, New York, NY *and*
Traumatic Stress Studies Division, Mount Sinai School of Medicine and Bronx Veterans Affairs Medical Center, New York, NY

Philip G. Zimbardo, PhD
Psychology Department, Stanford University, Stanford, CA

Joseph Zohar, MD
Psychiatry Department, Chaim Sheba Medical Center, Ramat Gan, Israel

I

The Psychology of Terrorism

1

The Psychology of Terrorism
Defining the Need and Describing the Goals

Bruce Bongar

Terrorism is about one thing: Psychology. It is the psychology of fear.
    Philip G. Zimbardo, personal communication, April 2004

The past decade has witnessed a dramatic transformation in the nature and use of terrorism. These changes have brought into high relief the need for better psychological and social responses to terrorism and man-made disasters. It is important to note that a major strategic intent of modern terrorists is to create huge numbers of secondary psychological casualties by means of large-scale physical attacks. The catastrophic acts of September 11, 2001, and their aftermath have forced military, medical, and psychological experts to re-evaluate their understanding of mass casualty terrorism. Given the relative newness of the discipline, we believe there is a great need for a text that covers aspects of psychology relevant to terrorism.

Definitional Issues

In 48 A.D., a Jewish sect called the Zealots carried out terrorist campaigns to force an insurrection against the Romans in Judea. These campaigns included the use of assassins—"sicarii," or dagger men—who would infiltrate Roman-controlled cities, stab Jewish collaborators or Roman legionnaires with a "sicae"(dagger), kidnap members of the staff of the Temple Guard to hold for ransom, or use poison on a large scale. These assassins were an eleventh-century offshoot of a Shia Muslim sect known as the Ismailis, who believed that dying in the process of their assault was an act of self-sacrifice and guaranteed them a pathway into heaven. By contrast, terrorist organizations today are often much larger, more loosely connected networks of full-time and part-time activists, and this anonymity removes inhibitions to inflict broad, indiscriminate damage (Hoffman, 2001).

The English word *terrorism* comes from the régime de la terreur that prevailed in France from 1793 to 1794, when a French revolutionary, Maximilian Robespierre, proclaimed that "Terror is nothing other than justice, prompt, severe, inflexible; it is therefore an emanation of virtue; it is not so much a special principle as it is a consequence of the general principle of democracy applied to our country's most urgent needs."

McDermott and Zimbardo (this volume) trenchantly point out that terrorism is not about war in any traditional sense of destroying the material resources of an enemy nation and taking over that country; instead, terrorism is fundamentally about psychology. Terrorist acts are designed strategically to incite terror and fright in civilian populations. They further note that terrorists in most instances are neither crazy nor irrational—though their acts may be evil in the extreme. Many authorities have also found that there is neither a specific terrorist psychological profile nor a singular psychopathological condition.

Crenshaw (2000) has emphasized this definitional dilemma and pointed out that the concept of terrorism is not well defined, that contradictions occur, that terrorism is a highly politicized term used to describe the behavior of oppositional forces, and that the category of terrorism includes diverse practices that range from kidnappings to bombings intended to create mass casualties. Furthermore, he notes that there is ongoing political pressure to define terrorist behavior in terms of psychopathology, and he clearly suggests that the lack of extensive, reliable interview data or empirical testing has made it difficult to draw dependable and valid inferences. He concludes that, despite the political climate, personality factors and psychopathologies are not specific to terrorists and there is little evidence of gender differences; instead, rather than individual factors, group dynamics within close units with shared ideologies and solidarity play a much larger role. In 2002 Shamir and Shikaki published the findings of their study, which examined the psychological processes applied by terrorists and terrorist organizations to justify their violence. They maintain that, "although there is no consensus over what terrorism is, most people seem to believe that terrorism is bad and should be eradicated" (541).

Contemporary Terrorism

The primary goal of terrorism is to disrupt society by provoking intense fear and shattering all sense of personal and community safety. The target is an entire nation, not only those who are killed, injured, or even directly affected.

> Hall, Norwood, Ursano, Fullerton,
> and Levinson, 2002

In a lengthy review on terrorism in the *Washington Quarterly,* Scott Atran (a research scientist at the National Center for Scientific Research in Paris and at the University of Michigan) has pointed out that most Americans currently feel no safer from terrorism, that they are more distrustful of many longstanding allies, and that they are increasingly anxious about the future. He cited a survey released in the early spring of 2004 by the nonpartisan Council for Excellence that found that more than three-quarters of Americans expect the United States to be the target of a major terrorist attack in the near future. A clear reality focus for such widespread anxiety and fear was noted:

> One distinct pattern in the litany of terrorist atrocities is that there has been an increasing interest in well-planned attacks designed to net the highest numbers of civilian casualties. Charting data from the International Policy Institute for Counter-Terrorism, Robert Axelrod, a political scientist at the University of Michigan, observes that a very few terrorist attacks account for a very large percentage of all casualties. Not only does this trend call for anticipating attacks with ever broader political, economic, and social effects, it also seems to point to an eventual suicide attack using chemical, biological, or nuclear weapons. Although that may take some time to plan effectively, long-term planning has proven to be Al Qaeda's hallmark. "God has ordered us to build nuclear weapons." (Atran, 2004, p. 70)

This extensive review also underscored a common misconception in the U.S. administration and media spin on the war on terrorism—namely, that terrorists are evil, deluded, or homicidal misfits who thrive in poverty, ignorance, and anarchy. Atran further stated that

> such a portrayal lends a sense of hopelessness to any attempt to address root causes because some individuals will always be desperate or deranged enough to conduct suicide attacks. Nevertheless, as logical as the poverty-breeds-terrorism argument may seem, study after study shows that suicide attackers and their supporters are rarely ignorant or impoverished. Nor are they crazed, cowardly, apathetic, or asocial. The common misconception underestimates the central role that organizational factors play in the appeal of terrorist networks. A better understanding of such causes reveals that the challenge is actually manageable: the key is not to profile and target the most despairing or deranged individual but to understand and undermine the organizational and institutional appeal of terrorists' motivations and networks. (Atran, 2004, p. 73)

It is also useful to remember that the attacks on September 11, 2001, were intended to cause far more deaths and injuries than they actually did. We know from the testimony of the 1993 World Trade Center bombers that terrorist planners believed the buildings would topple when attacked, not cascade down upon themselves; the original intent was to spread death and injury among countless inhabitants of Lower Manhattan and not merely among those who worked in the targeted skyscrapers. As British prime minister Tony Blair has observed, modern terrorists "have no moral inhibition on the slaughter of the innocent. If they could have murdered not 7,000 [sic] but 70,000 does anyone doubt they would have done so and rejoiced in it?" (Blair, 2001). The al-Qaeda leadership had met several years previously and explored attacking nuclear power facilities in the United States (but actually had some qualms about the terrorist act "getting out of control and decided not to do that for now" [Blair, 2001]). When directly queried by a journalist who interviewed them in Pakistan about what "for now" meant, a senior correspondent for Al Jazeera (an Arabic-language television station in Qatar) said, "for now, means for now!" (obviously leaving the door open for future planning for such assaults; Blair, 2001). Credible intelligence sources have also discovered that the same group responsible for 9/11 were at least actively trying to secure materials for either a radiological dispersion device and/or chemical or biological agents that could be used to attack U.S. targets (both in the United States and abroad).

In addition, terrorism authorities such as Ariel Merari of Tel Aviv University have been warning of the threat of "megaterrorism" since the early 1990s. The goal of megaterrorists is not to achieve political ends but simply to kill enormous numbers of "enemy" civilians. An example of this brand of terrorism is the May 23, 2002, attempt to detonate the Pi Gilot fuel depot in Tel Aviv; had the terrorists succeeded, an estimated 20,000–40,000 civilians living nearby would have been killed (Dunn, 2002). Given the practical and technological means—chemical, biological, nuclear, or explosive—a single act of megaterrorism could easily claim the lives of 100,000 innocent civilians.

This hyperhomicidal form of terrorism is not restricted to al-Qaeda operatives. In 1995 members of the apocalyptic cult Aum Shinrikyō managed to kill only 12 (and not 12,000) people in the Tokyo subway because of luck and inexperience, not moral or tactical constraint. This same organization had previously purchased a sheep farm in western Australia in order to mine uranium and construct a nuclear bomb (Stern, 1999). Only fortuitous intervention by Japanese law enforcement forestalled a much larger tragedy. Even after the dismantling of Aum Shinrikyō, a myriad of millennial cults that hope to provoke the apocalypse through terrorism remain in our midst (Lifton, 1999).

Psychological Impact

It is impossible to say anything that is able to give a true idea of it to those who did not see it, other than this, that it was indeed very, very, very dreadful, and such as no tongue can express.
Daniel Defoe, *Journal of the Plague Year*

The heinous events of September 11, 2001, have forever changed our awareness of the impact of mass casualty terrorism. Ariel Merari (personal communication, January 30, 2003) has stated that the only factors constraining the terrorists who seek to destroy us are practical and technical, not political or moral. Among the lessons learned by Merari and others on the front lines is that the strategic intent of modern terrorists is to create huge numbers of secondary psychological casualties by means of large-scale physical attacks. In the 1970s it was often repeated that terrorists "want a lot of people watching, not a lot of people dead"; today it is more accurate to say that terrorists want a lot of people dead—and even more people crippled by fear and grief.

Government and military officials acknowledge that we are currently unprepared to care for the large numbers of medical and psychological casualties that would result from an attack involving weapons of mass destruction (WMD) and/or bioterrorism. National authorities such as Leon E. Moores, a physician at the Walter Reed Army Medical Center, have calculated that the number of casualties from a WMD attack would be in the thousands but that the long-lasting psychological consequences would have a devastating affect on millions of people.

Military psychologists have long known that fear, stress, and exhaustion cause more casualties than do bombs and bullets. The ratios of psychological to physical casualties can be enormous; for every one death directly caused by an Iraqi Scud missile attack on Israel during the Gulf War, there were 272 hospital admissions resulting from clinical psychological emergencies. The March 20, 1995, sarin attack in the Tokyo subway killed 12 people and caused more than 4,000 nonaffected individuals to go to area hospitals, often with psychogenic symptoms of chemical injury (World Health Organization, 2001).

> Clearly, the impact on society can be much greater than initial casualty rates might imply. The long-term psychological impact of the use or even threat of WMD is difficult to predict. Changes in daily activity, depression and suicide rates, and economic impact can last for years or even decades, and current disaster experts have no models to predict the ultimate need for psychological assessment or treatment services. Many experts contend, based on the Israeli experience and other similar venues (e.g., Northern Ireland) that the strain on the medical resources and psychological strength of a society could potentially be crippling. (Moores, 2002)

At present, the psychological science needed to provide proper and effective treatment for victims of horrendous events such as September 11 and for future potential terrorist events (including the use of WMD) simply does not exist. Despite a wealth of information about psychological assessment and intervention following severe individual trauma (e.g., combat, rape), natural disasters, and airplane crashes, for example, there is no widespread scientific or clinical consensus regarding the efficacy of these treatment interventions with people who are directly affected by a terrorist attack. A similar scarcity of scientific data exists regarding appropriate treatments specifically designed for people not directly exposed to, but struggling to cope with, actual or threatened terrorist acts. Obviously, such effects are magnified by the 24/7 news cycle and the widespread availability of Internet connectivity.

Treatment of Victims of Terror

In the aftermath of September 11, an urgent need arose for the services of highly trained psychologists and other mental health professionals in treating thousands of victims, rescuers, and their families. Sadly, the effort to deliver quality mental health services was largely scattered, disorganized, and understaffed and involved mostly well- meaning but inadequately trained mental health professionals. The insufficient training of those who rushed to help was not entirely their own fault; little training is available in disaster mental health services (or in the psychological response to acts of terrorism), and even less (if any) training is available in treatment protocols that have scientific, empirical support for their efficacy. It is important—and chilling—to note that some authorities (Rose, Bisson, & Wessely, 2002; Van Emmerick, Kamphuis, Hulsbosch, & Emmelkamp, in press) have concluded that popular models of disaster mental health response (e.g., critical incident stress debriefing) are potentially harmful to victims of terrorist acts.

Critical Incident Stress Debriefing

Devilly and Cotton (2004) have critically reviewed the literature on critical incident stress debriefing (CISD) and made a powerful conclusion:

> It is surprising, perhaps, that CISD has become so universally accepted despite the fact that there is no data from randomized clinical trials demonstrating its efficacy as a clinical intervention. . . . Indeed, as noted earlier, two recent studies suggest that CISD is either ineffective or actually worsens PTSD [posttraumatic stress disorder] symptoms instead of preventing the later development of PTSD, as is generally believed. Obviously, much more research is needed. As we ask ourselves, however, . . . how CISD could have attracted so many strong adherents in the absence of convincing data, the answer may lie in the low prevalence of PTSD among individuals exposed to natural disasters. . . . If most people exposed to natural disasters will never develop PTSD, then most people exposed to natural disasters who receive CISD will never develop PTSD. The pertinent question, therefore, is whether individuals most at risk to develop PTSD following acute traumatization will have more favorable outcomes if they receive CISD. Clearly we must move beyond clinical impressions and descriptive studies to rigorous randomized trials

if we hope to learn whether CISD can actually prevent the later development of PTSD among acutely traumatized individuals.(p. 35)

In their critical review of CISD, Devilly and Cotton (2004) also extensively emphasized the work of Litz, Gray, Bryant, and Adler (2002) and Rose, Bisson, and Wessely (2002):

1. It appears that there is sufficient evidence to recommend that psychological debriefing not be provided to individuals immediately after trauma. . . . There is consensus, however, that providing comfort, information, support, and meeting people's immediate practical and emotional needs play useful roles in one's immediate coping with a highly stressful event (Litz et al., 2002).
2. There is no current evidence that psychological debriefing is a useful treatment for the prevention of posttraumatic stress disorder after traumatic incidents. Compulsory debriefing of victims of trauma should cease (Rose et al., 2002).

Devilly and Cotton carefully examined the reasons CISD might be harmful and found five major areas of concern:

1. the lack of choice
2. poor timing
3. retraumatizing the victim of terror
4. vicarious traumatization
5. superficiality (Devilly & Cotton, 2004, pp. 39–40)

Last, even given a more balanced observation drawing on the other side's more clinical material,

It seems that what can be definitively and strongly said is that the research done so far has not convincingly demonstrated that critical incident stress debriefings are useful in preventing posttraumatic stress disorder or other pathological reactions to trauma. A question that remains unanswered is whether or not debriefing has beneficial effects that to date have not been measured. (Devilly and Cotton, 2004, pp. 39–40)

Additional Research Issues

In 1999 the National Research Council and the Institute of Medicine, in an attempt to address the threat of chemical and biological attacks, produced several recommendations for the direction of future research. These organizations identified several "areas of concern" in which immediate progress was necessary. It is important to note that little, if any, meaningful work has so far been published in any of these areas (Table 1.1):

In 2005 the American Psychological Association's primary instrument for disseminating professional news (*APA Monitor,* February, 2005) reported on the outcome of a conference that convened in November of 2004, where more than 100 participants from federal, state, and local government Homeland Security and Defense entities and from major research institutions and universities came together to discuss the possible development of a curriculum in homeland security that would reflect the contributions of psychology and other behavioral sciences. Suggestions and discussion topics included the following:

1. risk assessment, perception, and communication
2. human behavior and social dynamics (e.g., motivation, culture, values) in disasters
3. human-centered design of the technologies involved in homeland security
4. decision-making dynamics such as crisis and stress management
5. the need for psychologists to study the content domains of homeland security from a behavioral and social science perspective
6. the realization that one's sense of security is a psychological state

Murphy has also proposed that

A true understanding of the psychology of terrorism includes: (1) advance knowledge of how and why individuals become attracted to terrorist groups and organizations and [the development of] interventions to reduce the likelihood that individuals will join such groups, (2) advance knowledge about the relationships between terrorists and terrorist groups and organizations, and [the] use [of] that knowledge to develop ways of influencing and disrupting the functioning of these groups, (3) [increasing] our understanding of the ways individuals and groups react to terrorist events, to the anticipation of terrorism and to counterterrorism strategies, with the goal of limiting the negative

Table 1.1. Recommendations of the National Research Council and the Institute of Medicine

Training: Identify resource material on chemical *and* biological agents, stress reduction after other traumas, and disaster response services; enlist the help of mental health professional societies in developing a training program for *their members.* The key to success in this attempt will be *in* offering continuing education credits and certification for mental health providers trained in chemical *and* biological attack response. (Breckenridge et al. 2003 have secured funding from the Office of the Surgeon General to provide training models, but this is still only one such funded training venue.)

Screening and Assessment: Identify suitable psychological screening methods for use by mental health providers and possibly first responders, differentiating adjustment reactions after chemical *and* biological attacks from more serious psychological illness (e.g., panic disorder, PTSD, psychosis, depression) and organic brain impairment from chemical or biological agents. *Conduct* research to identify trauma characteristics and behavior patterns that predict *whether* long-term disability *will* be necessary.

Communication: Develop health education and crisis response materials for the general public, including specific communication on chemical or biological agents. Additional information is needed on risk assessment *and* threat perception by individuals and groups and on risk communication by public officials, especially the roles of both the mass media and the Internet in the transmission of anxiety (or confidence). Some information is available in EPA studies of pollutants and toxic waste, but little or no systematically collected data *exist* on fears and anxieties related to the possibility of purposefully introduced disease.

effects of terrorism and negative reactions to counterterrorism efforts, (4) develop[ing] effective methods of communicating information about terrorism risks to policy makers, first responders and the public in ways that are consistent with the best underlying behavioral science (risk perception, communication techniques, social influence) and [developing materials] that are informative to and understood by recipients, and (5) build[ing] resilience among the potential targets of terrorism and develop[ing] methods of limiting the success of terrorists in spreading fear, anxiety and alarm. (2004, p. 5)

Furthermore, Murphy (2004) has pointed out that the most important weapon for a terrorist is not a gun or a bomb but rather the uncertainty, fear, and alarm that terrorist attacks and the threat of those attacks produce. He emphasizes that an important vulnerability of terrorists is not the technical wizardry of intelligence services but rather that fact that terrorists *always* depend on others—other members of their own groups, members of allied groups, the societies in which they live and operate, family, friends, acquaintances—and are therefore open to attack via the social networks that sustain them. Murphy concludes that, given the importance of social and psychological factors in understanding and combating terrorism and its effects, the potential importance of the behavioral and social sciences in the war on terror is clear.

The present book is the direct product of an international conference held in the fall of 2002.

This conference, which brought together some of the foremost national and international authorities on the psychology of terrorism (almost all of whom are authors of their respective chapters in this book) had the following as its goals:

1. designing a strategy and making recommendations on how to evaluate and deliver scientific, empirical treatment interventions for the victims of terrorism and their rescuers
2. training current and future mental healthcare professionals in the effective use of these treatments
3. conducting scientific research on the psychology of terrorism that will assist governmental and community agencies in preventing, preparing for, and recovering from mass casualty assaults
4. organizing and training rapid-response teams of professional clinicians that will respond immediately and effectively in the event of future national crises and emergencies
5. most importantly, emphasizing the role of psychological science (and not mere opinion) in our understanding of the psychological dimensions of acts of terror

Tactical and Strategic Perspectives

Psychology can also contribute to our understanding of terrorist motivations and recruitment techniques, which can provide a basis for innovative tactical and strategic-level counterterrorism programs. A comprehensive understanding of the psychology of terror will also help to establish a rational and defensible prioritization of potential terrorist targets in the United States and abroad based on the extent of the psychological impact created by an attack. In addition, there are preliminary indications that it may be possible to detect behavioral patterns and physical characteristics, such as gait and facial expression, of suicide bombers as they approach a target (Merari, personal communication, July 2004). These indicators could provide security forces at the intended site of attack with a brief warning and an opportunity for interdiction. Such research could also have broader prevention benefits and include knowledge of the terrorists' psychological makeup and motivations, which would provide a basis for information operations programs to dissuade them from volunteering for a mission or persisting in it. Such tactical programs based on initial results in Israel have already helped increase the number of suicide candidates who have aborted their mission.

From a strategic perspective, psychological research can advance the development of programs to decrease support for terrorist attacks within communities that generate such incidents. More generally, studies in the psychology of terrorism will support efforts by the United States to win "the war of ideas" and attack adversary recruitment efforts at the strategic level. It may also be possible to utilize technical means to detect potential terrorists, including suicide bombers, before they strike. Basic and applied research into the psychology of terrorism that examines behavioral patterns and physical characteristics may well lead to methods that directly support attack prediction and prevention (Atran, 2004).

Brief Perspective on the Israeli Experience

Pines (2004) has stated that "life in Israel is very stressful. Since its establishment in 1948, Israel has gone through five major wars. Even during times of peace, soldiers are killed while protecting the borders, and civilians live with a constant threat of terrorist activities. People's bags are checked whenever they enter public places and periodically

terrorist bullets are fired at civilians and bombs explode. In recent years suicide bombers started exploding themselves in populated areas causing death and injury" (p. 69).

Cowen (2005) has reported on the ideas of Danny Brom, the director of the Israel Center for the Treatment of Psychotrauma, who stated that "as to terrorism we are not talking about PTSD; we are talking about an attack on the fabric of society. . . . We have to develop resiliency-building services." Cowen says that Brom also suggested that the educational system could be an alternative delivery system for mental health services if proper testing and training are provided and that, at the end of the day, we will become a stronger society as the result of attempts to weaken us. Danieli, Brom, and Sills (2005) have also emphasized the importance of fostering a community's capacity for resilience, the centrality of traumatic grief, the need for multicultural understanding in services and treatment, and for proactive community organization in the face of terrorism.

Pines (2004) has further commented that "people who live in a country that was established on the ashes of the holocaust, who confront regularly the death and injury of young soldiers protecting its borders, and of civilians under terrorist attacks, are more acutely aware of death and consequently of the significance of their own life" (p. 70). She cites the work of Bleich, Gelkopf, and Solomon (2003), who found that Israelis reported lower levels of PTSD than do Americans living in New York City after the terrorist attack of September 11. She points out that the lowest levels of PTSD were reported among settlers in the occupied territories, who feel that living where they do is a calling. However, it is not the mere living in Israel but the existential significance attached to it that keeps them there (Pines, 2004, p. 75).

Prevention Issues

At a 2004 NATO conference on the prevention of suicide terrorism (organized by Scott Atran and Ariel Merari and sponsored by the NATO Office of Science and Technology), Simon Wessely of the British Institute of Psychiatry suggested that, when psychological weapons lose their novelty, they lose their primary potency. Wessely believes that it is vital that the public receive sound and sensible information that is accurate and reassuring. It is also potentially dangerous to (even inadvertently) amplify responses to biological and chemical weapons (e.g., investigators who are clad in "space suits") (Wessely, Hyams, & Bartholomew, 2001). Moreover, he contends that the public's general level of fear and anxiety may remain high for years, exacerbating preexisting psychiatric disorders (Wessely et al., 2001; Wessely, personal communication, June 2004). Hall et al. (2002) have described an additional role for psychological science and practice in preparing a community for possible terrorist attacks by focusing their attention on the risks of collective behaviors (e.g., panic and mass hysteria) or mass psychogenic illness. They maintain that psychologists can play a role in educating the authorities and the public about the risks and containment of panic.

Pape (2003) has argued that terrorism itself is not a form of psychopathology and, in fact, contends that terrorism—and in particular suicide terrorism—can be seen as a logical strategic decision by organizations. Pape drew this conclusion after examining information from all of the completed suicide terrorist attacks between 1980 and 2001 and then inferring that we can reasonably conclude that suicide terrorism results in the achievement of the desired outcomes and that it is therefore a mistake to assume that suicide terrorism is irrational.

Hall and his colleagues have posited that terrorism is the most disturbing kind of disaster because it is caused not by natural, technological, or accidental forces but by deliberate, human malevolence (Hall et al., 2002). They assert that the most psychologically taxing factor of terrorism is living in a heightened state of fear and alert that an indiscriminate and undetermined threat will strike without warning in the foreseeable future. Hoffman (2001) particularly mentions the work of Barbera, Macintyre, and De Atley (2001), who, after the sarin attack in the Tokyo subway, found that 73.9% of the 5,000 people seeking treatment were suffering from psychological effects such as shock, emotional upset, or a psychosomatic complaint. Hoffman (2001) further speculated on the limitations in our current understanding of terrorist behavior and stated that it is generally assumed that terrorist groups are more likely to imitate previous successful attacks than to develop innovative new ideas. However, no imitations of the Aum Shinrikyō attack have been attempted, perhaps because of the

challenges illustrated by the relative lack of success by even such a well-funded and well-trained terrorist group (Hoffman, 2001).

Flynn (2004) emphasizes that, although we currently have ideas about how to treat people's psychopathological responses, we do not yet have intervention strategies for dealing with nationwide stress reactions. Flynn further suggests that this lack of information resulted in a missed opportunity that could have "increased social support, promoted positive coping behavior, and built positive cohesion among diverse groups" (2004, p. 165). Flynn also says that, in the future, mental health professionals should be aware that our role involves an acceptance of the fact that pathologies are not the only area of study and that we should expand our scope to understand resiliency mechanisms.

Stein et al. (2004) have examined the relationship between psychology and terrorism and described the latter as essentially a psychological attack on a society's social capital: "In this way, terrorism is fundamentally different from other community-wide traumatic events.... The natural course of reactions following a terrorist attack may be broader and more prolonged than reactions to other disasters because a goal of terrorism is to create such reactions" (p. 106). Hoffman (2001) has stated that the true goal of terrorist attacks is to "rend the fabric of trust that bonds society" and to elicit "irrational, emotional," and repressive countermeasures. Terrorists seek not only to inflict physical damage to their victims but also to leverage that damage to accomplish broader political goals, ranging from specific policy changes to mass panic and public disaffection from existing government authorities. "The primary goal of terrorism is to disrupt society by provoking intense fear and shattering all sense of personal and community safety. The target is an entire nation, not only those who are killed, injured, or even directly affected" (Hall et al., 2002, p. 2).

It is also crucial not to extrapolate too broadly from the field of disaster mental health to the newly emerging area of the psychology of terrorism. Flynn has pointed out that "research is not nearly as extensive and complete as it needs to be and we are far too dependent on extrapolation from other types of traumatic events" (2004, p. 164).

An excellent example of how different warnings of terrorism are from the traditional warnings of impending natural disasters is presented by Zimbardo and Kluger (2003), who underscore the need for effective psychological science in examining the color-coded level of alert—green-blue-yellow-orange-red—employed by the U.S. government as an early warning system for the public. They have noted obvious flaws in the system—especially the fact that the current system creates anxiety without providing instruction on how to remain safe. Instead of being a useful warning device, the color-coded warning system, they maintain, has "a profoundly negative impact on our individual and collective mental health . . . a 'pre-traumatic stress syndrome' and its effect on our day-to-day lives is debilitating" (Zimbardo & Kluger, 2003, p. 34). Furthermore, that system is counterproductive in that it provides vague information, which serves only to increase fear in the public (which, ironically, is the goal of terrorism; Zimbardo & Kluger, 2003).

Conclusion

The emerging field of the psychology of terrorism thus ranges from first response to basic science, from the epidemiological to the cross-cultural to the case study, and from controlled clinical trials to rigorous qualitative methodologies. In the following chapters we address the goals of the various conferences and groups that have sought to define this newly emerging area. Within these chapters we present the newest findings on treatment and clinical response protocols. We also explore the theory and history of terrorism and examine the larger cultural and social psychological dimensions of this new field. The authors of the subsequent chapters also explore a wide range of subjects, such as the role of national, state, and local agencies and volunteer groups in responding to terrorist threats, military response, psychological consequences of terrorism, special populations, prevention, training, and research.

The hope is that this volume can fill the need for a comprehensive resource for mental health clinicians, medical care providers, researchers, educators, and others who respond to acts of terrorism. The primary audience will be mental health and primary care providers (specifically, psychologists, psychiatrists, emergency and primary care physicians, crisis intervention counselors, social workers, public sector nonprofit agencies such as the Red

Cross, and undergraduate and graduate-level college and university students. However, we also believe that there will be an important secondary audience that includes police departments, fire departments, emergency medical personnel, military personnel, local elected officials responsible for preparing for and responding to terrorist threats, and federal, state, regional, and local government agencies.

References

Asukai, N., & Maekawa, K. (2002). Psychological and physical health effects of the 1995 sarin attack in the Tokyo subway system. In J. M. Havenaar, J. G. Cwikel, & E. J. Bromet (Eds.), *Toxic turmoil: Psychological and social consequences of ecological disasters* (pp. 149–162). New York: Kluwer Academic/Plenum.

Atran, S. (2004, June). Mishandling suicide terrorism. *Washington Quarterly, 27*(3), 67–90.

———, and Merari A. (2004, June). NATO Office of Science and Technology Invitational Conference on the Prevention of Suicide Terrorism, Lisbon.

Blair, T. (2001, October). Part one of the speech by Prime Minister Tony Blair at the Labour Party conference. *Guardian Unlimited* (UK). Retrieved February 4, 2006, from http://politics.guardian.co .uk/speeches/story/0,11126,590775,00.html

Bleich A., Dycian, A., Koslowsky, M., Solomon, Z., & Wiener, M. (1992). Psychiatric implications of missile attacks on a civilian population. *Journal of the American Medical Association, 268,* 613–615.

Bleich, A., Gelkopf, M., & Solomon, Z. (2003). The psychological impact of ongoing terrorism and suicide bombing on Israeli society: A study of a national sample. *Journal of the American Medical Association, 260,* 612–620.

Cowen, D. (2005, March 16). Interview with Daniel Brom. *Canadian Jewish News,* 4

Crenshaw, M. (2000). The psychology of terrorism: An agenda for the 21st century. *Political Psychology, 21*(2), 405–420.

Danieli, Y., Brom, D., & Sills, J. (2005). The trauma of terrorism: Sharing knowledge and shared care, an international handbook. New York: Haworth.

Devilly, G. J., & Cotton, P. (2004). Caveat emptor, caveat venditor, and critical incident stress debriefing/management (CISD/M). *Australian Psychologist, 39,* 35–40.

Dunn, R. (2002, May 24). Bomb explodes at Israeli fuel depot. *Sydney Morning Herald.* Retrieved February 4, 2006, from http://www.smh.com.au/articles/ 2002/05/23/1022038458284.html

Flynn, B. W. (2004, Summer). Commentary on "A national longitudinal study of the psychological consequences of the September 11, 2001, terrorist attacks: Reactions, impairment, and help-seeking. Can we influence the trajectory of psychological consequences to terrorism?" *Psychiatry* 67(2), 164–166.

Giuliani, R., & Von Essen, T. (2003). Foreign Press Center briefing: New York City after September 11, 2001. Retrieved February 4, 2006, from http://fpc.state.gov/23971.htm

Hall, M. J., Norwood, A. E., Ursano, R. J., Fullerton, C. S., & Levinson, C. J. (2002). Psychological and behavioral impacts of bioterrorism. *PTSD Research Quarterly, National Center for Post-Traumatic Stress Disorder, 13*(4), 1–7.

Hassett, A. (2002, September). Unforeseen consequences of terrorism. *Archives of Internal Medicine (162)*, 1809–1813.

Hoffman, B. (2001). Change and continuity in terrorism. *Studies in Conflict and Terrorism, 24*, 417–428.

Lifton, R. J. (1999). *Destroying the world to save it: Aum Shinrikyō, apocalyptic violence, and the new global terrorism.* New York: Henry Holt.

Litz, B., Gray, M., Bryant, R., & Adler, A. (2002). Early interventions for trauma: Current status and future directions. *Clinical Psychology Science and Practice, 9*, 112–134.

Moores, L. (2002). Threat credibility and weapons of mass destruction. *Neurosurgical Focus, 12*, 1–3.

Murphy, K. (2004, December). Mission statement for a proposal for the establishment of a center for the behavioral and social science of counterterrorism. Meeting held at Pennsylvania State University.

Pape, R. A. (2003). The strategic logic of suicide terrorism. *American Political Science Review, 97*(3), 1–19.

Pines, A. (2004, June). Why are Israelis less burned out? *European Psychologist, 9*(2), 69–77.

Rose, S., Bisson, J., & Wessely, S. (2002, April 22). Psychological debriefing for preventing post-traumatic stress disorder (PTSD). *Cochrane Library, 1.* Oxford, UK: Update Software (CD-ROM).

Shamir, J., & Shikaki, K. (2002). Self-serving perceptions of terrorism among Israelis and Palestinians. *Political Psychology, 23*(3), 537–557.

Stein, B. D., Elliott, M. N., Jaycox, L. H., Collins, R. L., Berry, S. H., Klein, D. J., et al. (2004, Summer). A national longitudinal study of the psychological consequences of the September 11, 2001, terrorist attacks: Reactions, impairment, and help-seeking. *Psychiatry* 67(2), 105–117.

Stern, J. (1999). *The ultimate terrorists.* Cambridge, MA: Harvard University Press.

Stewart, J. B. (2002). *Heart of a soldier: A story of love, heroism, and September 11th.* New York: Simon & Schuster.

Van Emmerick, A. A. P., Kamphuis, J. H., Hulsbosch, A. M., & Emmelkamp, P. M. G. (in press). Single-session debriefing following psychotrauma, help or harm? A metaanalysis. *Lancet.*

Wessely, S. (2002). Protean nature of mass sociogenic illness. *British Journal of Psychiatry, 180*, 300–306.

———, Hyams, K., & Bartholomew, R. (2001). Psychological implications of chemical and biological weapons. *British Medical Journal, 323*, 878–879.

World Health Organization. (2001, October). *World health report 2001—Mental health: New understanding, new hope.* Geneva: Author.

Zimbardo, P., & Kluger, B. (2003, May/June). Phantom menace: Is Washington terrorizing us more than Al Qaeda? *Psychology Today, 3*, 34–36.

2

Psychological Issues in Understanding Terrorism and the Response to Terrorism

Clark McCauley

This chapter begins with a brief effort to put modern terrorism in context. Thereafter, the chapter is divided into two main sections. The first deals with psychological issues involved in understanding the perpetrators of terrorism, including their motivations and strategies. The second deals with the U.S. response to terrorism, including issues of fear and identity shift in reaction to the events of September 11, 2001. I cannot offer a full review of the literature related to even one of these issues, and for some of them there is so little relevant literature that I can only point in the general directions that research might take. In using a very broad brush, I apologize in advance to scholars whose knowledge and contributions are not adequately represented here. A little theory can be a dangerous thing, especially in the hands of a nonspecialist in the relevant theory. But the events of 9/11 warrant some additional risk taking in connecting psychological research to our understanding of the origins and effects of terrorism.

Terrorism as a Category of Violence

Violence and the threat of violence to control people is an idea older than history, but the use of the word *terror* to refer to political violence goes back only to the French Revolution of the 1790s. Threatened by resistance within France and foreign armies at French borders, the revolutionaries undertook a Reign of Terror to suppress the enemy within. This first violence to be called terrorism had the power of the state behind it. Terrorism today is usually associated with political violence perpetrated by groups without the power of the state. Few of these nonstate groups have referred to themselves as terrorists, although prominent exceptions include the Russian Narodnaya Volya in the late 1800s and the Zionist Stern Gang of the late 1940s. Most nonstate terrorists see themselves as revolutionaries or freedom fighters.

State terrorism was not only first, it also continues to be more dangerous. Rummel (1996) estimates that 170 million people were killed by government in the twentieth century, not including 34 million who died in battle. Most of the civilian victims were killed by their own government or, more precisely, by the government controlling the area in which the victims were living. Stalin, Mao, and Hitler were the biggest killers (42 million, 37 million, 20 million respectively), with Pol Pot's killing of 2 million Cambodians coming in only seventh in the pantheon of killers. By comparison, killing by nonstate groups is miniscule. Rummel estimates that 500,000 were killed in the twentieth century by terrorists, guerillas, and other nonstate groups. State terrorism is thus greater by a ratio of about 260 to 1. Worldwide, Myers (2001) counts 2,527 deaths from terrorism in the 1990s. Three thousand terrorist victims on September 11 is thus a big increment in the killing done by terrorists, but that event does not change the scale of the comparison: State terrorism is by far the greater danger.

Despite the origin of the term *terrorism* in reference to state terror and despite the preeminence of state terror in relation to nonstate terror, terrorism today is usually understood to mean nonstate terrorism. Nonstate terrorism includes both antistate terror and vigilante terror, but it is usually antistate terrorism that is the focus of attention—violence against recognized states by small groups without the power of a state. Most definitions of antistate terrorism also include the idea of violence against noncombatants, especially women and children, although the suicide bombing of the U.S. Marine barracks in Beirut in 1984 is often referred to as terrorism, as is the 9/11 attack on the Pentagon.

Antistate terrorism cannot be understood outside the context of state terrorism. Compared with the nineteenth century, the twentieth century saw massive increases in state power. The modern state reaches deeper into the lives of citizens than ever before. It collects more in taxes, and its regulations, rewards, and punishments push further into work, school, and neighborhood. The state culture is thus ever harder to resist; any cultural group that does not control a state is likely to feel in danger of extinction. But resistance to state culture faces state power that continues to grow. In the context of growing state power, those who would contest against the state are likely to feel increasingly desperate.

Much has been written about how to define antistate terrorism, but I generally agree with those who say the difference between a terrorist and a freedom fighter lies mostly in the politics of the beholder (see McCauley, 1991, and McCauley, 1993, for more on this issue). The psychological question is how members of a small group without the power of a state become capable of political violence that includes violence against noncombatants. In the remainder of this chapter I follow common usage in referring to antistate terrorism simply as "terrorism."

Terrorist Motivations

People become terrorists in many different ways and for many different reasons. Here I simplify in order to consider three kinds of explanation of the 9/11 attacks: They are crazy, they are crazed by hatred and anger, or they are rational within their own perspective. My argument is that terrorism is not to be understood as pathology and that terrorists emerge out of a normal psychology of emotional commitment to cause and comrades.

Terrorism as Individual Pathology

A common suggestion is that there must be something wrong with terrorists. They must be crazy or suicidal or psychopathological. Only someone devoid of moral feelings could do the cold-blooded killing that a terrorist does.

The Search for Pathology

Thirty years ago this suggestion was taken very seriously, but thirty years of research has found little evidence that terrorists are suffering from psychopathology. This research has profited by what now amounts to hundreds of interviews with terrorists. Some are captured and interviewed in prison. Some active terrorists can be found in their home neighborhoods, if the interviewer knows where to look. And some retired terrorists are willing to talk about their earlier activities, particularly if these were successful. Itzhak Shamir and Menachem Begin, for instance, moved from anti-Arab and anti-British terrorism to leadership of the state of Israel. Interviews with terrorists rarely find any disorder listed in the *Diagnostic and Statistical Manual of Mental Disorders*.

More systematic research confirms the interview results. Particularly thorough were the German studies of the Baader-Meinhof Gang. Although the terrorists had gone underground and their locations were undisclosed, their identities were known. Excellent German records provided a great deal of information about each member. Pre- and perinatal records, pediatric records, preschool records, lower-school records, grade-school records, high-school records, and university records (most had had some university education)—all of these were combed for clues to understanding the trajectory to terrorism. Family, neighbors, and classmates—all those who had known an individual before the leap to terrorism—were interviewed. A comparison sample of people from the same neighborhoods, matched for gender, age, and socioeconomic status, was similarly studied. The results of these investigations fill several feet of shelf space but are easy to summarize. The terrorists did not differ from the comparison group of nonterrorists in any substantial way; in particular, the terrorists did not show higher rates of any kind of psychopathology.

Terrorists as Psychopaths

Some have suggested that terrorists are *antisocial personalities* or *psychopaths*. Psychopaths can be intelligent and very much in contact with reality; their problem is that they are socially and morally deficient. They are law breakers, and they are deceitful, aggressive, and reckless in disregarding the welfare of others. They do not feel remorse for hurting others. Just as some people cannot see color, psychopaths cannot feel empathy or affection for others.

Explaining terrorism as the work of psychopaths brings a new difficulty, however. The 9/11 attackers were willing to give their lives in the attack. So far as I am aware, no one has ever suggested that a psychopath's moral blindness can take the form of self-sacrifice. In addition, psychopaths are notably impulsive and irresponsible. The mutual commitment and trust that is evident within each of the four groups of attackers and in the cooperation among the groups is radically inconsistent with the psychopathic personality.

It is possible that a terrorist group might recruit a psychopath for a particular mission if the assignment requires inflicting pain or death without the distraction of sympathy for the victims, but the undertaking would have to be a one-person job, something that requires little or no coordination and trust. And it would have to offer a reasonable chance of success without suicide.

The Case Against Pathology

Of course, there are occasional lone bombers or lone gunmen who kill for political causes, and such people may indeed suffer from some form of psychopathology. A loner like Theodore Kaczynski, the "Unabomber," who sent out letter bombs in occasional forays from his wilderness cabin, may suffer from psychopathology. However, terrorists who operate in groups, especially those that can organize successful attacks, are very unlikely to suffer from serious psychopathology.

Indeed, terrorism would be a trivial problem if only those with some kind of psychopathology were terrorists. Rather, we have to face the fact that normal people can be terrorists and that we ourselves are capable of terrorist acts under some circumstances. This fact is already implied in recognizing that military and police forces involved in state terrorism are all too capable of killing noncombatants. Few would suggest that the broad range of soldiers and police involved in such killing must all be suffering some kind of psychopathology.

Terrorism as Emotional Expression

On October 11, 2001, when asked at a press conference why people in the Muslim world hate the United States, President Bush expressed amazement and replied, "That's because they don't know us." President Bush is not the only one to accept the idea that the 9/11 attacks were an expression of hatred. "Why do they hate us?" has been the headline of numerous stories and editorials in newspapers and magazines. Despite the headlines, there has been little analysis of what hatred means or where it comes from.

Hatred and Anger

The surprising fact is that, although a few psychoanalysts have discussed hatred, very little psychological research has focused on hate or hatred. Gordon Allport (1954) briefly mentioned hatred in writing *The Nature of Prejudice,* and Marilyn Brewer (2001) has asked, "When does in-group love become out-group hate?" However, empirical research on hatred, particularly research that distinguishes it from anger, is notably absent. In contrast, there is a large and well-developed literature on the emotion of anger. Does hatred mean anything more than strong anger? An example suggests that hatred may be different. A parent can be angry with a misbehaving child, angry to the point of striking the child. Nevertheless, even caught up in that violence, the parent would not hate the child.

A few differences between anger and hatred show up in the way these words are used in everyday speech. Anger is hot, whereas hatred can be cold. Anger is a response to a particular incident or offense; hatred expresses a longer-term relation of antipathy. We sometimes talk about hatred when we mean only strong dislike, as in "I hate broccoli," but even this usage suggests the sense of a general and unwavering dislike, a dislike without exceptions, and perhaps even the wish that broccoli would be erased from every menu.

In *The Deadly Ethnic Riot,* Donald Horowitz (2001) offers a distinction between anger and hatred that is consistent with the language just considered. Horowitz quotes Aristotle as follows: "The angry man wants the object of his anger to suffer in return; hatred wishes its object not to exist" (p. 543). This distinction begs for a parallel distinction in offenders or offenses, one that can predict when an offense will lead to anger and when to hatred. One possibility (see also Brewer, 2001) is that an offense that includes long-term threat is more likely to elicit the desire to eliminate the offender. The emotional reaction to threat is fear. Thus hatred may be a compound of anger and fear, or, as Sternberg (2003) suggests, a variable blend of disgust, anger-fear, and contempt.

Another perspective is offered by Royzman, McCauley and Rozin (2004), who suggest that hate is not an emotion or a blend of emotions but rather an extreme form of negative identification. Negative identification means feeling bad about the successes of others; negative identification means feeling good about the successes of others. Thus the hater feels joy or pride when the target of hate is losing, hurting, or weakening, but feels anger, fear, or humiliation when the target of hate is winning, gaining, or strengthening. Similarly love is an extreme form of positive identification, and the lover can feel either positive or negative emotions depending on what is happening to the loved one. As extremes of the human capacity for identification, hate and love are the occasions of experiencing many different emotions depending on the situation of the one loved or hated.

Whether or not hate is an emotion, hate has some relation to anger and research on anger may be able to help us understand the behavior of terrorists.

The Psychology of Anger

Explanation of terrorism as the work of people blinded by anger is at least generally consistent with what is known about the emotion of anger. In particular, there is reason to believe that anger gets in the way of judgment. In *Passions within Reason,* Robert Frank (1988) argues that blindness to self-interest is the evolutionary key to anger. If each person acted rationally on self-interest, the strong could do anything they wanted to the weak. Both would realize that the weak cannot win, and the weaker would always defer to the stronger. However, anger can lead the weaker to attack the stronger despite the objective balance of forces. The stronger will win, but will suffer some costs along the way, and the possibility of these costs restrains the stronger and improves the bargaining position of the weaker.

This perspective suggests an evolutionary advantage for people for whom anger can conquer fear. The result should be a gradual increase in the proportion of those who are capable of anger. Everyday experience suggests that, under certain circumstances, most people are capable of anger. What are those circumstances, that is, what are the elicitors of anger?

There are basically two theories of anger (Sabini, 1995, pp. 411–428). The first, which comes to us from Aristotle, says that anger is the emotional reaction to insult—an offense in which someone is not accorded due respect or status. The second, which emerged from experimental research with animals, says that anger is the emotional reaction to pain, especially the pain of frustration. Frustration is understood as the failure to receive an expected reward. These theories obviously have a great deal in common. Respect that is expected but not forthcoming creates a painful frustration. For our purposes, the two theories differ chiefly in their emphasis on material welfare. Insult is subjective, a social judgment, whereas at least some interpretations of frustration include objective poverty and powerlessness as sources of frustration that can lead to anger. This interpretation of frustration-aggression theory was popular at the 2002 World Economic Forum, where many luminaries cited material deprivation as the cause (or at least an important cause) of violence aimed at the West (A. Friedman, 2002).

Individual Frustration and Insult

The immediate difficulty of seeing the 9/11 terrorists as crazed with anger is the fact, much cited by journalists and pundits, that they were not obviously suffering from frustration or insult. Mohammed Atta came from a middle-class family in Egypt, studied architecture in Cairo, traveled to Hamburg, Germany, for further studies in architecture, and had a part-time job doing architectural drawings for a German firm. His German thesis, on the ancient architecture of Aleppo, was well received. According to Thomas Friedman's (2002) inquiries, several of the other 9/11 pilot leaders came from comparable middle-class backgrounds with similar threads of personal success.

The origins of the 9/11 terrorist leaders are thus strikingly different from those of the Palestinian suicide terrorists that Ariel Merari studied in Israel for decades (Lelyveld, 2001). The Palestinians were young, male, poor, and uneducated. Their motivations were manifold but sometimes included the several thousand dollars awarded to the family of a Palestinian martyr. The amount is small by Western standards but enough to lift a Palestinian family out of abject poverty, including support for parents and aged relatives and a dowry for the martyr's sisters. It is easy to characterize these suicide terrorists as frustrated by poverty and hopelessness, with frustration leading to anger against Israel as the perceived source of their problems.

More recent studies, however, consistently conclude that terrorists and suicide terrorists are not generally poor or uneducated. Rather they have education and prospects at least average, often higher than average, in relation to the group they come from (Atran, 2003; Krueger & Maleckova, 2002; Pape, 2005). It seems that the middle-class origins of the 9/11 leadership are not unusual and that personal frustration associated with poverty, poor education, and unemployment is not a useful explanation of terrorism.

If not angry about personal frustrations and insults, terrorists may yet be angry about frustrations and insults their group has suffered.

Group Frustration and Insult

In the *Handbook of Social Psychology,* Kinder (1998) summarizes the accumulated evidence that political opinions are only weakly predicted by narrow self-interest and more strongly predicted by group interest. The poor do not support welfare policies more than others, young males are not less in favor of war than others, and parents of school-age children are not more opposed than others to busing for desegregation. Rather it is group interest that is the useful predictor. Sympathy for the poor predicts favoring increased welfare. Sympathy for African Americans predicts support for busing and other desegregation policies. Unless self-interest is exceptionally large and clear cut, voters' opinions are not self-centered but group centered.

Similarly, Kinder recounts evidence that political action, including protest and confrontation, is motivated more by identification with group interest than self-interest. "Thus participation of black college students in the civil rights movement in the American South in the 1960s was predicted better by their anger over society's treatment of black Americans in general than by any discontent they felt about their own lives.... Thus white working-class participants in the Boston antibusing movement were motivated especially by their resentments about the gains of blacks and professionals, and less by their own personal troubles" (Kinder, 1998, p. 831).

Group identification makes sense of sacrifice by people who are not personally frustrated or insulted. The mistake is to imagine that self-sacrifice must come from personal problems, rather than identification with group problems. This error rests in ignorance of the fact that many twentieth century terrorists have been people from comfortable circumstances, people with options. The Baader-Meinhof Gang in Germany, the Red Brigade in Italy, the Weather Underground in the United States—these and many other post–World War II terrorist groups consisted mostly of people with middle-class origins and middle-class skills honed by at least some university education (McCauley & Segal, 1987). Explaining self-sacrifice as a result of personal problems is no more persuasive for terrorists than for Mother Theresa or U.S. Medal of Honor winners.

The power of group identification is thus the foundation of intergroup conflict, especially for large groups, where self-interest is probably maximized by free riding, that is, by letting other group members pay the costs of advancing group welfare that the individual will profit from. Here I am briefly asserting what I elsewhere argue for in more detail (McCauley, 2001).

The explanation of terrorists' sacrifice as a fit of anger overcoming self-interest can now be reformulated in terms of anger over group insult and group frustration. The potential origins of such anger are not difficult to discern.

Insult and Frustration as Seen by Muslims (and Others)

From Morocco to Pakistan lies a belt of Muslim states in which governments have police and military power but little public support. The gulf between rich and poor is deep and wide in these countries, and government is associated with Western-leaning elites for whom government, not private enterprise, is the source of wealth. Political threat to the state is not tolerated; imprisonment, torture, and death are the tools of the state against political opposition. As the Catholic Church in Poland under Communism came to be the principal refuge of political opposition, so fundamentalist Muslim mosques are the principal refuge of political opposition to government in these states.

In this conflict between Muslim governments and Muslim peoples, the United States and other Western countries have supported the governments. When the Algerian government was about to lose an election to the Islamic Salvation Front in 1992, the government annulled the election, and Europeans and Americans were glad to accept the lesser of two evils. Western countries have supported authoritarian governments of Egypt, Jordan, and Pakistan with credits and military assistance. U.S. support for Israel against the Palestinians is only one part of this pattern of supporting power against people.

Al-Qaeda is an association of exiles and refugees from the political violence going on in Muslim countries. Long before declaring jihad against the United States, Osama bin Laden was attacking the house of Saud for letting U.S. troops remain in the holy land of Mecca and Medina after the Gulf War. Fifteen of the 9/11 terrorists originally came from Saudi Arabia, although most of them seem to have been recruited from the Muslim diaspora in Europe. The United States has become a target because it is seen as supporting the governments that created the diaspora. The United States has, in effect, stumbled into a family feud. If this scenario seems strained, consider the parallel between Muslims declaring jihad on this country for supporting state terrorism in Muslim countries, and the United States declaring war on any country that supports terrorism against it.

It is important to recognize that it is not only Arab and Muslim countries in which U.S. policies are seen as responsible for terrorist attacks against the United States. In an *International Herald Tribune*-Pew poll of 275 "opinion makers" in 24 countries, respondents were asked how many ordinary people think that U.S. policies and actions in the world were a major cause of the 9/11 attack (Knowlton, 2001). In the United States only 18% of respondents said that many people think this; in 23 other countries an average of 58% said most or many people hold this opinion. In Islamic countries 76% said most or many think this, and even in Western European countries 36% said most or many people agree. Americans do not have to accept the judgments of other countries, but we will have to deal with them.

Anger or Love?

If group identification can lead to anger as a result of frustrations and insults suffered by the group, it remains to be determined whether there is any evidence of such emotions in the 9/11 terrorists. Our best guide to the motives of those who carried out those attacks is the document found in the luggage of several of the attackers. Four of the five pages of this document have been released by the FBI, and Makiya and Mneimneh (2002) have translated and interpreted them. I am indebted to Hassan Mneimneh for his assistance in understanding this document.

The four pages are surprising for what they do not contain. There is neither a list of group frustrations and insults nor a litany of injustice to justify violence. "The sense throughout is that the would-be martyr is engaged in his action solely to please God. There is no mention of any communal purpose behind his behavior. In all of the four pages available to us there is not a word or an implication about any wrongs that are to be redressed through martyrdom, whether in Palestine or Iraq or in 'the land of Muhammad,' the phrase bin Laden used in the al-Jazeera video that was shown after September 11" (Makiya and Mneimneh, 2002, p. 21). Indeed, the text approvingly cites a story from the Hadith, the collection of sayings and actions attributed to the Prophet and his companions, about Ali ibn Abi Talib, cousin and son-in-law of the Prophet, who is spat upon by an infidel in combat. The Muslim holds his sword until he can master the impulse for vengeance—an individual and human motive—and strikes only when he can strike for the sake of God.

Rather than anger or hatred, the dominant message of the text is a focus on the eternal. There are many references to the Koran, and the vocabulary departs from seventh-century Arabic only for a few references to modern concepts such as airport and plane (and these modern words are reduced to one-letter abbreviations). To feel connection with God and the work of God and to experience the peace of submission to God's will—these are the imperatives and the promises of the text. Invocations and prayers are to be offered at every stage of the journey: the last night, the journey to the airport, boarding the plane, takeoff, seizing control of the plane, and welcoming death. The reader is reminded that fear is an act of worship due only to God. If killing is necessary, the language of the text makes the killing a ritual slaughter with vocabulary that refers to animal sacrifice, including the sacrifice of Isaac that Abraham was prepared to offer.

Judging from this text, the psychology of the 9/11 terrorists is not one of anger or hatred or vengeance. The terrorists are not righting human wrongs but acting with God and for God against evil. In the most general terms, this is a psychology of attachment to the good rather than a psychology of hatred for evil. Research with U.S. soldiers in World War II found something similar; hatred of the enemy was a minor motive in combat performance, whereas attachment to buddies and not wanting to let them down was a major motive (Stouffer et al., 1949). This resonance with the psychology of combat—one that is usually treated as normal psychology—again suggests the possibility that terrorism and terrorists may be more normal than we usually recognize.

Terrorism as Normal Psychology

The trajectory by which normal people become capable of doing terrible things is usually gradual, perhaps imperceptible to the individual. This is among other things a moral trajectory, such as Sprinzak (1991) and Horowitz (2001) have described. In too-simple terms, terrorists kill for the same reasons that groups have killed other groups for centuries. They kill for cause and comrades, that is, with a combination of ideology and intense small-group dynamics. The cause that is worth killing for and dying for is not abstract but personal—a view of the world that makes sense of

life and death and links the individual to some form of immortality.

The Psychology of Cause

Most people believe in something more important than life. We have to because, unlike other animals, we know that we are going to die. We need something that makes sense of our life and our death, something that makes our death different from that of a squirrel lying by the side of the road. The closer and more immediate death is, the more we need the group values that give meaning to life and death. These include the values of family, religion, ethnicity, and nationality—the values of our culture. Dozens of experiments have shown that thinking about death—especially their own—leads people to embrace the values of their culture more strongly (Pyszcznski, Greenberg, & Solomon, 1997).

These values do not have to be explicitly religious. Many of the terrorist groups since World War II have been radical-socialist groups with purely secular roots: the Red Brigade in Italy, the Baader-Meinhof Gang in Germany, the Shining Path in Peru, the Tamil Tigers in Sri Lanka. Animal rights and environmental issues can be causes that justify terrorism. For much of the twentieth century, atheistic communism was such a cause. Thus there is no special relation between religion and violence; religion is only one kind of cause in which people can find an answer to mortality.

What is essential is that the cause should have the promise of a long and glorious future. History is important in supporting this promise. A cause invented yesterday cannot easily be seen to have a glorious and indefinite future. Moreover, the history must be a group history. No one ever seems to have had the idea that she or he alone will achieve some kind of immortality. Immortality comes as part of a group: family group, cultural group, religious group, or ideological group. A good participant in the group, one who lives up to its norms and contributes to the group, will to that extent live on after death as part of the group. The meaning of the individual's life is the future of the cause, embodied in the group that goes on into the future after the individual is dead.

The Psychology of Comrades

The group's values are focused to a personal intensity in the small group of like-minded people who perpetrate terrorist violence. Most people belong to many groups—family, coworkers, neighborhood, religion, country—and each of these has some influence on individual beliefs and behavior. Different groups have different values, and the competition of values reduces the power of any one group over its members. However, members of an underground terrorist cell have put this group first in their lives, dropping or reducing every other connection. The power of this one group is now enormous and extends to every kind of personal and moral judgment. This is the power that can make violence against the enemy not just acceptable but necessary.

Every army aims to do what the terrorist group does: link a larger group cause with the small-group dynamics that can deliver individuals to sacrifice. Every army cuts trainees off from their previous lives so that the combat unit can become their family, their fellow soldiers become their brothers, and their fear of letting down their comrades becomes greater than their fear of dying. The power of an isolating group over its members is not limited to justifying violence. Many nonviolent groups also gain power by separating individuals from groups that might offer competing values. Those that use this tactic include religious cults, drug treatment centers, and residential schools and colleges. In brief, the psychology behind terrorist violence is normal psychology; it is abnormal only in the intensity of the group dynamics that link cause with comrades.

Some commentators have noted that the 9/11 terrorists, at least the pilot leaders, spent long periods of time dispersed in the United States. How could the intense group dynamics typical of underground groups be maintained in dispersal? There are two possible answers. The first is that physical dispersal is not the same as developing new group connections. It seems that the dispersed terrorists lived without close connections to others outside the terrorist group. They did not take interesting jobs, become close to coworkers, or develop romantic relationships. Although living apart, they remained connected to and anchored in only one group—their terrorist group.

The second possibility is that group dynamics can be less important to the extent that the cause—its ideology—is more important. As noted previously, the pilot leaders of the 9/11 terrorists were not poor or untalented; they were men with a

middle-class background and education. For educated men, the power of ideas may substitute to some degree for the everyday reinforcement of a like-minded group. Indeed, the terrorist document referred to earlier is a kind of manual for using control of attention to control behavior, and this kind of manual should work better for individuals familiar with the attractions of ideas. Probably both possibilities—a social world reduced to one group despite physical dispersal and a group of individuals for whom the ideology of cause is unusually important and powerful—contributed to the cohesion of the 9/11 perpetrators.

The Psychology of Cult Recruiting

Studies of recruiting for the Unification Church (UC) provide some insight into differences in vulerability to the call of cause and comrades (McCauley & Segal, 1987). Galanter (1980) surveyed participants in UC recruiting workshops in Southern California and found that the best predictor of who becomes a member was the answer to a question about how close the person feels to people outside the Unification Church. Those with outside attachments were more likely to leave, whereas those without outside connections were more likely to join. This is the power of comrades.

Barker (1984) surveyed participants in Unification Church recruiting workshops in London and found that the best predictor of who becomes a member was the answer to a question about goals. Those who said they were looking for "something but I don't know what" were more likely to join. This is the power of cause, a group cause that can give meaning to one's life. Terrorist groups, like cult groups, cut the individual off from other contacts and are particularly attractive to those without close connections and the meaning that comes with group anchoring. Only those who have never had the experience of feeling cut off from family, friends, and work will see this kind of vulnerability as a type of pathology. The rest of us will feel fortunate that we did not at this point in our lives encounter someone recruiting for a cult or terrorist group.

The Psychology of Crisis

The psychology of cause and comrades is multiplied by a sense of crisis. Many observers have noted an apocalyptic quality in the worldview of terrorists. Terrorists see the world precariously balanced between good and evil, at a point where action can bring about the triumph of the good. The "end times" or the millennium or the triumph of the working class is near or can be made near by right action. Action—extreme action—is required immediately for the triumph of the good and the defeat of evil. This "ten minutes to midnight" feeling is part of what makes it possible for normal people to risk their lives in violence.

Consider the passengers of the hijacked flight that crashed in western Pennsylvania. The passengers found out from their cell phones that hijacked planes had crashed into the World Trade Center. They had every reason to believe that their plane was on its way to a similar end. Unarmed, they decided to attack the hijackers and sacrificed their lives in bringing the plane down before it could impact its intended target, which was probably the Pentagon or the White House. When it is ten minutes to midnight, there is little to lose and everything to gain.

The sense of crisis is usually associated with an overwhelming threat. In the case of the 9/11 terrorists it seems to be fear that fundamentalist Muslim culture is in danger of being overwhelmed by Western culture. The military and economic power of the West and the relative feebleness of once-great Muslim nations in the modern era are submerging Muslims in a tidal wave of individualism and irreligion. It is attachment to a view of what Muslims should be—and fear for their future—that are the emotional foundations of the terrorists. They do not begin from hatred of the West but from love of their own group and culture, which they believe is in danger of extinction from the power of the West.

Similarly, the United States, mobilized by President Bush for a war against terrorism, does not begin from hatred of al-Qaeda but from love of country. Mobilization includes a rhetoric of crisis and of impending threat from an evil enemy or, more recently, an "axis of evil." America's anger toward al-Qaeda, and perhaps more broadly toward Arabs and Muslims, is not an independent emotion but a product of patriotism combined with a crisis of threat.

The Psychology of the Slippery Slope

The sense of crisis does not spring full blown upon a person. It is the end of a long trajectory to terrorism, a trajectory in which the person moves slowly toward an apocalyptic view of the world and a correspondingly extreme behavioral commitment. Sprinzak (1991) has distinguished three stages in this trajectory: a *crisis of confidence,* in which a group protests and demonstrates against the prevailing political system with a criticism that yet accepts the system's values; a *conflict of legitimacy,* in which the group loses confidence in reform and advances a competing ideological and cultural system while moving to angry protest and small-scale violence; and a *crisis of legitimacy,* in which the group embraces terrorist violence against the government and everyone who supports it. Whether as someone joining an extreme group or as a member of a group that becomes more extreme over time, the individual becomes more extreme in a series of steps so small as to be nearly invisible. The result is a terrorist who may look back at the transition to terrorism with no sense of ever having made an explicit choice.

Psychology offers several models of this kind of slippery slope (see McCauley & Segal, 1987, for more detail). One is Milgram's obedience experiment, in which 60% of subjects are willing to deliver the maximum shock level ("450 volts XXX Danger Strong Shock") to a supposed fellow subject in a supposed learning experiment. In one variation of the experiment, Milgram had the experimenter called away on a pretext, and another supposed subject came up with the idea of raising the shock one level with each mistake from the "learner." In this variation, 20% went on to deliver maximum shock. The 20% yielding cannot be attributed to the authority of the experimenter and is most naturally understood as the power of self-justification acting on the small increments in shock level. Each shock delivered becomes a reason for giving the next higher shock because the small increments mean that the subject has to see something at least a little wrong with the last shock if there is something wrong with the next one. A clear choice between good and evil would be a shock generator with only two levels, 15 volts and 450 volts, but the 20% who go all the way never see a clear choice between good and evil.

Another model of the terrorist trajectory is more explicitly social psychological. Group extremity shift, which is the tendency for group opinion to become more extreme in the direction initially favored by most people, is currently understood in terms of two mechanisms: relevant arguments and social comparison (Brown, 1986, pp. 200–244). Relevant arguments theory explains the shift as a result of individuals hearing new arguments in discussion that are biased in the initially favored direction. Social comparison theory explains the shift as a competition for status in which no one wants to fall behind in supporting the group-favored direction. In the trajectory to terrorism, initial beliefs and commitments favor action against injustice, and group discussion and in-group status competition move the group toward more extreme views and more extreme violence.

The slippery slope is not something that happens only in psychology experiments and foreign countries. Since 9/11, there have already been suggestions from reputable people that U.S. security forces may need to use torture to get information from suspected terrorists. This is the edge of a slope that leads down and away from the rule of law and the presumption of innocence.

Terrorism as Strategy

Psychologists recognize two kinds of aggression: emotional and instrumental. Emotional aggression is associated with anger and does not calculate long-term consequences. The reward of emotional aggression is hurting someone who has hurt you. Instrumental aggression is more calculating—it involves the use of aggression as a means to other ends. The balance between these two in the behavior of individual terrorists is usually not clear and might usefully be studied more explicitly in the future. The balance may be important in determining how to respond to terrorism: emotional aggression should be less sensitive to objective rewards and punishments, and instrumental aggression more sensitive.

Of course, the balance may be very different in those who perpetrate the violence than in those who plan it. The planners are probably more instrumental because they are usually thinking about what they want to accomplish. They aim to inflict long-term harm to their enemy and to gain lasting advantage for themselves.

Material Damage to the Enemy

Terrorism inflicts immediate damage in destroying lives and property, but terrorists hope that the long-standing costs will be much greater. They want to create fear and uncertainty far beyond the victims and those close to them. They want their enemy to spend time and money on security. In effect, the terrorists aim to lay an enormous burden on every aspect of the enemy's society, one that transfers resources from productive purposes to antiproductive security measures. The costs of increased security are likely to be particularly high for a country like the United States, where an open society is the foundation of economic success and a high-tech military.

The United States is already paying enormous taxes of this kind. Billions more dollars are going to the FBI, the CIA, the Pentagon, the National Security Agency, and a new bureaucracy for the Department of Homeland Security. Billions are going to bail out the airlines, to increase the number and quality of airport security personnel, and to pay the National Guard stationed at airports. The costs to business activity are perhaps even greater. Long lines at airport security points and fear of air travel have cut both business and holiday travel. Hotel bookings are down, urban restaurant business is down; in short, all kinds of tourist businesses are down. Long lines of trucks at the Canadian and Mexican borders are slowed for more intensive searches, and the delays necessarily contribute to the cost of goods transported. The Coast Guard and the Immigration and Naturalization Service now focus on terrorism and have decreased their attention to the drug trade. I suspect that the expenses of increased security and the war on terrorism will far outrun the costs of the losses at the World Trade Center and the reparations to the survivors of those who died there.

Political Damage to the Enemy

In the longer term, the damage terrorism does to civil society may be greater than any dollar costs (see McCauley, this volume). The response to terrorism inevitably builds the power of the state at the expense of the civil society. The adage that "war is the health of the state" is evident to anyone who tracks the growth of the federal government in the United States. The Civil War, World War I, World War II, the Korean War, the Vietnam War, the Gulf War, and now the war against terrorism—in every war the power of government grows in direction and extent never recovered when the conflict is over.

Polls taken in the years preceding the terrorist attack on September 11 indicate that about half of adult Americans saw the federal government as a threat to the rights and freedoms of ordinary citizens. No doubt fewer would say so in the aftermath of those attacks, a shift consistent with the adage that "war is the health of the state." If more security could ensure the safety of a nation, however, the Soviet Union would still be with us. It is possible that bin Laden had the Soviet Union in mind in an interview broadcast by CNN. "Osama bin Laden told a reporter with the Al Jazeera network in October that 'freedom and human rights in America are doomed' and that the U.S. government would lead its people and the West 'into an unbearable hell and a choking life' " (Kurtz, 2002).

Mobilizing the In-Group

Terrorists particularly hope to elicit a violent response that will assist them in mobilizing their own people. A terrorist group is the apex of a pyramid of supporters and sympathizers. The base of the pyramid is composed of all those who sympathize with the terrorists' cause even though they may disagree with the violent means they use. In Northern Ireland, for instance, the base of the pyramid is all those who agree with "Brits out." In the Islamic world, the base of the pyramid is all those who agree that the United States has been hurting and humiliating Muslims for fifty years. The pyramid is essential to the terrorists for cover and for recruits. They hope that a clumsy and overgeneralized strike against them will hit some of those in the pyramid below them. The blow will enlarge their base of sympathy, turn the sympathetic but unmobilized to action and sacrifice, and strengthen their own status as leaders at the apex.

Al-Qaeda had reason to be hopeful that U.S. strength could help them. In 1986, for instance, the United States attempted to reply to Libyan-supported terrorism by bombing Libya's leader, Khaddafi. The bombs missed Khaddafi's residence but hit a nearby apartment building and killed numerous women and children. This mistake was downplayed in the United States but was a public relations success for anti-U.S. groups across North Africa. In 1998, the United States attempted to reply to al-Qaeda's attacks on U.S. embassies in Africa by sending cruise missiles against terrorist camps in Afghanistan and against a supposed bomb factory in Khartoum. It appears now that the "bomb factory" was in fact producing only medical supplies.

A violent response to terrorism that is not well aimed is a success for the terrorists. The Taliban did their best to play up U.S. bombing mistakes in Afghanistan but were largely disappointed. It appears that civilian casualties of U.S attacks in Afghanistan number somewhere between 1,000 and 3,700, depending on who is estimating (Bearak, 2002). Although Afghan civilian losses may thus approach the 3,000 U.S. victims of 9/11, it is clear that U.S. accuracy has been outstanding by the standards of modern warfare. Al-Qaeda could still hope to profit by perceptions of a crusade against Muslims if the United States extended the war on terrorism to Iraq, Iran, or Somalia. In 2006, as this chapter goes to press, the U.S. presence in Iraq seems to have done all that Al-Qaeda could hope for.

U.S. Reaction to 9/11: Some Issues of Mass Psychology

In this section I consider several psychological issues raised by the U.S. reaction to the terrorist attacks of September 11, 2001. Has the United States been terrorized? What kinds of identity shifts may have occurred after 9/11?

Fear After 9/11

There is little doubt that the events of 9/11, soon followed by another plane crash at Rockaway Beach, made Americans less willing to fly. In early 2002, air travel and hotel bookings were still significantly below the levels recorded in the months before the attacks. Beyond the fear of flying, Americans evidently became generally more anxious and insecure. At least some law firms specializing in the preparation of wills and trusts saw a big increase in business after 9/11. Gun sales were up in some places after that date, suggesting a search for increased security broader than the threat of terrorism. Owning a gun may not be of much help against terrorists, but, at least for some people, a gun can be a symbol and reassurance of control and personal safety. Pet sales were also reported up in some places after the September attacks. Again, a pet is not likely to be of much help against terrorists, but, at least for some, a pet may be an antidote to uncertainty and fear. A pet offers both an experience of control and the reassurance of unconditional positive regard (Beck & Katcher, 1996).

It is tempting to interpret a big decrease in air travel as evidence of a substantial increase in fear, but it may be that even a small increase in fear can produce a large decrease in the willingness to fly. When the stakes are high, a small change in risk perception can trigger a large decrease in one's inclination to bet. Indeed, decreased willingness to fly need not imply any increase in fear. Some may already have been afraid of flying and found 9/11 not a stimulus to increased fear but a justification for acting on fears had previously been ridiculed and suppressed. Thus it may be only a minority who felt an increased fear of flying after 9/11.

Myers (2001) has offered four research generalizations about perceived risk that can help explain the increased fear of flying after 9/11. We are biologically prepared to fear heights, we particularly fear what we cannot control, we fear immediate more than long-term and cumulative dangers, and we exaggerate dangers represented in vivid and memorable images. All of these influences can help explain the fear of flying, but only the last one can explain the reason that fear of flying increased after 9/11. Fear of heights preceded 9/11. On entering a plane, every passenger gives up control, and the immediate risk of climbing on a plane is little affected by four or five crashes in a brief period of time.

Myers notes, however, that the risks of air travel are largely concentrated in the minutes of takeoff and landing. This is a framing issue: Do air travelers see their risk in terms of deaths per passenger mile—which makes air travel much safer than driving—or do they see the risk as deaths per minute of takeoff and landing? With the latter perspective, air travel may be objectively riskier than driving.

Still, Myers may be correct in focusing on the importance of television images of planes slicing into the World Trade Center, but the importance of these images may have more to do with control of fear and norms about expressing it than with the actual level of fear. Myers reports a 1989 Gallup poll concerning commercial aviation that indicates that, even before 9/11, 44% of those willing to fly were willing to admit they felt apprehensive about flying. It is possible that this anxiety is controlled

by a cognitive appraisal that flying is safe, and the images of planes crashing interfere with this appraisal. This interpretation is similar to the "safety frame" explanation of how people can enjoy the fear arousal associated with riding a roller coaster or watching a horror film (McCauley, 1998b).

If the safety frame is disturbed, the fear controls behavior, and, in the case of air travel, people are less willing to fly. One implication of this interpretation is that, for at least some people, government warnings of additional terrorist attacks in the near future would make no difference in the level of trepidation experienced—vivid crash images may release the latent fear no matter what the objective likelihood of additional crashes.

Acting on the uneasiness experienced is a separate issue. Warnings of future terrorist attacks may affect the norms of acting on a fear of flying, that is, the warnings may reduce social pressure to carry on business as usual and lessen ridicule for those who are afraid of flying. Fear of flying is an attitude, and social norms undoubtedly have much to do with determining when attitudes are expressed in behavior (Ajzen & Fishbein, 1980).

Indeed, the impact of government warnings and increased airport security are very much in need of investigation. President Bush was in the position of trying to tell Americans that they should resume flying and that new airport security measures made flying safe again, even as security agencies issued multiple warnings of new terrorist attacks. These warnings had the peculiar quality of being completely unspecific about the nature of the threat or what to do about it. The possible downside of such warnings is suggested by research indicating that threat appeals are likely to be repressed or ignored if they do not include specific and effective action to avoid the threats (Sabini, 1995, pp. 565–566). Even the additional airport security measures may be of dubious value. It is true that many Americans seemed reassured to see army personnel with weapons stationed in airports, although the objective security value of troops with no training in security screening is by no means obvious. But if there is any value to the framing interpretation of increased anxiety, then adding military security at airports may actually increase travelers' apprehension. Vivid images of armed troops at airports may actually undermine rather than augment the safety frame that controls the fear of flying.

Differences in security procedures from one airport to another can also exacerbate fear. A journalist from Pittsburgh called me not long after new security procedures were introduced at U.S. airports. His newspaper had received a letter to the editor written by a visitor from Florida, a letter excoriating the Pittsburgh airport for inadequate security. The writer had been frightened because she was asked for identification only once on her way to boarding her return flight from Pittsburgh, whereas, in boarding the Florida flight to Pittsburgh, she had been stopped for identification five times.

Fear of flying is not the only apprehension to emerge from 9/11. Survivors of the attacks on the World Trade Center (WTC), those who fled for their lives that morning, may still be fearful of working in a high-rise building and afraid even of all of the parts of Lower Manhattan that were associated with commuting to and from the WTC. Many corporate employees who escaped the WTC returned to work in new office buildings in northern New Jersey. In these new settings, some may have been retraumatized by frequent fire and evacuation drills that associated their new offices and stairwells with the uncertainties and fears of the same environment at the WTC. For these people, the horror of the WTC may have been a kind of one-trial traumatic conditioning experiment, with follow-up training in associating their new work place with the old one. Their experience and their fears deserve research attention.

A small step in this direction was a December 2001 conference at the University of Pennsylvania's Solomon Asch Center for the Study of Ethnopolitical Conflict. The conference brought together eight trauma counselors from around the United States who had been brought in to assist WTC corporate employees returning to work in new office spaces. Several potentially important issues emerged at the conference. Perhaps most important is that the counselors were selected and directed by corporate employee assistance programs with more experience in physical health than mental health problems. Thus the counselors were all contracted to use critical incident stress debriefing techniques with everyone they assisted; at least officially, no room was left for a counselor to exercise independent judgment about what approach might best suit a particular situation.

Similarly, because the counselors were seen as interchangeable resources, a counselor might be sent to one corporation on one day and to a different corporation the next day, even as another counselor experienced the reverse transfer. The importance of becoming familiar with a particular corporate culture and setting, the personal connection between individual counselor and the managers that control that setting, and the trust developed between counselors and people needing assistance and referral in that setting—these were given little attention in the organization of counseling assistance. It appears that the experience of the counselors working with WTC survivors has not yet been integrated with the experience of those working with survivors of the Oklahoma City bombing (Pfefferbaum, Flynn, Brandt, & Lensgraf, 1999). There is a long way to go before we are able to develop anything like a consensus on "best practice" for assisting survivors of such attacks.

In sum, fear after 9/11 includes a range of fear reactions, including fear of flying by those with no personal connection to the WTC, more general anxieties associated with death from uncontrollable and unpredictable terrorist attacks, and specific workplace fearfulness among those who escaped the WTC attacks. These reactions offer theoretical challenges that can be of interest to those interested in understanding the relation between risk appraisal and fear (Lazarus, 1991), as well as to those who are interested in the commercial implications of public fears.

Cohesion After 9/11: Patriotism

After 9/11, all over the United States, vehicles and homes were decorated with the U.S. flag. Walls, fences, billboards, and emails were emblazoned with "God bless America." Clearly, the immediate response to the attacks was a sudden upsurge in patriotic expression. The distribution of this phenomenon across the country could be a matter of some interest. Was the new patriotism greater in New York City than elsewhere? Did it decline in concentric circles of distance from New York? Was it greater among blue-collar than white-collar families? Was it greater for some ethnic groups than for others? Was it stronger in cities, possibly perceived as more threatened by future terrorist attacks, than in suburbs and small towns?

The attacks of 9/11 represent a natural experiment relevant to two prominent approaches to conceptualizing and measuring patriotism. In the first approach, Kosterman and Feshbach (1989) distinguish between patriotism and nationalism. Patriotism is love of country and generally considered a good thing; nationalism is a feeling of national superiority that is regarded as a source of intergroup hostility and conflict. Schatz, Staub, and Lavine (1999) offer a distinction between critical and uncritical patriotism. Critical patriotism refers to love of country expressed as willingness to criticize its policies and its leaders when these go wrong; uncritical patriotism refers to love of country coupled with a rejection of criticism—"my country right or wrong." Critical patriotism is accounted the good thing, and uncritical patriotism the danger.

Thus both approaches distinguish between good and bad forms of patriotism, and both offer separate measures of these forms. That is, there is a scale of patriotism and a scale of nationalism, and there is a scale of critical patriotism and a scale of uncritical patriotism. In both approaches, there is some evidence that the two scales are relatively independent. Some people score high on patriotism, for instance, but low on nationalism. Similarly, some people score high on critical patriotism and also score high on uncritical patriotism (an inconsistency that seems to bother those taking the scale less than it bothers theorists).

What happened to these different aspects of patriotism among Americans after 9/11? Since increased cohesion is known to increase conformity and pressure on deviates, one might expect that patriotism, uncritical patriotism, and nationalism increased, whereas critical patriotism decreased. Another possibility is that scores on these measures were unchanged after 9/11 but that identification with the country increased in relation to other directions of group identification. That is, Americans rating the importance of each of a number of groups—country, ethnic group, religious group, family, school—might rate country higher in relation to other groups.

It seems likely that both kinds of patriotism increased, both scores on the patriotism scales and ratings of the relative importance of country. If so, additional questions arise. Did nationalism and uncritical patriotism increase more or less than the "good" forms of patriotism? Was the pattern of change different according to geography, education, or ethnicity?

Cohesion After 9/11: Relations in Public

News reports immediately after 9/11 suggested a new interpersonal tone in New York City. Along with shock and fear came a new tone in public interactions of strangers, a tone of increased politeness, helpfulness, and personal warmth. Several reports suggested a notable drop in crime, especially violent crime, in the days that followed 9/11.

It would be interesting to know whether these reports can be substantiated with more objective measures of social behavior in public places (McCauley, Coleman, & DeFusco, 1978). Did the pace of life in NYC slow after the attacks? That is, did people on the streets walk more slowly? Did eye contact between strangers increase? Did commercial transactions (e.g., with bus drivers, postal clerks, supermarket cashiers) include more personal exchanges? Did interpersonal distance in interactions between strangers decrease? This research will be hampered by the absence of relevant measures from NYC in the months before 9/11, but measures taken now could lay the foundation for assessing change if the U.S. suffers future terrorist attacks.

Cohesion After 9/11: Minority Identity Shifts

A few reports have suggested that minority groups experienced major changes of group identity after 9/11. Group identity is composed of two parts: private and public identity. Private identity is the way in which the individuals think of themselves in relation to groups they belong to. Public identity is how people believe others perceive them.

Public Identity Shift for Muslims and Arabs

The attacks of 9/11 produced an immediate effect on the public identity of Arabs, Muslims, and those, like Sikhs, who can be mistaken by Americans for Arab or Muslim. Actual violence against members of these groups seems mercifully to have been rare, with 39 hate crimes reported to the New York City Police Department in the week ending September 22 but only one a week by the end of December (Fries, 2001). Much more frequent has been the experience of dirty looks, muttered suggestions to "go home," physical distancing, and discrimination at work and school (Sengupta, 2001). Many Arab Americans and Muslims say they have been afraid to report this kind of bias.

Americans' reactions to Muslims and Arabs after 9/11 pose a striking theoretical challenge. How is it that the actions of 19 Arab Muslims can affect Americans' perceptions of the Arabs and Muslims that they personally encounter? The ease with which the 19 were generalized to an impression of millions should amaze us; "the law of small numbers" (Tversky & Kahneman, 1971), in which small, unrepresentative samples are accepted as representative of large populations, has not been observed in research on stereotypes. Indeed, the difficulty of changing stereotypes has often been advanced as one of their principal dangers.

Of course, not every American accepted the idea that all Arabs are terrorists, but even those who intellectually avoided this generalization sometimes found themselves fighting a new unease and suspicion toward people who looked Arabic. Whether on the street or boarding a plane, Americans seem to have had difficulty controlling their emotional response to this newly salient category. It seems unlikely that an attack by 19 Congolese terrorists would have the same impact on perceptions of African Americans. Why not?

One possible explanation of the speed and power of the group generalization of the 9/11 terrorists is that humans are biologically prepared to essentialize cultural differences of members of unfamiliar groups. Gil-White (2001) has suggested that there was an evolutionary advantage for individuals who recognized and generalized cultural differences so as to avoid the extra costs of interacting with those whose norms do not mesh with local norms. This perspective suggests that we may have a kind of default schema for group perception that makes it easy to essentialize the characteristics of a few individuals encountered from a new group. To essentialize means to see the unusual characteristics of the new individuals as the product of an unchangeable group nature or essence. Previous familiarity with the group, a preexisting essence for the members, could interfere with this default; consequently, African terrorists would not easily lead to a generalization about African Americans.

It would be useful to know more about the experience of Muslims and Arabs in the United States after 9/11, not least because those who experience bias may become more likely to sympathize with terrorism directed against the United States. Interviews and polls might inquire not only about the respondents' personal experiences of bias but also about their perception of what most of the members of their group experienced. As elaborated earlier, the motivation for violence may have more to do with group experience than personal problems.

Public Identity Shift for African Americans

The attacks of 9/11 may also have produced an effect on the public identity of African Americans. Their sharing in the costs and threats of terrorist attack may have strengthened their public status as Americans. Several African Americans have suggested that the distancing and unease they often feel from whites they interact with was markedly diminished after 9/11. The extent and distribution of this feeling of increased acceptance by white Americans could be investigated in interviews with African Americans. Again, the distinction between personal experience and perception of group experience may be important in estimating the political impact of 9/11 on African Americans.

Finally, an issue of great practical importance is that of understanding the public identity of Muslim African Americans as a minority within a minority. This group is likely to have faced conflicting changes after 9/11, with increased acceptance as African Americans on the one hand and decreased acceptance as Muslims on the other. The distinctive attire of African American Muslims, particularly that of the women of this community, makes them readily identifiable in public settings. With the attire goes a community lifestyle that also sets this minority apart from other African Americans. Thus, public reactions to Muslim African Americans should be very salient in their experience, and researchers with entrée to their community could investigate this experience. Again, the distinction between the personal experiences of individual respondents and perceived group experience may be important.

One way to learn about shifts in the public identities of minorities is to study changes in the mutual stereotyping of majority and minority. Stereotypes are today generally understood as perceptions of probabilistic differences between groups, differences that may include personality traits, abilities, occupations, physique, clothing, and preferences (McCauley, Jussim, & Lee, 1995). Thus, researchers might ask both minority and majority group members about whether and how 9/11

changed their perceptions of the differences between majority and minority.

Perhaps even more important for understanding the public identity of minorities would be
research that asks about *metastereotypes*. Metastereotypes are perceptions of what "most people"
believe about group differences. Although little
studied, metastereotypes may be more extreme than
personal stereotypes; there is some evidence that
individuals believe that most people see more
marked differences between in-groups and out-
groups than they do (Rettew, Billman, & Davis,
1993). The public identity of the minority might
thus be measured as the average minority individual's perception of what "most people" in
the majority group see as the differences between
minority and majority. Related metastereotypes
might also be of interest: the average minority individual's perception of what most minority members believe about majority-minority differences,
the average majority member's perception of what
most majority members believe about these differences, and the average majority member's perception of what most minority members believe
about these differences.

The attacks of 9/11 and their aftermath offer
a natural experiment in conflicting pressures on
public identity. Research on the public identities
of minorities could enliven theoretical development even as the research contributes to gauging
the potential for terrorist recruitment in groups—
Muslim Arabs in the United States, Muslim African
Americans—that security services are likely to
see as being at risk for terrorist sympathies. In
particular, public identity shifts for Muslim African
Americans will be better understood by comparison with whatever shifts may obtain for African
Americans who are not Muslim.

Private Identity Shifts

Private identity concerns the beliefs and feelings
of an individual about a group that person is part
of. The most obvious shifts in private identity are
those already discussed as shifts in patriotism. Patriotism is a particular kind of group identification,
that is, identification with country or nation, and
increases in patriotism are a kind of private identity
shift. This obvious connection between national
identification and patriotism has only recently become a focus of empirical research (Citrin, Wong,
& Duff, 2001; Sidanius & Petrocik, 2001).

Here I want to focus on shifts in the private
identities of minorities. As with public identity
shifts, the three minority groups of special interest
are Muslim Arabs living in the United States,
African Americans, and Muslim African Americans. For each group, research can focus on
changes since 9/11 in their feelings toward the
United States and feelings toward their minority
group. What is the relation between changes in
these two private identities? It is by no means
obvious that more attachment to one identity
means less attachment to others, but in terms of
behavior there may be something of a conservation
principle at work. Time and energy are limited,
and more behavior controlled by one identity may
mean less behavior controlled by others. We have
much yet to learn about the relation between more
particularistic identities, including ethnic and religious identities, and overarching national identity.

Group Dynamics Theory and Political Identity

Public reaction to terrorist attacks is strikingly
consistent with results found in research with
small face-to-face groups. In the group dynamics
literature that began with Festinger's (1950) theory of informal social influence, cohesion is attachment to the group that comes from two kinds
of interdependence. The obvious sort of interdependence arises from common goals of material
interest, status, and congeniality. The hidden interdependence arises from the need for certainty
that can be obtained only from the consensus of
others. Agreement with those around us is the
only source of certainty about questions of value,
including questions about good and evil and
what is worth living for, working for, and dying
for.

It seems possible that identification with large,
faceless groups is analogous to cohesion in small
face-to-face groups (McCauley, 2001). A scaled-up
theory of cohesion leads immediately to the implication that group identification is not one single
thing but a number of related things. Research has
shown that different sources of cohesion lead to
different types of behavior. Cohesion based on
congeniality, for instance, leads to groupthink,
whereas cohesion based on group status or material interest does not (McCauley, 1998a).

Similarly, various sources of ethnic identification may lead to different behaviors. Individuals who care about their ethnic group for status or material interest may be less likely to sacrifice for the group than members who care about their group for its social reality value—for the moral culture that makes sense of the world and the individual's place in it. Research on the effects of 9/11 on group identities might try to link various measures of group identification with different behaviors after 9/11: giving blood or money, community volunteer work, will revisions, changed travel plans, and more time spent with one's family. The distinctions between patriotism and nationalism and between critical and uncritical patriotism are steps in this direction.

Research on group dynamics has shown that shared threat is a particularly potent source of group cohesion; similarly, the threat represented by the 9/11 attacks seems to have heightened feelings of patriotism and national identification in the United States (Moskalenko, McCauley, & Rozin, 2006). Research also shows that high cohesion leads to an acceptance of group norms, respect for group leaders, and pressure on deviates (Duckitt, 1989). Similarly, the U.S. response to the 9/11 attacks seems to have included a new respect for group norms (less crime, more politeness), new respect for group leaders (President Bush, Mayor Giuliani), and a new willingness to sanction deviates (hostility toward those who sympathize with Arabs and Muslims; Knowlton, 2002).

Conclusion

In the first part of this chapter, group dynamics theory was the perspective brought to bear in understanding the power of cause and comrades in moving normal people to terrorism. In particular I suggested that the power of a group to elicit sacrifice depends upon its terror-management value, which is another way of talking about the social reality value of the group.

Group dynamics research and the psychology of cohesion also provide a useful starting point for theorizing the origins and consequences of group identification, including many aspects of public reaction to terrorism. Terrorism is a threat to all who identify with the group targeted, and at least the initial result of an attack is always increased

identification—heightened cohesion—in the group attacked. The nonobvious quality of this idea is conveyed by the many unsuccessful attempts to use air power to demoralize an enemy by bombing its civilian population (Pape, 1996).

In sum, I have argued that both origins and effects of terrorist acts are anchored in group dynamics. Along the way I have tried to suggest how the response to terrorism can be more dangerous than the terrorists.

References

Ajzen, I., & Fishbein, M. (1980). *Understanding attitudes and predicting behavior.* New York: Prentice Hall.

Allport, G. W. (1954). *The nature of prejudice.* Cambridge, MA: Addison Wesley.

Atran, S. (2003, March 7). Genesis of Suicide Terrorism. *Science, 299,* 1534–1539.

Barbera, J., Macintyre, A. G., & De Atley, C. A. (2001, October). Ambulances to nowhere: America's critical shortfall in medical preparedness for catastrophic terrorism. BCSIA Discussion Paper 2001-15, ESDP Discussion Paper ESDP-2001-07, John F. Kennedy School of Government, Harvard University.

Barker, E. (1984). *The making of a Moonie: Choice or brainwashing?* London: Basil Blackwell.

Bearak, B. (2002, February 11). Afghan toll of civilians is lost in the fog of war. *International Herald Tribune,* pp. 1, 8.

Beck, A., & Katcher, A. (1996). Between pets and people: The importance of animal companionship. West Lafayette, IN: Purdue University Press.

Brewer, M. (2001). Ingroup identification and intergroup conflict: When does ingroup love become outgroup hate? In R. D. Ashmore, L. Jussim, & D. Wilder (Eds.), *Social identity, intergroup conflict, and conflict reduction* (pp. 17–41). New York: Oxford University Press.

Brown, R. (1986). *Social psychology, the second edition.* New York: Free Press.

Citrin, J., Wong, C., & Duff, B. (2001). The meaning of American national identity: Patterns of ethnic conflict and consensus. In R. D. Ashmore, L. Jussim, & D. Wilder (Eds.), *Social identity, intergroup conflict, and conflict reduction* (pp. 71–100). New York: Oxford University Press.

Duckitt, J. (1989). Authoritarianism and group identification: A new view of an old construct. *Political Psychology, 10,* 63–84.

Festinger, L. (1950). Informal social communication. *Psychological Review, 57,* 271–282.

Frank, R. L. (1988). *Passions within reason: The strategic role of the emotions.* New York: Norton.

Friedman, A. (2002, February 5). Forum focuses on "wrath" born of poverty. *International Herald Tribune,* p. 11.

Friedman, T. (2002, January 28). The pain behind Al Qaeda's Europe connection. *International Herald Tribune,* p. 6.

Fries, J. H. (2001, December 22). A nation challenged: Relations; complaints of anti-Arab bias crimes dip, but concerns linger. *New York Times,* p. B8.

Galanter, M. (1980). Psychological induction into the large group: Findings from a modern religious sect. *American Journal of Psychiatry, 137,* 1574–1579.

Gil-White, F. (2001). Are ethnic groups biological "species" to the human brain? *Current Anthropology, 42,* 515–554.

Horowitz, D. L. (2001). *The deadly ethnic riot.* Berkeley: University of California Press.

Kinder, D. (1998). Opinion and action in the realm of politics. In D. T. Gilbert, S. Fiske, & G. Lindzey (Eds.), *The handbook of social psychology, Vol. 2* (4th ed., pp. 778–867). New York: McGraw-Hill.

Knowlton, B. (2001, December 20). How the world sees the U.S. and Sept. 11. *International Herald Tribune,* pp. 1, 6.

———. (2002, February 12). On U.S. campuses, intolerance grows. *International Herald Tribune,* pp. 1, 4.

Kosterman, R., & Feshbach, S. (1989). Towards a measure of patriotic and nationalistic attitudes. *Political Psychology, 10,* 257–274.

Krueger, A. B., & Maleckova, J. (2002). Education, poverty, political violence, and terrorism: Is there a causal connection? *Working Paper 9074.* Cambridge, MA: National Bureau of Economic Research. Retrieved on March 8, 2006, from http://papers.nber.org/papers/w9074.pdf.

Kurtz, H. (2002, February 2–3). America is "doomed," bin Laden says on tape. *International Herald Tribune,* p. 5.

Lazarus, R. S. (1991). Cognition and motivation in emotion. *American Psychologist, 46,* 352–367.

Lelyveld, J. (2001, October 28). All suicide bombers are not alike. *New York Times Magazine,* pp. 48–53, 62, 78–79.

Makiya, K., & Mneimneh, H. (2002, January 17). Manual for a "raid." *New York Review of Books, 49,* pp. 18–21.

McCauley, C. (1991). Terrorism research and public policy: An overview. In C. McCauley (Ed.), *Terrorism research and public policy* (pp. 126–144). London: Frank Cass.

———. (1998a). Group dynamics in Janis's theory of groupthink: Backward and forward. *Organizational Behavior and Human Decision Processes, 73,* 142–162.

———. (1998b). When screen violence is not attractive. In J. Goldstein (Ed.), *Why we watch: The attractions of violent entertainment* (pp. 144–162). New York: Oxford University Press.

———. (2001). The psychology of group identification and the power of ethnic nationalism. In D. Chirot & M. Seligman (Eds.), *Ethnopolitical warfare: Causes, consequences, and possible solutions* (pp. 343–362). Washington, DC: APA Books.

———. (2003). Making sense of terrorism after 9/11. In R. S. Moser & C.E. Frantz (Eds.), *Shocking violence II: Violent disaster, war and terrorism affecting our youth* (pp. 10–32). Springfield, IL: Charles C. Thomas.

———, Coleman, G., & DeFusco, P. (1978). Commuters' eye contact with strangers in city and suburban train stations: Evidence of short-term adaptation to interpersonal overload in the city. *Environmental Psychology and Nonverbal Behavior, 2,* 215–255.

———, Jussim, L. J., & Lee, Y.-T. (1995). Stereotype accuracy: Toward appreciating group differences. In Y.-T. Lee, L. J. Jussim, & C. R. McCauley (Eds.), *Stereotype accuracy: Toward appreciating group differences* (pp. 293–312). Washington, DC: APA Books.

———, & Segal, M. (1987). Social psychology of terrorist groups. In C. Hendrick (Ed.), *Review of personality and social psychology, Vol. 9* (pp. 231–256). Beverly Hills: Sage.

Moskalenko, S., McCauley, C., & Rozin, P. (2006). Group identification under conditions of threat: College students' attachment to country, family, ethnicity, religion and university before and after September 11, 2001. *Political Psychology, 27*(1), 77–98.

Myers, D. G. (2001). Do we fear the right things? *American Psychological Society Observer, 14*(10), 3, 31.

Pape, R. A. (1996). *Bombing to win: Air power and coercion in war.* Ithaca, NY: Cornell University Press.

———. (2005). *Dying to win: The strategic logic of suicide terrorism.* New York: Random House.

Pfefferbaum, B., Flynn, B. W., Brandt, E. N., & Lensgraf, S. J. (1999). Organizing the mental health response to human-caused community disasters with reference to the Oklahoma City bombing. *Psychiatric Annals, 29*(2), 109–113.

Pyszcznski, T., Greenberg, J., & Solomon, S. (1997). Why do we need what we need? A terror management perspective on the roots of human social motivation. *Psychological Inquiry, 8,* 1–20.

Rettew, D. C., Billman, D., & Davis, R. A. (1993). Inaccurate perceptions of the amount others stereotype: Estimates about stereotypes of ones' own group and other groups. *Basic and Applied Social Psychology, 14,* 121–142.

Royzman, E., McCauley, C., & Rozin, P. (2004). From Plato to Putnam: Four ways of thinking about hate. In R. Sternberg (Ed.), The psychology of hate (pp. 3–35). Washington, DC: APA Books.

Rummel, R. J. (1996). *Death by government.* New Brunswick, NJ: Transaction Publishers.

Sabini, J. (1995). *Social psychology* (2d ed.). New York: Norton.

Schatz, R. T., Staub, E., & Lavine, H. (1999). On the varieties of national attachment: Blind versus constructive patriotism. *Political Psychology, 20,* 151–174.

Sengupta, S. (2001, October 10). A nation challenged: Relations; Sept. 11 attack narrows the racial divide. *New York Times,* p. B1.

Sidanius, J., & Petrocik, J. R. (2001). Communal and national identity in a multiethnic state: A comparison of three perspectives. In R. D. Ashmore, L. Jussim, & D. Wilder (Eds.), *Social identity, intergroup conflict, and conflict reduction* (pp. 101–129). New York: Oxford University Press.

Sprinzak, E. (1991). The process of delegitimization: Towards a linkage theory of political terrorism. In C. McCauley (Ed.), *Terrorism research and public policy* (pp. 50–68). London: Frank Cass.

Sternberg, R. J. (2003). A duplex theory of hate: Development and application to terrorism, massacres, and genocide. *Review of General Psychology, 7*(3), 299–328.

Stouffer, S. A., et al. (1949). *The American soldier: Vol. 4. Combat and its aftermath.* Princeton, NJ: Princeton University Press.

Tversky, A., & Kahneman, D. (1971). Belief in the law of small numbers. *Psychological Bulletin, 2,* 105–110.

3

The Need for Proficient Mental Health Professionals in the Study of Terrorism

Larry E. Beutler
Gil Reyes
Zeno Franco
Jennifer Housley

The disciplines of psychology that are devoted to the understanding of terrorism and the treatment of victims of terrorism are new and generally rely on extrapolation of knowledge from related fields. However, while this strategy is effective in beginning the process of illuminating this poorly researched domain, it is also problematic. Not only have many of the conventional treatments used with victims and responders proven to be less effective than conventionally thought when applied to trauma generally (Litz, Bryant, & Adler, 2002), but serious questions have also been raised about whether treatments that work for those exposed to civil, natural, or even military-related disasters will work equally well with someone who has been exposed to the systematic and planned acts of terrorists.

For example, incidence rates of symptoms that are suggestive of posttraumatic stress disorder (PTSD) seem to be quite situation specific and vary from one type of trauma to another. The most widely cited figure representing PTSD in military populations derives from the National Vietnam Veterans Readjustment Study (NVVRS), which determined the likelihood of PTSD among those who served during the Vietnam years to be about 30%, regardless of whether they were exposed to combat (Marlowe, 2001; Wessely & Jones, in press). In contrast, the most reliable figures representing PTSD in the general population, following the terrorist attack of September 11, 2001, places the incidence rate at about 4%, which indicates virtually no effect from 9/11. The incidence rates of PTSD-like symptoms are higher in areas that were directly affected by the terrorist attacks. In the New York City area, the estimated rates hover at about 11% and are noticeably lower in Washington, DC (Schlenger, Caddell, Ebert, Jordan, Rourke, et al., 2002). These latter results suggest that the prevalence rates approximate those reported by the NVVRS studies only in the immediate aftermath of 9/11 and among those directly affected. Even here, the rates of PTSD symptoms decline quickly over time, returning to normative levels within 6 months to a year (Galea et al., 2003; Resnick, Acierno, Holmes, Dammeyer, & Kilpatrick, 2000).

Because of such disparities between terrorist-initiated trauma and other forms of civilian and military trauma, many questions have been raised in the field of trauma response about whether established treatments for civilian PTSD are appropriate for terrorist-initiated traumas. These concerns also stimulate questions about who might then provide the treatment. Is it sufficient for one to have been trained in the use of widely practiced treatments for civil and military PTSD? An affirmative answer to this question fails to consider both the fundamental differences present in the nature of response to terrorism as a particular traumatic event and the associated differences that terroristic events may portend in the required treatment regimens.

This chapter explores what is currently known about how terrorism impacts victims in unique and probably more profound ways than other forms of catastrophic disaster, builds a theoretical framework that explores the way in which terrorism specifically impacts traumatization and recovery, and considers the effective treatment of victims of and first responders to terrorist attacks. From these starting points, we then identify the particular skills that constitute expertise in this arena, an approach that contrasts with the more common procedure of evaluating one's expertise on the basis of training, experience, and knowledge. The objective of these considerations is to question the nature of expertise and training that might be advantageous for those who treat the victims of terrorist attacks. The comprehensive view of terrorism and related trauma presented here form a foundation for the creation of expertise that may be central for mental health professionals working in this field. Such a foundation of knowledge should begin to guide both clinical practice and research.

Terrorism Versus Disasters: Differential Psychological Response

The intentionality of an act of terrorism serves as a signal contributor, differentiating the responses of victims of a natural disaster from those of victims of a terrorist attack. The implication of intentional malevolence, which can neither be effectively predicted nor prevented, and the concomitant feelings of uncertainty, distrust, and loss of control that follow are fundamentally different from the experience of fear associated with a naturally occurring disaster—even if the disaster is serious and large scale. Whereas one can prepare for an earthquake or a hurricane, the nature of a terrorist act is likely uncertain and defies effective preparation. The most insidious forms of terrorism, such as the use of biological weapons, may be impossible to detect even after an attack occurs, leaving one

fearful of an almost omnipresent danger in the environment. The fear generated by terrorist attacks extends into the most basic reaches of the human mind, activating systems that have been fundamental to our survival but long unused, and this may cause reactions that undermine one's emotional and mental well-being.

One of the difficulties of developing the ability to predict and manage victims' responses to terrorism is the unavailability of systematic, empirical research on the events that immediately follow a terrorist attack (Neria, Suh, & Marshall, 2004). By nature these attacks are infrequent and unexpected events and do not provide researchers with an opportunity to systematically observe the response of victims and create well-designed studies to examine effective treatment. Instead, behavioral scientists who are interested in the aftereffects of this form of violence have two basic options. They can respond with a hurriedly constructed inquiry immediately following a mass-casualty event. Alternatively, they can search for analogous events that have a higher base rate of occurrence and greater predictability and thus offer greater experimental control. In order to bridge this gap between the available information and the knowledge that is needed to illuminate this developing area in psychology, we present findings drawn from both the relatively small body of literature dealing specifically with the psychological sequelae of terrorist attacks, as well as a broader range of findings from other events that have been carefully selected to be as analogous to terrorism as possible.

Psychological Responses to Terrorism

A few large-scale studies examining the fear and psychological symptoms associated with the distress caused by the 9/11 attacks have been published. Additionally, findings from incidents that share the fundamental elements of terrorism, including malevolent intent, unpredictability, the threat of future attack, and the possibility of environmental contamination, provide insight into this unique area of study. Analogous events run the gamut from very serious incidents involving numerous casualties and mass panic (e.g., the cesium 137 release and panic in Goiania, Brazil, in 1987), in-garrison military incidents (e.g., the attack on Pearl Harbor), and individual or small-group events (e.g., domestic and gang violence) to the absurd (e.g., the panic caused by the "War of the Worlds" broadcast in 1938). These comparable incidents allow us to examine the ways in which the fear produced by terrorism differs from "fated" events such as natural disaster.

To understand psychological distress and the symptoms associated with trauma, we must first understand the fundamental psychological processes that underlie fear and threat assessment. Exposure to any disaster, whether generated by humans or occurring naturally, can be expected to deeply impact the cognition, affect, and physical functioning of those who are in the path of the catastrophe. However, we suggest that the intentional nature of terrorism essentially alters these perceptions. We argue that these differences are seen in the development of causal attributions that are employed to explain the event, in the heuristics that may bias perception of it, and in risk assessments that assist us in estimating ongoing and future threats.

It appears that terrorist attacks differ systematically across each of these domains when compared to natural disasters or accidental traumatization. Moreover, preexisting vulnerabilities, as well as peritrauma and posttrauma risk factors, are central to predicting which people will recover normally from a terrorist event and which will experience interrupted or delayed recovery. These elements are developed in the following sections, and later in the chapter they are integrated into a model that describes threat assessment and its relationship to psychological trauma.

Causal Attributions

The sense of causal understanding found after many natural disasters is often absent in the wake of a terrorist attack. The dynamics of a hurricane, tornado, accidental plane crash, or earthquake represent events that are easily understood by the public. Furthermore, clear causal attributions about the event can be drawn, and expectations about the location, progression, and duration of the event are generally known or can be reasonably estimated (Slovic, 2002). Based on experience of or prior education about the disaster, first responders and potential victims can typically consider an impending event with a sense of what to expect and the actions they can perform to mitigate the situation. In the worst-case scenario, an evacuation plan can be devised. Importantly, the lack of

malicious intent allows even those who are directly impacted to gradually delimit the event and to understand it as an unpleasant, though fundamentally "normal," part of life.

Conversely, the causal attributions drawn from a terrorist event are much less orderly. Almost by definition, these acts are designed to invoke a pervasive fear of an unknown, unpredictable, yet intentional threat. Where a naturally occurring disaster is almost always bound by time or geographic location, terrorism is not similarly delimited. Paul Slovic (2002), an expert in the field of risk perception, notes that the most feared forms of terrorism, such as chemical or biological attack, are "emergencies [that] contaminate in ways that never seem to end" (p. 425). To the victims, the event has no apparent closure.

Further, whereas natural disasters are generally understood as the work of "fate" or an "act of God," the only causal attributions that can be drawn from terrorist activity is the malevolent intent of a human agent, and often this agent is unknown to the victims. Thus, the exact message and rationale for the assault are usually unclear to the immediate victims, and the intended message is generally not meant for them specifically. Rather, the objective of the assailants is to incite fear in the general population in order to draw the attention of political leaders (Pfefferbaum, Pfefferbaum, North, & Neas, 2002). The immediate causal attributions are based on the limited knowledge that the event is deliberately caused and malevolent in nature. Thus, a victim's abilities to understand, anticipate, plan for, and delimit the event are seriously impaired.

Without the availability of clear event contingencies, victims are faced with several key questions for which no clear answers are immediately available, such as (1) Who was the intended target? (2) Do I fit the target profile? (3) What is the likelihood of another attack? And, if so, (4) What further attack methods may be employed? Without the ability to explain the event and without clear answers to questions used to evaluate immediate personal danger, a victim or witness to a terrorist event is left with little sense of personal control or agency. The result may be a profound sense of helplessness and defeat.

Heuristics

Because of the salience of the event and the unpredictability of terrorism, both direct victims and those secondarily exposed are likely to respond disproportionately to event-related stimuli, placing them at greater risk for increased fear, anxiety, and possible psychological difficulty. The analysis of risk, formally referred to as *risk assessment* by researchers in this field, is a function that humans have instinctively performed long before recorded history (Slovic, 2002). Natural selection produced a refined system that enabled people to incorporate information of many types, analyze it based on past experiences, and produce an affective reaction capable of governing our behavior. This form of risk assessment, called *experiential risk assessment,* is considered to be "intuitive, automatic, and fast" (Slovic, 2002, p. 425). Research on fear-related stimuli has demonstrated that people preconsciously attend to threatening information (Ohman, Flykt, & Esteves, 2001). Operating largely outside of consciousness and relying primarily on recalled visual information and associative thoughts, experiential risk assessment produces simple emotions—a "gut feeling" about a given event (Slovic, 2002, p. 425).

This form of reasoning is a powerful and generally useful behavioral motivator. However, the emotionally charged images, feelings, physical consequences, and media attention that are typical outcomes of terrorist events may create an overwhelming fear and anxiety in both the direct victims and those secondarily exposed through the media (Pfefferbaum et al., 2002). Because experiential risk assessment is rapid and largely automatic, it relies on the availability heuristic and is vulnerable to the base rate fallacy, giving more weight to recent, easily imagined, and highly arousing events and overestimating their future likelihood (Chapman & Harris, 2002; Slovic & Weber, 2002). Although these systems may initially play a vital role in a person's survival, the salience of the stimuli related to terrorism also plays into a fundamental signal-processing bias in human risk assessment that may short-circuit the system, resulting in the elicited fears and anxieties continuing beyond the point of utility and potentially putting the victim at risk for PTSD or other serious psychological difficulties.

Risk Assessment

Currently, very few models exist that specifically describe the factors involved in risk perception as applied to terrorism. Initial efforts to provide a

model of fear in these situations suggest that two factors may be central to understanding how people assign affective values to terrorist incidents. The first factor can be described as *dread risk,* a continuum beginning with low-dread events, which are seen as controllable, not catastrophic, decreasing in risk over time, and generating little risk for future generations (Slovic & Weber, 2002). Conversely, high-dread events are viewed as having a high mortality rate, being globally catastrophic and inescapable, and increasing in risk over time.

A second factor is *unknown risk,* which begins at the low-risk level with well-understood, observable, non-novel events (Slovic & Weber, 2002). If an event is high on the unknown risk dimension, it is characterized by having delayed or persisting effect and being a novel threat that is poorly understood (Slovic & Weber, 2002). Using this model, Slovic and Weber provide a two-dimensional chart with unknown risk on the Y axis and dread risk on the X axis. Earlier research by Slovic allows a wide variety of different threatening events to be placed in this two-dimensional space, in which events that fall in quadrant I are viewed as the most threatening. Examples of things found at the extreme end in quadrant I include DNA technology, radioactive waste, nuclear reactor accidents, and nuclear fallout (earlier work by Slovic as cited in Slovic & Weber, 2002).

Because we are most concerned with the psychological consequences of these events and the role of mental health response in combating sequelae such as PTSD, depression, and drug abuse following a mass-casualty event, it may be helpful to translate the model proposed by Slovic and Weber (2002) into terminology that is typically used by disaster psychologists and first responders. Doing so helps us determine what constitutes an "expert" who can provide discriminating help to the victims of mass terrorism.

In addition to the factors already proposed by Slovic, we also suggest an additional factor that has not been carefully explored—the role of perceived malevolent intent—to round out this matrix and to lend further assistance to the professional who attempts to establish priorities for effective intervention. In analyzing the psychological risk involved in a terrorist attack, psychologists, social workers, other mental health professionals, and first responders may be assisted by evaluating the following dimensions: (1) the scale of the attack (dread risk); (2) proximity to the attack (dread risk); (3) perceived personal threat (dread risk); (4) the type of weapon used (unknown risk); (5) duration of threat (unknown risk); and (6) the nature of the malevolent intent (adapted from Slovic & Weber, 2002). In general, as the value of each of these dimensions increase, the risk of psychological harm also rises.

Terrorism and Traumatization

Throughout this chapter we address concerns related to different two populations: the general public exposed to a major terrorist event and the first responders, including firefighters, police officers, emergency medical technicians, military personnel, and other relief workers. Although some of the considerations for each distinct population overlap, we approach them as having fundamental differences in training, expectations, and support systems that cause them to differ in initial response, later assessment of trauma symptoms, and final recovery. Some of the key concepts that describe the process of traumatization may serve as an underpinning for understanding what first responders experience. However, when undertaking to treat first responders, clinicians should incorporate the information that is specific to this population in the assessment, planning, and delivery of treatment.

General Public

One of the keys in understanding the variations in anxiety created by external events is the understanding of the adaptive and evolutionary significance of these responses. Wakefield (1992) emphasizes the role of evolutionary events as a central theme in behavior. This perspective asserts that every behavior has evolutionary significance. That is, it increases the probability of the survival of the species. In the case of anxiety, arousal likely serves to motivate and activate an organism to prepare itself for danger and thus reduces the chances of premature death. Various levels of arousal promote vigilance and reflect the levels of danger expected by the organism.

However, at some point, when the danger is unpredictable and uncontrollable, as in the case of terrorism, the result may be a level of arousal that is no longer adaptive but rather is dysfunctional.

The resulting panic no longer ensures survival and instead actually places the organism at risk for self-injury and accident by virtue of the disorganized, goal-directed behavior that accompanies this hyperaroused state. Hyperarousal caused by a terrorist attack may dispose the majority of the exposed population to an initial adaptive fear response. However, a smaller number of people may begin showing symptoms of acute stress disorder (ASD), and a subset of this group may progress to PTSD. In fact, research performed after the Oklahoma City bombing demonstrated that feeling nervous or afraid immediately following the bombing was the best single affective predictor of later PTSD onset (Tucker, Pfefferbaum, Nixon, & Dickson, 2000).

A powerful example of how we respond to risk assessments that seem particularly threatening and how these assessments play into maladaptive hyperarousal can be drawn from the Israeli experience during the Gulf War. Two retrospective studies of the rates of physical and psychological illness during 18 discreet attacks involving 39 missile explosions in Israel (Bleisch, Dycian, Koslowsky, Solomon, & Wiener, 1992) have shown that 27% of hospital admissions were due to unnecessary atropine (a chemical warfare antidote) injections, presumably due to stress reaction or mishandling of the atropine injectors. Additionally, a substantial increase in acute anterior wall myocardial infarction and sudden out-of-hospital deaths (as compared to five control periods) was also noted (Meisel et al., 1991). Hospital staff determined that about 43% of hospital admissions during this time were for psychological rather than physical symptoms (Bleisch et al., 1992). Interestingly, the rates of heart attack and sudden death attenuated rapidly after the initial attacks, suggesting that most people had adjusted to the new threat fairly rapidly (Meisel et al., 1991).

The SCUD missile attacks in Israel were initially feared to contain chemical weapons, but only conventional warheads were actually used (Bleisch et al., 1992). Even though the media overly dramatized the likelihood of mass exposure to chemical or biological agents in Israel, it is critical that disaster mental health providers and first responders view the use and even the threat of nonconventional weapons as a special situation that may elicit a particularly strong fear response in the public (Slovic & Weber, 2002), generate a great many psychological casualties, produce a high rate of false positive reports of exposure (Pastel, 2001), and rapidly overwhelm public health resources. The risk of evoking a particular type of fear-generated response, known as outbreaks of multiple unexplained symptoms (OMUS), tends to increase when unconventional weapons are introduced into the threat matrix (Pastel, 2001).

The concept of OMUS reflects a modern interpretation of the more traditional descriptions of "mass psychogenic illness" and "mass hysteria" (Pastel, 2001, p. 44). In general, OMUS occur in response to an unobservable environmental contagion, real or imagined, and are denoted by a host of somatic symptoms with no apparent physical cause (Pastel, 2001). Unlike classic mass panic, OMUS occur relatively frequently (Small, Propper, Randolph, & Eth, 1991) and can be very costly to both the government and private sectors. The effects of OMUS are often reinforced by mass media, rumor, and highly visible response interventions and subsequent investigation. Examples of OMUS include those that surfaced at Three Mile Island and during the Alar-poisoning panic (Pastel, 2001). In each of these cases, broadcast and/or print media played a central role in inciting fear.

While most cases of OMUS yield comparatively harmless results, the picture becomes much more complex in the event of a bona fide terrorism act or an accident involving a chemical, biological, radiological, or nuclear (CBRN) device. For example, the radiological poisoning of 249 people in Goiania, Brazil, in 1987 from contact with scrap metal that was contaminated with cesium 137 resulted in more than 5,000 unexposed people (of the 125,800 screened) demonstrating physical symptoms (Pastel, 2001). The symptoms these 5,000 unexposed people exhibited were very similar to those of the much smaller number of people who were sickened by actual radiation poisoning. This phenomenon made it difficult to differentiate between the two groups. In the case of a possible CBRN incident, the previously used terms for OMUS (e.g., mass hysteria) seem particularly inappropriate since the syndrome may be viewed as a powerful self-protective mechanism that encourages flight from an area containing an unknown pathogen. It is plausible that OMUS and their concomitant social components, such as "psychological contamination" (Pastel, 2001), may have an evolutionary component that served to generate fear and stimulate flight in the event of unexplained illness or death.

In addition to the fear and anxiety produced by a mass-casualty event, by creating an event that is unbounded by time (and potentially unbounded by geography), terrorism also removes factors that are assumed to be central to healthy mental functioning, such as a sense of predictability, agency, and control. Research on Holocaust survivors has demonstrated that victims made considerably fewer attributions of internal control and many more external control attributions as compared to similar control participants (Suedfeld, 2003). In more recent disasters, including the Chernobyl reactor accident and the Loma Prieta earthquake, even those who were not directly victimized experienced a degradation of the optimistic bias that many researchers believe to be important in maintaining mental health (Weinstein, Lyon, Rothman, & Cuite, 2000). Similarly, people who were close to large-scale tornado damage but were not directly impacted show significantly lower usage of self-protecting biases, many more intrusive thoughts about future tornados, a lowered perception of control over the damage caused by these events, increased feelings of personal vulnerability, and more feelings of anxiousness and depression in response to related stimuli (Weinstein et al., 2000).

So far we have primarily considered the affective and cognitive components of trauma in response to terrorism. While closely related to the perception of anxiety, the physical aspects of a terrorist attack—including both physical exposure and immediate somatic response—must also be considered by practitioners who seek to assist victims effectively in the aftermath of such an event. Clear evidence was found demonstrating that physical injury was one of the most predictive factors in later onset of PTSD following the Oklahoma City bombing (Tucker et al., 2000). The immediate physical response of those directly exposed, such as increased heart rate and trembling, has also been shown to be substantially correlated with PTSD and subclinical PTSD symptoms (Tucker et al., 2000).

Although we generally assume that proximity to and the magnitude of an event are related to the likelihood of later psychological difficulty (Weinstein et al., 2000), PTSD symptoms following large-scale events are evidently not correlated with proximity to the worst levels of destruction or exposure to greater loss of life (Goenjian et al., 2001). In a study of PTSD symptoms and depression in adolescent victims following Hurricane Mitch in Nicaragua, investigators found that the majority of victims' subjective exposure ratings "did not follow a dose-of-exposure pattern" (Goenjian et al., 2001, p. 792). Moreover, no significant correlation was found between those in the most badly damaged city where the greatest loss of life had occurred and victims in a nearby city that was not as severely impacted (Goenjian et al., 2001). The authors of this study suggest that a ceiling effect may occur when the severity of the event is sufficiently great, with the result that physical proximity becomes a less important factor in the development of mental health problems.

While the precise mechanisms through which human intent to cause harm operates on risk perception and fear have not been fully explicated, the events of 9/11 and other intentional tragedies clearly differ from both natural disaster and unintended mass-casualty events. Paul Slovic states that "a startling feature of the September 11 attacks and the subsequent anthrax exposures and deaths is the degree to which a handful of determined individuals, in a very short time, so greatly disrupted the world's most powerful nation" (2002, p. 425).

Any major disaster, whether caused by nature, unintentional human error, or intentional malevolence, is likely to result in profound physical injury, immediate fear, and potential long-term psychological difficulties. However, we argue that the combination of the perception of human intentionality, the lack of ability to generate a coherent set of expectations, the persistence of an unknown threat, and the ubiquity of the threat all serve to differentiate terrorism from other mass-casualty events. These differences fundamentally alter human perceptions of the event, increasing their salience and heightening their arousal components. In view of this, we suggest that the fear generated by terrorism may be more persistent and more potent in generating psychological sequelae than other forms of disaster.

First Responders

Thus far we have addressed victims and their treatment. However, first responders can, and probably should, be included in what we refer to as victims of terrorist attacks. To a large extent, they cannot be distinguished from the immediately targeted bystanders who are the usual victims. Next to the immediate victims of an attack, first responders are the first to see its aftermath and are those who are called upon immediately to manage the situation and treat those affected. However, just because they may not be directly affected by the initial terrorist action, they are still susceptible to the aftermath and thus suffer many of the same illnesses and symptoms that the victims they are treating may develop.

The first responder population is broad. Generally speaking, they are the professionals and volunteers who arrive first on the scene following a terrorist attack or are on the front line in caring for victims. Some obvious examples include police officers, firefighters, and ambulance personnel. Others include emergency room staff, hazmat teams, military personnel, utility crews, and volunteers.

Both victims and first responders share certain characteristics within the context of terrorist events. First responders, like the general population, are subject to the unpredictability of the event and the difficulty in simulating an exact replica during training exercises and, of course, can experience strong emotional reactions. Each population utilizes an array of coping strategies to deal with the trauma they witness. Treatments for psychological conditions resulting from exposure to trauma overlap between the general population and the first responders. Additionally, just as there are different cultures present among the general population, different cultures are present among first responders. These features contribute to how a terrorist event is appraised, what coping style is used, and how frequently treatment is sought if psychological harm is identified.

Moreover, each first responder population has a "culture" that is unique to their profession and that is shaped both by the services they provide and by their level of investment in these services. These factors contribute to the type of psychological impacts that result from emergency scenes. For example, although firefighters and police officers both respond to emergency scenes, there are fundamental differences in their roles. A firefighter's role is acute in nature and medically oriented; they have little opportunity for ongoing contact with victims following an emergency.

In contrast, because the role that police officers play extends beyond the emergency scene, they may have more contact with victims in postcrisis situations. Thus firefighters have a culture that centers around the acute care of victims, whereas that of police officers centers around continual exposure.

Key differences between populations of victims and first responders must be considered by the knowledgeable professional who intervenes. First responders have responsibilities in disaster situations, whereas victims may not. For example, first responders must identify and address the effects of disasters on the general population and may utilize coping strategies that are unique to their trades both in type and intensity. The health and safety of others depend on the health and skill of the first responders. This charge carries with it emotions such as the fear of failure, which in turn can affect the way in which first responders deal with trauma situations.

Addressing each population based on its unique culture can assist us in identifying barriers to predicting susceptibility to mental health difficulties, determining which method of prevention might be most useful, choosing an effective approach to mental health education and training, and learning which type of intervention may be called for.

The Effects of Exposure to Terrorism

In this section we build upon the topics presented in the prior two portions of the chapter to round out a model that helps explain the fundamental psychological differences between intentional acts of terrorism and natural disasters and how they set the stage for either normal or interrupted recovery. A more comprehensive perspective on the psychological sequelae of terrorism and their treatment will enable us to begin constructing effective mental health measures and allocate limited resources in an emergency more efficiently, as well as manage the incredibly high cost of response to and recovery from terrorism. We argue that the basic psychological and physical responses to terrorism, such as the affective components of fear, are later processed through an increasingly complex matrix involving causal attributions, heuristics, and risk assessment. These more complex activities rely

heavily on cognition and memory and, as such, may be deeply impacted by preexisting risk factors that cue trauma-related recollections. In the following sections, we consider both preexisting and posttrauma risk factors that influence the development of psychological effects following a terrorist attack.

Risk Factors: General Public

Several vulnerability factors have been associated with higher rates of PTSD-like symptoms in retrospective studies and include prior exposure, particularly early in life, to violence or other major traumatic events, gender (females are at greater risk for chronic PTSD), age (younger victims are generally at greater risk), intelligence, concurrent mood disorder, neuroticism, and a low level of social support (Litz, Gray, Bryant, & Adler, 2002; McNally, Bryant, & Ehlers, 2003). Several attempts have been made to demonstrate that these vulnerability factors cause higher levels of PTSD symptoms through prospective studies, and the results have largely supported the initial retrospective findings (McNally et al., 2003). These results have largely been derived from pre- and post-deployment testing of troops and have demonstrated that those with more serious PTSD symptoms scored lower on IQ tests (and that IQ does not change after deployment), were more likely to have personality traits of hypochondriasis, psychopathic deviate, paranoia, and femininity based on Minnesota Multiphasic Personality Inventory (MMPI) scores, and exhibited more negativism toward their deployment (McNally et al., 2003). Litz et al. (2002, p. 114) state that "It has become axiomatic that prior exposure to potentially traumatizing events (PTEs) is a risk factor for chronic PTSD stemming from a subsequent PTE." Prior exposure is represented in affect laden memories that are activated by a current event or trauma, and then serve to exacerbate and sensitize the individual to that event. These incipient, internal cues from memory may be important features that reduce the capacity for adapting and resilience.

For example, in determining which factors precipitate PTSD and explain why some people develop it and others, similarly exposed, do not, Dalgleish (2004) concludes that PTSD is a joint function of at least three separate aspects of cognitive representation. These include the presence of associative networks in which prior stressors activate remembered and rehearsed cognitive pathways; verbal or prepositional representations; and schemas or preexisting beliefs about oneself and others. Memories and associational pathways alone are insufficient to account for the variations in response. Also needed is a language system through which these events are processed and the activation of self-related schemas that lend themselves to feelings of helplessness and hopelessness.

In addition to the risk factors that may be present prior to a traumatic event, several factors have been identified that may serve as peri- and posttraumatic markers for future psychological difficulty:

1. People with many or very severe ASD symptoms that appear 1–2 weeks following a traumatic event. Particular attention should be given to these people if these symptoms are comorbid with high rates of rumination. This appears to be one of the best, simplest, and most straightforward screening methods currently available.
2. People who experience high levels of physical symptoms, such as a rapid heart rate, after having been removed from the trauma stimulus. These types of measures may be particularly useful for Emergency Medical Technicians (EMTs) and physicians.
3. People who experience ASD or PTSD symptoms in conjunction with signs of clinical depression are at higher risk for developing chronic PTSD.
4. People who display a high level of active avoidance or precautionary symptoms
5. People who make maladaptive attributions about their symptoms
6. People with serious physical injuries as result of the trauma event
7. People with low levels of social support?

(list adapted from Litz et al., 2002; McNally et al., 2003).

Risk Factors: First Responders

Again, the risk factors for the general public serve as a foundation for understanding the vulnerabilities of first responders. However, a number of specific psychological risk factors should be considered for members of special response teams, including characteristics of the event itself, such as type, timing, and the destructive agent used. These can affect the stress level of first responders in different ways. For example, because they are considered more preventable, human-induced events precipitate stronger feelings of anger and blame than natural disasters. Paton (1996) states that events that occur during nighttime hours are perceived as more threatening than those that occur during the day.

Another factor related to timing is the degree of uncertainty associated with a threat. The events of 9/11 can serve as an example since it was unclear whether additional attacks were forthcoming. A related stressor has to do with whether there was warning before the disaster. In addition, Paton states that "invisible" threats, such as chemical or radiation hazards, may elicit more reaction than visible threats such as flooding. Finally, the greater the number of threats associated with the disaster, the greater the reaction felt by emergency workers. The 9/11 catastrophe illustrates how one incident can yield multiple threats. Fires, the collapse of buildings, death, suffering, and health hazards were just a few of the many threats that both victims and first responders faced during that incident.

A second grouping of the stressors identified by Paton (1996) involves the perceptions of the events by the first responders and the way in which their ability to do their jobs is affected. Having insufficient opportunity for effective action, knowing the victims and/or their families, receiving additional job-related responsibilities, and having to meet increased emotional, physical, and time demands can all trigger additional stress for first responders. Lack of adequate resources can negatively affect their ability to perform their jobs and can thus also result in stress. In addition, unrealistic expectations can make recovery from trauma more difficult (McCammon, Durham, Jackson, & Williams, 1988). Another complicating factor is the degree and duration of emotion suppression following an emergency situation (McCammon et al., 1988).

The third group of stressors relays the importance of the organizational structure in which the first responders are working. Changes to this structure can result in additional stress. For example, interagency coordination difficulties, conflicts, or failure can have adverse effects on the emotional and functional capabilities of emergency workers, and feelings of inadequacy and help-lessness can ensue. Emotions such as these can hamper workers' ability to perform their job successfully and efficiently. There are many roles that need fulfilling in disaster situations, and constantly having to change roles, such as going from saving someone's life to speaking with the media, can put extra strain on first responders as well.

Although there may be little one can do to affect the time, type, or nature of a future terrorist attack or other unforeseen disaster situation, some of these stressors can likely be reduced through training and preparedness work. For example, establishing firm roles and responsibilities, providing sufficient resources, ensuring adequate levels of staffing for shift rotations, and requiring additional preparatory training may all contribute to supporting a first responder in the line of duty and assisting in reducing the degree of stress felt in such a situation.

A Proposed Model of Threat Assessment and Trauma

Based on the more detailed understanding of fear and threat assessment developed in the preceding sections, we suggest a model of terrorist response that addresses six major factors grouped into three time categories:

1. Peritrauma and immediate posttrauma phase
   Factor 1. initial (objective) threat assessment
   Factor 2. immediate physical response
   Factor 3. immediate affective response
2. Assessment phase (posttrauma)
   Factor 4. mediators (prior traumatization, other risk factors, training, etc.) (these impact factor 5)
   Factor 5. cognition and memory (these impact factor 6)
   Factor 6. subjective threat assessment
3. Resolution phase (continuing)
   Either the individual continues to feel threatened and experiences ongoing symptoms, or the threat is downgraded and the symptoms begin to abate.

By being familiar with these factors, a practitioner can begin to categorize the experiences a victim has had and construct a comprehensive treatment plan in case the person's natural recovery process fails. To synthesize the information presented earlier and to explain the model, we suggest the following hypothetical timeline:

First, immediately following a terrorist attack, affected individuals must assess the objective threats in the environment, including personal physical injury, exposure, physical symptoms of shock, observing injury to others, witnessing death, and fearing for the survival of one's family members.

Second, both during and after a mass-casualty event, these objective threats may generate the immediate affective responses of fear and anxiety. As people move from the experience of the traumatic event into recovery, they begin to process the event more deeply. During this assessment phase, risk factors for PTSD, such as exposure to prior trauma, become increasingly salient and may deeply impact the cognitions and memories related to the event. Similarly, resiliency factors may be important at this stage in shielding the individuals from what otherwise might lead to problematic thought and memory patterns revolving around the event. It is also at this assessment stage that causal attributions and heuristics may be applied, both of which rely heavily on cognitive and memory processes. Thus, mediators such as risk and resiliency factors, along with cognition and memory, are central to a victim's subjective (or secondary) threat assessment. Terrorist attacks may be particularly powerful in influencing the secondary appraisal of fear-related stimuli because they elicit thoughts that revolve around threat persistence (unboundedness), malevolence, and fear of the unknown (CBRN devices, etc.).

Finally, in the resolution phase, a victim's fear and psychological symptoms either begin or abate as their subjective threat assessment wanes. However, if the subjective threat assessment does not decrease, the individual may be at risk for developing ASD or PTSD.

Normal Versus Interrupted Recovery

Practitioners should remain aware that, even in normal recovery, many psychological and physical symptoms associated with the traumatic event may be present and can persist for some time (Litz et al., 2002). However, if one's response to the trauma is normal and the individual has the usual sources of support and resilience, recovery may be relatively rapid, and the victim may return to baseline in days or weeks. Alternatively, the assessments, modulators, and risk factors may dispose a person to be traumatized to such a degree that resilience is impaired, and the normal restoration of mental health may be delayed or interrupted.

Furthermore, research on disaster victims has not always shown congruent symptoms across all event types (Brewin, Andrews, Rose, & Kirk, 1999; Goenjian et al., 2001; Morgan, Grillon, Lubin, & Southwick, 1997), and differences in correlations between the age of the adults and distress in victims and first responders have also proven difficult to pin down. Some studies have found that older rescue workers and victims tend to be more resilient in the face of disaster, while others have found that older victims are most at risk, and still others have demonstrated that those in their middle years are most likely to be affected (Tucker et al., 2000). Similarly, we can expect that different types of terrorist attacks will result in nuances in healthy and pathological recovery.

The types of psychological trauma and other after effects that are associated with major mass-casualty events include PTSD, ASD, major depressive disorder (MDD), burnout, anxiety, sleep disorders, and drug and alcohol abuse. In some rare instances the practitioner should also be prepared to handle OMUS (Bleisch et al., 1992; Pastel, 2001; Tucker et al., 2000). We briefly describe the clinical diagnostic criteria for each of these disorders (or theoretical formulations for trauma-related syndromes not listed in the *Diagnostic and Statistical Manual of Mental Disorders (DSM-IV-TR)*) as well as how they manifest in postdisaster situations.

However, the majority of what remains of this chapter focuses on treating acute stress disorder and preventing chronic PTSD since these two associated conditions encapsulate the central problems associated with the trauma exposure with which mental health practitioners must deal and are the general focus of the literature on the psychology of catastrophic events. We also highlight these disorders because their treatment among victims of mass-casualty events is poorly understood and because the efficacy of the treatments that have been used to date are hotly debated by researchers and theorists in the field of trauma psychology.

Specific Disorders Associated With Mass-Casualty Terrorist Events

The following descriptions of psychological disorders that may occur after exposure to a mass-casualty event are drawn from the *DSM-IV-TR,* except where noted, and we have used the language employed there in order to ensure congruity between these paraphrased descriptions and the actual diagnostic criteria for the disorders. The descriptions are intended for informational purposes only. We refer the reader to the *DSM-IV-TR* for more details, specific symptoms, and formal diagnostic procedures.

PTSD

According to the *DSM-IV-TR,* posttraumatic stress disorder may occur following exposure to an extremely traumatic stressor when a person has directly witnessed situations that result in actual or threatened mortality or physical injury and the individual's response to this situation includes a strong affective component of intense fear, helplessness, and/or horror. One or more cardinal symptoms of reexperiencing, three or more symptoms of avoidance and/or numbing, and two or more symptoms of increased arousal are needed to meet the full clinical criteria. The symptoms must be present for at least 1 month and are considered to be acute if the symptoms last for less than 3 months; they are considered chronic if they persist for more than 3 months. Children may present slightly differently, especially with regard to reexperiencing, with repetitive play that is thematically related to the trauma event and nightmares with no specific content. Trauma reenactment in younger children may be common.

ASD

Acute stress disorder is largely similar to PTSD but is shorter in duration and focuses more on the dissociative symptoms than PTSD does (Brewin et al., 1999). The *DSM-IV-TR* suggests that ASD "is the development of characteristic anxiety, dissociative, and other symptoms that occur within one month after exposure to an extreme stressor." Symptoms must last at least 2 days before diagnosis can be made. As with PTSD, the victim must both witness an event that threatened or resulted in serious physical harm to the victim or others and present an intense affective response including fear, helplessness, or horror. Three or more dissociative symptoms must be present, one or more reexperiencing symptoms must occur, and notable avoidance, anxiety, or arousal symptoms are required for this diagnosis

Depression

A major depressive episode is diagnosed following a period of 2 or more weeks in which an individual reports a depressed mood or anhedonia toward most normal activities. Depression is generally associated with a set of vegetative symptoms, such as sleeping difficulties and lethargy. Thoughts about personal worthlessness and suicide often occur. Especially in mass-casualty situations, symptoms related to bereavement should be separated from a potential diagnosis, and treatment should specifically address bereavement concerns if the individual has lost close relatives or friends. Depression has frequently been reported among those who were subjected to the terrors of 9/11 (Galea et al., 2002).

Burnout

Although not a *DSM-IV-TR* category, burnout can nonetheless result from high-stress occupational situations and can detrimentally affect job performance. It is helpful to consider burnout as both a process and a result. A person who experiences burnout may progress through different stages, and the symptoms are similar to those of stress, anxiety, and depressive disorders. Eventually, after experiencing prolonged levels of high stress and anxiety, an individual may socially withdraw and become apathetic and possibly resentful. Following this stage, the person may become depressed and exhibit many of the classic signs of depression. In addition to anxiety and depression, substance abuse is also associated with burnout. Burnout is preventable and can often be identified by the individual once provided with education about the condition.

Anxiety

Subclinical anxiety symptoms may be quite common after a mass-casualty event. Evidence suggests that feeling afraid or anxious immediately after a large-scale disaster may increase the risk for an onset of PTSD. However, the clinical diagnosis of generalized anxiety disorder (GAD) requires that the symptoms be present most of the time during a 6-month period. Those who suffer from GAD find it difficult to control their worry and exhibit at least three of the following symptoms: restlessness, fatigue, impaired concentration, irritability, muscle tension, sleep disturbance (either in falling asleep, staying asleep, or sleeping restfully). In children, only one of these symptoms is necessary to meet clinical diagnostic criteria.

Sleep Disorders

A diagnosis of primary insomnia is indicated when an individual has difficulty falling or staying asleep or experiences nonrestorative sleep for a period of 1 month or more. Primary insomnia causes serious distress in important life functions and is not due to biologically based sleep problems such as apnea or circadian rhythm upset. In trauma-exposed people, nightmare disorder may also occur. This is typified by repeated awakenings from sleep with detailed recall or extended and extremely frightening dreams, usually involving threats to personal survival, security, or self-esteem. The nightmares must cause significant difficulty in some aspect of life functioning to meet clinical criteria and must not occur during the course of another disorder, such as PTSD.

Drug Abuse and Dependence

Because of the wide variety of drugs that may be abused or for which dependence may develop, we concentrate here on the general criteria for substance abuse and dependence. Clinicians who suspect specific forms of drug use in trauma-exposed clients should refer to the *DSM-IV-TR* for further information. Due to the ubiquity of and ease in obtaining alcohol, clinicians should be particularly alert for signs of alcohol abuse in trauma victims. The criteria for substance abuse include a maladaptive pattern of substance use that leads to one or more of the following domains: failure to fulfill major obligations at work, school, or home; recurrent use of the substance when its ingestion puts the individual at risk for physical harm; legal difficulties related to the use of the substance; and continued use of the substance despite social or relational problems associated with intoxication. These criteria must be met within the space of a

12-month period. As with depression, drug abuse is particularly likely to increase following terror attacks, judging from the results of follow-ups on 9/11 victims (Vlahov et al., 2002).

OMUS

Outbreaks of multiple unexplained symptoms are not part of the *DSM-IV-TR* taxonomy of psychological disorders. Instead, this is a phenomenon that has been periodically observed in response to specific environmental factors. OMUS has been referred to as "mass anxiety" or "mass hysteria" in earlier formulations; however, because the phenomenon is probably an evolutionary response to a potential unknown, invisible pathogen, it should not be viewed as an inherently dysfunctional response (Pastel, 2001). OMUS may generate real somatic symptoms, including vomiting, diarrhea, rashes, and breathing difficulty, which are difficult to distinguish from symptoms of actual exposure to a CBRN device (Pastel, 2001). The phenomenon is also denoted as "psychological contamination" or the "social transmission" of symptoms (Jones, Craig, Hoy, & Gunter, 2000; Small et al., 1991). Typically, OMUS occur in environments where a potential pathogen causes one person to feel ill; then a number of other people report similar symptoms without being similarly exposed (Small et al., 1991). The phenomenon is viewed as a social and psychological response to potential environmental contamination, often in the absence of actual threat or personal exposure, resulting in somatic symptoms that quickly spread through the affected population and are usually transient but may recur with exposure to the location of the initial illness (Small et al., 1991).

Current Intervention Approaches and Myths of Treatment

The most frequently used model for reducing trauma in an attempt to prevent PTSD and other serious psychological consequences is critical incident stress debriefing (CISD) (Litz & Gray, 2004). This model was developed by Jeffery Mitchell in the early 1980s and was originally designed to provide comprehensive stress management approaches for use with first responders (Mitchell, 1983). The system later evolved into a broader

individual and community intervention framework known as critical incident stress management (CISM) (Litz & Gray, 2004). The CISD system has been used as the sole treatment intervention for numerous police and fire departments throughout the country for the better part of the last two decades (Litz & Gray, 2004).

With the increasing popularity of CISD, the absence of alternative treatments, and the purported benefits of the intervention, many government agencies, not-for-profit relief organizations, and private corporations felt compelled to offer it following traumatic incidents and often made attendance compulsory for victims. Thus, CISD evolved from an intervention specific to emergency responders to one that became the standard of care for nearly all victims of disasters, even though it was not originally designed for use with the general public. Mitchell argues that it is not appropriate for civilian casualties who have been directly impacted by a disaster (those with serious injury or who have experienced the death of a relative), and there is little empirical evidence to support its use in this more general context (Litz & Gray, 2004).

As originally formulated, CISD was intended to be a single-session group intervention. Within the treatment group, a mental health professional trained in CISD leads a discussion that follows a seven-step progression: (1) introduction; (2) fact phase (in which the event is re-created through the participants' stories); (3) thought phase (in which the participants describe their thoughts during the crisis); (4) reaction phase (in which the participants may experience catharsis); (5) symptom phase (in which each participant's current symptoms are discussed); (6) teaching phase (in which symptoms are normalized through psychoeducation); and (7) reentry phase (event closure; referrals are given as necessary) (Everly & Mitchell, 1999). The CISD model suggests that the intervention should take place as soon as possible following a traumatic event, typically within 24–72 hours.

The treatment model focuses primarily on talking through the trauma and reliving the emotional experiences of the event in a protected environment (Litz & Gray, 2004). When conducted with police officers, firefighters, or other first responders, the CISD groups are usually formed with prestanding units who experienced the same event. The theoretical framework of CISM suggests that the sharing of the experience assists in the normalization of symptoms and provides a framework for reliving the event through the multiple perspectives of the participants.

Myth: Talking It Through Prevents Traumatization

Until recently, common wisdom within the trauma treatment community held that ventilating the victim's emotions immediately following the event was requisite in preventing the later onset of PTSD. However, there is increasing empirical evidence to suggest that early treatment for trauma may interfere with the mind's natural healing processes (Gist & Lubin, 1999; Litz et al., 2002; McNally et al., 2003; Rose, Bisson, & Wessley, 2001). In fact, there is some suggestion that interventions that focus heavily on the emotional reliving of the event in the days immediately following the tragedy may actually put people who might otherwise recover normally at increased risk for PTSD (Rose et al., 2001). After a traumatic event, an individual typically experiences dissociative symptoms, such as emotional numbing, detachment, reduced awareness, derealization, and depersonalization. These symptoms may actually be normal, healthy reactions to highly stressful events (McNally et al., 2003). Dissociation may in fact serve as a temporary buffer, allowing an individual to process stressful information without attending to the events in consciousness. However, the CISD model encourages mental health professionals to pierce this protective veil and reintroduce the powerful emotional reaction to the trauma as soon as possible.

The CISD intervention model has recently come under increased scrutiny for several reasons. Litz & Gray (2004) list a number of concerns with the CISD approach. First, at a theoretical level, the debriefing seems to not consider the natural course of psychological healing that takes place for most people following trauma. Second, most of the studies examining the CISD model have been authored by the group that developed it and have not been replicated in other settings. Third, the majority of the studies of CISD suffer from critical methodological flaws. Fourth, the CISD model was originally developed for the treatment of first

responders, and the originator of the CISD intervention has suggested that it may not be appropriate for the general public. Finally, alternative approaches have not been extensively developed and empirically examined as comparisons to the CISD model.

As a result of this increased interest, three major meta-analyses of the CISD treatment system were undertaken and have recently been published (Litz & Gray, 2004). These reviews examine the relatively few randomized controlled trials (RCTs) probing the efficacy of CISD that are available. We consider two of these meta-analyses in detail. The first was conducted by Rose, Bisson, & Wessely in 1998 as part of a Cochrane Review. This study was subsequently updated in 2001 and served as the first major review of RCTs of the efficacy of the CISD treatment system.

Using established search criteria, the authors of the Cochrane Review identified 11 studies that involved the use of single-session psychological debriefing with participants who had recently been exposed to a trauma. All of the interventions used a variation of emotional recounting of the event. The authors of the review also noted that the quality of most of the studies was poor (Rose et al., 2001). The Cochrane Review poses some compelling and disturbing questions about the use of CISD and related treatment systems.

These meta-analyses found no quantitative support for the contention that single-session debriefing leads to a reduction in PTSD risk. The report also entertains the possibility that this type of early intervention may instead hinder recovery and increase the risk of chronic PTSD. Two of the long-term follow-up studies included in the review found that those receiving a single treatment following a traumatic event had worse prognoses for mental health difficulty as compared to the controls. Further, Rose and his colleagues found that debriefing did not reduce other psychological difficulties associated with exposure to trauma, including depression and anxiety (Rose et al., 2001). The authors of the review suggest that single-session psychological debriefing treatments may suffer from the following problems that reduce this intervention's efficacy: (1) The interventions may be too short; (2) the follow-up may be too short to show results; (3) the treatment timing may be incorrect; and (4) the idea of debriefing may have been incorporated into contemporary culture, rendering formalized intervention unnecessary. Each of these possibilities warrants further investigation.

The review by Rose et al. (2003) hypothesizes reasons for the observed negative or null outcomes with single-treatment interventions. The first is the suggestion that those who experience shame or guilt reactions in response to a traumatic event may be at risk when only a single, emotion-laden treatment is provided and further exploration of these emotions is not offered. Second, psychological debriefing may attach an unnecessary stigma to the normal recovery symptoms observed in trauma victims. Rose and colleagues note that "Debriefing, by increasing awareness of psychological distress, may paradoxically induce distress in people who would otherwise not have developed it" (Rose et al., 2003, p. 9). Finally, the authors of this review argue that psychological debriefing may be problematic because it subscribes to the dubious notion that all victims experience the traumatic event and progress through recovery in a fairly uniform manner. These hypotheses should serve as the basis for future research examining both the efficacy and the possible dangers of single-session, emotion-driven treatment systems for trauma.

A second set of meta-analyses performed by Litz and his colleagues (2002) sought to confirm and expand upon the findings of the Cochrane Review. These analyses examined the results of six RCTs involving psychological debriefing. The inclusion criteria for this meta-analysis differ somewhat from those found in the review by Rose et al. (2001). However, the same pattern of results emerged. The findings confirmed that psychological debriefing provided no more relief of symptoms than could be expected with natural recovery over time. A small difference in effect size indicated that psychological debriefing may result in greater levels of PTSD symptoms following treatment. However, Litz and colleagues caution against interpreting these findings or those of the study by Rose et al. (2001) as providing definitive evidence of negative side effects with the use of this treatment approach (Litz et al., 2002).

As a result of the mounting evidence showing that CISD may not be as effective as hoped, one of the leading researchers in the field of acute stress treatment has concluded that, "Contrary to the conclusions of advocates of CISD/CISM, there is no sufficiently rigorous empirical support for the use of CISD/CISM in the secondary prevention of chronic PTSD. Controlled studies reveal it to be therapeutically inert when applied to individuals" (Litz & Gray, 2004, p. 101). In light of these findings, a conference convened by the National Institute of Mental Health concluded that CISD should not be used as an intervention with trauma victims, a view seconded by the British National Health Service (Litz & Gray, 2004). In response, dramatic shifts in the world of trauma intervention have begun to occur as several major insurance agencies have discouraged large organizations from hiring CISD counselors to provide this intervention because it is increasingly viewed as prior art, no longer the standard of care, and a lawsuit risk (Yandrick, 2004).

Myth: Most People Are at Risk

One of the common misconceptions about terrorism and trauma is the expectation that a large proportion of the affected population will develop full-blown PTSD symptoms in the months following the event (McNally et al., 2003). In fact, the general public and even direct victims appear to be surprisingly resilient. In the wake of what was arguably the most significant act of terrorism in peacetime, the events of September 11, 2001, surprisingly few people used the psychological and other support services offered by the 9,000 professional and paraprofessional counselors who were rushed to New York following the tragedy (McNally et al., 2003). The Project Liberty program, a federally funded initiative designed to provide counseling to affected New Yorkers, estimated that 25% of the city's inhabitants would need counseling and prepared to meet the need for psychological services for a staggering 2.5 million victims, yet just slightly more than half a million city residents used these services (McNally et al., 2003).

In fact, in summarizing PTSD prevalence data gathered by several researchers following the 9/11 attacks, McNally and colleagues (2003) stated that, while predictions of significant distress surged, the actual rates of PTSD symptoms ranged from just 7.5% to 20% in the general public who had been near Ground Zero at the time of the attacks. Four months later, a similar study with participants living near the World Trade Center site found that the proportion of the population experiencing PTSD-like symptoms dropped to 1.7% (McNally et al., 2003). One national study of PTSD prevalence following 9/11 found slightly higher numbers, with 17% of the sample meeting criteria 8 weeks after the attacks and falling to 5.8% after 6 months (Litz & Gray, 2004). Similarly, estimates of PTSD rates in Israeli civilians (ostensibly due to ongoing terrorist activity) found that between 2.7% and 9.4% of respondents met the criteria for PTSD (depending on the stringency of the inclusion criteria). Only 5.3% felt they needed to seek professional treatment for stress related to terrorist activity, while more than 60% of the participants reported feeling that their lives were threatened (Bleisch, Gelkopf, & Solomon, 2003).

Several studies following the 9/11 tragedy found similar results, and a number of researchers in the field have suggested that, even though many people may initially exhibit stress symptoms, this is a fundamentally normal process, and most people recover from the trauma without the high rate of chronic psychological illness that was initially predicted (Litz et al., 2002; McNally et al., 2003). Furthermore, while a high proportion of people who were representatively sampled across the nation endorsed items indicating that they had experienced stress-related symptoms following the events of 9/11, there is little evidence to suggest that the majority of those who were exposed through the media were at risk for developing PTSD (Pfefferbaum et al., 2002). Moreover, those with severe symptoms immediately after a major traumatic event are no more likely to develop chronic PTSD than those who experience lesser symptoms (McNally et al., 2003). These findings, as well as the progression of recovery they suggest, should be central to our understanding of the human response to intentional mass-casualty events.

What Mental Health Professionals Need to Know About Intervention

Based on mounting evidence that single-session psychological debriefing treatments provide no benefit and may even hinder the recovery process, researchers and clinicians have become increasingly interested in developing and using alternative treatment systems with disaster-traumatized

individuals. These interventions differentiate between immediate response, which occurs in the hours following a terrorist event, and the more long-term treatment of people who have residual symptoms. Together they compose the content of the knowledge that mental health practitioners should apparently have as they anticipate providing care to survivors.

Do's and Don'ts in the Immediate Aftermath of Terror

Mental health professionals must be trained to respond to disasters such as terrorist attacks with a broader range of skills than that required in the office practice of psychotherapy. Various initiatives have been set in motion to provide them with the tools they need to treat these victims.

Various recommendations have been made for how best to intervene with those at psychological risk following terrorist events. CISD is no longer a treatment intervention one should use lightly or simply because one has been instructed to do so. Newer approaches derived from empirically based treatments are becoming available for the emergency mental health responder. In the remainder of this chapter, we present a brief overview of current recommendations. However, additional research-based information is forthcoming and practitioners should view this effort as an initial effort to build the ground work for future work. Mental healthcare workers should actively seek out new information as it becomes available because of the fledgling nature of this field. For example, the area of psychological first aid (PFA) appears to be gaining strength as an alternative to CISD, and research findings in this area should inform practice as they become available.

Emerging treatments focus on the unique aspects of victims of terrorism. Thus, treatment conceptualizations are becoming more specific and refined. For example, despite the developing belief among researchers in this field that early psychological intervention may be contraindicated, this does not imply that no support should be offered to individuals immediately following a trauma event. To the contrary, social support has been repeatedly shown to help prevent chronic PTSD, and, perhaps more importantly, negative social contacts immediately following a critical incident appear to increase the risk of PTSD (McNally et al.,

2003). Further, feelings of nihilism and despair that are associated with chronic PTSD are best addressed by assisting the client to build (or rebuild) a strong social support network through reengagement in social activities (Miller, 2002).

Psychological First Aid

Borrowing from a model developed to treat refugees, it appears that the most important first step in psychological treatment is to reestablish a sense of safety and to provide basic services such as food, shelter, and contact with loved ones. Miller (2002) states that, immediately after a trauma event, "Physical care is psychological care." This approach, termed "psychological first aid," is not envisioned as a treatment program (Litz et al., 2002). Psychological first aid differs from psychological debriefing models in that its primary focus is the provision of physical comfort and psychoeducation to normalize symptoms; in short, it puts in place a referral system for people who feel the need for more assistance. Also contrary to the CISD model, Litz and his colleagues (2002) state that "This position recognizes that most people do not suffer from PTSD [or more accurately ASD] in the immediate days after an event; rather the majority of people will have transient stress reactions that will remit with time" (p. 128).

Through the use of psychological first aid, the practitioner is also able to strengthen preexisting social networks that may encourage more natural debriefing (e.g., with family members or co-workers), approaches that have been found to often be more effective and better received than overt, practitioner-led debriefing (Gist & Lubin, 1999). Finally, this approach also allows the psychologist, social worker, or other mental health professional to passively monitor the progression of recovery and to enable them to flag those who are at high risk for PTSD, monitor them, and step in as needed.

While psychological first aid provides an appropriate framework for general intervention, Bryant & Harvey (2000, p. 84) note that "There is now convergent evidence that approximately 80% of individuals who are diagnosed with ASD subsequently suffer chronic PTSD." In light of this finding, effective, early interventions are needed for the subset of victims who fail to recover naturally. If a reduction in symptoms is not apparent after an appropriate period of time, which is assumed to be 1–2 weeks (Litz & Gray, 2004), the practitioner should begin considering more aggressive intervention.

Minimum Intervention Guidelines for Responding to Victims and Rescuers During Crises

It is imperative that the ways in which we help crisis victims reflect the best scientific knowledge available. However, because of the nature of science, what we know and what we can recommend are always changing. Because of the way that scientific information accumulates, we are likely to find out more quickly when something does not work than when it does. Thus, we have learned many things from scientific research that we initially believed *should* have been helpful, yet some have turned out to be ineffective and even harmful (Gist & Woodall, 2000; Litz et al., 2002; Rose, Bisson, & Wessely, 2001; Rose, Brewin, et al., 1999; Rose, Wessely, & Bisson, 1998). At the same time, we are finding that many of the commonsense procedures and fundamental ways of providing assistance are surprisingly helpful to people in crisis.

Despite the extensive instruction that is frequently offered and the treatments that are accepted as if their use represents factual and scientifically derived knowledge, actual scientifically generated and supported knowledge about what best to do in the immediate wake of trauma is quite limited. There are, however, some general guidelines that can be derived from research studies. We have compiled these into a straightforward list of basic do's and don'ts for the clinician who is seeking to assist victims and rescuers in the first hours and days following a major community crisis. These recommendations represent the best knowledge that is available at the present time.

Things to Do

The following points offer some guidance as to specific actions and approaches a clinical practitioner can engage in to provide effective support following a terrorist attack or similar mass-casualty event:

1. Remember that effective first response comes not from your role as a healer but rather from your role as one who provides comfort, direct support, and useful information. You are most

effective as a source of accurate information, immediate guidance, and direct assistance with the needs and demands of the present. If victims have lost their home, it is far more important to reduce the immediate feelings of stress by providing shelter than it is to listen empathically to the feelings of helplessness that loss entails. In the face of loss and threat, it is also more effective to provide immediate calming and instrumental care than to encourage early ventilation and catharsis.

2. Get your hands "dirty"—get into the field—in order to make sure that physical and medical needs are addressed. It is very helpful in later contacts to have met people first in these settings and to have initially provided immediate and pragmatic forms of help before attempting to offer more personal levels of support.

3. Provide information and guidance at very practical levels. Arm yourself with as much information as you can garner and communicate it clearly and systematically to those you encounter. Relate your information clearly, using only fully authoritative sources (do not be a vehicle for rumors and misinformation).

4. Establish a working relationship with the client. Make sure that your role is understood and that the client has given permission for you to assist. Make known your identity, credentials, relationships to other organizations (e.g., Red Cross, employer of rescue personnel) very clearly, and establish the objectives for the encounter. Do not proceed unless the individual is willing to accept your help.

5. Ensure that physical and safety needs (e.g., medical, shelter, food) are provided before addressing the emotional impacts of the trauma. Keep the initial focus on meeting basic needs and preserving stamina.

6. Provide a clearly defined objective and end point for the contact and relationship. Tell people what to expect. Most of the time, you will need to provide one or more direct referrals for subsequent assistance. Ensure that the options your provide reflect a wide range of possibilities.

7. Emphasize the client's strengths rather than weaknesses or deficits. Provide reassurance ("this will pass"; "you will get through this") and maintain a sense of calm. If handouts or written information are used, these materials should be carefully structured to promote expectations of resilience and recovery rather than providing laundry lists of pitfalls and symptoms.

8. Direct victims and rescuers to community resources that offer comfort and assistance. Connect victims with sources of aid that will provide direct and continuing support (e.g., family, community, faith-based resources).

9. Rescuers are critically affected by the tendency to identify with victims and to the effects of exhaustion—help them to establish and maintain boundaries, pace their efforts and expectations, and control emotions during protracted encounters.

10. Work with a companion whenever possible, and let the coworker help you maintain perspective and objectivity.

Things to Avoid

The following points offer some guidance as to specific actions and approaches a clinician should avoid following a terrorist attack or similar mass-casualty event:

1. Emotion-focused debriefing in the immediate aftermath of trauma—by its many labels, including psychological debriefing (PD), CISD, and multiple stressor debriefing (MSD)—has not been shown to be effective in preventing later difficulties and may even cause problems to become entrenched or more severe over time. "Debriefing," as used here, includes any approach that involves (a) revisiting and reconstructing the details and feelings associated with the traumatic event and any of the following additional procedures: (b) encouragement to explore and deepen one's reexperiencing of the emotion-laden events; (c) normalization of reactions, especially elements of negative feelings; and (d) education regarding the signs and symptoms of PTSD. While doing these things often seem to be a good idea, the evidence is strong and accumulating that these are aspects of help giving that should be avoided during the initial stages of trauma reaction.

2. Some examples of other treatments that are frequently used but whose effects have not yet been demonstrated scientifically to be helpful include reexposure therapy, eye movement

desensitization and reprocessing (EMDR), thought field therapy (TFT), acupuncture, and various patent remedies. Cognitive therapy (CT) has been found to be effective in high-risk populations and in those whose problems persist beyond the initial reaction, but even this approach should be avoided during the immediate aftermath period. Any continuing "treatment" should be used only if indicated by careful evaluation.

3. Avoid being the primary focus for the provision of assistance and emotional or social support. Healthy resolution may ultimately depend on fostering a sense of self-efficacy and mastery of the threat and challenge. The greatest risk to helpers and clinicians may be "overhelping," or what some have called "the tyranny of urgency." This is the tendency to go too far in helping people do what they need to do for themselves or even doing for them what can best be done by their own families and reference groups.

4. The vast majority of those who are exposed to even severe trauma will not experience PTSD and will recover through their own resources and in their own time. Thus, it is important to respect the natural recovery process and to avoid presuming that someone needs professional mental health assistance. Be "invisibly supportive." People recover at different rates and by different means. Let victims set their own pace, talk about things that are important to them, and seek their own space. Some people need a period of withdrawal; beyond this, it is important that victims feel empowered to take some steps on their own in order to gain a sense of personal agency. Do not push them to discuss—before they are ready—or to do something that they are reluctant to do.

5. Do not be too formal. Don't carry or wear the badges of distance, such as a clipboard or a white coat, which might mark you as a "removed," clinical observer. Respect the client's privacy and keep the relationship open.

Follow-Up Treatment

In the weeks following a traumatic incident, most people will recover in response to psychological first aid and the minimalist treatment. Most people

are very resilient and do not need long-term assistance. However, during the first days and weeks following a crisis it is difficult to reliably distinguish those who will have prolonged difficulty and those who will not. A clinician should not attempt to make formal mental health assessments until 2 or more weeks have passed. Nonetheless, a brief, initial screening, as long as it does not interfere with providing immediate physical and medical assistance, along with support, encouragement, and comfort, might help identify those who should be recontacted after a few weeks and considered for more prolonged treatment.

Initial Screening

Screening of risk factors can be accomplished with four basic, relatively unobtrusive queries:

1. Have the individuals experienced other intense exposures or instances of trauma (has anything like this happened before)?
2. Is there any history of prior mental health treatment or of circumstances for which the individuals or others thought treatment should have been sought?
3. Do the individuals have at least one other person with whom they can talk and share their problems? Has doing so seemed productive and helpful in the past?
4. Were the individuals exposed (in their judgment) to particularly gruesome or disturbing aspects of this event?

Follow-Up Evaluation

Persons experiencing lingering difficulties after the initial impact has passed (generally 2–6 weeks) should be evaluated for further mental health assistance within the context of an established professional relationship. These services are generally best provided by agencies and professionals within the local community, where enduring therapeutic relationships can be developed.

Where further treatment is indicated, empirically supported, conservative approaches such as CT spread across four or five sessions should be among the primary considerations. Therapists attempting longer-term interventions should seek specific training and supervision in these approaches and especially in their application to traumatic exposure. Case management that includes social work and systems advocacy should also be considered as a critical adjunct to ensure that continuing or emergent instrumental needs continue to be supportively addressed. If more intensive follow-up is indicated by the persistence of debilitating anxiety after a few weeks, there are several treatments that have been found to be useful for restoring normal functioning.

Prolonged Exposure

While the CISD model relies on a single-exposure intervention, more rigorously constructed short-term interventions involving imaginal exposure over a number of sessions have demonstrated significant reductions in PTSD symptoms (Bryant & Harvey, 2000). These findings were identified in studies of traumatic reactions to sexual and nonsexual assault, and lowered rates of PTSD were found during a 3-month follow-up after cessation of treatment. However, although this intervention approach appears to be effective in reducing symptoms for some people, initial studies indicate that these results occur in only about half of the victims who are treated (Bryant & Harvey, 2000). Based on preliminary findings, in vivo exposure may also be an effective treatment for PTSD prevention; however, little systematic research has been undertaken in this area (Bryant & Harvey, 2000). Prolonged exposure (PE) techniques are typified by recalling the traumatic event for a period of not less than 50 minutes. The approach aims to completely activate the fear-related memories of the event long enough to cause habituation to the stimulus (Bryant & Harvey, 2000).

Cognitive Behavioral Therapy

Based on the limited literature currently available, elements of cognitive behavioral therapy (CBT) and PE appear to be the most appropriate tools in the reduction of initial stress symptoms and ASD symptoms and in the prevention of chronic PTSD (Litz et al., 2002). The key features of CBT and PE treatment that may assist a trauma victim typically include elements from PE and include imaginal exposure to trauma-related memories, graduated in vivo exposure to avoided situations, cognitive restructuring, and homework tasks to support the therapeutic process (Bryant & Harvey, 2000; Litz et al., 2002). One of the critical components of this approach is that the intervention is carried out

multiple times over several weeks, allowing a supported processing of the event (Litz & Gray, 2004). Under the watchful eye of a trained practitioner, serious issues that may be left unidentified and unresolved in a single session may be detected and addressed. Initial controlled trials have demonstrated that when CBT and PE techniques are used with ASD patients, the intervention dramatically reduces PTSD rates at follow-up, with only 15% of the participants continuing to meet criteria, compared to 67% in a supportive counseling control condition (Bryant & Harvey, 2000). While CBT combined with PE is perhaps the best approach currently known, care should be taken if the patient is acutely traumatized, suicidal, experiencing concomitant mental health problems, or under stress because of continued exposure. The powerful effects of exposure therapy may overwhelm these clients, leading them to drop out of therapy (Bryant & Harvey, 2000).

Other Treatment Considerations

The field of trauma treatment has received increasing attention from a wide variety of researchers and theorists in psychology and related fields since the events of September 11, 2001. While much of the research currently under way will explore the efficacy of various components of psychological debriefing, CBT, and other "talk therapies," pharmacological interventions are also being examined. Some research has pointed to continued physical arousal symptoms following the removal of victims to safety as an indicator of risk for PTSD onset. Based on this model, some have suggested that pharmacological interventions that suppress the sympathetic nervous system response, such as propranolol (a beta-blocker), may be effective in disrupting the immediate fear response and, in turn, serve to lower the risk of PTSD. While this is just one emerging treatment model, it illustrates that practitioners need to remain vigilant as new research informs a changing standard of care.

Special Considerations for First Responders

A common perception of emergency personnel is that they are somehow stronger people, both emotionally and physically, than most and that this strength allows them to do their jobs and remain unaffected by the tragedy and trauma they witness. Their attraction to their professions seems to suggest a solid personality that responds quickly and appropriately in emergency situations. However, even if these perceptions are rooted in fact, emergency response workers are still subjected to repeated stress. Exposure to mass-casualty incidents, repeated exposure to stressful situations, and always being on alert for the next call can contribute to potential psychological injury over the course of a career or in the aftermath of a disaster. These adverse effects can come in various forms and include emotional, cognitive, and somatic effects. However, there are certain identified resilience mechanisms and coping strategies that can assist in buffering against such adverse effects.

Efforts to assist first responders have emphasized intervention techniques, but attention should also be focused on preparatory strategies to promote adaptation and minimize impact prior to a mass-casualty event (Paton, 1996). Emergency response workers are often involved in repeated training for various aspects of their jobs. Two of the goals of training are practice and preparation—practice in using problem-solving abilities in novel situations and preparation for doing one's job and for knowing what to expect while doing it.

Training is often considered in the functional perspective of engaging in and practicing job-related duties. But performing these responsibilities sometimes extends beyond one's capacity to accomplish functional tasks, such as starting an intravenous (IV) injection. A professional must be mentally able to follow through with those tasks in a disaster situation and maintain a state of psychological health over the long term in order to ensure an extended career in the emergency response field.

Predisaster psychology training could benefit emergency response workers, for example, by helping them determine what psychological stressors they are susceptible to and learn how to recognize when victims, their coworkers, or they themselves are experiencing adverse psychological effects. Such instruction can also help them learn to communicate effectively with others and to practice coping mechanisms to deal with such stress. Also, training provided to desensitize emergency response personnel to situations they might encounter could provide benefits through increasing their familiarity with the associated environmental factors and emotional reactions. For example, prebriefings on what to expect were associated with adaptive capabilities in FEMA workers and assisted in mitigating the stress of understanding what they were about to go through in responding to an emergency (García, 2003). This implies that briefing first responders on what to expect at an emergency scene could assist by desensitizing them and therefore reduce the stress associated with responding to an emergency scene. Additional training might include educating response workers about the mental health resources available through their employer and in their community.

While those who do not work in the field of trauma or death and dying may find the humor of emergency personnel morbid and distasteful, it serves a valuable purpose in relieving stress and helping them transition from one call to the next. Studies on the use of humor by emergency personnel have shown that, among experienced paramedics, humor was ranked higher than other coping mechanisms, including talking with friends and family, socializing, going out, and exercising (Rosenberg, 1991). Pretrained subjects in Rosenberg's study stated that humor relieved tension and served as a tool by which they could cognitively and emotionally refocus themselves to regain perspective and even transcend a situation. Experienced paramedics said that humor provides a mental break and assists them in returning to a normal state of mind. In addition, those paramedics who used humor less showed higher levels of stress. Subjects of this study also communicated that humor has limits and that overreliance on it to the exclusion of other coping mechanisms is counterproductive.

In a study on leisure coping used by police and emergency response workers, it was found that leisure coping and both short- and long-term stress coping are positively related (Iwasaki, Mannell, Smale, & Butcher, 2002). This relationship extends beyond the benefits of general coping. Coping with short-term stress includes stress reduction, and coping with long-term stress includes benefits associated with both physical and mental health. Leisure activities also seem to benefit emergency response workers through mood regulation, temporary escape from job-related stress, companionship with friends and family, and the fostering of feelings of empowerment, perceived control, and a positive attitude toward life.

Firefighters and police officers, as well as other emergency response professionals, experience a strong bond both within individual departments and across the country. When the news that firefighters in New York City had perished during the 9/11 crisis reached firefighters on the West Coast, the emotions felt for their "fallen brothers" were profound. Many tears were shed among this group of tough workers, and those who were not sent to Ground Zero confronted feelings of helplessness, grief, and despair. Departments around the country implemented "boot collections" (using fire boots to hold the donations) at public places to send money to the families of their "brothers." Departments held moments of silence for the firefighters who had lost their lives. The bond felt between professionals in their respective fields is arguably a strong one, and it may assist emergency response professionals in coping with trauma in that they rarely experience it alone.

McCammon and colleagues (1988) questioned emergency response workers about the frequency with which they used particular coping mechanisms in response to two disaster situations. In the case of an explosion at an apartment building, behaviors they deemed helpful included reminding themselves that things could be worse, looking at the situation realistically, being more helpful to others, thinking about the meaning of life following the event, and talking to others about the incident.

Acknowledgments. This research was performed while the third author (Zeno Franco) was on appointment as a U.S. Department of Homeland Security (DHS) fellow under the DHS Scholarship and Fellowship Program, a program administered by the Oak Ridge Institute for Science and Education (ORISE) for DHS through an interagency agreement with the U.S. Department of Energy (DOE). Oak Ridge Associated Universities ORISE is managed by DOE contract number DE-AC05-000R22750.

All of the opinions expressed in this chapter are the authors' and do not necessarily reflect the policies and views of DHS, DOE, or ORISE.

References

American Psychiatric Association. (2000). *Diagnostic and statistical manual of mental disorders: DSM-IV-TR* (4th ed.). Washington, DC: Author.

Bleisch, A., Dycian, A., Koslowsky, M., Solomon, Z., & Wiener, M. (1992). Psychiatric implications of missile attacks on a civilian population. *Journal of the American Medical Association, 268*(5), 613–615.

Bleisch, A., Gelkopf, M., & Solomon, Z. (2003). Exposure to terrorism, stress-related mental health symptoms, and coping behaviors among a nationally representative sample in Israel. *Journal of the American Medical Association, 290*(5), 612.

Brewin, C., Andrews, B., Rose, S., & Kirk, M. (1999). Acute stress disorder and posttraumatic stress disorder in victims of violent crimes. *American Journal of Psychiatry, 156*(3), 360–366.

Bryant, R., & Harvey, A. (2000). *Acute stress disorder: A handbook of theory, assessment, and treatment.* Washington, D.C.: American Psychological Association.

Chapman, C., & Harris, A. (2002). A skeptical look at September 11th: How we can defeat terrorism by reacting to it more rationally. *Skeptical Inquirer, 26*(5), 29–34.

Dalgleish, T. (2004). Cognitive approaches to posttraumatic stress disorder: The evolution of multirepresentational theorizing. *Psychological Bulletin, 130,* 228–260.

Everly, G., & Mitchell, J. (1999). *Critical incident stress management (CISM): A new era and standard of care in crisis intervention* (2d ed.). Ellicott City, MD: Chevron.

Galea, S., Ahern, J., Resnick, H., Kilpatrick, D., Bucuvalas, M., Gold, J., et al. (2002). Psychological sequelae of the September 11 terrorist attacks in New York City. *New England Journal of Medicine, 346,* 982–987.

Galea, S., Vlahov, D., Resnick, H., Ahern, J., Susser, E., Gold, J., et al. (2003). Trends of probable posttraumatic stress disorder in New York City after the September 11 terrorist attacks. *American Journal of Epidemiology, 158,* 514–524.

García, E. (2003). Supporting the Federal Emergency Management Agency rescuers: A variation of critical incident stress management. *Military Medicine, 168*(2), 87–91.

Gist, R., & Lubin, B. (Eds.). (1999). *Response to disaster: Psychosocial, community, and ecological approaches.* Philadelphia: Taylor & Francis.

Gist, R., & Woodall, S. (2000). There are no simple solutions to complex problems. In J. M. Violanti & P. Douglas (Eds.), *Posttraumatic stress intervention: Challenges, issues, and perspectives* (pp. 81–95). Springfield, IL: Charles C. Thomas.

Goenjian, A., Molina, L., Steinberg, A., Fairbanks, L., Alvarez, M., Goenjian, H., et al. (2001). Posttraumatic stress and depressive reactions among Nicaraguan adolescents after Hurricane

Mitch. *American Journal of Psychiatry, 158*(5), 788–794.

Iwasaki, Y., Mannell, R. C., Smale, B. J., & Butcher, J. (2002). A short-term longitudinal analysis of leisure coping used by police and emergency response service workers. *Journal of Leisure Research, 34*(3), 331–339.

Jones, T., Craig, A., Hoy, D., & Gunter, E. (2000). Mass psychogenic illness attributed to toxic exposure at a high school. *New England Journal of Medicine, 342*(2), 96–101.

Litz, B., & Gray, M. (2004). Early intervention for trauma in adults. In B. Litz (Ed.), *Early intervention for trauma and traumatic loss.* New York: Guilford Press.

———, Bryant, R., & Adler, A. (2002). Early intervention for trauma: Current status and future directions. *Clinical Psychology: Science and Practice, 9*(2), 112–134.

Marlowe, D. H. (2001). *Psychological and psychosocial consequences of combat and deployment.* Santa Monica: RAND.

McCammon, S. L., Durham, T. W., Jackson, E. J., & Williams, J. E. (1988). Emergency workers' cognitive appraisal and coping with traumatic events. *Journal of Traumatic Stress, 1*(3), 353–372.

McNally, R., Bryant, R., & Ehlers, A. (2003). Does early psychological intervention promote recovery from posttraumatic stress? *Psychological Science in the Public Interest, 4*(2), 45–79.

Meisel, S., Kutz, I., Dayan, K., Pauzner, H., Chetboun, I., Abrel, Y., et al. (1991). Effect of Iraqi missile war on incidence of acute myocardial infarction and sudden death in Israeli civilians. *Lancet, 338*(8788), 660–661.

Miller, L. (2002). Psychological interventions for terroristic trauma: Symptoms, syndromes, and treatment Strategies. *Psychotherapy: Theory/Research/Practice/Training, 39*(4), 283–296.

Mitchell, J. (1983). When disaster strikes . . . the critical incident stress debriefing process. *Journal of Emergency Medical Services, 8,* 36–39.

Morgan, C., Grillon, C., Lubin, H., & Southwick, S. (1997). Startle reflex abnormalities in women with sexual assault–related posttraumatic stress disorder. *American Journal of Psychiatry, 154*(8), 1076–1080.

Neria, Y., Suh, E. J., & Marshall, R. D. (2004). The professional response to the aftermath of September 11, 2001, in New York City: Lessons learned from treating victims of the World Trade Center attacks. In B. Litz (Ed.), *Early intervention for trauma and traumatic loss* (pp. 201–215). New York: Guilford.

Ohman, A., Flykt, A., & Esteves, F. (2001). Emotion drives attention: Detecting the snake in the grass. *Journal of Experimental Psychology: General, 130*(3), 466–478.

Pastel, R. (2001). Collective behaviors: Mass panic and outbreaks of multiple unexplained symptoms. *Military Medicine, 166*(12), 44–46.

Paton, D. (1996). Training disaster workers: Promoting well-being and operational effectiveness. *Disaster Prevention and Management, 5*(5), 11–18.

Pfefferbaum, B., Pfefferbaum, R., North, C., & Neas, B. (2002). Does television viewing satisfy criteria for exposure in posttraumatic stress disorder. *Psychiatry, 65*(4), 306–309.

Resnick, H., Acierno, R., Holmes, M., Dammeyer, M., & Kilpatrick, D. (2000). Emergency evaluation and intervention with female victims of rape and other violence. *Journal of Clinical Psychology, 56,* 1317–1333.

Rose, S., Bisson, J., & Wessely, S. (2001). Psychological debriefing for preventing post traumatic stress disorder (PTSD) (Cochrane Review). *Cochrane Library, 3.* Oxford University Press: Update Software.

Rose, S., Brewin, C. R., Andrews, B., & Kirk, M. (1999). A randomized controlled trial of individual psychological debriefing for victims of violent crime. *Psychological Medicine, 29,* 793–799.

Rose, S., Wessely, S., & Bisson, J. (1998). Brief psychological interventions ("debriefing") for trauma-related symptoms and prevention of posttraumatic stress disorder (Cochrane Review). *Cochrane Library, 2.* Oxford University Press: Update Software.

Rosenberg, L. (1991). A qualitative investigation of the use of humor by emergency personnel as a strategy for coping with stress. *Journal of Emergency Nursing, 17*(4), 197–202.

Schlenger, W. E., Caddell, J. M., Ebert, L., Jordan, B. K., Rourke, K. M., Wilson, D., et al. (2002). Psychological reactions to terrorist attacks: Findings from the National Study of Americans' Reactions to September 11. *Journal of American Medical Association, 288,* 581–588.

Slovic, P. (2002). Terrorism as hazard: A new species of trouble. *Risk Analysis, 22*(3), 425–426.

———, & Weber, E. (2002, April). Perceptions of risk posed by extreme events. Paper presented at the Risk Management Strategies in an Uncertain World, April 12–13, Palisades, New York.

Small, G., Propper, M., Randolph, E., & Eth, S. (1991). Mass hysteria among student performers: Social relationship as a symptom predictor. *American Journal of Psychiatry, 148*(9), 1200–1205.

Suedfeld, P. (2003). Specific and general attributional patterns of Holocaust survivors. *Canadian Journal of Behavioural Science, 35*(2), 133–141.

Tucker, P., Pfefferbaum, B., Nixon, S., & Dickson, W. (2000). Predictors of post-traumatic stress symptoms in Oklahoma City: Exposure, social support, peri-traumatic responses. *Journal of Behavioral Health Services and Research, 27*(4), 406–416.

Vlahov, D., Galea, S., Resnick, H., Ahern, J., Boscarino, J. A., Bucuvalas, M., Gold, J., & Kilpatrick, D. (2002). Increased use of cigarettes, alcohol, and marijuana among Manhattan residents after the September 11th terrorist attacks. *American Journal of Epidemiology, 155,* 988–996.

Wakefield, J. C. (1992). The concept of mental disorder: On the boundary between biological facts and social values. *American Psychologist, 47,* 373–388.

Weinstein, N., Lyon, J., Rothman, A., & Cuite, C. (2000). Changes in perceived vulnerability following natural disaster. *Journal of Social and Clinical Psychology, 19*(3), 372–395.

Wessely, S., & Jones, E. (in press). Psychiatry and the "lessons of Vietnam": What were they, are they still relevant? *War and Society.*

Yandrick, R. M. (2004). *Traumatic event debriefings getting second thoughts.* Crisis Management International. Retrieved April, 2004, from http://www.cmiatl.com/news_article59.html

4

War Versus Justice in Response to Terrorist Attacks

Competing Frames and Their Implications

Clark McCauley

Often lost in discussion of the September 11, 2001, attacks on the World Trade Center (WTC) is the fact that a very similar attack, with similar motivation and related perpetrators, occurred eight years earlier. On February 16, 1993, a truck bomb in the basement parking garage of the WTC killed six, injured hundreds, and damaged property to the extent of half a billion dollars. The bomb was designed to topple one of the towers into the other and to bring both towers down. The man behind this plan, Ramzi Yousef, noted regretfully that if he had had a little more funding his design would have succeeded and killed tens of thousands (Kirk, 2002). The U.S. response to this attack was police work and prosecution. After trials and convictions, six Arab men are in U.S. prisons, and a seventh person is still being sought.

On September 11, 2001, a second attack on the World Trade Center brought down the Twin Towers and caused nearly 3,000 deaths. The 9/11 perpetrators were similar in origins and motivation to the 1993 perpetrators; indeed one of the planners of the 9/11 attacks, Khalid Shaikh Mohammed, is Ramzi Yousef's uncle. Despite the similarity of the attacks, the U.S. response was strikingly different. Rather than criminal justice proceedings, the U.S. response was a war on terrorism. "On September the 11th, enemies of freedom committed an act of war against our country. . . . Our war on terror begins with al Qaeda, but it does not end there. It will not end until every terrorist group of global reach has been found, stopped and defeated" (Bush, 2001).

Within the rhetoric of war, however, there has been frequent recourse to the rhetoric of criminal justice. "Whether we bring our enemies to justice or justice to our enemies, justice will be done. . . . We will come together to give law enforcement the additional tools it needs to track down terror here at home" (Bush, 2001; White House Press Office, 2003).

The rhetoric of justice and the rhetoric of war may appear complementary, as in the often-debated qualifications of "just war." But closer inspection indicates that these two kinds of rhetoric instantiate two very different frames for understanding the nature of the terrorist threat and the appropriate response to it. In this chapter I explore the inconsistent and even contradictory implications of these frames, and I suggest that more emphasis on the criminal justice frame offers some important advantages for what all of us agree will be an extended U.S. effort to secure itself from terrorist attacks.

Framing and Human Judgment

The power of framing effects has been demonstrated in two decades of research in psychology and economics. Perhaps the most famous demonstration is Tversky and Kahneman's (1981) "Asian disease problem." Several hundred people were randomly divided into two groups, so that the two groups would on average be very similar. Each group was given a different problem.

> **Problem 1.** Imagine that the United States is preparing for an outbreak of an unusual Asian disease, which is expected to kill 600 people. Two alternative programs to combat the disease have been proposed. Assume that the exact scientific estimates of the consequences of the programs are as follows:
> **Program A:** If Program A is adopted, 200 people will be saved.
> **Program B:** If Program B is adopted, there is a one-third probability that 600 people will be saved and a two-thirds probability that no one will be saved.
> *Which of the two programs would you favor?*

Tversky and Kahneman (1981) found that 72% of the group reading Problem 1 favored Program A. The prospect of saving 200 lives with certainty was more attractive than the probability of a one-in-three chance of saving 600 lives.

> **Problem 2.** The second group read the same story of the threat of Asian disease but with different program options.
> **Program C:** If Program C is adopted, 400 people will die.
> **Program D:** If Program D is adopted, there is a one-third probability that nobody will die and a two-thirds probability that 600 people will die.
> *Which of the two programs would you favor?*

Surprisingly, 78% of the group reading Problem 2 favored Program D. The prospect of 400 people lost for certain was worse than the probability of a two-in-three chance of losing 600. The surprise value of the difference in the results for the two problems is that they offer exactly the same alternatives, except that Problem 1 is framed as gain (people will be saved) and Problem 2 is framed as loss (people will die). The results indicate that the participants in this study preferred certainty to risk when comparing gains but preferred risk to certainty when comparing losses.

These results opened a gold rush of studies to learn more about when and how different frames can affect human judgment in ways that are, statistically at least, mysterious or even irrational (Shafir & Le Boeuf, 2002). One indication of the significance of this research is that Kahneman's work on framing effects was cited in the award of his Nobel Prize in economics in 2002. The demonstrated power of framing effects is the foundation for the argument of this chapter, namely, that war and justice may have importantly different implications for how the United States responds to terrorist threats.

A Framing Analysis of the Difference Between 1993 and 2001

One way to think about the results of the Asian disease problem is that most people prefer a sure gain to a chance of larger gain ("risk averse for gain") but prefer a chance of losing nothing to a certainty of losing something ("risk seeking for loss"). This understanding can be applied to the problem of terrorism if we assume that, after 9/11, terrorism was expected to kill 600 American civilians the following year. As with most applications of formal models, this analysis excludes many complications, including the loss of lives—both foreign civilians and U.S. military—associated with the war on terrorism. In defense of this exclusion, it might be argued that U.S. leaders and U.S. citizens do not weigh these lives as heavily as civilian deaths in the United States.

If we translate 600 lives threatened by Asian disease into 600 lives threatened by terrorism, the effect of framing as gain versus framing as loss will be as follows. Two antiterrorism programs are available: criminal justice and war. Presented in terms of saving lives, criminal justice promises for certain to save 200 lives from terrorism, whereas war has a chance of saving all 600 lives. Presented in terms of lives lost, criminal justice gives up 400 lives for certain, whereas war offers a chance of losing no lives to terrorism. If we focus on saving lives and if we are risk averse for gains, we will prefer criminal justice to war as the response to terrorism. However, if we focus on lives lost and if we are risk seeking for loss, we will prefer war to criminal justice.

One might argue about how the probabilities should change as we move from the Asian disease threat to the terrorist threat, but the point survives that framing the response to terrorism in terms of saving lives is likely to favor criminal justice, whereas framing it in terms of lives lost is likely to favor war. It is not difficult to see how, immediately after 9/11, with 3,000 deaths fresh and personalized in the televised suffering of relatives and friends of the dead, the predominant framing was in terms of lives already lost and lives to be lost in future terrorist attacks. This framing in turn favored war as the response to the 9/11 attacks.

In contrast, the six deaths caused by the 1993 attack on the WTC did not rise out of the everyday death toll of car accidents and homicides. As attention to the 1993 deaths was small, the framing of the response to terrorism was less about lives lost and more about saving lives by bringing the terrorists to justice.

Thus research on framing can help explain why criminal justice was the predominant frame for the U.S. response to the terrorist attack on the WTC in 1993, but war was the predominant frame for the response to a 9/11 terrorist attack similar to the one in 1993 in all but the death toll. Nevertheless, the rhetoric of bringing enemies to justice remains available in public discourse in the United States, mixed with and sometimes submerged in the rhetoric of the war on terrorism (Bush, 2005), and it is useful to draw out the divergent implications of these two frames. Whereas Roth (2004) brought a human-rights framework to this comparison, I focus on the psychological implications of war and criminal justice in response to terrorism.

Justice Versus War: In the Beginning

The beginning of a criminal justice response to terrorism is the specification of a violation of the criminal code. Charges are brought against defendants, if necessary against criminals unknown until investigation uncovers the identity of the perpetrators. Once identified, the criminal defendants are brought to trial, and a jury determines their guilt or innocence.

In the case of the 1993 attack on the WTC, four suspects were apprehended within a month of the blast. They went on trial in a federal court on September 13, 1993. The trial lasted 6 months, with the presentation of 204 witnesses and more than 1,000 pieces of evidence. On March 4, 1994, the jury convicted the four defendants— Mohammed Salameh, Nidal Ayyad, Mahmud Abouhalima, and Ahmad Ajaj—on all 38 counts against them. On May 25, 1994, a judge sentenced each defendant to 240 years in prison and a $250,000 fine.

On February 7, 1995, authorities in Pakistan arrested Ramzi Yousef, who was then extradited to the United States. On November 12, 1997, Yousef was found guilty of masterminding the 1993 bombing, and on January 8, 1998, he was sentenced to life in prison without parole. In a related case, Sheikh Omar Abdul Rahman, a blind cleric who preached at mosques in Brooklyn and Jersey City, was sentenced to life imprisonment on October 1, 1995, for conspiracy to bomb New York City landmarks (not specifically for the 1993 WTC bombing, however).

In contrast, the beginning of a war is typically a declaration from one government to another that a state of war exists between them. The casus belli does not usually require investigation or discovery; an attack or ultimatum is typically the clear occasion of war. In the case of al-Qaeda, the declaration of war against the United States is usually identified with a May 26, 1998, news conference in which Osama bin Laden appeared with the two sons of Sheik Omar Abdul Rahman, the spiritual leader of those convicted of the 1993 attack on the World Trade Center. Within 11 weeks of the declaration, al-Qaeda attacked U.S. embassies in Kenya and Tanzania with bombs that killed 224 people, including 12 Americans.

The U.S. response was not a declaration of war against al-Qaeda but a campaign to kill al-Qaeda members and to destroy their bases, notably by cruise missile attacks on al-Qaeda bases in Afghanistan. It was only after the 9/11 attacks that Pres. George W. Bush declared war on terrorism, not just on al-Qaeda but on all terrorists with international reach. The logic of the extension was that any terrorist group with international reach was an ally or a potential ally of al-Qaeda.

The expansive definition of enemies in the war on terrorism points to a notable difference between war and criminal justice. The beginning of a criminal justice response to war is precise and limited in requiring the specification of criminal code violations and of particular individuals accused of these violations. Even conspiracy charges have to be substantiated by evidence of some material link between the conspirator and a criminal act, planned or accomplished. In contrast, a declaration of war designates a group enemy—typically a nation—and often more than one nation joins the list of enemies as alliances come into play. The war on terrorism is larger than a war on al-Qaeda, and the expansion of enemies is typical after a declaration of war.

In sum, those who were sought for the 1993 WTC attack were individuals; those who were sought for the 2001 WTC attack were an ill-defined group of Arabs and Muslims—al-Qaeda—and terrorist groups everywhere.

Criminals Versus Combatants

This difference in specificity leads immediately to another difference: the labeling of the enemy. The targets of criminal justice are criminals, that is, lawbreakers, norm breakers, individuals who are not generally seen as typical of the group they come from. The United States has criminal gangs, including those that are predominantly Italian, predominantly Colombian, predominantly Russian, and predominantly Chinese. It is true that some prejudicial association between such gangs and their larger ethnic group is often made in public images and occasionally found even in political discourse, but in general the association is weak. Americans do not generally feel hostility toward or discriminate against Italians because there is a Cosa Nostra.

In contrast, war is typically declared on a state that is seen to represent a people or a nation. The last war formally voted by the U.S. Congress was against Germany and Japan. When it is not easy to specify a nation-representing state, even violence that looks like war does not get a formal declaration of war. The U.S. military presence in Korea was formally a "police action" under UN auspices, the Vietnam War was properly the "Vietnam Conflict" insofar as the U.S. Congress never declared war, and the U.S. intervention in Panama in 1989 was to safeguard 35,000 American citizens there from a drug-trafficking tyrant, Gen. Manuel Noriega. The war-making power of the U.S. president as commander in chief no longer requires a formal declaration of war from the U.S. Congress. Never-

theless, the rhetoric of war calls on the ideal case in which the enemy is a state and its people.

When enemy combatants represent a national or ethnic group, that whole group is seen as the enemy or at least as having a tendency and potential to serve the enemy. After the United States declared war on Japan, Japanese civilians could be rounded up without trial and put in detention camps for years. Similar if lesser actions were taken against Italian Americans after the United States declared war on Italy in World War II. In England, World War I made it expedient for the royal family to give up its identity as the House of Hanover to become the House of Windsor.

There is a parallel in the war on terrorism. After identification of the 9/11 attackers as Muslim Arabs, a wave of hostility and even occasional violence was visited on many in the United States who were identified (in some cases incorrectly—Sikhs, for instance) as Arab or Muslim (Arab American Institute, 2002; Kaplan, 2006). This hostility contributed to the war on terrorism insofar as it helped support the roundup and imprisonment, without charges, hearing, or habeas corpus, of nearly a thousand Arab and Muslim noncitizens living in the United States (Parker & Fellner, 2004). In another way, however, this group-level attribution of suspicion and responsibility was counterproductive: It hindered U.S. security forces seeking information and assistance against terrorists from Arab and Muslim citizens of the United States.

Thus the difference between criminal and combatant is clear in this respect: Criminals are atypical and soldiers are representative. Criminals act in their own interest; soldiers act for their nation. It is an irony of the war on terrorism that war implies combatant status for the terrorists and responsibility for terrorist acts to those the terrorists claim to represent. Understood as criminals, terrorists represent only themselves, and those they claim to represent can be asked to help apprehend them.

Small Versus Large Enemy

Along with the difference between criminal and combatant comes an implication about the size of the enemy. In war, an enemy state usually represents millions of citizens and commands significant armed forces. Thus a declaration of war is a declaration against a very large enemy. The argument for war against terrorism is that even a small number of terrorists can use modern technology (fully fueled aircraft in the case of the 9/11 attacks) to inflict horrendous damage. Without denying this argument, it is important to note that the war on terrorism can give an exaggerated impression of the size of the terrorist enemy.

Even if we think of al-Qaeda as more a franchise than a state or corporation, it probably does not amount to more than 5,000 people worldwide. Perhaps 18,000 went through the al-Qaeda training camps in Afghanistan before these were destroyed, and perhaps one-quarter of these are still alive, connected, and committed to violence (Robb, 2004). A network of 5,000 would be large for a criminal conspiracy (such as the Cosa Nostra in the United States perhaps), but tiny by the standards of wartime enemies. Declaring war on terrorism conduces to seeing terrorism as larger than it actually is. This bias plays well for the terrorists, raising their self-esteem and their status among those who sympathize with the cause they claim to advance.

Competing Priorities Versus Survival

A declaration of war is a declaration of mortal threat, an announcement of the utmost danger that calls for the utmost sacrifice. A criminal justice procedure is business as usual. Violent criminals are indeed a threat to society but not one that calls for national mobilization. One implication of declaring war on terrorism is that the threat to the United States is a danger to national interest that can go as far as endangering the survival of the nation.

This difference is important because engaging a mortal threat brings a massive shift in priorities. A declaration of war implies that, until it is won, the war has top priority. All other values and priorities are put on the back burner until the war is over. The public agenda is fighting the war, and any cost is acceptable in the context of asking young people to pay the ultimate price. The war gets first and unlimited call on resources of money, time, and talent; political preferences are formed around policies and personalities in terms of their perceived value for prosecuting the war. The predictable result of external threat is an increase in

patriotism that is experienced as the exhilarating warmth of unity, common values, common purpose, and common sacrifice (LeVine & Campbell, 1972, pp. 31–32).

In contrast, the criminal justice system has to compete with many other public interests and priorities. Even if the public perceives that crime is a major and escalating problem, criminal justice does not automatically take first place in the allocation of public resources. Political leaders often compete on the basis of what they promise to do about crime and criminals and what resources the criminal justice system should have. However, they seldom claim, at least in the United States, that crime is the only problem. It is almost always linked to problems of education, jobs, housing, and welfare policy, and these issues compete with the criminal justice system for resources in responding to crime.

It is difficult in a democracy to maintain a state of war indefinitely. Other priorities begin to reassert themselves; the mobilizing advantage of war sooner or later begins to fade. This has been the fate, in the United States, of the "war on poverty" and the "war on drugs." Thus the war on terrorism is ill adapted to a long-term strategy against terrorism. Unfortunately, there is every reason to believe that terrorism is a long-term problem. It is not a group or a cause but a strategy, one that has been around for millennia (e.g., the Jewish sicarii of the first century AD). No one is predicting how long the war on terrorism will take, only that it will last as long as it takes.

Police Work Versus Combat: Expertise

War on terrorism asserts a military response to terrorism. This has implications with regard to the expertise deployed. Military forces are trained to fight an enemy military: Find them, fix them, destroy them. From the evidence of Napoleon's campaigns, von Clausewitz developed his famous treatise, *On War:* "To sum up: of all the possible aims in war, the destruction of the enemy's armed forces always appears as the highest" (von Clausewitz, 1989, p. 99). This perspective encouraged a clear distinction between combatants, men in uniform, and noncombatant civilians—a distinction that has been eroding since the French Revolution (McCauley, 2005).

Here the focus is on military expertise. Modern armed forces are composed of highly specialized components with a ratio of tail to tooth that is perhaps ten to one, that is, ten people in logistics and coordination for each one at risk in combat. Land, sea, and air forces depend on complex information systems to focus intricate and powerful weapon systems against the enemy. These systems are essential in fighting another modern army but relatively ill suited for fighting terrorists who emerge from and disappear back into civilian populations. The difficulties of even the best-trained army in fighting terrorism and insurgency are evident in the U.S. experience in Afghanistan and Iraq. In both places, overwhelming military power has not yet been able to find and destroy the enemy.

Fighting terrorism effectively is more like police work than military combat. Effective police work requires understanding a local culture, knowing the details of social and physical geography in a local area, developing local relationships, and cultivating local sources of information. This kind of expertise is very different from integrated arms and large-scale logistics. It is no disgrace to a modern army to recognize that it is ill prepared for police work or the kind of economic and community development work that can support effective police work. At a minimum, effective police work requires speaking the local language, but learning foreign languages is not typically a high priority in military training.

Beyond the local level, the story is similar. International cooperation is crucial for fighting international terrorists. Putting together patterns of individual behavior and networks of contacts requires sharing intelligence across borders—something at least as difficult as sharing between the FBI and the CIA within the United States. International police cooperation is a better model of this kind of sharing than international military cooperation; police and security services are more likely than the military to have useful information about individual terrorists and terrorist groups.

It is worth noting briefly that, along with the difference in expertise of those fighting crime and those fighting war, there is also a difference in the expertise of those studying crime and those studying war. Researchers who focus on crime are generally based in sociology and criminology, whereas researchers who study war are more often from political science and psychology. In particular,

the criminal justice framing of response to terrorism points to untapped potential in understanding terrorism with data and theory from criminology (LaFree & Dugan, 2004).

Police Work Versus Combat: Values

Procedurally, the criminal justice system has to deal explicitly with the values of privacy and civil rights. Police and district attorneys can always imagine how their work would be forwarded and public safety improved by changes in procedure or law that would give them greater access to citizens' financial, health, telephone, and travel records or greater leeway in interrogation and use of the results of interrogations. Defense attorneys can always imagine how clients' rights can be enlarged or protected against the procedures sought by police and district attorneys. Judges are required to imagine both sides. Perhaps the most important aspect of the criminal justice system is that it brings people from the same training—law school—to an institutionalized competition of public interest in security with private interest in individual rights. Indeed, many lawyers have the opportunity to work both sides of this competition during their professional careers—as prosecuting attorney at one time and as defense attorney at another time.

In contrast, the military has no professional experience of balancing competing values. The military hierarchy is consistent and unidimensional. Winning is the only value. MacArthur's *Message From the Far East,* memorized by every West Point cadet, is paradigmatic: "From the Far East I send you one single thought, one sole idea—written in red on every beachhead from Australia to Tokyo—There is no substitute for victory!" In the U.S. military, it is a kind of cross-cultural experience to work with another branch of the armed services: army officers working with air force or navy officers, for instance. There is no parallel to the competition of perspectives that exists for attorneys; there is no career path for officers to serve first in fighting U.S. enemies and then to serve the enemy fighting the United States.

The criminal case against the perpetrators of the 1993 WTC bombing brought prosecuting and defense attorneys to a contest in which both sides came from the same professional preparation, and the contest included a negotiation of individual rights versus the public's right to security. The war against terrorism has no such balancing act; the officers who plan and command and the soldiers who follow are little practiced in representing the perspective or rights of the enemy. This, in brief, is the story of the violations of human rights of prisoners at Abu Ghraib and likely of prisoners at Guantanamo as well. Police are required to practice every day the rights of suspects; soldiers are not similarly practiced in the rights of prisoners.

Nor are soldiers drilled in the rights of non-combatants. The distancing phrase for civilian casualties of military campaigns is "collateral damage." The U.S. military in Afghanistan was, by modern standards, unusually successful in avoiding civilian casualties. Yet approximately 3,000 civilians were killed in the U.S. campaign that defeated and dispersed the Taliban and its al-Qaeda allies in Afghanistan (Herald, 2002). It is not only fire power that kills civilians. Increased mortality associated with the U.S.-led embargo of Iraq between 1990 and 1998 is estimated to have included at least 100,000 deaths among Iraqi children under 5 years of age (Garfield, 1999). Modern war would be impossible if killing noncombatants were strictly proscribed and prosecuted.

In short, war brings a unidimensional scale of value in which nothing can compete with the value of winning, whereas criminal justice brings an institutionalized and well-practiced competition of values. In time of war, talk about money cost or opportunity cost or human-rights cost is unpatriotic; in the criminal justice system, these costs can be counted in the balance of competing values and priorities.

Judicial Error Versus Collateral Damage

Terrorism is the warfare of the weak, the strategy of those who cannot win by conventional means and who see their cause as sinking toward extinction (McCauley, 2002). Terrorists have many goals: publicity for their cause, a recovered sense of power and agency against the power that is crushing them, and revenge and justice against those who have done terrible things to their friends and their cause. Less commonly recognized is the terrorist goal that is essential for the survival of a terrorist group: mobilization of sympathizers to increased support

and increased action for the cause the terrorists claim to represent. A terrorist group is only the apex of a pyramid in which the base is all who agree with the terrorist aims even if they do not agree with the attacks on civilians that are the hallmark of terrorism (McCauley, 2002). For the Irish Republican Army, for instance, the base of the pyramid has been all those who agree with "Brits out." Ascending in the pyramid, numbers decrease but commitment, risk taking, and support for killing civilians increase.

The terrorists cannot survive without the cover, information, money, and new recruits that come from the pyramid. Anything that cuts off the terrorists from the pyramid is a mortal threat; anything that increases mobilization of the base of the pyramid behind terrorist leadership is a success. Here is where the strategy of jujitsu politics enters the contest between terrorists and the state. The best scholars (Crenshaw, 2002) and the most thoughtful terrorists (Marighella, 1970) recognize that a crucial terrorist goal is to provoke a state response that will mobilize the uncommitted among those who sympathize with the terrorists' goals. As jujitsu is the art of using the opponent's strength against him, so jujitsu politics is the art of provoking the enemy to a response that will mobilize support against them.

For terrorists, the promise of a military response is that military values do not give much attention to collateral damage. In *Bombing to Win*, Robert Pape (1996) reviews twentieth-century military thinking about using aerial bombing to destroy the morale of enemy civilians. Sometimes this thinking goes as far as explicitly aiming for the mass killing of civilians; sometimes it goes only so far as recognizing the impossibility of avoiding killing them. Such thinking has not disappeared, as mentioned earlier in relation to the civilian casualties in Afghanistan. Such casualties continue as the U.S. occupation of Afghanistan continues. Similarly, the U.S. occupation of and war on terrorism in Iraq cannot avoid civilian casualties. The increase in hostility toward the United States in polls in Islamic countries provides the foundation for increased support and more recruits for al-Qaeda.

In contrast, the criminal justice response to the 1993 bombing brought five of six indicted perpetrators to trial but provided no warrant for punishing their friends and neighbors. The criminal justice system also makes mistakes, but these are more likely to lead to imprisoning the wrong people than to killing the wrong people. A criminal justice response to terrorism offers terrorists a much smaller opening for jujitsu politics.

Justice Versus War: In the End

As war has an official and explicit beginning, so it should have an official and explicit end. There is unconditional surrender (World War II) or negotiated surrender (World War I) or at least a truce agreement to mark the end of war. Even wars that are described as police actions or humanitarian interventions have an end. The Korean War stalemate ended in a truce, and the Vietnam War ended with a peace treaty, the withdrawal of U.S. troops, and the fig leaf of an international control commission to ensure the peace. It is worth noting that the Vietnam War was the longest the United States has fought, enduring from 1964 to 1973.

In contrast, the criminal justice system faces a problem without end. No one expects that crime will be exhausted or beaten or that it will surrender. No one expects that crime will sign a peace treaty or even a truce. There has never been a society without rules or one without sanctions for violation of those rules. What it lacks in mobilizing power the criminal justice system makes up in staying power. Police, prosecuting attorneys, defense attorneys, judges, and prisons together constitute a criminal justice system that is expected to go on indefinitely into the future, along with the criminal acts that they respond to.

The criminal justice response to the 1993 attack on the WTC continues today. One of the suspects, Abdul Rahman Yasin, was interviewed shortly after the bombing, provided useful information, was released, took flight to Iraq, and has not been seen since. He is still a wanted man, as the criminal justice response to the 1993 attack grinds on. The war on terrorism that began after 9/11 also continues. It remains to be seen how long this war can be maintained before competing interests and values undermine its vigor.

Conclusion

It is time to summarize the implications of war and justice with a view toward evaluating the relative strengths and weaknesses of these two frames for the U.S. response to a continuing terrorist threat.

War has a clear beginning and a clear and not-too-distant end; criminal justice is a never-ending effort to control and ameliorate a problem that will not go away. War targets a unified enemy group—a people or a nation; criminal justice targets individual perpetrators of criminal acts. War recognizes the enemy as large and dangerous; criminal justice makes the enemy small and tawdry. War puts every other public interest and value on the back burner; criminal justice has to compete for resources year after year in the national scale of priorities. War puts the military in charge of response; criminal justice puts lawyers and police in charge.

The differences between legal and military subcultures bring other important differences. Military professionals are focused on winning as the single scale of value; police, prosecutors, defense attorneys, and judges are experienced in balancing the public's right to security against individual and civil rights. Military mistakes often get people killed, including enemy civilians; criminal justice mistakes put the wrong people behind bars but seldom put innocents into coffins. Military mistakes mobilize terrorist sympathizers behind terrorist leadership; criminal justice mistakes are smaller and can be redressed with retrial and compensation. The collateral damages from military strikes and military occupation of foreign lands are a rich contribution to jujitsu politics; criminal justice operations and mistakes offer less opportunity for advancing the terrorist cause.

Despite its limitations, war offers unique advantages over criminal justice as a response to terrorism. War produces the warmth and direction of national unity behind national leaders. War brings resources against terrorism that are difficult to justify or funnel through the criminal justice system. War brings at least the perception that everything possible is being done to prevent future terrorist attacks. In general, war has the status of a heroic response to a mortal threat; criminal justice is government business as usual. War can reach directly and quickly to foreign bases and foreign support for terrorism that cannot be reached—or only slowly reached—with the forces of criminal justice.

Unfortunately, no one today predicts that the war on terrorism will end anytime soon. The command and control capacity of al-Qaeda has been degraded as the leadership has been killed, captured, or driven into deep hiding places. The current and continuing dangers of terrorist attack are more a matter of local franchise operations in a corporation that has lost its headquarters. Under these conditions, some of the advantages of the war on terrorism have begun to fade. The attention and priority given to the war on terrorism cannot last indefinitely, military occupations in foreign lands cannot be maintained indefinitely, blank checks of support to foreign governments for attacks on their own "terrorists" cannot be honored indefinitely, and the government's reach into the lives of U.S. citizens cannot deepen indefinitely. In sum, war is not an effective response to a chronic problem.

This is a lesson that the United States has had multiple opportunities to learn. Previous efforts to harness the rhetoric and unity of war against chronic problems have been notably unsuccessful. The U.S. war on poverty never came to victory or even truce, and the gap between rich and poor may even be growing. The U.S. war on drugs went so far in military stylistics as to appoint a commander in chief or czar, but drug trafficking and drug abuse are not vanquished and perhaps not even weakened.

Against a chronic threat of terrorist attack, the U.S. response might usefully give increased salience to the criminal justice frame. Criminal justice does not glorify the terrorists and their cause. Criminal justice does not stereotype an ethnic or religious group as the enemy and avoids losing the cooperation of the communities the terrorists claim to represent. Criminal justice does not undermine the balance of public security and civil rights in the United States and thus preserves a civil society worth defending from terrorism (Hirshon, 2002). Perhaps most important, criminal justice does not lead to the collateral damages and foreign occupations that are the lifeblood of terrorist mobilization against the United States.

Some movement in this direction may be visible. In Germany, Mounir el Motassadeq was convicted in 2003 of involvement in the 9/11 plot, but his verdict was overturned when an appeals court ruled that his trial was unfair because the United States refused to produce testimony from terrorism suspects in U.S. custody. In August 2005, el Motassadeq was sentenced to seven years in prison as a member of a terrorist organization. And in Spain, twenty-four Muslim men suspected of being members of Al Qaeda went on trial in April 2005, three of them accused of providing support for the 9/11 attacks. Prison terms were handed down in September 2005, though charges related to 9/11 were not sustained. Zacarias Moussaoui, the only person facing trial in the United States in connection with the 9/11 attacks, pleaded guilty to participating in an al-Qaeda conspiracy. The penalty phase of his trial is going on as this chapter goes to press in March 2006.

It appears, then, that the criminal justice systems of Western countries are capable of engaging al-Qaeda's terrorists. Criminal justice may be slower than the war on terrorism, but it may be surer in reaching terrorist perpetrators.

For many, however, the crucial argument against a criminal justice response to terrorism is that criminal justice failed miserably on 9/11. Premise: Bringing the 1993 perpetrators to trial, conviction, and incarceration did not save the United States from the attacks of 9/11. Conclusion: The war on terrorism is the stronger medicine required. The answer to this argument is straightforward. Criminal justice has not failed when crime is not eliminated; it fails only when crimes are not solved and criminals are not put away. No one argues that the war on terrorism has failed because terrorist alerts continue. To a modern democratic state, terrorist threat is not a mortal peril, not like a severe acute respiratory syndrome (SARS) epidemic but more like a recurring flu. Criminal justice can be the treatment of choice for a chronic terrorist threat.

Acknowledgments.   I thank Gary LaFree for his careful reading of this chapter and suggestions for improving it. I am grateful also for research opportunities provided by Bryn Mawr College and the Solomon Asch Center for Study of Ethnopolitical Conflict at the University of Pennsylvania. Preparation of this chapter was supported by the United States Department of Homeland Security through the National Consortium for the Study of Terrorism and Responses to Terrorism (START), grant number N00140510629. However, the opinions expressed in this chapter are those of the author and do not necessarily reflect views of the U.S. Department of Homeland Security.

References

Arab American Institute. (2002). Healing the nation: The Arab American experience after September 11: A first anniversary report by the Arab American Institute. Retrieved September 15, 2004, from http://www.aaiusa.org/PDF/healing_the_nation.pdf

Bush, G. W. (2001). Address to a joint session of the American Congress and the American people. Retrieved September 15, 2004, from http://www.whitehouse.gov/news/releases/2001/09/20010920–8.html

———. (2005). President thanks U.S. troops at Wiesbaden Army Airfield Base. Retrieved April 2, 2005, from http://www.whitehouse.gov/news/releases/2005/02/20050223–8.html

Crenshaw, M. (2002). The causes of terrorism. In C. Besteman (Ed.), *Violence: A reader* (pp. 99–118). New York: New York University Press.

Garfield, R. (1999, July). Morbidity and mortality among Iraqi children from 1990 through 1998: Assessing the impact of the Gulf War and economic sanctions. Retrieved September 15, 2004, from http://www.casi.org.uk/info/garfield/dr-garfield.html

Herald, M. W. (2002). A dossier on civilian victims of United States' aerial bombing of Afghanistan: A comprehensive accounting [revised]. Retrieved September 15, 2004, from http://www.cursor.org/stories/civilian_deaths.htm

Hirshon, R. E. (2002, February 15). Military tribunals *Wall Street Journal* letter to the editor. Retrieved April 20, 2005, from http://www.abanet.org/leadership/wallstreet_letter.htm

Kaplan, J. (2006). Islamophobia in America?: September 11 and Islamophobic hate crime. *Terrorism and Political Violence, 18,* 1–33.

Kirk, M. (2002, October 3). The man who knew. Transcript of Public Broadcasting System *Frontline* program #2103. Retrieved September 15, 2004, from http://www.pbs.org/wgbh/pages/frontline/shows/knew/etc/script.html

LaFree, G., & Dugan, L. (2004). How does studying terrorism compare to studying crime? In M. Deflem (Ed.), *Terrorism and counter-terrorism: Criminological perspectives* (pp. 53–75). Oxford, UK: Elsevier Science.

LeVine, R. A., & Campbell, D. T. (1972). *Ethnocentrism: Theories of conflict, ethnic attitudes, and group behavior.* New York: Wiley.

Marighella, C. (1970). Minimanual of the urban guerrilla. In C. Marighella, *For the liberation of Brazil* (pp. 61–97; J. Butt & R. Sheed, Trans.). Havana: Tricontinental.

McCauley, C. (2002). Psychological issues in understanding terrorism and the response to terrorism. In C. Stout (Ed.), *The psychology of terrorism: Vol. 3. Theoretical understandings and perspectives* (pp. 3–30). Westport, CT: Praeger.

———. (2005). Terrorism and the state: The logic of killing civilians. In James J. F. Forest (Ed.), *The making of a terrorist: Recruitment, training and root causes, Volume three root causes* (pp. 238–253). Westport, CN: Praeger Security International.

Pape, R. A. (1996). *Bombing to win: Air power and coercion in war.* Ithaca, NY: Cornell University Press.

Parker, A., & Fellner, J. (2004). Above the law: Executive power after 9/11 in the United States. Retrieved September 15, 2004, from the Human Rights Watch website: http://hrw.org/wr2k4/8.htm

Robb, J. (2004, May). Journal: An estimate of al-Qaeda's current strength. Retrieved September 15, 2004, from http://globalguerrillas.typepad.com/globalguerrillas/2004/05/journal_an_esti.html

Roth, K. (2004, January–February). The law of war in the war on terror. *Foreign Affairs, 83,* 2–7.

Shafir, E., and Le Boeuf, R. A. (2002). Rationality. *Annual Review of Psychology, 53,* 491–517.

Tversky, A., & Kahneman, D. (1981, January). The framing of decisions and the psychology of choice. *Science, 211*(30), 453–458.

von Clausewitz, C. (1989). *On war* (M. Howard & P. Paret, Eds. and Trans.). Princeton, NJ: Princeton University Press.

White House Press Office. (2003, May 16). President Bush vows to bring terrorists to justice: Remarks by the president upon departure for Camp David, the South Lawn. Retrieved September 15, 2004, from http://www.whitehouse.gov/news/releases/2003/05/20030516–15.html

Terrorism

II

Terrorism

5

The Staircase to Terrorism

A Psychological Exploration

Fathali M. Moghaddam

Despite notorious disagreements about the definition of terrorism (Cooper, 2001) and claims that "one person's terrorist is another person's freedom fighter," there is general agreement that terrorism has become a monstrous problem in many parts of the world and that every effort must be made to end it. For the purposes of this discussion, terrorism is defined as *politically motivated violence that is perpetrated by individuals, groups, or state-sponsored agents and intended to bring about feelings of terror and helplessness in a population in order to influence decision making and to change behavior.* Terrorism is depicted in this discussion as a problem, especially because many major international terrorist groups work to weaken rather than to strengthen democracy and because terrorism distracts people and resources from paths blazed by growing grassroots pro-peace, pro-democracy movements in different parts of the world. Contemporary terrorism is particularly dangerous because terrorists might gain access to weapons of mass destruction (Gurr & Cole, 2002). Terrorism is often strongly influenced by ideology, but it can also be carried out for material gain (to benefit one's family, for example).

Psychologists have a vitally important responsibility in combating terrorism because, first, the actions of terrorists are intended to bring about

specific psychological experiences—terror and helplessness (Moghaddam & Marsella, 2004); second, terrorism often has harmful psychological consequences (Danieli, Engdahl, & Schlenger, 2004; Wessells, 2004); and third, subjectively interpreted values and beliefs often serve as the most important basis for terrorist action (Bernholz, 2004). Psychologists are contributing in important ways to a better understanding of terrorism, as well as more effective coping with its individual and communal health consequences (Crenshaw, 2000; Danieli, Brom, & Waizer, in press; Galea, Ahern, Resnick, Kilpatrick, Bucuvalas, et al., 2002; Horgan & Taylor, 2003; Moghaddam & Marsella, 2004; North, Nixon, Shariat, Mallonee, McMillen, et al., 1999; North, Tivis, McMillen, Pfefferbaum, Spitznagel, et al., 2002; North & Pfefferbaum, 2002; Pyszczynski, Solomon, & Greenberg, 2003; Robbins, 2002; Schlenger, Caddell, Ebert, Jordan, Rourke, et al., 2002; Schuster, Stein, Jaycox, Collins, Marshall, et al., 2001; Silke, 2003; Silver, Holman, McIntosh, Poulin, Gil-Rivas, 2002; Stephenson, 2001; Stout, 2002). However, there is an urgent need for greater attention to the social and psychological processes that lead to terrorist acts.

A better understanding of terrorism is essential for the development of more effective policies to combat this global problem. Critical assessments of the available evidence suggest that there is little validity in explanations of terrorism that assume a high level of psychopathology among terrorists (Ruby, 2002) or that terrorists come from economically deprived backgrounds or have little education (Atran, 2003). Clearly, explanations intended to reduce the causes of terrorism to dispositional, intrapersonal factors are too simplistic, despite the serious efforts made to profile terrorists (e.g., Fields, Elbedour, & Hein, 2002), as are explanations that are founded only on the material conditions in which terrorism takes place, despite attempts to identify demographic and socioeconomic factors associated with terrorism (e.g., Ehrlich & Liu, 2002). The present discussion is intended as a modest contribution toward a more dynamic, comprehensive account of the social and psychological processes leading to terrorism. A central proposition is that terrorism can best be understood through a focus on the *psychological interpretation* of material conditions and the options *seen* to be available to overcome *perceived* injustices, particularly injustices in the procedures through which decisions are made (Tyler & Huo, 2002).

The Stairway to the Terrorist Act

Toward a more in-depth understanding of terrorism, it is useful to envisage a narrowing stairway leading to a terrorist act at the top of a building. The stairway leads to higher and higher floors, and whether people remain on a particular floor depends on the doors and spaces that they imagine open to them on that floor. The fundamentally important feature of the situation is not only the actual number of floors, stairs, rooms, and so on but more importantly, in some contexts, how people perceive the building and the doors they think are open to them. As people climb the stairway, they see fewer and fewer choices, until the only possible outcome is the destruction of others, or oneself, or both. This kind of "decision tree" conceptualization of behavior has proved to be a powerful tool in psychology. For example, Latané and Darley (1970) conceptualized helping behavior as the outcome of five choice points that lead an individual to either help or not help others in an emergency.

Two points need to be clarified at the outset about the staircase metaphor. First, the metaphor is intended to provide a general framework within which to organize current psychological knowledge and to help direct future research and policy; it is not intended as a formal model to be tested against alternatives. Metaphors have proven highly useful in psychological science (e.g., in conceptualizing intelligence; see Sternberg, 1990) and can play a constructive role in better understanding the roots of terrorism. Second, the staircase metaphor is intended to apply only to behavior encompassed by terrorism as defined earlier in this discussion; it is not intended to apply to other types of minority influence tactics.

Ground Floor: Psychological Interpretation of Material Conditions

A puzzle arises when the economic and educational backgrounds of terrorists are considered: Poverty and lack of education become problematic as explanations for terrorist acts. In the West Bank and Gaza, support for armed attacks against Israeli targets tends to be greater among Palestinians with more years of education (Krueger & Maleckova, 2002). A British army document discussing the Provisional Irish Republican Army (PIRA) in 1978, at a time when armed attacks by the PIRA had reached a peak, stated that "there is a stratum of intelligent, astute and experienced terrorists who provide the backbone of the organization. . . . Our evidence of the calibre of rank and file terrorists does not support the view that they are mindless hooligans drawn from the unemployed and unemployable" (in Coogan, 2002, p. 468). Similarly, poverty and lack of education were not found to be characteristic of captured terrorists associated with al-Qaeda in Southeast Asia (Singapore Ministry of Home Affairs, 2003) or of Osama bin Laden or the al-Qaeda members who perpetrated the tragedy of 9/11 (Bodansky, 2001). Clearly, absolute material conditions do not account for terrorism; otherwise, acts of terrorism would be committed more by the poorest people living in the poorest regions, and this is not the case.

Psychological research points to the fundamental importance of *perceived* deprivation. The seminal research of Stouffer and others on military personnel during World War II demonstrated that there is not necessarily an isomorphic relationship between material conditions and subjective experience: Members of the U.S. Army Air Corps expressed less satisfaction with military life compared to some other units, despite the higher rate of promotions in that branch of the military (Stouffer, Suchman, De Vinney, Star, & Williams, 1949). Similarly puzzling was the fact that African American soldiers stationed in the North often expressed less satisfaction than those stationed in the South. The concept of relative deprivation was introduced to explained such trends: The higher rate of promotions in the air corps raised expectations and created more dissatisfaction for those who were not promoted, and African Americans in the North had higher expectations about equal treatment. Half a century of psychological research underlines the importance of subjective perceptions of feelings of deprivation (Collins, 1996).

Particularly relevant to terrorism is Runciman's (1966) distinction between *egoistical* deprivation, in which individuals feel deprived because of their position within a group, and *fraternal* deprivation, which involves feelings of deprivation that arise because of the position of an individual's group in comparison with other groups. Research evidence suggests that fraternal deprivation is under certain conditions a better predictor of feelings of discontent among minorities than is egoistical deprivation (Dion, 1986; Guimond & Dubé-Simard, 1983), and in some cases such feelings translate to collective action (Martin, Brickman, & Murray, 1984). Gurr's (1970) theoretical formulation and subsequent research (e.g., Crosby, 1982) suggest that fraternal deprivation is more likely to arise when group members feel their path to a desired goal—one that their group deserves and others possess—has been blocked. For example, in the case of terrorism, especially important could be a *perceived* right to independence and the retention of indigenous cultures for a society, a perception that other societies have achieved this goal, and a feeling that, under present conditions, the path to this goal has been obstructed (by Americans, for example). Of course, such perceptions may be influenced by deep prejudices (Moghaddam, 1998, ch. 10).

The literature on collective mobilization also underlines the importance of subjective perceptions (Taylor & Moghaddam, 1994). From the French Revolution (Schama, 1989) to the Iranian Revolution (Arjomand, 1988) and other collective uprisings in modern times, it is perceived and relative injustices rather than absolute deprivation that coincide with collective nonnormative action (Miller, 2000). Perceptions of injustice may arise for a variety of reasons, including economic and political conditions and threats to personal or collective identity (Tajfel & Turner, 1986; Taylor, 2003). Perceived threat to identity is of central importance in the case of religious fundamentalists because of the unique ability of religion to serve identity needs (Seul, 1999) and the feeling that increasing globalization, secularization, and Westernization are undermining traditional non-Western ways of life. Identity threat is also of deep concern to broader segments of non-Western populations, particularly the youth, who often grapple with the "good copy problem" (Moghaddam & Solliday, 1991), the feeling that the very best they can achieve is to become a "good copy" of the Western model of women and men propagated by the international media—a "good copy" that can never become as good as the original.

Minority groups have different resources available for meeting the challenge of the good copy problem (for example, the development of alternative media and educational systems, political opposition groups, or cultural institutions that allow for the evolution of alternative identities). However, in most Islamic societies of the Near and Middle East, local dictators have shut down all of these possibilities, and the only remaining avenue for the development of alternative identities is the mosque. It is only in the mosque that alternative political and cultural voices, as well as religious ones, can find an outlet, and it is only in the mosque that the young can meet the challenge of the good copy problem.

Radical elements have also been attracted to the mosque, using the monopoly of the mosque to gain privileged access to the young. Not surprisingly, the source of the greatest number of terrorist attacks against the West are the two countries where the mosque has a monopoly and where national identity is most directly positioned as Islamic: Saudi Arabia, the home of Islam's holiest sites, and Pakistan, which gained independence from India in 1947 on the basis of its "Islamic character." Thus, in these societies particularly, the only institution available for voicing dissatisfaction and trying to overcome the good copy problem is the mosque.

At the "foundational" ground floor, then, what matters most is perceptions of fairness. Someone may be living in extremely poor, crowded conditions in Bombay and not feel unjustly treated despite the opulent living conditions of others in the city; however, another person may be living in relatively comfortable conditions in Riyadh but feel very unjustly treated. A number of those who feel unjustly treated become motivated to search further for options to address their grievances.

First Floor: Perceived Options to Fight Unfair Treatment

People climb to the first floor and try different doors in search of solutions to what they perceive as unjust treatment. Two psychological factors shape their behavior on the first floor in major ways: first, perceived possibilities for personal mobility to improve their situation (Taylor & Moghaddam, 1994) and, second, perceptions of procedural justice (Tyler, 1994).

A first key question is, are there doors that could be opened by talented persons motivated to make progress up the societal hierarchy? Plato (*The Republic*, book three, 415b–d) warned of the inevitable collapse of a society that does not allow for the rise of talented people to the top of the social hierarchy and correspondingly the downward mobility of those who lack talent but are the offspring of those in power. This idea received elaboration in elite theory (Pareto, 1935) and is central to modern psychological theories of intergroup relations (Taylor & Moghaddam, 1994). Evidence suggests that the survival of even apparently rigid hierarchical systems, such as the cast system of India, is aided by some level of social mobility, albeit informal (Scrinivas, 1968). A variety of research evidence suggests that when paths to individual mobility are seen to be open, there is far less tendency to attempt nonnormative actions (e.g., Tyler, 1990; Wright, Taylor, & Moghaddam, 1990).

This is probably because of a strong human tendency to want to believe that the world is just and that one's personal efforts will be rewarded fairly (Lerner, 1980). Research on equity theory endorses the view that people strive for justice and feel distressed when they experience injustice (see the classic work of Adams, 1965, and Walster, Walster & Berscheid, 1978, as well as more recent

formulations such as Brockner & Wiesenfeld, 1996). However, the equity tradition also underlines the vital role of psychological interpretations of justice and the need for policy makers to understand local cultural practices and ideas—"the native's point of view"—in justice. When local cultural interpretations lead to a view that the in-group is being treated fairly, there is greater likelihood of support for central authorities.

The availability of avenues for participating in decision making is a key factor in perceived justice and support for authorities (Tyler, 1994). Independent of the outcomes of judicial processes (distributive justice) and the explanations that authorities provide for their decisions and the considerations they show to the recipients of decisions (interactional justice), the research of Tyler (Tyler, 2001; Tyler & Huo, 2002) demonstrates that the major factor in perceived legitimacy and willingness to abide by government regulations is how fair people perceive the decision-making process to be (procedural justice). Although much of the research on procedural justice has been conducted in Western societies, there is solid evidence in support of basic universals in perceived rights and duties (Doise, 2002; Moghaddam & Riley, in press) and strong reasons to believe that procedural justice also plays a central role in many and perhaps all major non-Western societies.

A primary influence on procedural justice is participation in decision making (Tyler & Huo, 2002). Opportunities for voice and participation in decision making are lacking in many parts of the world, as evidenced by UN "human development" reports (e.g., "The spread of democratization appears to have stalled, with many countries failing to consolidate and deepen the first steps toward democracy and several slipping back into authoritarianism. Some 73 countries—with 42% of the world's people—still do not hold free and fair elections, and 106 governments still restrict civil and political freedoms"; United Nations Development Programme, 2002, p. 13). It is clear that low income is no obstacle to democracy and that a region with an enormous deficit in democracy is the Middle East and North Africa. The democratic movements that have influenced the lives of hundreds of millions of people in Latin America and parts of Africa and Asia have yet to have a serious impact on Islamic societies of the Middle East and North Africa. There is general agreement that options for voice, mobility, and participatory democracy are particularly lacking in Saudi Arabia, the country of origin for many of the most influential terrorist networks currently active on the world stage (Schwartz, 2002).

This is not, of course, a justification for attempting the wholesale transplantation of Western-style democracy to non-Western societies, but there is a need to support *contextualized democracy,* a sociopolitical order that allows participation in decision making and social mobility through the utilization of local, culturally appropriate symbols and strategies. Contextualized democracy needs to proceed with attention to the details of the cultural context in non-Western societies (see Moghaddam, 2002, particularly Chapters 2 and 3), such as that of Shi'a Islam (Moghaddam, 2004). Contextualized democracy should be given the highest priority in countries such as Saudi Arabia, where a combination of repression and corruption (see, for example, Aburish, 1995) leaves minimal options for any kind of public expression of dissatisfaction and participation in meaningful decision making. Psychological theories (Taylor & Moghaddam, 1994) suggest that a range of possible interpretations will arise among people in this situation, including displacement of aggression; those who vehemently blame others (e.g., "America—the Great Satan") for their perceived problems climb the stairs to the second floor.

Second Floor: Displacement of Aggression

Terrorism involves acts of violence against civilians and others who are only indirectly involved in the power struggle among the terrorists, governmental authorities, and others. Attacks on civilians often involve displaced aggression. Of course, displaced aggression can be verbal and indirect. Most of the people who climb up to the second floor do not undertake physical aggression; rather, they limit themselves to verbal attacks. However, some of them go beyond verbal displacement of aggression, often through the influence of their leaders.

Such displacement of aggression was discussed extensively by Freud (1921, 1930) and has a uniquely important role in his account of intergroup relations (see Taylor & Moghaddam, 1994, ch. 2). The explanatory power and contemporary relevance of displaced aggression are underlined by ongoing research (Marcus-Newhall, Pederson, Carlson, & Miller, 2000; Miller, Pederson, Earlywine, & Pollock, 2003). According to Freud, the role of displaced aggression must be understood in the larger context of intergroup processes.

Freud's account of displaced aggression in intergroup relations gives particular importance to three factors, the first of which is the role of leaders. In Freud's group psychology, leaders play an important role in redirecting negative emotions within the group onto others outside the group. He argued that it is always possible to "bind together a considerable number of people in love as long as there are other people left over to receive the manifestations of their aggressiveness" (1930, p. 114). Second, Freud gives importance to the targets of displacement. Such targets are not randomly selected; rather, according to Freud, they are dissimilar outsiders. Third, Freud points to the in-group cohesion that results from out-group threat. By highlighting threats from dissimilar outsiders, leaders increase in-group cohesion and strengthen their own support base.

Related to Freud's analysis, a strategy widely adopted by leaders for dealing with dissatisfactions among populations in some part of the world is anti-Americanism (e.g., see Atran, 2003, p. 1538). For example, Rushdie (2002) has argued that anti-Americanism is serving to deflect criticism away from governments in the Middle East:

> As always, anti-US radicalism feeds off the widespread anger over the plight of the Palestinians. . . . However . . . anti-Americanism has become too useful a smokescreen for Muslim nations' many defects—their corruption, their incompetence, their oppression of their own citizens, their economic, scientific and cultural stagnation.

In such contexts, those who develop a readiness to physically displace aggression and actively seek out opportunities to do so eventually climb the stairs to the third floor in search of ways to take action.

Third Floor: Moral Engagement

Terrorist organizations arise as a parallel or shadow world, with a parallel morality that justifies "the struggle" to achieve the "ideal" society by any means possible. From the perspective of the mainstream, terrorists are "morally disengaged," particularly because of their willingness to commit acts of violence against civilians. However, from the perspective of the morality that exists within terrorist organizations, terrorists are "morally engaged," and it is the government and its agents who are "morally disengaged." The terrorist organization becomes effective by mobilizing sufficient resources (McCarthy & Zald, 1977) to persuade recruits to become disengaged from morality as defined by governmental authorities (and often by the majority in society) and morally engaged in the way morality is constructed by the terrorist organization (for a related discussion, see Bandura, 2004). In the context of the Islamic world, terrorist organizations have fed on interpretations of Islam that laud what outsiders see as acts of terrorism but terrorists depict as martyrdom (Davis, 2003; Gold, 2003; Rashid, 2002). While the struggle for control over the "correct" interpretation of Islam is for the most part public (Donnan, 2002), the terrorist organizations that have evolved according to an ideology of martyrdom are secretive.

Recruits are persuaded to become committed to the morality of the terrorist organization through a number of tactics, the most important of which are isolation, affiliation, secrecy, and fear. Studies of terrorist organizations and their networks (e.g., Alexander & Swetman, 2002; Coogan, 2002; Kaplan & Marshall, 1996; Rapoport, 2002; Sageman, 2004) reveal that, even when terrorists continue to live their "normal" lives as members of communities, their goal is to develop their parallel lives in complete isolation and secrecy. Recruits are trained to keep their parallel lives a secret even from their wives, parents, closest friends, and all others around them. The illegal nature of their organization, perceived harsh governmental measures against them, and perceived lack of openness in society all contribute to their continued isolation and the sense of affiliation with other in-group members. In essence, terrorist organizations become effective by positioning themselves at two levels: at the macrolevel, as the only option toward reforming society (they point to alleged government repression and dictatorship as proof of their assertion), and at the microlevel, as a "home" or in-group for disaffected individuals (mostly young, single males), some of whom are recruited to carry out the most dangerous missions through programs that often have a very fast turnaround.

Fourth Floor: Categorical Thinking and the Perceived Legitimacy of the Terrorist Organization

After a person has climbed to the fourth floor and entered the secret world of the terrorist organization, there is little or no opportunity to leave alive. In most cases new recruits in the first category, who will be relatively long-term members, become part of small cells, typically of four or five persons each, with access to information only about the other members in their own cell. In the second category, the foot soldiers who are recruited to carry out violent attacks and to become suicide bombers, the entire operation of recruitment, training, and implementation of the terrorist act may take no more than 24 hours. Within those 24 hours, the recruited member is typically given a great deal of positive attention and treated as a kind of celebrity, particularly by the recruiter (who stays by his side constantly) and by a charismatic cell leader.

The cell structure of terrorist organizations may have first been widely adopted among guerilla forces fighting dictatorships in Latin America in the mid-twentieth century and is designed to limit infiltration and discovery by antiterrorist agents. By the late 1960s and early 1970s, the cell structure was being copied by most terrorist organizations, including those operating in Western societies (e.g., Coogan, 2002, p. 466). Often it is informal friendship networks and a need to belong that binds people to such cells (Sageman, 2004). Immersion in secret small-group activities leads to changes in perceptions among recruits: a legitimization of the terrorist organization and its goals, a belief that the ends justify the means, and a strengthening of the categorical "us versus them" view of the world.

Social categorization is a powerful psychological process (McGarty, 1999) that can lead to in-group favoritism and out-group discrimination even when the basis of categorization is trivial in a real-world context (Taylor & Moghaddam, 1994, Chapter 4). A categorical "us versus them" view of the world is one of the hallmarks of terrorist organizations and the people attracted to them (Pearlstein, 1991; Taylor, 1988). Western psychological literature has identified right-wing authoritarians as having a categorical viewpoint (Altemeyer, 1988a, 1988b), but in the world context, religious fundamentalism may be more directly related to an "us versus them" viewpoint among both Easterners (Alexander, 2002) and Westerners (Booth & Dunne, 2002). Just as Islamic fundamentalists have labeled the United States the "Great Satan," leading evangelist Christians in the United States have backed the view that "Islam was founded by . . . a demon-possessed pedophile" (Cooperman, 2002). This "us versus them" thinking from the West has played into the hands of fundamentalists abroad, particularly Saudi Wahhabism (Gold, 2003) and the radical form of Shi'i Islam, as represented by Hizballah in Iran and Lebanon, for example (Shapira, 2000). Of course, a categorical "us versus them" viewpoint is not sufficient to lead to terrorism; another important element is a belief in the terrorist organization as a just means to an ideal end.

Commitment to the terrorist cause strengthens as the new recruit is socialized into the traditions, methods, and goals of the organization. More than a century of research on social influence (Moghaddam, 1998, Chapters 6 and 7) suggests that conformity and obedience are very high in the cells of terrorist organizations, where the cell leader represents a strong authority figure and nonconformity, disobedience, and disloyalty receive the harshest punishments. The recruits at this stage face two uncompromising forces: From within the organization, they are pressured to conform and to obey in ways that will lead to violent acts against civilians (and often against themselves); from outside the organization, especially in regions such as the Middle East and North Africa, they face governments that do not allow even minimal voice and democratic participation in addressing perceived injustices. These dictatorial governments are seen as puppets of world powers, particularly the United States—a perception endorsed by a variety of international critics (Scranton, 2002).

During their stay on the fourth floor, then, individuals find their options have narrowed considerably. They are now part of a tightly controlled group that they cannot exit from alive.

Fifth Floor: The Terrorist Act and Sidestepping Inhibitory Mechanisms

Terrorism involves acts of violence against civilians, often resulting in numerous deaths. The experiences of professional military units demonstrate the intensive programs required to train soldiers to kill enemy soldiers (Grossman, 1995) and raise the question as to how terrorist organizations train their members to carry out the act that kills innocent civilians. The answer is found in two psychological processes that are central to intergroup dynamics (Brown & Gaertner, 2001). The first involves social categorization (of civilians as part of the out-group), and the second involves psychological distance (through exaggerating differences between the in-group and the out-group).

First, the categorization of civilians as part of the out-group matches the pattern of secrecy practiced by terrorist organizations; recruits to terrorist organizations are trained to treat everyone, including civilians, outside their tightly knit group as the enemy (Sageman, 2004). Newspaper headlines such as "terrorist blast kills three innocent bystanders" have little meaning from the perspective of terrorist organizations because of the particular way in which they have categorized the world into "us" and "them" and because of their perception that anyone who is not actively resisting the government is a legitimate target of violence. Besides, by attacking civilian targets, social order might be disrupted, and the terrorist act could serve as a spark to get people to "recognize the truth" and revolt against authorities (this was even assumed by the Oklahoma City bombers; see Linenthal, 2001). Thus, from the point of view of terrorist organizations, acts of violence against civilians are justified because civilians are part of the enemy, and only when civilians actively oppose the targeted "evil forces" will they no longer be the enemy. The perception of civilians as part of the enemy helps explain how terrorists sidestep what Lorenz (1966) termed "inhibitory mechanisms."

Lorenz (1966) has argued that inhibitory mechanisms serve to limit intraspecies killing. For example, when two wolves fight, it usually becomes clear fairly soon that one of them is stronger, with the result that the weaker wolf signals defeat by moving back and showing signs of submission. The aggression of the winner is inhibited by the signals of submission; thus the winner does not continue to attack and attempt to seriously injure or kill the loser. Inhibitory mechanisms also evolved to influence human behavior; crime statistics (Federal Bureau of Investigation, 2002) show that most killings of humans by humans take place through the use of guns and other weapons that allow killing from a distance and enable the sidestepping of inhibitory mechanisms potentially triggered through eye contact, pleading, crying, and other means (also see discussion of weapons and homicide in Smith & Zahn, 1999). Lorenz (1966) argued that among humans, inhibitory mechanisms have been bypassed through modern weapons, which allow an attacker to destroy a target from a long distance away.

The case of terrorist attacks suggests that inhibitory mechanisms can also be effectively circumvent by psychological distance, perhaps similar to the distancing that takes place between a rapist and the victim, particularly through the rapist's adoption of cultural myths about rape (see Burt, 1980, and readings in Searles & Berger, 1995). Terrorists often operate in tight physical proximity to their human targets, particularly in the case of suicide bombers, so they could potentially be influenced by the kinds of pleading and other signals that typically trigger inhibitory mechanisms. However, two key factors serve to sidestep these mechanisms during terrorist attacks. First, by categorizing the target, albeit civilians, as "the enemy" and exaggerating differences between ingroup and out-group, terrorists psychologically distance themselves from the other humans they intend to destroy. Second, the victims seldom become aware of the impending danger before the attack actually occurs, so they do not have an opportunity to behave in ways that might trigger inhibitory mechanisms.

Some Policy Implications

In this final section I highlight four important policy implications arising from the stairway metaphor.

1. Prevention Must Come First

The stairway metaphor has an overarching policy implication that is familiar to psychologists who are researching and practicing in mental health: Prevention is the long-term solution to terrorism. This is in line with a model of mental health that is integral to a larger public health care system and that provides broad-based services.

Policies to combat terrorism should concentrate on changing conditions for people situated at the foundation level of the stairway, with the aim of achieving a situation in which the general population rightly feels that it lives in a just society. This long-term policy should go hand in hand with short-term strategies to deal with the small number of individuals who have already climbed to the top of the stairway and are active in terrorist organizations. However, there needs to be a shift away from an almost complete preoccupation with secretive counterterrorism units and measures, away from a total concern with hunting for the "bad apples," and away from a naive reliance on improved technology and superior military might as the way to defeat terrorism. Such a policy shift may appear risky, but in practice it provides the best long-term safeguard against terrorism.

2. Procedural Justice Toward Contextualized Democracy

Psychological research clearly highlights the important role that procedural justice can play in bringing about contextualized democracy. Local cultural practices and symbolic systems need to be incorporated and used to enable more legal opportunities for voice and mobility, as well as to influence perceptions of these opportunities. Such policies must include women and other minorities in the decision-making process. It is particularly in this regard that support is needed for democratic processes even when they contradict local traditions, such as a tradition of allowing only a very limited role for women in the public sphere (as is still the case in much of the Middle East and North Africa). In this regard, special attention must be given to the relationship between educational avenues and opportunities for voice and mobility.

3. Educating Against Categorical "Us Versus Them" Thinking

In order to help bring about greater voice and mobility in societies such as those in the Middle East and North Africa, it is important to appropriately frame the fight against terrorism and particularly the way in which we categorize the social world. As people climb up the stairway, their categorization of the world into "us versus them," "the forces of good versus the forces of evil," and so on becomes more prominent and rigid. The challenge is to prevent such an inflexible style of categorization from becoming the norm at the foundation level, where most of the people are situated. A starting point for implementing this policy is to avoid—and indeed to combat—a categorization of the world into "us versus them" and "good versus evil." Such categorization only endorses the views of fundamentalists and increases the probability of more people climbing up the stairway to commit terrorist acts. This requires a major policy shift in a number of countries. In the United States, despite assurances by some members of the Bush administration that "there is no war against Islam," the rhetoric of "you are either with us or against us" has played into the hands of fundamentalists.

4. Interobjectivity and Justice

To strengthen a shared worldview on justice, rights, and duties, we must implement policies to influence *interobjectivity*, the understandings shared within and between cultures (Moghaddam, 2003). These policies can build on a foundation of probable psychological universals in justice but must also take into consideration the perceptions among many non-Western people that their indigenous identities are threatened as a result of increasing globalization and Western influence. These types of policies with global implications require working through—and being supportive of—international organizations such as the United Nations.

Concluding Comment

Ultimately, terrorism is a moral problem with psychological underpinnings; the challenge is to prevent disaffected youth and others from becoming engaged in the morality of terrorist organizations. A lesson from the history of terrorism in the Middle East and other parts of the world is that this moral problem does not have a technological solution and is therefore at odds with the contemporary tendency to try to find technological solutions to moral dilemmas (Moghaddam, 1997). More sophisticated technology and increased force will not end terrorism in the long term. Despite the often-repeated declaration that the "war on terror will be a long one," policies for ending terrorism have been more short-term strategies, often driven

by political needs rather than by scientific understanding. The focus of policies for the most part has been on people who have climbed all the way up the stairway and are already committed to carrying out terrorist acts. Policies aimed at these individuals do not address the foundational problem at the bottom of the stairway, involving the vast majority of people. Basic issues at the foundational level need to be addressed by guiding principles, including how the majority perceive fairness, openness, and voice opportunities in their societies and how they are influenced by leaders to see the source of their problems as external and to displace aggression onto out-group targets. As part of a policy shift, a categorization of the world into "us versus them" needs to be avoided.

Acknowledgments. I am grateful to anonymous reviewers for comments made on an earlier draft of this chapter.

References

Aburish, S. K. (1995). *The rise, corruption, and coming fall of the House of Saud.* New York: St. Martin's Press.

Adams, J. S. (1965). Inequality in social exchange. In L. Berkowitz (Ed.), *Advances in experimental social psychology: Vol. 2* (pp. 267–299). New York: Academic Press.

Alexander, Y. (2002). *Palestinian religious terrorism: Hamas and Islamic Jihad.* Ardsley, NY: Transnational Publishers.

———, & Swetman, M. (2002). *Usama bin Laden's al-Qaeda: Profile of a terrorist network.* Ardsley, NY: Transnational Publishers.

Altemeyer, B. (1988a). *Enemies of freedom: Understanding right-wing authoritarianism.* San Francisco: Jossey-Bass.

———, B. (1988b, March/April). The good soldier, marching in step: A psychological explanation of state terror. *Sciences,* 30–38.

Arjomand, S. A. (1988). *The turban for the crown: The Islamic revolution in Iran.* New York: Oxford University Press.

Atran, S. (2003). Genesis of suicide terrorism. *Science,* 299, 1534–1539.

Bandura, A. (2004). The role of selective moral disengagement in terrorism and counterterrorism. In F. M. Moghaddam & A. J. Marsella (Eds.), *Understanding terrorism: Psychosocial roots, causes, and consequences* (pp. 121–150). Washington, DC: American Psychological Association.

Bernholz, P. (2004). Supreme values as the basis for terror. *European Journal of Political Economy, 20,* 317–333.

Bodansky, Y. (2001). *Bin Laden: The man who declared war on America.* New York: Random House.

Booth, K., & Dunne, T. (Eds.). (2002). *Worlds in collision: Terror and the future of global order.* New York: Palgrave Macmillan.

Brockner, J. M., & Wiesenfeld, B. M. (1996). An integrative framework for explaining reactions to decisions: Interactive effects of outcomes and procedures. *Psychological Bulletin, 120,* 189–208.

Brown, R., & Gaertner, S. L. (Eds.). (2001). *Blackwell handbook of social psychology: Intergroup processes.* Oxford: Blackwell.

Burt, M. R. (1980). Cultural myths and supports for rape. *Journal of Personality and Social Psychology, 38,* 217–230.

Collins, R. L. (1996). For better or worse: The impact of upward social comparison on self-evaluations. *Psychological Bulletin, 116,* 457–475.

Coogan, T. P. (2002). *The IRA.* New York: Palgrave.

Cooper, H. H. A. (2001). The problem of definition revisited. *American Behavioral Scientist, 44,* 881–893.

Cooperman, A. (2002, June 20). Anti-Muslim remarks stir tempest. *Washington Post,* A3.

Crenshaw, M. (2000). The psychology of terrorism: An agenda for the 21st century. *Political Psychology, 21*(2), 405–420.

Crosby, F. (1982). *Relative deprivation and working women.* New York: Oxford University Press.

Danieli, Y., Brom, D., & Waizer, J. (Eds.). (in press). *The trauma of terror: Sharing knowledge and sharing care.* New York: Haworth Press.

Danieli, Y., Engdahl, B., & Schlenger, W. E. (2004). The psychosocial aftermath of terrorism. In F. M. Moghaddam & A. J. Marsella (Eds.), *Understanding terrorism: Psychosocial roots, consequences, and interventions* (pp. 223–246). Washington, DC: American Psychological Association.

Davis, J. (2003). *Martyrs: Innocence, vengeance, and despair in the Middle East.* New York: Palgrove Macmillan.

Dion, K. L. (1986). Responses to perceived discrimination and relative deprivation. In J. M. Olson, C. P. Herman, & M. P. Zanna (Eds.), *Relative deprivation and social comparison: The Ontario symposium: Vol. 4* (pp. 159–180). Hillsdale, NJ: Erlbaum.

Doise, W. (2002). *Human rights as social representations.* London: Routledge.

Donnan, H. (Ed.). (2002). *Interpreting Islam.* London: Sage.

Ehrlich, P. R., & Liu, J. (2002). Some roots of terrorism. *Population and Environment, 24,* 183–191.

Federal Bureau of Investigation. (2002). *Uniform crime reports for the United States.* Washington, DC: U.S. Government Printing Office.

Fields, R. M., Elbedour, S., & Hein, F. A. (2002). The Palestinian suicide bomber. In C. E. Stout (Ed.), *The psychology of terrorism: Vol. 2* (pp. 193–223). Westport, CT: Praeger.

Freud, S. (1921). Group psychology and the analysis of the ego. In J. Strachey (Ed. and Trans.), *The standard edition of the complete psychological works: Vol. 18* (pp. 69–143). London: Hogarth.

———. (1930). Civilization and its discontents. In J. Strachey (Ed. and Trans.), *The standard edition of the complete psychological works: Vol. 21* (pp. 59–145). London: Hogarth.

Galea, S., Ahern, J., Resnick, H., Kilpatrick, D., Bucuvalas, M., Gold, J., et al. (2002). Psychological sequelae of the September 11 terrorist attacks in New York City. *New England Journal of Medicine, 346,* 982–987.

Gold, D. (2003). *Hatred's kingdom: How Saudi Arabia supports the new global terrorism.* Washington, DC: Regnery.

Grossman, D. (1995). *On killing: The psychological cost of learning to kill in war and society.* New York: Little, Brown.

Guimond, S., Dubé-Simard, L. (1983). Relative deprivation theory and the Quebec nationalist movement: The cognition-emotion distinction and the person-group deprivation issue. *Journal of Personality and Social Psychology, 44,* 526–535.

Gurr, N., & Cole, B. (2002). *The new face of terrorism: Threats from weapons of mass destruction.* New York: I. B. Tauris.

Gurr, T. R. (1970). *Why men rebel.* Princeton: Princeton University Press.

Horgan, J., & Taylor, M. (2003). *The psychology of terrorism.* New York: Frank Cass.

Kaplan, D. E., & Marshall, A. (1996). *The cult at the end of the world: The terrifying story of the Aum doomsday cult, from the subways of Tokyo to the nuclear arsenals of Russia.* New York: Crown.

Krueger, A., & Maleckova, J. (2002, July). Education, poverty, political violence, and terrorism: Is there a causal connection? NBER Working Paper no. W9074, National Bureau of Economic Research, Cambridge, MA. Retrieved January 7, 2006, from http://papers.nber.org/papers/W9074

Latané, B., & Darley, J. M. (1970). *The unresponsive bystander: Why doesn't he help?* Englewood Cliffs, NJ: Prentice Hall.

Lerner, M. J. (1980). *The belief in a just world: A fundamental delusion.* New York: Plenum.

Linenthal, E. T. (2001). *The unfinished bombing: Oklahoma City in American memory.* New York: Oxford University Press.

Lorenz, K. (1966). *On aggression* (M. Wilson, Trans.). New York: Harcourt, Brace, World.

Marcus-Newhall, A., Pederson, W. C., Carlson, M., & Miller, N. (2000). Displaced aggression is alive and well: A meta-analytic review. *Journal of Personality and Social Psychology, 78,* 670–689.

Martin, J., Brickman, P., & Murray, A. (1984). Moral outrage and pragmatism: Explanations for collective action. *Journal of Experimental Social Psychology, 20,* 484–496.

McCarthy, T. D., & Zald, M. N. (1977). Resource mobilization and social movements: A partial theory. *American Journal of Sociology, 82,* 1212–1241.

McGarty, C. (1999). *Categorization in social psychology.* Thousand Oaks, CA: Sage.

Miller, D. L. (2000). *Introduction to collective behavior and collective action* (2nd ed). Prospect Heights, IL: Waveland.

Miller, N., Pederson, W. C., Earlywine, M., & Pollock, V. E. (2003). A theoretical model of triggered displaced aggression. *Personality and Social Psychology Review, 7,* 75–97.

Moghaddam, F. M. (1997). *The specialized society: The plight of the individual in an age of individualism.* Westport, CT: Praeger.

———. (1998). *Social psychology: Exploring universals in social behavior.* New York: Freeman.

———. (2002). *The individual and society: A cultural integration.* New York: Worth.

———. (2003). Interobjectivity and culture. *Culture and Society, 9,* 221–232.

———. (2004). Cultural continuities beneath the conflict between radical Islam and pro-Eastern forces: The case of Iran. In Y. T. Lee, C. McCauley, F. M. Moghaddam, & S. Worchel (Eds.), *The psychology of ethnic and cultural conflict* (pp. 115–132). Westport, CT: Praeger.

———, & Marsella, A. J. (Eds.). (2004). *Understanding terrorism: Psychosocial roots, consequences, and interventions* (pp. 223–246). Washington, DC: American Psychological Association.

Moghaddam, F. M., & Riley, C. J. (in press). Toward a cultural theory of rights and duties in human development. In N. Finkel & F. M. Moghaddam (Eds.), *The psychology of rights and duties: Empirical contributions and normative commentaries.* Washington, DC: American Psychological Association.

Moghaddam, F. M., & Solliday, E. A. (1991). "Balanced multiculturalism" and the challenge of peaceful coexistence in pluralistic societies. *Psychology and Developing Societies, 3,* 51–72.

North, C. S., Nixon, S. J., Shariat, S., Mallonee, S., McMillen, J. C., Spitznagel, et al. (1999). Psychiatric disorders among survivors of the Oklahoma City bombing. *Journal of the American Medical Association, 282,* 755–762.

North, C. S., & Pfefferbaum, B. (2002). Research on the mental health effects of terrorism. *Journal of the American Medical Association, 288,* 633–636.

North, C. S., Tivis, L., McMillen, J. C., Pfefferbaum, B., Spitznagel, E. L., Cox, J., et al. (2002). Psychiatric disorders in rescue workers after the Oklahoma City bombing. *American Journal of Psychiatry, 159,* 857–859.

Pareto, V. (1935) *The mind and society: A treatise in general sociology.* 4 vols. New York: Dover.

Pearlstein, R. M. (1991). *The mind of the political terrorist.* Wilmington, DE: Scholarly Resources.

Plato. (1987). *The republic* (D. Lee, Trans.). Harmondsworth, UK: Penguin.

Pyszcznski, T., Solomon, S., & Greenberg, J. (2003). *In the wake of 9/11: The psychology of terror.* Washington, DC: American Psychological Association.

Rapoport, D. C. (Ed.). (2002). *Inside terrorist organizations* (2d ed.). London: Frank Cass.

Rashid, A. (2002). *Jihad: The rise of militant Islam in Central Asia.* New Haven: Yale University Press.

Robbins, S. (2002). The rush to counsel: Lessons of caution in the aftermath of disaster. *Families in Society: Journal of Contemporary Human Services, 83,* 113–116.

Ruby, C. L. (2002). Are terrorists mentally deranged? *Analysis of Social Issues and Public Policy, 2,* 15–26.

Runciman, W. G. (1966). *Relative deprivation and social justice: A study of attitudes to social inequality in twentieth-century England.* Berkeley: University of California Press.

Rushdie, S. (2002). Anti-Americanism has taken the world by storm. *Guardian.* Retrieved January 7, 2006, from http://www.guardian.co.uk/afghanistan/comment/story/0,11447,645579,00.html

Sageman, M. (2004). *Understanding terror networks.* Philadelphia: University of Pennsylvania Press.

Schama, S. (1989). *Citizens: A chronicle of the French revolution.* New York: Vintage.

Schlenger, W. E., Caddell, J. M., Ebert, L., Jordan, B. K., Rourke, K. M., Wilson, D., et al. (2002). Psychological reactions to terrorist attacks: Findings from the national study of Americans' reactions to September 11. *Journal of the American Medical Association, 288,* 581–588.

Schuster, M. A., Stein, B. D., Jaycox, L. H., Collins, R. L., Marshall, G. N., Elliott, M., et al. (2001). *New England Journal of Medicine, 345,* 1507–1512.

Schwartz, S. (2002). *The two faces of Islam: The house of Saud from tradition to terror.* New York: Doubleday.

Scranton, P. (Ed.). (2002). *Beyond September 11: An anthology of dissent*. London: Pluto Press.

Scrinivas, M. N. (1968). Mobility in the caste system. In M. Singer & B. S. Cohen (Eds.), *Structure and change in Indian society* (pp. 189–200). Chicago: Aldine.

Searles, P., & Berger, R. J. (Eds.). (1995). *Rape and society: Readings on the problem of sexual assault*. Boulder, CO: Westview Press.

Seul, J. R. (1999). "Ours is the way of God": Religion, identity, and intergroup conflict. *Journal of Peace Research, 36,* 553–569.

Shapira, S. (2000). *Hizballah between Iran and Lebanon*. Tel Aviv: Kakibbutz Hameuchad.

Silke, A. (Ed.). (2003). *Terrorism, victims, and society: Psychological perspectives on terrorism and its consequences*. Hoboken, NJ: Wiley.

Silver, R. C., Holman, E. A., McIntosh, D. N., Poulin, M., & Gil-Rivas, V. (2002). Nationwide longitudinal study of psychological responses to September 11. *Journal of the American Medical Association, 288,* 1235–1244.

Singapore Ministry of Home Affairs. (2003, January 9). White paper: The Jemaah Islamiyah arrests and the threat of terrorism. Retrieved April 19, 2006, from http://www2.mha.gov.sg/mha/detailed.jsp?artid=667&type=4&root=0&parent=0&cat=0&mode=arc.

Smith, M. D., & Zahn, M. A. (Eds.). (1999). *Studying and preventing homicide: Issues and challenges*. Thousand Oaks, CA: Sage.

Stephenson, J. (2001). Medical, mental health communities mobilize to cope with terror's psychological aftermath. *Journal of the American Medical Association, 286,* 1823–1825.

Sternberg, R. J. (1990). *Metaphors of mind: Conceptions of the nature of intelligence*. Cambridge: Cambridge University Press.

Stouffer, S. A., Suchman, E. A., De Vinney, L. C., Star, S. A., & Williams, R. M. (1949). *The American soldier: Adjustment during army life: Vol. 1*. Princeton: Princeton University Press.

Stout, C. E. (Ed.). (2002). *The psychology of terrorism*. 4 vols. Westport, CT: Praeger.

Tajfel, H., & Turner, J. C. (1986). The social identity theory of intergroup behavior. In S. Worchel & G. Austin (Eds.), *Psychology of intergroup relations* (pp. 2–24). Chicago: Nelson-Hall.

Taylor, D. M. (2003). *The quest for identity*. Westport, CT: Praeger.

———, & Moghaddam, F. M. (1994). *Theories of intergroup relations: International social psychological perspectives*. Westport, CT: Praeger.

Taylor, M. (1988). *The terrorist*. London: Brassey's Defence Publishers.

Tyler, T. R. (1990). *Why people obey the law*. New Haven: Yale University Press.

———. (1994). Governing amid diversity: The effect of fair decision-making procedures on the legitimacy of government. *Law and Society Review, 28,* 809–831.

———. (2001). Trust and law abidingness: A proactive model of social regulation. *Boston University Law Review, 81,* 361–406.

———, & Huo, Y. J. (2002). *Trust in the law*. New York: Russell Sage Foundation.

United Nations Development Programme. (2002). *Human development report 2002: Deepening democracy in a fragmented world*. New York: Oxford University Press.

Walster, E., Walster, G. W., & Berscheid, E. (1978). *Equity: Theory and research*. Boston: Allyn & Bacon.

Wessells, M. G. (2004). Terrorism and the mental health and well-being of refugees and displaced people. In F. M. Moghaddam & A. J. Marsella (Eds.), *Understanding terrorism: Psychosocial roots, consequences, and interventions*. Washington, DC: American Psychological Association.

Wright, S. C., Taylor, D. M., & Moghaddam, F. M. (1990). Responding to membership in a disadvantaged group: From acceptance to collective protest. *Journal of Personality and Social Psychology, 58,* 994–1003.

6

Terrorism and the Media

Joel N. Shurkin

The media find themselves in a dysfunctional position relative to terrorism. On the one hand, they must report terrorist attacks as they happen. On the other, they are part of the reason these incidents occur in the first place. For members of the media, the situation raises interesting, difficult, and complex professional and ethical problems. The fact is that the media are crucial in determining the general community's reaction to terrorism. Fortunately, the media seem to understand that.

When the World Trade Centers were attacked on September 11, 2001, the common refrain among journalists was that nothing like this had happened before and that the usual journalistic procedures and rules were inadequate. Undoubtedly, like most Americans, they were stunned. The story had astounding scope. A quick visit to an almanac would show that on any business day as many as 20,000 people could be in the two buildings at one time. The number of casualties was beyond imagination or more than the heart could bear, as the mayor of New York said. It was the first attack on U.S. soil since Pearl Harbor, but this time it was not on a Hawaiian island but in Manhattan, the media center of the country—if not the Western world—and it was seen live—on television.

The attack was planned on exactly that premise—that the media would cover the story with the immediacy it deserved. That's probably why the attack was in two parts. The first plane hitting the first building got everyone's attention. When the second plane struck, the cameras were on, and billions of people watched it live in their homes. While later replays of the event were edited somewhat, those watching live saw bodies fall from the towers, people who had jumped or been pushed, tumbling in space against the beautiful autumn sky. No one knew how many people were still in the building when they so gracefully and awfully collapsed. The sight could not have been more horrible. That, of course, was exactly what the terrorists wanted, but the television networks could not turn off the cameras, photographers could not avert their lenses, and reporters could not turn away. Whatever else anyone can say of the attacks, they were brilliantly conceived with the media in mind.

This dichotomy made the attacks perhaps the most difficult reporting assignments in modern journalistic history. That the media did as well as they did is a tribute to them—and a lesson.

Most of the media believed that what happened that day had no precedent. In fact, it did have. Although the nuclear accident at Three Mile Island was *not* terrorism, many of the same issues were raised then. And if journalists thought it would be a while before they were confronted with the same issue, they were mistaken.

Handmaiden to Terrorism

Without the media, there would likely be no modern terrorism. Palestinian terrorists know that the Israeli and the world press will cover every bombing, particularly of civilian targets. If it did not, there would be no political point in blowing up a bus. Historically, the terrorists do not fancy themselves murders but martyrs for a cause, although with the rise of the new religious fanaticism that may well be changing (Council on Foreign Relations, 2004). In a free society that almost guarantees that publicity, the dominant image requires publicity and the media.

Studies agree that a symbiotic relationship exists between the terrorists and the media. In its most cynical form, the image is of terrorists using the media as a conduit for their message and the media using the terrorists for dramatic stories (Lockyer, 2003). Terrorism has been called political "theater," and that's how terrorists view it. A nineteenth-century anarchist called it "propaganda by deed" (Council on Foreign Relations, 2004). If terrorism can be defined as violence that is designed to deliver a message, the media are the messenger. Experts are divided on whether the publicity always helps the terrorists' cause, with some pointing out that their message plays differently to different audiences. As the Palestinians have discovered, in public opinion the method overshadows the message after a while.

It goes without saying that virtually all editors and reporters would rather not have these stories to cover, and all of them understand they are being used. They are aware that the language they employ in these stories is crucial—politicizing language was not an idea invented by George Orwell. Words have meanings beyond those found in the dictionary. Janny de Graaf (Schmid and de Graaf, 1982) has argued that, when journalists interview subjects, they are more inclined to use the subject's wording, whether it comes from a terrorist cell or a government. For instance, when is a "terrorist" a "guerilla"? Who is a "murderer" and who a

"freedom fighter"? Israelis view Palestinian bombers as terrorists, while Palestinians point out that Menachem Begin, a former prime minister of Israel and something of a national hero, used a similar technique against the British to win Israel's independence. The difference is who won and who got to write the history.[1]

Three Mile Island and the Precedent of Reporting the Threat of Disaster

From a journalistic point of view, there was precedent for 9/11, a huge story that could have been made worse by the media if they had acted irresponsibly. The precedent was set 33 years earlier at Three Mile Island, a nuclear power plant in Pennsylvania. No terrorism was involved, merely human incompetence, but the media were placed in the awesome position of having to report a complex story with insufficient information and having to get it right.

I was science editor of the *Philadelphia Inquirer* at the time and faced the problem head on. The confusion we confronted easily matches the confusion reporters faced on 9/11—confusion that had been deliberately created. And, if we got the story wrong, there might be unwarranted panic or people would be placed in danger that could have been avoided.

Three Mile Island sits on an actual island in the middle of the Susquehanna River, south of Harrisburg, Pennsylvania. It was operated by a medium-sized utility, Metropolitan Edison, which in retrospect was probably too small for the responsibility of running a nuclear power plant. On March 28, 1979, because of operator error, the plant began a partial meltdown.

The Associated Press relayed the first word of the incident after the company reported a minor radioactive release from the plant. Throughout the morning, news from the company continued to portray the event as minor, but after a few hours it was clear that something unusual was happening.

The media, including the *Inquirer,* were unprepared for the event. Like many science reporters, I had avoided writing about nuclear energy because, after a subconscious cost-benefit analysis, I had concluded that the aggravation created by proponents and opponents of nuclear energy—on the phone and in the mail—outweighed the benefits of doing the stories.[2] Hence, although I had written about how these plants worked and knew something of the technology, I was about to be blindsided by a story well beyond my expertise.

When I reported for work that morning and asked one of the editors whether he needed any help, I was told the political reporters at the state capital could handle the story. I was skeptical but went back to my seat and waited. Within a few hours, the reporters in Harrisburg were screaming for help. They had no idea what was happening at the plant and were getting no information from the company. I was sent to Middletown, Pennsylvania, the community nearest to the plant. When I got there, I found that every other newspaper was going through a similar process, with editors assuming the story was a simple one, requiring no expertise and only later shipping out their science writers.

The most serious problem was a lack of reliable and creditable information. At first, Metropolitan Edison simply refused to be of any help, at least in part because the officials there had no clue what was happening within the containment vessels of the reactors. Then the lawyers apparently took over, and the company's small information machinery simply shut it down. The *Inquirer* even tape-recorded a conversation that took place between the company and the employees of a public relations firm, Hill and Knowlton, which had been brought in to help them with the emergency, as they conspired to prevent information from leaking. They produced a press kit that contained nothing useful and set up a telephone number that was specifically designed to be eternally busy.

Even the federal government played along. The Nuclear Regulatory Commission (NRC) set up a trailer outside the press center, and the information officer set up a system so he would *not* have to give out information. Not only was the press excluded from information, but so was the state government, which had the final responsibility for the public's safety.

In one of history's great ironies, 13 days before the incident at Three Mile Island, Hollywood had released a film starring Jane Fonda, *The China Syndrome,* in which a reactor goes wild and threatens everything around it.[3] The movie was playing in Middletown at the time. In the film, a character says the meltdown could wipe out most of central Pennsylvania. And that is exactly the problem that was facing the media at Three Mile Island.

Richard Thornburg, then governor of Pennsylvania, called the president of the United States and demanded that someone produce information that he could use—and, by extension, that the press could use. The NRC sent a man named Harold Denton to Middletown to act as a conduit between the public and the government. The information—such as it was—finally began to flow.[4]

Still, reporters faced serious questions. The extent of the danger from the radiation was controversial in the extreme in the scientific community, one of the reasons the stories were so contentious. Some reputable scientists held that any radiation at all imposed a danger of cancer on the public; others said that only a certain level was dangerous. As a competent reporter, you could predict the answers you would get by knowing whom to call. So, whom *do* you call?

Several days into the accident, a bubble of hydrogen built up in the reactor and threatened to explode—a calamity in the making, one that could indeed have endangered most of central Pennsylvania. No one could predict what would then happen. What do you say? If you report that the reactor is likely to explode, you will set off a panic. And what if it didn't explode? If you say everything is under control or the danger is minimal and it then blows up, a lot of people who could have fled would be in the path of the radiation.

The general, unspoken consensus was that we had to play it straight and with moderation, giving the information we had clearly and calmly and with as much context as possible, and let people decide for themselves what to do. I called experts on radiation I knew to be moderates who would give me unruffled, measured responses. This in itself was a problem. Readers, who apparently expected experts to have answers, began flooding the newspaper editors with complaints about our less-than-specific information. They wanted experts who told them whether something was dangerous; they did not want stories that straddled the fence. In 35 years of journalism, it was the most profound professional decision I ever had to make. We actually sat, discussed the matter, and decided how to write the stories (Sandman & Paden, 1979a, 1979b). That almost never actually happens in the field. Reporters usually act on instinct.

I suspect that similar discussions occurred in newsrooms all over the country on 9/11 and for the same reasons. Because information was scarce and unreliable, it was difficult for everyone to comprehend exactly what was happening, only that it was gigantic and the potential enormous. What other buildings were being attacked and by whom? Word came quickly of the attack at the Pentagon, but rumors of another at the State Department proved untrue even after they were reported in the major media. How many planes were still in the sky carrying terrorists? The FAA had reports of dozens; in fact, there was only one. Was the United States under a general attack, or were New York and Washington the only targets? Should people panic? Were they safe? With billions of viewers—including a vast proportion of the American public—watching, reporters had to think before they wrote in ways they had not often done before.

Anthrax and the Media as the Target

It happened again quickly. This time the media were the target, and it *was* terrorism. Again obstructions were placed between reporters and the information they needed. As with Three Mile Island, this new development became a primer for the government on how *not* to handle terrorism (Ricchiardi, 2001).

Within weeks of 9/11, a terrorist struck again. To this day, no one knows who the perpetrator was, but the first victim was Robert Stevens, 63, a photo editor at a supermarket tabloid published by American Media in Florida. The official response only fueled the panic, especially after Stevens died. Part of the difficulty was that the weapon of choice was anthrax, a disease so obscure that virtually no one knew much about it.

That most of the targets were in the media was a cunning ploy. As Ricchiardi wrote, "If you want to scare the wits out of America, scare journalists first." The attacks were brought by the U.S. mail right into newsrooms.

"If you were a terrorist with only a small amount of anthrax, you want to send it to the people who would get you on the evening news—people at the news tabloid, a news anchor, a politician," said Kyle Olson, a terrorism expert (quoted in Ricchardi, 2001).

Once the disease was identified, all of the information was shut down. NBC's Robert Bazell said, "all the government agencies including NIH and CDC were told not to talk. They were trying to develop a model where all the information came from a central source (Thomas, 2003). Meanwhile, of course, no information was getting out. Rick Weiss of the *Washington Post* was less kind. He described the policy as "One department, one voice. But that one voice is busy right now, so please leave a message" (quoted in Thomas, 2003). The process was similar to that adopted by the NRC and Metropolitan Edison: Pretend you are giving out information when in fact you are doing nothing of the sort.

Information was the first casualty. Confusion reigned. The Bush administration urged Americans to go about their business; meanwhile, the FBI was predicting new attacks.

Journalists had "no precedent, no strategy to deal with rapid-fire breaking news of infection by killer germs, no ready-made pool of experts" (Ricchiardi, 2001,). Part of the problem was a lack of personnel, with one public relations person initially assigned to answer questions. That person recorded more than 135 messages a day, and there likely were still more calls that were simply not logged. Between October 4 and October 18, the media office reported 2,229 calls. Many more (an average of 230 calls a day) went unreported. By October 14, five more public information officers (PIOs) had been brought in to handle the load.

Getting one of the PIOs on the phone did not solve reporters' problems, however. They were usually referred elsewhere and then to CDC in Atlanta—an unproductive circle. Meanwhile, as the attacks spread by mail to other news media, including the office of NBC's Tom Brokaw, and as the U.S. Postal Service gradually shut down, coverage exploded. Some of the cable news channels went "all anthrax all the time" (Thomas, 2003). At this juncture, another plague erupted, just as it had on 9/11, and many instant experts appeared, many (if not most) of whom had no idea what they were talking about. One channel produced an "expert" who repeatedly referred to the anthrax "virus," when a bacillus in spore form is actually what causes anthrax.

By October 15 it was obvious to everyone that the public needed more information—and needed it accurately and quickly. CDC brought in another 10 PIOs. By October 18 it was able to produce an extensive, multipurpose press release confirming that a postal worker in New Jersey had contracted the disease. Information went up on the Web and in Spanish. Real information began to replace bad; Gresham's Law of Journalism had been reversed.

The next time we might not be so lucky. Anthrax is a disease that is relatively hard to spread. Had it been variola, the smallpox virus, we would not have had several weeks to get our act in order. The anthrax attack killed 5 of the 11 people who became infected. More than 2,000 hoaxes and false reports emptied government buildings and shut down post offices. Most of the terrorism experts feared that the worst could come at any moment.

"I think the press has been prudently cautious in reporting the story and therefore helped the country understand that there is no need to be panic-stricken about this," said Robert Giles, curator of the Nieman Foundation, when the scare was over (quoted in Ricchiardi, 2001).

How Did the Media Do?

In these difficult episodes, the American media did surprisingly well. Even the most free swinging sobered up. The main problem they had was not of their making; rather, it was bureaucracies—government and industrial—that were keeping information they needed from them. Of course, in the case of 9/11, reporters were confronting a situation that was so gigantic that useful information was impossible to ascertain.

A study by the Pew Research Center for the People and the Press, made after 9/11, showed that the press's image was improved by the coverage it provided of the attacks (Pew Research Center for the People and the Press, 2001). However, there was some unhappiness with a number of the practices the press had engaged in, and the somewhat mellow attitude of the public has probably wafted away (Pew Research Center for the People and the Press, 2002). According to the 2001 study, the Pew Center reported that, after the attack, 47% of respondents thought news organizations were politically biased, compared with 59% in early September. Additionally, more people thought the media tried not to be biased (26% after the attack versus 35% in early September). More than half still thought the media had tried to cover up their mistakes, however. More than a third believed jour-

nalists and reporters help society solve its problems, and half felt the media get in the way.

The study also found that the public could not get enough of the news.

Another effect of 9/11 was that the media, in some regard, sobered up. Before the attack, with news coverage sliding inexorably toward trivia, celebrity news, and junk medicine at the cost of reporting serious news—particularly international news—one result was a reversal of that trend, at least for a while.

Rosenstiel reported that, right after the attack, "the war on terrorism has caused a colossal shift in the news people see on network television" (Rosenstiel, 2001). The networks were producing more traditional hard news than they had in decades. The news agenda on the networks was more reminiscent of the 1970s than the 1990s, but that expansion was limited. The new interest was in the war on terrorism, not in the broad world beyond that subject. Even Rosenstiel admitted, however, that the sobering up might be just a temporary reaction. A year later, Althaus reported that everything was unfortunately back to normal (Althaus, 2002).

Notes

1. Part of the problem may be the lack of neutral words to describe these acts. The Israeli government and many Zionists have been in a decades-long battle with the British Broadcasting Company over the terminology the BBC uses to describe events in the Middle East (Honest Reporting, 2004) Thirty years ago in New York I had a similar battle as news editor for Reuters, when the London office removed the word "terrorist" from every story about airplane hijackers, claiming it was politically charged and inappropriate for customers in the area.

2. That there are stories like that is one of the great secrets of journalism. Abortion is another example. All that printing stories does is excite the readers and viewers who care passionately one way or the other. They do not change anyone's mind. Hence, many reporters do the stories only when they have to.

3. The "China syndrome" is an engineering construct in which a nuclear reactor melts down through the floor of the containment vessel and keeps going. It would, in theory, eventually hit groundwater and explode. But, taken to the extreme, it would then keep going—all the way to China.

4. Thornburg eventually recommended that pregnant women leave the area.

References

Althaus, S. (2002, September). American news consumption during times of national crisis. *PS: Political Science and Politics, 35*(3), 517–521.

Council on Foreign Relations. (2004). Islam in a changing world. Retrieved April 19, 2006, from http://www.cfr.org/publication/7533/islam_in_a_changing_world.html.

Honest Reporting. (2004, January 14). BBC's selective sensitivity. Retrieved April 19, 2006, from http://www.honestreporting.com/articles/45884734/critiques/BBCs_Selective_Sensitivity.asp.

Lockyer, A. (2003, August 18). The relationship between media and terrorism. Canberra: Australian National University. Retrieved April 19, 2006, from http://rspas.anu.edu.au/papers/sdsc/viewpoint/paper_030818.pdf.

Pew Research Center for the People and the Press. (2001, November 28). Terror coverage boosts news media's image. Retrieved April 19, 2006, from http://people-press.org/dataarchive/.

———. (2002, August 4). News media's improved image proves short lived. Retrieved April 19, 2004, from http://people-press.org/reports/display.php3?ReportID=159.

Ricchiardi, S. (2001, December). The anthrax enigma. *American Journalism Review, 23*(10), 18–23.

Rosenstiel, T. (2001, November). Before and after: How the war on terrorism has changed the news agenda, network television, June to October 2001. Retrieved January 8, 2006, from http://www.journalism.org/resources/research/reports/agenda/default.asp.

Sandman, P., & Paden, M. (1979a, July–August). At Three Mile Island. *Columbia Journalism Review,* 43–58.

———. (1979b, July–August). The "Inquirer" goes for broke. *Columbia Journalism Review* (sidebar), 48–49.

Schmid, A. P., & de Graaf, J. (1982). *Violence as communication: Insurgent terrorism and the Western news media.* London: Sage.

Thomas, P. (2003, Spring). The anthrax attacks: A journalist assesses what went wrong in coverage of this story. *Nieman Reports,* 11–14.

7

What Is Terrorism?

Key Elements and History

Scott Gerwehr
Kirk Hubbard

Laqueur (1987) defines terrorism as the illegitimate or extranormal use of violence against noncombatants to achieve political ends. Although there are innumerable definitions of terrorism, they all bear some resemblance to Laqueur's definition, and particularly this notion that the ends cannot be reached directly by the means. Indeed, a key difference between military activities (e.g., guerrilla or special operations) and acts of terror is that terrorism takes place "on a stage" with an audience in mind (Rubin & Friedland, 1986; Jenkins, 1975). Unlike most guerrilla attacks or special operations, an act of terrorism is usually of little military value but instead "sends a message" to the target audience, for example, in drawing attention to a historical grievance or discrediting hated authorities (Schmid, Jongman, & Stohl, 1988). Even the most horrific of recent terrorist acts—Kenya and Tanzania in 1998, Washington and New York in 2001, Madrid in March 2004—are insignificant in military terms. They are, however, powerful and vivid messages from terrorist groups writ in blood and carnage.[1]

Delivering such a message in a shocking, sensational fashion is meant to catalyze political change, and it is inarguable that dramatic political change has been spawned by these acts. Terrorism can therefore be seen as a form of social influence, employing acts of extranormal violence (instead of leaflets or loudspeakers, for example) to influence a target population's emotions, motives, objective reasoning, perceptions, and ultimately, behavior. Social influence is normally instantiated in tools and techniques such as rumor, social proof, radio and television broadcasts, posters, and graffiti. However, violence itself can be a dramatic medium for changing attitudes and perceptions. Nothing in the definition of social influence prohibits the consideration of extranormal violence as a tool of attitude and behavioral change. Thus a well-timed bit of sabotage that disables a banking system may bolster an effort to worsen an already shaky economic situation. Similarly, direct action that prevents police or fire-fighting personnel from responding to an explosion may help discredit those two agencies. In sum, virtually any form of violence may be pressed into the service of social influence so long as the goal is to manipulate a target audience's perceptions, cognitions, and actions. Terrorism fits the description. Hoffman (1998) states:

> Terrorism is specifically designed to have far-reaching psychological effects beyond the

immediate victim(s) or object of the terrorist attack. It is meant to instill fear within, and thereby intimidate, a wider "target audience" that might include a rival ethnic or religious group, an entire country, a national government or political party, or public opinion in general. . . . Through the publicity generated by their violence, terrorists seek to obtain the leverage, influence and power they otherwise lack to effect political change on either a local or an international scale.

Sudden, shocking acts of extranormal violence are the medium for producing these psychological effects, and this is a potent means of communicating. There is ample historical precedent to support this assertion (Bell, 1978; Downes-Le Guin & Hoffman, 1993). For example, the Reagan administration felt compelled to facilitate the release of more than 700 Shiite prisoners from Israeli prisons in exchange for the 39 Americans aboard TWA 847, which was hijacked in 1985. Why? After more than 2 weeks of intense coverage by the news media, there was widespread support among the American public for a nonviolent quid pro quo ending. This domestic pressure (a deliberate and explicit goal of the hijackers) proved irresistible to the Reagan administration.

There are many such historical examples of terrorism producing political change through social influence, and these examples will ineluctably lead to future imitators. The presence of so many potential targets, civilians, and news media is a powerful attractant to would-be terrorists, and they are virtually guaranteed a wide audience both domestically and internationally for their message.

Social Influence Campaigns

Four hostile newspapers are more to be feared than a thousand bayonets.
    General Burnod, *Military Maxims of Napoleon*

For our purposes, we may state that a social influence campaign is generally characterized by the following features:

• One individual, group, or government (A) communicates with another person, group, or government (B) on multiple occasions.

• The communications from A to B are purposive: They are meant to galvanize specific changes in attitudes and behaviors. That said, they may operate directly or indirectly (i.e., propagated in some fashion through a third party or mediated through another cognitive process).

• The communications from A to B are discrete and finite and can be characterized by a channel or medium of communication.

Although widespread understanding and appreciation of the importance of social influence campaigns spans the historical record, their scientific study dates from the pioneering work of Carl Hovland and his colleagues during and after World War II (the famous "Yale model" of persuasion, based on learning theory). Since that time much excellent work has been done, and we draw on it in examining the particulars of historical terrorism. The Yale model of social influence can serve at least as a broad-strokes description of the structure of a large-scale persuasion attempt (for how an audience internalizes and processes it, we incorporate more recent scientific work, such as Petty and Cacioppo's Elaboration Likelihood Model). As the following discussion points out, many terrorist campaigns can be usefully thought of in these terms, and specific acts of terrorism can be thought of as the individual communications in the course of a social influence campaign. A noteworthy qualifier to this characterization is the fact that these communications have decidedly different intentions and are meant to reach multiple populations.

There are two broad dimensions of the Yale model: the process of persuasion and the variables of persuasion. As the Yale model suggests (Hovland, Janis, & Kelley, 1953; many subsequent reports), a look at the process of any social influence attempt will reveal six stages (exposure, attention, comprehension, acceptance, retention, and translation) that must be navigated to successfully persuade a target audience. When examining the outcomes of the persuasion attempt, there will be four types of independent variable (source, message, target, and channel).

A Process View of Social Influence

• *Exposure.* The first stage required to translate influence into desired action is exposure. In general, exposure requires that the message reach the audience; for example, an elaborate radio campaign is useless if the target audience does not listen to the station that broadcasts the communication. To achieve the intended psychological objectives, a communicator must transmit the persuasive message through the correct channel to the appropriate audience (by appropriate, we mean the audience that can directly or indirectly produce the desired response).

* *Attention.* Even if the message is transmitted through the correct channels, the appropriate audience still might not notice it. Attention can sometimes be difficult to achieve. The world is a noisy place: New messages compete with contradictory information and sheer background noise, which can drown out an otherwise persuasive communication.[2] The message should be crafted to pierce this surrounding noise and suit the channel through which it is transmitted (Klapper, 1960).

* *Comprehension.* An influence campaign must ensure that the intended audience understands the persuasive communication. This requires the communicator to craft and deliver the message in a culturally appropriate manner, employing syntax, images, words, concepts, and intentions that are tailored to the audience. Notably, a message that is linguistically or idiomatically ill suited will likely fail and may even be counterproductive (Eagly, 1974). This stage poses a significant hurdle for terrorism in terms of social influence.

* *Acceptance.* The target audience must not only comprehend the message but also accept it. Indeed, a well-crafted message can be transmitted, noticed, and comprehended but still trigger instant rejection by audiences if it is not articulated to gain their acceptance (Chaiken, 1987; Chaiken, Liberman, & Eagly, 1989; Petty and Cacioppo, 1986). One example of how this rejection might occur involves the inappropriate use of schemas.[3] A widely disseminated message advertising a bounty on a wanted fugitive might seem entirely reasonable to the sender, but to a target audience the very notion of a bounty (i.e., the "bounty" schema) may invoke all manner of negative—even taboo—associations relating to hospitality norms, kinship ties, and group affiliation,

which in turn leads to quick and decisive rejection of the message. This stage is perhaps the single most important obstacle in the way of terrorism as a vector of social influence.

* *Retention.* Even an influential message must have a durable effect on the target audiences; "durable" here means that the audience remembers the persuasive message long enough for the desired behavior to emerge at a propitious time (Hovland, Lumsdaine, & Sheffield, 1949). Notably, the retention requirements of an influence campaign depend on its objectives. A few minutes may be long enough to galvanize the surrender of a hostage taker holed up in a barricaded house, but a few years may be needed to reduce monetary support to a government or a popular social movement. In the context of terrorism, a clear example of success in navigating the retention stage is the train bombings in Madrid in March 2004. This act of terror took place 3 days before a national election and utterly eclipsed all other issues in the race for the following 3 days. The shocking and horrific acts, which the public interpreted as a punishment for Spanish support of the U.S. invasion of Iraq, indisputably affected the outcome of the election.

* *Translation.* Translation entails cognitive change leading to behavioral change or the translation of perception into action. For translation to occur, an unobstructed path must exist for a changed attitude to result in altered behavior (see, for example, Darley & Batson, 1973). The target audience may truly experience a change in attitude, yet be restrained by repressive societies and/or authoritarian leaders. The literature on social psychology indicates that circumstances strongly influence actual decision making.[4] Thus, influence attempts have a greater possibility of success if they are conducted in an environment that facilitates the translation of changes in attitude into changed behavior.

This sequence represents a view of the *process* of a social influence campaign. Another view of social influence comes from Smith, Lasswell, and Casey (1946), who state that the outcomes of any persuasion attempt are dependent upon the characteristics of four types of independent variable: source, recipient, message, and medium. There is significant interplay between these categories and the particulars of the process described earlier.

- *Source.* The apparent origin of a message can matter significantly in how it is received by an audience. Relevant data about the originator of the communication include factors such as credibility (Kelman & Hovland, 1953; Husek, 1965), authority (McGuire, 1969; Bochner & Insko, 1966), likeability and attractiveness (Chaiken, 1979), similarity to the recipient (Byrne, 1971; Goethals & Nelson, 1973), trustworthiness (Andreoli & Worchel, 1978), and perceived profit motive (Hovland & Mandell, 1952).
- *Recipient.* Several characteristics of a target audience can weigh heavily in how the message is perceived and processed. These variables include motivation (Petty, Harkins, & Williams, 1980), issue involvement (Petty & Cacioppo, 1979), and culture (Eagly & Warren, 1976).
- *Message.* As many of these sequential steps imply, the content and nature of a message will figure prominently in its ultimate effect. The relevant qualities of a message can include salience and vividness (Taylor & Fiske, 1975), emotional content (e.g., fear; see Janis & Feshbach, 1953; Leventhal, 1970), the number of arguments (Calder, Insko, & Yandell, 1974; Norman, 1976), and others.
- *Medium.* The medium plays an important role in delivering and mediating the effects of the actual message. Some media are particularly effective vectors of persuasive communications, while others lend themselves less to this function. Among the characteristics that matter in the choice of medium are style (e.g., audio versus video; see Chaiken & Eagly, 1976), setting (e.g., one on one versus group; see Burnstein & Vinokur, 1977), and nonverbal accompaniment (Harper, Weins, & Matarazzo, 1978).

In the following sections we highlight social influence variables in historical cases of terrorism to help us understand when and how terrorism is effective. Our argument is that the requirements for effective social influence are virtually identical to those for successful terrorism (in the sense of achieving the stated political aims).

Terrorism as Social Influence

Kill one, warn a thousand.
  Chinese proverb

It is not possible to adequately treat all historical terrorism within a single section of a single chapter. Moreover, the very word *terrorism* was coined by Edmund Burke to describe state terror: the government's "reign of terror" in revolutionary France (1793–1794). In fact, Robespierre opined that "Terror is nothing other than justice, prompt, severe, inflexible; it is therefore an emanation of virtue." These views clearly differ quite markedly from how the word is commonly used today (to denote a criminal atrocity perpetrated against noncombatants for political and/or ideological ends). In this chapter we do not embrace either view of terrorism. Instead we examine terrorism as a persuasive instrument of marginal, revolutionary, or nonstate groups seeking significant political change (not perpetuating the status quo). We sample the space of historical terrorism for illustrations of the violence-as-social-influence theme, and we argue that this perspective on terrorism is applicable and fruitful in helping us to understand the rise and fall of terrorist campaigns in all times and places.

Terrorist acts by definition include some key aspects of persuasive communication, as we have already outlined:

- *Transmission and propagation.* The nature of the international news media virtually guarantees that target audiences will be *exposed* to the terrorists' message (step 1 of the Yale model). The proliferation of and competition among news outlets has created a 24-hour news cycle in order to satisfy the public's appetite for sensational news and competitive advantage (i.e., items not possessed by competitors). This means that, day or night, virtually anywhere in the world, there will be a near-instantaneous transmission of news of terrorist acts to millions of viewers, listeners, and readers—with a subsequent multiplication as coverage continues or is rebroadcast.
- *Vividness.* By their shocking nature, terrorist acts capitalize on the salience effect (Nisbett & Ross, 1980), ensuring that target audiences pay *attention* to the message (step 2 of the Yale model).

• *Fear Content*. Horrifying acts of murder and mayhem are exemplars of fear-based communication. A fear-based message can be very persuasive when calibrated correctly (Leventhal, 1970; Rogers & Mewborn, 1976; Rogers, 1983): It must clearly depict the possible consequences of not heeding the message and the likely avoidance of those consequences if the message is heeded; moreover, the audience must perceive itself as able to act upon the message. Terrorists can often raise or lower the level of fear at will (e.g., by phoning or not phoning in a threat before setting off a bomb), which gives them control over most of these factors.

• *Dual processing*. Terrorist acts are both simple and complex messages: The violence is usually accompanied by lengthy manifestos or statements advocating the terrorist group's ideology (e.g., Osama bin Laden's 1996 declaration of jihad against the United States). The terrorist act and any accompanying statement may be processed both by peripheral and central routes (the Elaboration Likelihood Model of Petty and Cacioppo [1996]). By this we mean that an act of terrorism can be a persuasive communication whether it is thought about systematically (e.g., reading a terrorist manifesto and evaluating its merits) or heuristically (e.g., witnessing an act of terror on TV and interpreting it as evidence of the current government's fragility and illegitimacy). This greatly furthers the goal of communicating with multiple audiences through a single discrete act.

• *Credibility and power*. Terrorism usually occurs at the initiative of a terrorist group. By this we mean that the terrorist group can turn the violence on or off and choose the timing, place, and manner of attacks. This is probably sufficient to establish the group as a credible source and thus an important contributor to the persuasiveness of its message among those who are processing it peripherally.[5]

• *Authority and legitimacy*. Wielding the power of life and death can place the terrorist group in the same cognitive frame as the government it opposes, a goal uppermost in the minds of many terrorist groups. They would like to be seen as an authority equivalent-but-adversary to the organization they oppose (and thus the agent of the people they purport to represent), while those same governments or authorities would like to depict the terrorists as criminal lunatics at the fringes of society, representing no one. This is not an idle struggle: With a perception of authority comes very real power to persuade (Hofling, Brotzman, Dalrymple, Graves, & Pierce, 1966; Milgram, 1974; Peters & Ceci, 1982; Blass, 1991, 1999).

• *Stoking "avoidant" motivation*. To the target audience among whom political change is to be catalyzed, the message of terrorism is one that emphasizes loss and suffering (e.g., obey us, or we will wreak more havoc and carnage upon you). Persuasion attempts that emphasize loss are more effective than those highlight gain (Meyerowitz & Chaiken, 1987). Seeking to prevent losses—"avoidant motivation"—is a powerful force for attitude change and action.

The Means of Communication: Bullets, Not Ballots

Not all violent acts constitute terrorism. For example, neither armed robbery nor mercenary activity would typically qualify as terrorism. The key element in defining an act as terrorist or not is its *instrumentality*. Is the violence meant to express an idea or serve a political/social/theological movement, and does it do so by harming civilians? If so, then, by most definitions, it is terrorism. When terrorist groups are deciding on a violent course of action, they always calculate the expressive or instrumental value of the violence.

Among the types of violent actions that can be considered terrorist are assassinations, bombings, kidnapping, torture, and intimidatory violence (e.g., kneecapping), arson, lynchings, and virtually any use of weapons of mass destruction (WMD) against a civilian populace. Aside from considering how the audience might receive the "message" of a violent act, terrorist groups are greatly interested in the milieu and how it might affect the processing of the meaning. This is not an idle concern. Much scientific work has been done on environmental factors and how they mitigate the transmission and impact of persuasive messages. This can include cognitive load and ambient noise (Brünken, Steinbacher, Plass, & Leutner, 2002), countermessages (Papageorgis & McGuire,

1961; McGuire, 1964), social proof and conformity (Latané & Darley, 1970; Latané & Nida, 1981; Tesser, Campbell, & Mickler, 1983; Wooten & Reed, 1998), and time pressure (Petty, Wells, & Brock, 1976).[6] Terrorist groups go to great lengths to exert control over the environment in which their message is transmitted and received; for example, they provide journalists with firsthand videotapes of attacks in order to ensure that their version—not the government's version—of events dominates the airwaves. All in all, with regard to other forms of social influence, it is the variables associated with the target audience that matter most in the psychological effect of terrorism.

The Target Audiences: At Whom Is Terrorism Aimed?

There will always be multiple audiences for any act of terrorism. In broad theoretical terms, these can be thought of in two distinct categories: the group on whose behalf the act is carried out (the constituency) and the group against whom the act is directed (the enemy). In practice, there will be some nuances and third-party effects, which is to say that some audiences may be proxies for others (e.g., attacking McDonald's as a symbol of the United States) or mediate the message in some way (e.g., attacking the UN to intimidate a wide array of international actors). That said, the effectiveness of a terrorist campaign—as is the case in any social influence campaign—is directly related to how well the author of the violent communication knows the target audience. Specifically, the critical knowledge is the way in which the target audience processes information and acts upon it.

The Constituency: The Group or Population for Whom the Terrorism Is Conducted

Virtually every group engaged in a campaign of terror draws support from a broad base of active and passive supporters; this is Fraserand Fulton's pyramidal model (1984). The number of full-time operatives (the acme of the pyramid) is quite small compared to the number of people needed to provide money, intelligence, safe haven, forged documents, munitions, transportation, and the like (the base of the pyramid). Moreover, beyond the active supporters are the vast numbers of like-minded people necessary to sustain the group over

time and propel the revolutionary movement from the margins of power to the center. This large population is perceived as the *constituency* of any terrorist group, which desires that the constituency view the acts of terror in a positive way. Indeed, the acts of terror are intended to be seen as blows struck on behalf of the constituency, in its name and for its betterment. For the Liberation Tigers of Tamil Elaam, the constituency is the 3–4 million Tamils chafing under Sinhalese rule on the island of Sri Lanka. For the Provisional Irish Republican Army, the constituency is the Catholic majority living in Northern Ireland. For al-Qaeda, the constituency is Muslims around the world, particularly Sunnis. Examples of simple messages aimed at the constituency in acts of terror are the following:

- Only through violent resistance can we accomplish our ends. Negotiation is capitulation to tyranny.
- Witness that our enemies are not invulnerable and that we are capable of injuring them.

Terrorist groups usually live or die based upon how well they communicate with their constituency; it would be fair to state that the power and resilience of any terrorist group greatly reflects the effectiveness of the social influence campaign used on its constituency. As Martha Crenshaw has pointed out (1981, 1991), when terrorist groups alienate, fail to motivate, or misread the mandate of the constituency, they are very likely to wither and dissolve. For example, alienation can occur when the acts of terror are excessively or wantonly brutal (such as a white supremacist shooting up a Jewish preschool and killing several children). Failure to motivate might take the form of simply receiving insufficient money or recruits from the constituency: The appeal for support is falling on deaf ears, as has been the case for Communist terrorist groups in Europe in recent years. Misreading the mandate of the constituency is a classic mistake; since the acts of terror are vicarious blows struck on behalf of the constituency, they must be aimed where the constituency would like them to fall. Bombings that kill the constituency's children are obviously in danger of misreading the mandate of the constituency (particularly among secular groups).

The Enemy: The Group or Population Against Whom the Terrorism Is Conducted

Since terrorist groups are almost always incapable of achieving the military defeat of their adversaries, the acts of terror must aim at one of Clausewitz's "centers of gravity," namely, the political will of the opposition. In practice this means creating sufficient pain, aversion, or disincentive on the part of the decision makers in the enemy authority to elicit political change and even revolution. This is clearly a tall order, though not at all impossible. In fact, there are many cases of campaigns of terror accomplishing this very thing (e.g., in Palestine [1948], Algeria [1962], Lebanon [2000], Sri Lanka [2001], and Spain [2004]). For two reasons it is usually easier to accomplish this goal in democratic societies than in authoritarian ones. First, it is easier to inflict harm on a population than on its leadership. Second, the leadership of democratic societies is more responsive and subject to the will of the population than authoritarian societies. Thus, when terrorism occurs and the population is injured, it is democratic leaders who generally must concern themselves most with the consequences.

A cunning terrorist group uses acts of violence to create or exploit fault lines between enemy decision makers and the population they control. This form of social influence campaign is almost the exact inverse of the campaign aimed at the terrorist group's constituency: In the former, the group is attempting to fracture and fragment support for the ruling authority and its political positions (e.g., maintaining a colonial outpost in a distant land), while in the latter case the group is trying to draw support from and unify often diverse groups and interests (e.g., to eject a colonial power from native territory). Examples of simple messages aimed at the enemy in acts of terror may include the following:

- The colonial government is weak and cannot control its possessions.
- You can expect more of this. The resistance will continue to kill colonial representatives until they depart.
- Since you have placed us all under your yoke, *all* of the members of the colonial empire will be made targets.

As we mentioned earlier, the durability and capability of terrorist groups is often based directly upon the social influence campaign aimed at their constituency. The success or failure of the terrorism depends upon the effectiveness of the social

influence campaign aimed at the enemy. This seems obvious, but it is often eclipsed by other concerns: technology, criminality, rationality, body counts, and so forth. These elements are important, but they do not determine the outcome of terrorist campaigns.

Historical Terrorism

In the following historical survey we highlight some of the key elements identified in the previous section, specifically those that are critical to the outcomes of terrorist campaigns. For a more comprehensive and detailed view of terrorism, there are excellent textbooks and monographs covering all aspects of historical terrorism, and interested readers will find some suggested readings in the bibliography.

Terrorism From Antiquity to World War II

Terrorism as acts of violence by marginal or revolutionary movements has ancient roots, and, though the particulars—the weapons and the causes—have changed, the fundamental nature of terrorism has not.

A group that would certainly be considered terrorist by today's prevailing standards were the Zealots of first-century Judea. They opposed Roman rule and conspired to topple it. Extreme elements among the Zealots assassinated Romans and Roman collaborators in order to catalyze both a reluctance among the indigenous populace to work for or with the Romans and to effect a Roman withdrawal in the long run. What makes these assassinations terrorist acts and social influence as we have defined them is the choice of location: densely populated public areas, such as marketplaces. Without a printing press (much less radio, TV, the Internet, and the like), the only sure way of quickly communicating a shocking act of violence to a large number of people was to carry them out in crowded public spaces. The Zealots knew that their assassinations would never amount to a telling or even a painful military blow to the Roman occupation, but they hoped the acts would nevertheless bring about the desired political change.

As we have already stated, there is often more than one audience for terrorist action; that is, terrorists usually attempt to influence more than one group at a time with a single violent action. Zealot violence was a medium of communicating with distinct target audiences—Romans, their actual and potential Jewish collaborators, and other Jews yearning to be relieved of the imperial yoke. For the Romans, the message was a statement of dedicated resistance and defiance; for actual and potential collaborators it was a frightening warning; for other Jews it was an invitation to rally and a vicarious act of insurrection. The simplicity and ardor of the message, delivered in a violent and shocking manner, elevated the status of the Zealots from fringe group to leading element of the revolt against Rome (A.D. 66–70).

The prototype for modern terrorism and terrorists is found in the Narodnaya Volya (People's Will) movement of Tsarist Russia in the latter part of the nineteenth century. The Narodnaya Volya was composed of anarchists who followed in the footsteps of prominent antitsarist revolutionaries such as Mikhail Bakunin and Sergey Nechaev. While many socialists and anarchists believed in (peaceful) revolutionary change, Bakunin and those who followed him felt that violence was the key to beginning a powerful wave of political chaos that would shatter the government.

The Narodnaya Volya carried out numerous assassinations (including that of Tsar Alexander II) to produce such an effect among the masses and state agencies; it was not the violence, but rather its psychological effect, that was their objective. How was such an outcome to be produced? Just as a key instrument of terrorism—dynamite—was a product of the late nineteenth century, so too was the second requisite component of terrorism: the rotary press and the ability to mass-produce inexpensive pamphlets and newspapers for public consumption. As Schmid and de Graaf have noted (1982), for marginal groups bent on catalyzing political change, the debut of mass media created an opportunity for "expressive violence," in which the savagery and its immediate consequences were the instrument to an end. In the case of terrorism, the end is always an extreme form of social influence: radical change in attitudes and behaviors.

From the Zealots to the Narodnaya Volya, what makes the terrorist is the terrorism: This is not an attempt at glibness but rather a recognition that it is the "expressive" component of "expressive violence" that transforms terrorism into an act of persuasive communication. It is "propaganda by the deed," as nineteenth-century revolutionary Paule Brousse termed it in an 1877 article of the same name. This communication is no less than a campaign of social influence.

Proxy, Anticolonial, and International Terrorism: World War II to 1980

Terrorism became commonplace in the decades following World War II. The major forces driving this evolution were the Cold War, anticolonialism, and the growth of international, televised media.

As a result of the Cold War, direct confrontation between the competing superpowers of the East Bloc and the West was avoided for the obvious reason of preventing a battle that might escalate to a nuclear conflict. This led to a booming market in proxy battles around the globe, replete with a massive flow of monies and weaponry. Besides installing and equipping murderous despots with the means to engage in state terror (e.g., U.S. support to the shah of Iran), it also led to the establishment of insurgent armed groups throughout Latin America, Africa, Europe, and Asia (e.g., Red Army Faction, Red Brigades). Many of these groups engaged in a full range of terrorist actions in the course of their struggles as they sought to sever the existing government's relationship with its supporters in the general population while building their own base of support and legitimacy. As proxies for the United States and the Soviets, these groups were able to generate international shock waves and gain political ground among the larger populace as a sure means of gaining continued support from their sponsor (key constituency).

Closely linked to the advent of the Cold War was the dissolution of colonial empires and the founding of nationalist groups seeking to expel foreign masters. In colonial outposts in Latin America, Africa, the Middle East, and Asia, the French, English, German, Japanese, and other empire-building nations suddenly found the natives restless. In the case of the Germans and the Japanese, the issue was who would devour the pieces of their dismembered dominions. For nationalist, anticolonial groups seeking to restore sovereignty or seize power in their own countries, the time was ripe, but their resources were limited, and conventional warfare against the countries that had survived World War II was out of the question. Hence the resort to terrorism. Terrorist acts would be used to force the colonial powers to rethink the price of ownership while rallying indigenous support to the cause.

The final ingredient to the rise of terrorism in the Cold War/post–World War II period was the explosion in international media. In the early nineteenth century, the fastest a message could be carried depended on the speed of a horse, and its reach was constrained by the number and range of the riders. By the late nineteenth century, messages were propagated instantaneously by wireless. With the advent of mass radio and then television broadcasting in the twentieth century came the ability to inform large numbers of people quickly. Moreover, the driving force behind much of the new mass media was a profit motive—and with it a need to grab and hold audiences. As the journalistic adage goes, "Bad news is good news, good news is bad news, and no news is also bad news." Terrorist acts are sensational and decidedly bad news and thus perfect fodder for media outlets seeking sales, readers, listeners, and viewers.

A prime example of terrorism in this period is that used by the Zionist groups in Palestine. As Menachem Begin has recounted in his autobiography, *The Revolt* (1972), Zionist groups studied the British government's decision-making process in the battle against Irish separatism and decided that a campaign of terror in the post–World War II environment would weaken domestic British support for a colonial presence in Palestine. Further, these acts of terror would both galvanize the Jewish population in the quest for a sovereign Jewish state and drive fearful Arab residents (Palestinians) into exile. The Zionist groups reasoned that a campaign of terror would be broadcast to a British public that was weary of conflict and war and eager to be relieved of a distant colonial outpost of little obvious value to the nation. The Zionists believed that the public would ultimately pressure the government to pull out. Indeed, British authorities turned to the UN for a solution that would relieve them of the increasing human costs of colonial control and thus became midwife to the civil war that brought about the state of Israel.

Other examples of terrorist tactics in the post–World War II period include the urban warfare fought by the Algerian Front de Libération Natio-

nale (FLN) against their French colonial masters (1954–1962) and by the Viet Cong against U.S. invaders during the Vietnam War (1962–1975). In both cases, small cells of insurgents planted bombs and threw grenades into areas crowded with combatants and noncombatants alike in order to exact a heavy human toll on the foreign occupiers. This price would never grow to an amount that the military decision makers could ill afford, but they were not the population targeted for influence. Rather, the cost in human lives brought about by the terrorism would be transmitted by the international media to the French and U.S. populations respectively, who in turn would exert pressure on their leaders to forego further loss.

The Rise of Religious Terror: 1980 to the Present

Conventional terrorism is violent communication aimed at a constituent population as well as an enemy population, but religious terrorism adds another audience: God. Under this model, terrorist acts are considered holy acts that are performed in the name of religious devotion, often to fulfill sacred edicts or bring about apocalyptic scenarios. This changes the calculus of terrorism significantly: Many of the constraints or earthly concerns that attempted to match the deed to the audience's perceptions and cognitions are removed, eclipsed by the absolutism of religious piety. As Hoffman has noted (1995), secular or nationalist terrorist groups act within the prevailing international political framework and wish to replace the existing order with another one. Since earthly audiences are involved, secular terror necessitates some degree of adherence to international norms relating to proportionality and precision of violence. Not so for religious terror. "Winning" is not measured in earthly (political, social, or economic) terms but rather in theological terms, which tend to be absolute, uncompromising, and not subject to normative constraints.[7] To religious terrorists, killing is a sacred act, not a political act.

Terrorism of the religious sort still very much includes a social influence component, but because the objective of political or social change is reduced and the element of religious change (martyrdom, apocalypse) is introduced, the aspect of social influence is generally narrowed to polarization and rallying. That is, the rhetoric of religious terrorism is uncompromising and divisive, resulting in faith-based, simplistic, good-versus-evil arguments. For the faithful or potential recruits this is an opportunity to join the forces of good; for those not swayed by the appeal, there is only confrontation or acquiescence—compromise is not possible. Consider, for example, the difference between two large, accomplished terrorist groups: the Liberation Tigers of Tamil Eelam (LTTE) and Hamas. As a predominately secular, ethnonationalist group, the LTTE is willing to negotiate with the Sri Lankan government; as a strictly religious and anti-Zionist group, Hamas is rarely able or inclined to find common ground with the Israeli government.

One superb example of religious terrorism today is Aum Shinrikyō. Between 1989 and 1995, this Japanese group murdered roughly 100 people and injured thousands, with the explicit intention of starting an apocalyptic war that would kill millions. Their goal was to usher in a new era that would see existing civilization destroyed, creating a blank slate that Aum could then use to create a utopian successor society. By the time Japanese authorities bestirred themselves to act against Aum, it had acquired thousands of zealous members, finances in excess of $100 million, extensive media operations, as well as businesses and land holdings in numerous countries. Aum scientists and engineers had developed, weaponized, and attacked civilians with anthrax bacillus, botulinum bacillus, and several types of nerve gas, poisons, and mind-altering drugs. Moreover, they had avidly been pursuing nuclear weaponry in the former republics of the Soviet Union. The leader and founder of Aum Shinrikyō was Shoko Asahara (born Chizuo Matsumoto), an undisputed and all-powerful guru, a self-styled prophet and messiah with an eschatological worldview and an unshakable grip on his followers. The acts of terror conducted by Aum members were constrained only by the will and approbation of God (as interpreted and related by Asahara).

Of course, no discussion of contemporary religious terrorism can or should avoid al-Qaeda and its affiliates. To understand the polarizing ideology, language, and actions of al-Qaeda, one should examine the lengthy treatises and polemics issued by Osama bin Laden and others, including his "declaration of jihad against the United States" (1996), and Ayman Zawahiri's "Knight Under the Prophet's Banner" (2001). An example of this language from bin Laden's 1998 *fatwa* (an opinion issued by a Muslim scholar) suffices to illustrate the principles outlined earlier, namely, that earthly audiences and norms no longer establish the appropriate guidelines for action:

> The ruling to kill Americans and their allies—civilians and military—is an individual duty for every Muslim who can do it in every country in which it is possible to do it. . . . We—with God's help—call on every Muslim who believes in God and wishes to be rewarded to comply with God's order to kill the Americans and plunder their money wherever and whenever you can find them.

There is clearly little room for empathy, negotiation, compromise, or hesitation in bin Laden's message. Al-Qaeda and its affiliates use sacred violence as an instrument of social influence, but the message and its parameters are inflexible and divisive. This means the constituency is limited to Muslims who accept bin Laden's authority and reasoning; the enemy population will be everyone else (most of whom are demonized or devalued under al-Qaeda's ideology). The third audience—the divine—is characterized by al-Qaeda's theology as sanctioning exactly this sort of dichotomous worldview and the unfettered violence that springs from it.

Conclusion: The "Persuasiveness" of Terrorist Acts

Terrorism works. It works the way advertising and marketing work; when an effective social influence campaign is well designed and well executed and when externalities do not interfere with or supersede the persuasion attempt, audiences react as desired. From the constituency audience, terrorist groups receive recruits, money, and a wide variety of logistical support. From the enemy audience, terrorist groups can directly or indirectly wrest political change, ranging from legitimacy and negotiation to utter revolution. So, outside of hoping that terrorists will undo their own cause by overreaching or be hindered by an environment that disrupts their campaign, is there anything else that can be done?

The answer is "yes." Terrorism and terrorist groups are vulnerable the way other forms of social influence campaigns and their originators are vulnerable. Consider the hundreds of billions of dollars that are spent each year on advertising and marketing campaigns within the United States alone; some campaigns are poorly constructed, and some are lost in the noise of the marketplace, but others are mitigated or effectively neutralized by competition and countercampaigns. For example, the six largest cigarette manufacturers together spent more than $11 billion on domestic advertising in 2001 ("FTC Cigarette Report for 2001," 2003). While they clearly do not employ violence as an instrument of social influence, their goals are not unlike those of terrorist groups in that they both perceive an enemy audience and a constituency audience. Blum (1989) has aptly summarized these goals of the cigarette manufacturers' advertising (social influence) campaigns:

- Recruit new smokers (constituency)
- Sustain existing smoking "membership" (constituency)
- Obtain protection and facilitation from legislators and opinion leaders (constituency)
- Associate smoking with positive values and social goods such as personal independence and self-sufficiency (constituency)
- Pull former smokers back in (constituency), or neutralize them as adversaries (enemy)
- Neutralize antismoking forces such as journalists and hostile legislators (enemy)

As powerful and pervasive as cigarette companies' social influence campaigns are, they can be undone by countercampaigns and milieu control (e.g., legislative action). These countermeasures can work at every step of the Yale process model (exposure, attention, comprehension, acceptance, retention, and translation) and each of the Yale independent variables (source, target, message, and medium). For example, countercampaigns can

- use fear-based messages (regarding health) to get smokers to quit and nonsmokers to never start (Insko, Arkoff, & Insko, 1965)
- affect the baseline social norms to prevent prosmoking campaigns from controlling the milieu (Worden & Flynn, 2002)
- parasitize pro-smoking ads to reduce their effectiveness (Cialdini, Demaine, Barrett, Sagarin, & Rhoads, in preparation). By "parasitize," we mean employ similar motifs and formats

(e.g., the Marlboro Man) but with reversed messages.
- reduce the credibility and likeability of the cigarette companies and, by association, their products (Goldman & Glantz, 1998).

These are just a few examples of countercampaigns that can be employed against the juggernaut of cigarette advertising. They are made possible by a careful analysis of the social influence elements manipulated by cigarette advertising and marketing campaigns, followed by the subsequent crafting of disruptive countermeasures suited to the analysis. We contend that a careful analysis of terrorism as social influence campaigns will yield a foundation for psychological countermeasures that can mitigate or thwart the psychological effects of terror as they propagate through the population and the media. These countermeasures can take the form of more effective risk communication by governmental agencies, better reporting by journalists, increased resilience in the population as a whole, better education of opinion leaders, a discrediting of terrorist groups, and many others.

To illustrate these principles with an example from successful counterterrorism campaigns, consider the last bullet point above on potential countercampaigns: reducing the credibility and likeability of the adversary and, by extension, its activities and products. This tactic has been used, albeit somewhat crudely and nonscientifically, in the past against terrorist groups:

Emilio Aguinaldo, who headed an insurrection against occupying U.S. forces in the Philippines at the start of the twentieth century, was captured and induced to sign an oath of loyalty to the United States. This greatly reduced his stature among his constituents, and the insurrection sputtered soon thereafter.

Abdullah Ocalan, who led the Kurdistan Workers Party (Partiya Karkeran Kurdistan [PKK]; 1984–1999) in terrorist acts against Turkey in order to create an autonomous Kurdish state, was captured. Turkish authorities induced him to publicly plead for a ceasefire and for his own life, which diminished his stature and credibility. As a result, the PKK's campaign soon ground to a halt.

Abimael Guzmán, who, during the 1980s, was the leader of the powerful Sendero Luminoso

(Shining Path) group of Peru, was captured in 1992. Paraded before the public in a cage and induced by the authorities into publicly pleading for his life and a ceasefire, Guzmán suffered a tremendous loss of authority and credibility among his constituency. Within 2 years of his arrest, thousands of Shining Path guerrillas had turned themselves in under a government amnesty program.

Notes

1. We use the term "terrorist group" to mean simply any group or institution that carries out acts of terrorism as we have defined them here. It is the act and not the ideology that makes terrorists. Moreover, terrorist acts are aimed at noncombatants alone. Many governments label assaults against them or their militaries as "terrorism," but this is inaccurate and propagandistic: Attacks on governmental or military targets are guerrilla warfare, not terrorism.

2. For more information, see Drolet and Aaker (2002).

3. Schemas are mental arrays of associated ideas, characteristics, and perceptions. They are used as cognitive shortcuts to reduce the burden of deep thinking and to quicken reactions. This peripheral (versus central) processing of information can have great utility—quickly associating smoke with fire has survival value—but can also be problematic (Hass, 1981). Racial or ethnic stereotypes are common examples of harmful schemas.

4. For more information on the how the environment affects decision making, see Asch (1953); Lasswell (1948); Janis (1982); and Petty and Cacioppo (1986).

5. Source credibility is among the most complex variables that figure in the outcome of persuasion attempts. A careful summary of the issues and research can be found in Petty and Cacioppo (1996).

6. "Cognitive load" is the significant encumbrance of an individual's working memory. "Ambient noise" refers to a low signal-to-noise ratio.

7. In an excellent example of this point, White (2002) points to the lesson taught by the biblical story of Joshua in the siege of Ai (Joshua 8:24–28). God orders Joshua to kill first the warriors of Ai and then every inhabitant of the city—young and old, male and female.

References

Andreoli, V., & Worchel, S. (1978). Effects of media, communicator, and position of message on attitude change. *Public Opinion Quarterly, 42*(1), 59–70.

Asch, S. (1953). Effects of group pressure upon the modification and distortion of judgments. In D. Cartwright & A. Zander (Eds.), *Group dynamics: Research and theory* (pp. 607–623). Evanston, IL: Peterson.

Begin, M. (1972). *The revolt.* Los Angeles: Nash.

Bell, J. B. (1978). *A time of terror: How democratic societies respond to revolutionary violence.* New York: Basic Books.

bin Laden, Osama. (1998, February 23). "Fatwa." *Al Quds al 'Arabi.* n. p.

Blass, T. (1991). Understanding behavior in the Milgram obedience experiment. *Journal of Personality and Social Psychology, 60,* 398–413.

———. (1999). The Milgram paradigm after 35 years: Some things we know about obedience to authority. *Journal of Applied Social Psychology, 29,* 955–978.

Blum, A. (1989). The targeting of minority groups by the tobacco industry. In L. A. Jones (Ed.), *Minorities and cancer* (pp. 153–163). New York: Springer.

Bochner, S., & Insko, C. (1966). Communicator discrepancy, source credibility, and opinion change. *Journal of Personality and Social Psychology, 4,* 614–621.

Brünken, R., Steinbacher, S., Plass, J. L., & Leutner, D. (2002). Assessment of cognitive load in multimedia learning using dual-task methodology. *Experimental Psychology, 49,* 109–119.

Burnstein, E., & Vinokur, A. (1977). Persuasive argumentation and social comparison as determinants of attitude polarization. *Journal of Experimental Social Psychology, 13,* 315–332.

Byrne, D. (1971). *The attraction paradigm.* New York: Academic Press.

Calder, B., Insko, C., & Yandell, B. (1974). The relation of cognitive and memorial processes to persuasion in a simulated jury trial. *Journal of Applied Social Psychology, 4,* 62–93.

Chaiken, S. (1979). Communicator physical attractiveness and persuasion. *Journal of Personality and Social Psychology, 3,* 1387–1397.

———. (1987). The heuristic model of persuasion. In M. P. Zanna, J. M. Olson, & C. P. Herman (Eds.), *Social influence: The Ontario symposium: Vol. 5* (pp. 3–39). Hillsdale, NJ: Erlbaum.

———, & Eagly, A. (1976). Communication modality as a determinant of message persuasiveness and message comprehensibility. *Journal of Personality and Social Psychology, 34,* 605–614.

Chaiken, S., Liberman, A., & Eagly, A. (1989). Heuristic and systematic information processing within and beyond the persuasion context. In J. S. Uleman & J. A. Bargh (Eds.), *Unintended thought* (pp. 212–252). New York: Guilford Press.

Cialdini, R. (1993). *Influence: Science and practice* (3d ed.). New York: HarperCollinsCollegePublishers.

———, Demaine, L. J., Barrett, D. W., Sagarin, B. J., & Rhoads, K. (in preparation). The poison parasite defense: A strategy for sapping a stronger opponent's persuasive strength.

Crenshaw, M. (1981). The causes of terrorism. *Comparative Politics, 13*(4), 379–399.

———. (1991). How terrorism declines. *Terrorism and Political Violence, 3*(1), 69–87.

Darley, J. M., & Batson, C. D. (1973). From Jerusalem to Jericho: A study of situational and dispositional variables in helping behavior. *Journal of Personality and Social Psychology, 27*(1), 100–108.

Downes-Le Guin, T., & Hoffman, B. (1993). *The impact of terrorism on public opinion, 1988–1989.* Santa Monica: RAND.

Drolet, A., & Aaker, J. L. (2002). Off target? Changing cognitive-based attitudes. *Journal of Consumer Research, 12*(1), 59–68.

Eagly, A. (1974). Comprehensibility of persuasive arguments as a determinant of opinion change. *Journal of Personality and Social Psychology, 29,* 758–773.

———, & Warren, R. (1976). Intelligence, comprehension, and opinion change. *Journal of Personality, 44,* 226–242.

Federal Trade Commission Cigarette Report for 2001. (2003). Washington, DC: Federal Trade Commission. Retrieved February 21, 2006, from http://www.ftc.gov/os/2003/06/2001cigreport.pdf.

Fraser, J., & Fulton, I. (1984). Terrorism counteraction. FC-100–37. Fort Leavenworth, KS: U.S. Army Command and General Staff College.

Goethals, G., & Nelson, R. (1973). Similarity in the influence process: The belief-value distinction. *Journal of Personality and Social Psychology, 25,* 117–122.

Goldman, L., & Glantz, S. (1998). Evaluation of antismoking advertising campaigns. *Journal of the American Medical Association, 279*(10), 772–777.

Harper, R., Weins, A., & Matarazzo, J. (1978). *Nonverbal communication: The state of the art.* New York: Wiley.

Hass, R. G. (1981). Effects of source characteristics on cognitive response and persuasion. In R. E. Petty, T. M. Ostrom, & T. C. Brock (Eds.), *Cognitive responses in persuasion* (pp. 141–172). Hillsdale, NJ: Erlbaum.

Hoffman, B. (1995). Holy terror: The implications of terrorism motivated by a religious imperative. *Studies in Conflict and Terrorism, 18,* 271–284.

———. (1998). *Inside terrorism.* New York: Colombia University Press.

Hofling, C., Brotzman, E., Dalrymple, S., Graves, N., & Pierce, C. (1966). An experimental study of nurse-physician relationships. *Journal of Nervous and Mental Disease, 143,* 171–180.

Hovland, C., Janis, I., & Kelley, H. (1953). *Communication and persuasion.* New Haven, CT: Yale University Press.

Hovland, C., Lumsdaine, A., & Sheffield, F. (1949). *Experiments on mass communication.* Princeton, NJ: Princeton University Press.

Hovland, C., & Mandell, W. (1952). An experimental comparison of conclusion-drawing by the communicator and by the audience. *Journal of Abnormal and Social Psychology, 47,* 581–588.

Hovland, C., & Weiss, W. (1951). The influence of source credibility on communication effectiveness. *Public Opinion Quarterly, 15,* 635–650.

Husek, T. (1965). Persuasive impacts on early, late, or no mention of a negative source. *Journal of Personality and Social Psychology, 2,* 125–128.

Insko, C. A., Arkoff, A., & Insko, V. M. (1965). Effects of high and low fear-arousing communications upon opinions toward smoking. *Journal of Experimental Social Psychology, 1,* 256–266.

Janis, I. (1982). *Groupthink: Psychological studies of policy decision.* Boston: Houghton Mifflin.

———, & Feshbach, S. (1953). Effects of fear-arousing communications. *Journal of Abnormal and Social Psychology, 48,* 78–92.

Jenkins, B. (1975). *International terrorism: A new mode of conflict.* Los Angeles: Crescent.

Kelman, H., & Hovland, C. (1953). "Reinstatement" of the communicator in delayed measurement of opinion change. *Journal of Abnormal and Social Psychology, 48,* 327–335.

Klapper, J. (1960). *The effects of mass communication.* Glencoe, IL: Free Press.

Laqueur, W. (1987). *The age of terrorism.* Boston: Little, Brown.

Lasswell, H. (1948). The structure and function of communication in society. In L. Bryson (Ed.), *The communication of ideas* (pp. 32–51). New York: Harper & Row.

Latané, B., & Darley, J. (1970). *The unresponsive bystander: Why doesn't he help?* New York: Appleton-Century-Crofts.

Latané, B., & Nida, S. (1981). Ten years of research on group size and helping. *Psychological Bulletin, 89,* 308–324.

Leventhal, H. (1970). Findings and theory in the study of fear communications. In L. Berkowitz (Ed.), *Advances in experimental social psychology: Vol. 5* (pp. 119–186). New York: Academic Press.

McGuire, W. J. (1964). Inducing resistance to persuasion. In L. Berkowitz (Ed.), *Advances in experimental social psychology: Vol. 1* (pp. 192–229). New York: McGraw-Hill.

———. (1968). Personality and attitude change: An information-processing theory. In A. G. Greenwald, T. C. Brock, & T. M. Ostrom (Eds.), *Psychological foundations of attitudes* (pp. 171–196). San Diego: Academic Press.

———. (1969). The nature of attitudes and attitude change. In G. Lindzey & E. Aronson (Eds.), *The handbook of social psychology, Vol. 3* (2d ed.; pp. 372–398). Reading, MA: Addison Wesley.

Meyerowitz, B., & Chaiken, S. (1987). The effect of message framing on breast self-examination attitudes, intentions, and behavior. *Journal of Personality and Social Psychology, 52,* 500–510.

Milgram, S. (1974). *Obedience to authority: An experimental view.* New York: Harper & Row.

Nisbett, R., & Ross, L. (1980). *Human inference: Strategies and shortcomings of social judgment.* Englewood Cliffs, NJ: Prentice Hall.

Norman, R. (1976). When what is said is important: A comparison of expert and attractive sources. *Journal of Experimental Social Psychology, 12,* 294–300.

Papageorgis, D., & McGuire, W. J. (1961). The generality of immunity to persuasion produced by pre-exposure to weakened counterarguments. *Journal of Abnormal and Social Psychology, 62,* 475–481.

Peters, D., & Ceci, S. (1982). Peer-review practices of the psychological journals: The fate of published articles, submitted again. *Behavioral and Brain Sciences, 5,* 187–195.

Petty, R., & Cacioppo, J. (1977). Forewarning, cognitive responding, and resistance to persuasion. *Journal of Personality and Social Psychology, 35,* 645–655.

———. (1979). Issue involvement can increase or decrease persuasion by enhancing message-relevant cognitive responses. *Journal of Personality and Social Psychology, 37,* 1915–1926.

———. (1981). *Attitudes and persuasion: Classic and contemporary approaches.* Dubuque, IA: W. C. Brown.

———. (1986). *Communication and persuasion: Central and peripheral routes to attitude change.* New York: Springer.

———. (1996). *Attitudes and persuasion: Classic and contemporary approaches.* Boulder, CO: Westview Press.

Petty, R., Harkins, S., & Williams, K. (1980). The effects of group diffusion of cognitive effort on attitudes: An information-processing view. *Journal of Personality and Social Psychology, 38,* 81–92.

Petty, R., Wells, G., & Brock, T. (1976). Distraction can enhance or reduce yielding to propaganda: Thought disruption versus effort justification. *Journal of Personality and Social Psychology, 34,* 874–884.

Rogers, R. (1983). Cognitive and physiological processes in fear appeals and attitude change: A revised theory of protection motivation. In J. Cacioppo & R. Petty (Eds.), *Social psychophysiology: A sourcebook* (pp. 153–176). New York: Guilford Press.

———, & Mewborn, R. (1976). Fear appeals and attitude change: Effects of a threat's noxiousness, probability of occurrence, and the efficacy of coping responses. *Journal of Personality and Social Psychology, 34,* 54–61.

Rubin, J., & Friedland, N. (1986). Theater of terror. *Psychology Today, 20*(3), 18–28.

Schmid, A., & de Graaf, J. (1982). *Violence as communication.* Newbury Park, CA: Sage.

Schmid, A., Jongman, A., & Stohl, M. (1988). *Political terrorism: A new guide to actors, authors, concepts, data bases, theories, and literature.* New York: North-Holland.

Smith, B., Lasswell, H., & Casey, R. (1946). *Propaganda, communication, and public opinion.* Princeton, NJ: Princeton University Press.

Taylor, S. E., & Fiske, S. T. (1975). Point of view and perceptions of causality. *Journal of Personality and Social Psychology, 32,* 439–445.

Tesser, A., Campbell, J., & Mickler, S. (1983). The role of social pressure, attention to the stimulus, and self-doubt in conformity. *European Journal of Social Psychology, 13,* 217–233.

Wooten, D., & Reed, A. (1998). Informational influence and the ambiguity of product experience: Order effects on the weighting of evidence. *Journal of Consumer Research, 7,* 79–99.

Worden, J., & Flynn, B. (2002). Using mass media to prevent cigarette smoking. In R. C. Hornik (Ed.), *Public health communication: Evidence for behavior change* (pp. 23–33). Mahwah, NJ: Erlbaum.

Zimbardo, P G., & Leippe, M. R. (1991). *The psychology of attitude change and social influence.* Boston: McGraw-Hill.

8

Psychological Aspects of Suicide Terrorism

Ariel Merari

By a strict definition, a suicide terrorist attack is an assault that is intended to achieve a political objective and is performed outside the context of a conventional war, in which the assailant intentionally commits suicide while killing others. The self-immolation element makes this form of terrorism substantially different in both its psychological foundations and potential consequences from other terrorist attacks that involve high risk for the perpetrators.

Suicide terrorism constitutes a political and strategic problem of considerable import. This observation seems obvious after the September 11, 2001, attacks in the United States. Yet even prior to the attacks in New York and Washington, suicide attacks had, on some occasions, far-reaching political consequences. In 1983, attacks against U.S. and French forces and diplomatic missions in Lebanon resulted in the evacuation of the Multinational Force from that country. This step enabled the Syrian de facto takeover of the country and, in the following years, had a vast influence on Lebanese domestic and international politics. In another arena, Palestinian suicidal terrorist attacks in Israel in 1996 resulted in a change of government and had a major deleterious impact on the Middle Eastern peace process.

Suicide terrorist attacks attract much public interest and concern. This phenomenon has always been surrounded by mystery and fear. The fact that, unlike ordinary self-immolation, terrorist suicide has been murderous and often directed against the random public, naturally augments the feeling of cryptic danger and the need to understand it. In the absence of empirical research on this phenomenon, the explanations offered have been quite speculative. The most common explanations have emphasized cultural factors. Islamic religious fanaticism has been particularly popular in this context (Taylor, 1988; Israeli, 1997; Hoffman, 1998). Taylor, for example, typically included the analysis of suicidal terrorism in a chapter titled "fanaticism." He finds the roots of this behavior in the tradition of the Assassins and attributes suicidal terrorism to Shiite fanaticism in particular: "The forces that gave rise to the Assassins remain and influence the Shi'ites today" (p. 109). Similarly, "the behaviours which we find so difficult to understand (suicide bombing, for example) have their origins in the kind of religious practice which characterises Islamic fundamentalism, and especially shi'iteism" (p. 110).

Taylor, however, extends his account to include political suicides of other societies, notably

Western, such as those by members of the German Red Army Faction in prison in the 1970s, the Irish hunger strikes in Maze Prison in 1980 and 1981, and the Jonestown mass suicide in 1978. His broader explanation attributes this phenomenon to social pressure and conformity that characterize certain societies: "Both contemporary Shi'ite society, and the Japanese society of the time, show many attributes of intense control, with restrictions on extra-societal influences. In many respects they are as 'psychologically' closed as the prisons which sustained both the Baader-Meinhof and the IRA suicides" (p. 120).

Raphael Israeli (1997) finds the basic explanation of this phenomenon in the Islamic frame of mind: "Turning to an Islamic frame of reference for a definition, and perhaps a diagnosis, would then appear imperative if we are to comprehend the underlying motives of this sort of unparalleled mode of self-sacrifice" (p. 107). However, he maintains (with no empirical evidence to support his claim) that personality factors also play a role in the making of a suicide terrorist. Specifically, he speculates that suicide bombers share three common characteristics: They are young and have few life responsibilities; they are unsuccessful or are shunned by their family and society, so that they feel isolated; and they have low self-esteem. Suicide terrorists, according to Israeli, "may be somewhat depressed and in search of easy solutions to their problems. Unsuccessful, perhaps self-despising, they find solace in becoming martyrs, thus almost instantly and mythically transforming frustration into glory, failure into victory and self-depreciation into public adoration" (p. 106).

Other explanations ascribed the phenomenon to indoctrination, even brainwashing, in the sense of persuading "uninformed youth" to commit suicide in the service of their advocated cause (Post, 2001). In an earlier study (Merari, 1990) I attributed politically motivated suicide, particularly cases of group suicide such as Massada (AD 73) and the Irish chain suicide of 1980 and 1981, to situational factors, notably group pressure, group commitment, and the influence of a charismatic leader, as well as to personality factors. These explanations are not entirely compatible with factual evidence that has accumulated on suicide terrorism.

Prevalence

Several writers have maintained that suicide terrorism is an ancient phenomenon, claiming that it was used by groups such as the Jewish Sicarii of the first century and the Muslim *hashashin* (Order of Assassins) of the eleventh through the thirteenth centuries (Sprinzak, 2000; Schweitzer, 2001; Atran, 2003). This claim is erroneous since these groups carried out attacks that involved great risk for the perpetrators, sometimes their almost sure death, but they were not suicide in the strict sense of self-immolation. As much as recorded evidence is concerned, true suicide terrorist attacks, in which the attackers kill themselves while killing others, are a modern phenomenon. The first recorded case of a suicide terrorist attack was the car bombing of the Iraqi embassy in Beirut on December 15, 1981, although as a methodical terrorist tactic, they were first used in Lebanon in 1983 by radical Islamic groups that later formed Hizballah.

A simple count of suicide attacks around the globe shows an alarming rise in recent years (see Figure 8.1). Of the 583 suicide attacks that were carried out around the world from 1981 to 2004, 435 of them (75%) took place between 2000 and 2004.

Indeed, since the first wave of suicide attacks carried out in Lebanon by Hizballah in 1983, this tactic has been espoused by many other groups around the globe. These include eight groups in Lebanon (six of them Lebanese and two Palestinian), four Palestinian groups in Israel's occupied territories, two Egyptian groups, the Kurdish Labor Party (PKK), the Turkish Revolutionary People's Liberation Front (a left-wing group), Chechen rebels, the Tamil Tigers (LTTE), Islamic militant groups in Kashmir, al-Qaeda, a militant Islamic group in Morocco, and anti-American groups in Iraq. Most of these have carried out only a small number of suicide assaults. Only a few have embarked on a systematic campaign of suicide attacks as a central method in their armed struggle. Table 8.1 shows the number of suicide attacks by country from 1981 through April 2005. The table also shows the number of people who committed terrorist suicide, as some attacks have involved multiple suicide attackers.

So far, suicide attacks have taken place in 30 countries. However, the great majority—nearly

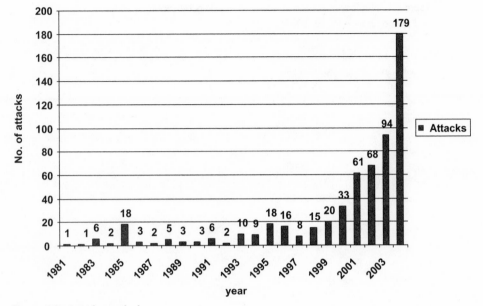

Figure 8.1. Suicide attacks by year.

88%—have been carried out in only 6 countries: Lebanon, Sri Lanka, Israel, Turkey, Russia, and Iraq. In fact, 73% of the world's tally have taken place in only 3 countries, namely Sri Lanka, Israel, and Iraq, and Israel and Iraq alone account for 63% of the world's total. These facts highlight an important characteristic of the nature of the spread of suicide terrorism as a terrorist tactic. Although the overall frequency of suicide attacks has been on the rise since this tactic first appeared in Lebanon in the 1980s, suicide terrorism does not spread in a fashion similar to the growth rate of the use of new technologies, such as the Internet or cellular phones. Rather, it is restricted to places where acute, violent conflicts are being waged, and in these places, it is limited to the duration of the acute struggle. It is true, however, that the likelihood that suicide attacks will be adopted as a tactic in an insurgent struggle is greater today than ever before. In this sense it seems that this tactic has become a trend, especially (but not exclusively) among militant Islamic groups.

Nevertheless, as demonstrated by the 9/11 events, the frequency of attacks is not the most important factor in creating the impact of suicide terrorism. Extremely large numbers of casualties result when the suicide method is coupled with other characteristics of the group, namely, the ability to acquire and use a large quantity of explosives (or other means of causing mass casualties), the selection of densely populated targets, and smart planning that makes it possible for the group to devise original modes of attack and circumvent defenses.

The Profile of Suicide Terrorists

Descriptions of the profiles of suicide terrorists relate to two types of data: demographic details and psychological characteristics. Whereas the demographic descriptors, such as age and gender, are relatively easy to obtain, psychological features, notably personality traits and motivations, are not readily accessible.

The numerous descriptions of the psychological (as distinguished from demographic) characteristics of suicide bombers offered so far have by and large been speculative, conjecturing from biographical details (e.g., Hudson, 1999; Weinberg, Pedahzur, & Canetti-Nisim (2003); Cronin, 2003; Kimhi & Even, 2004; Holmes, 2005; Ricolfi, 2005). Very few of the reports have been based on interviews with would-be suicide bombers or with their families (Andoni, 1997; Hassan, 2001).

Table 8.1. Number of suicide attacks and attackers by country and period, as of April 30, 2005

Country	Period	No. of Suicide Attacks	No. of Suicide Attackers
Afghanistan	2001–2004	6	7
Argentina	1992–1994	2	2
Bangladesh	2001	2	4
Bolivia	2004	1	1
China	1998–2002	3	3
Croatia	1995	1	1
Egypt	1993–2005	5	6
India	1991–2001	9	9
Indonesia	2002–2004	4	5
Iraq	1988–2005	256	291
Israel	1988–2005	175	195
Kenya	1998–2002	2	4
Kuwait	1983–1985	2	2
Lebanon	1981–1999	41	41
Morocco	1995–2003	6	13
Pakistan	1995–2004	15	20
Philippines	2003	1	1
Portugal	1983	1	5
Qatar	2005	1	1
Russia/Chechnya	2000–2004	33	40
Saudi Arabia	2001–2004	8	15
Spain	2004	1	7
Sri Lanka	1987–2004	68	113
Tanzania	1998	1	1
Tunisia	2002	1	1
Turkey	1996–2004	25	26
Uganda	1998	1	1
USA	2001	5	20
Uzbekistan	2004	4	6
Yemen	2000–2002	2	4
Total	1981–2005	682	845

Note: Counts of the number of suicide attacks in Sri Lanka vary considerably, presumably because of differences in the definition of a suicide attack.

Interviews with would-be suicide bombers were conducted by nonpsychologists and have not utilized psychological tests. The common conclusion that suicide bombers are psychologically "normal" should be treated with caution. Whereas acute psychosis (e.g., schizophrenia or depression) would probably be detected by a layperson, diagnosing more subtle personality disorders requires thorough clinical interviews and personality tests. The presence of these kinds of disorders is not likely to be revealed in an interview by nonprofessionals.

Psychological data on suicide terrorists of most groups have not been published. Since 1983 I have collected data on suicide terrorism around the globe from a variety of sources, mainly media reports that included demographic and biographical details of suicides, sometimes based on interviews with the suicides' families. Valuable information was gained from interviews with jailed would-be suicides. Particularly useful as a basis for psychological autopsy was a systematic set of data on 34 of the 36 Palestinian suicide terrorists from 1993 to 1998. These data were based on interviews with family members (parents and siblings) of the suicides. Other data included interviews with people who attempted to carry out suicide attacks but failed and with Hamas and Palestinian Islamic Jihad (PIJ) trainers of suicide bombers. Data on suicide terrorists in Israel after 1998 and on suicide attackers in Lebanon from 1983 to 1989 (almost all of the suicide attacks in Lebanon took place within this time frame) are based mainly on media sources (and include some demographic characteristics), as well as on interviews with jailed would-be suicides.

Demographic Characteristics

Age

The mean age of the Lebanese suicide bombers was 21, and the age range was 16–28. The mean age of the Palestinian suicides prior to the second intifada was 22, with a range of 18–38. The age range of the Palestinian suicides in the current intifada was somewhat broader (17–53), but the average remained the same: 22. Two-thirds of them were between 18 and 23 years old. Pape (2005:208) reported that the average age of the LTTE suicides was 21.9. The age range of the female PKK suicides was 17–27, and the males were 18–40 years old. The mean age of the actual and would-be male suicides combined was 27 (Ergil, 2001). The age range of the al-Qaeda 9/11 suicides was reported as 20–33 (Schweitzer and Shay, 2002).

Marital Status

Data for the Lebanese sample are lacking, but clearly almost all of the suicides were single. In the 1993–1998 Palestinian sample, 31 (91%) were single (moreover, none of them was engaged to be married), and three were married (only one of them had children). During the second intifada (which started on September 29, 2000, and is still going on at the time of this writing), the proportion of married suicide bombers remained below 10%. By the 1997 Palestinian Authority (PA) census, the median age at first marriage was 23 (Palestinian Central Bureau of Statistics, 1997). The fact that almost all of the suicides have been single may suggest that unmarried

persons are more willing to volunteer for suicide missions.

However, in the Palestinian case, it has also been the policy of the organizations to refrain from recruiting married people for such missions. In a study of the demographic characteristics of Hizballah members killed in action (most of them were not suicides), Hurwitz (1999) found that, of those whose marital status was known, only 45% were single. Hurwitz notes, however, that Hizballah's leadership preferred to recruit unmarried youth, but this policy was incongruent with the Lebanese Shiite custom of marrying young. Martin Kramer (1991) has also noted that Hizballah's "window of opportunity" for recruiting a youngster for military activity was rather narrow because the Lebanese custom of marrying young allows the organization only a few years for training and participation in operations. Thus, although the willingness to embark on suicide missions is presumably higher among young, unmarried people, both marital status and age of the suicides seem to reflect Hizballah's policy.

Gender

In the Lebanese case, 38 of the suicides were males, and 7 were females (all of the latter were sent by secular groups). All of the Palestinian suicides prior to the second intifada were males. This, however, was a result of the fact that, until recently, the Palestinian organizations that used suicide attacks were religious groups, which objected to the use of women in combat missions. During the second intifada the secular groups of Fatah and the Popular Front for the Liberation of Palestine (PFLP) also espoused suicide attacks. After Fatah started using women (as well as men) for suicide missions, the religious PIJ and Hamas followed suit in a few cases. Nevertheless, the percentage of females among Palestinian suicide bombers remained very small, less than 4%. It is noteworthy that left-wing Turkish and Kurdish groups, as well as the Tamil Tigers, have used women as often as men for suicide attacks. In the PKK, 11 of the 15 terrorist suicides between 1995 and 1999 were women (Ergil, 2001). In the LTTE there is a special women's suicide unit, called "Birds of Freedom" (Joshi, 2000), and about one-third of the suicide attacks have been carried out by women (Schweitzer, 2001; Chandran, 2001). Thus, the greater number of male suicides in the

Lebanese and Palestinian cases reflects only the preference of religious Islamic groups.

Socioeconomic Status

Reliable data are available only for the 1993–1998 Palestinian sample. In this study, the economic level of the suicides' families was assessed by the interviewer on the basis of her extensive acquaintance with the living conditions of the Palestinians in the West Bank and the Gaza Strip. In general, the economic status of the Palestinian suicides' families represents a cross-section of the Palestinian society in the Palestinian Occupied Territories. In the 1993–1998 sample, the 34 families were distributed as follows: very poor, 12%; poor, 21%; lower middle class, 26%; middle class, 32%; upper class, 9%.

Education

The education level of the suicides at the time of their suicidal attack was higher than that of the general Palestinian society. Of the suicides studied, 26% had at least a partial university education. In comparison, according to the Palestinian Central Bureau of Statistics (2002) data, 11.9% of the general Palestinian population had some education beyond high school. Table 8.2 shows the distribution of the suicides' education level.

Refugees Versus Nonrefugees

Whereas 21% of the Palestinian population in the Territories live in refugee camps (Arzt, 1997, p. 60; Shavit and Banna, 2001), prior to the second intifada they were responsible for 56% of the suicides, more than twice their proportion in the population. Thus, living in a refugee camp should be regarded as an important contributing factor to the likelihood of committing a suicide attack. This phenomenon is true for both the West Bank and the Gaza Strip: In each of these regions, refugee camps' residents are represented among the suicides at more than twice their share of the general population. Because no relationship has been found between economic status and participation in suicide attacks, the influence of being a refugee is presumably not due to the greater economic hardship associated with the refugee status. Rather, it probably reflects the greater militancy of refugees' descendents and the greater support for Hamas and Islamic Jihad among them.

Religion

Suicide attacks in Lebanon were initially carried out by the radical Shiite groups, which eventually formed Hizballah. For this reason the phenomenon of suicide terrorism, especially the Middle Eastern brand, has been associated in public perception with religious fanaticism. This notion has also permeated academic writings. However, by 1986 it became clear that nearly two-thirds of the suicide attacks in Lebanon were carried out by secular groups (Merari, 1990).

Prior to the second intifada, suicide attacks by Palestinians were carried out only by militant religious groups (two-thirds of them by Hamas and one-third by the Palestinian Islamic Jihad). In the second intifada ("al-Aqsa intifada"), two secular groups—Fatah and the PFLP—have also resorted to suicide attacks. By April 2005, these two secular groups combined had been responsible for 27% of the suicide attacks in the second intifada.

The conclusion that religious fanaticism is neither a necessary nor a sufficient factor in suicide terrorist attacks gains further support from the fact that several other nonreligious groups have resorted to this tactic. Thus, the Tamil Tigers (LTTE), a group that has carried out numerous suicide attacks, is composed of Hindus and motivated by nationalist-separatist sentiments rather than by religious fanaticism (Hopgood, 2005:47–48). Suicide attacks have also been carried out by Marxist (and therefore clearly nonreligious) groups such as the Kurdish PKK and the Turkish Revolutionary People's Liberation Front.

Table 8.2. Education level of Palestinian suicides and of the general Palestinian population (percentage)

Education	No schooling	Partial elementary	Elementary	High school	Partial university	Full university
Suicides	0	2.9	8.8	62	23.5	2.9
General Population	10.5	29.2	25.3	23.0	11.9	

Revenge for Personal Suffering

Some observers have suggested that the suicides have been motivated by the wish to inflict revenge for suffering that they had personally experienced (Joshi, 2000; Fisk, 2001). Whereas this explanation is clearly incorrect in the case of the September 11 attackers, it may still be true with regard to suicide attacks in most other places, such as Lebanon, Israel, Turkey, and Sri Lanka. This question was directly examined in the study of the 1993–1998 Palestinian suicides. In that study, the suicides' families were asked about events that could presumably provide a reason for a personal grudge. These included the killing of a close family member by Israeli forces, the killing of a friend, the wounding or beating of the suicide in clashes with Israeli soldiers, and the arrest of the suicide.

Analysis of the results suggests that a personal grudge has not been a necessary factor and apparently not even a major one in initiating the wish to embark on a suicide mission, although in all probability it was a contributing factor in some of the cases. Thus, in only 1 of the 34 cases, a close family member of the suicide had been killed by Israeli forces; however, in 15 cases the interviewees mentioned that a friend of the suicide had been killed prior to the suicide mission. In 7 cases a close family member (a father or a brother) had been jailed. With regard to the suicide's personal encounters, in 16 of the cases the suicide had been beaten or wounded in clashes with Israeli forces during demonstrations. Eighteen of the suicides had been jailed, most of them for short periods of time for minor charges, such as participation in violent demonstrations.

In assessing these findings as indicative of personal trauma, one should remember that most of the Palestinian youth were involved in various aspects of the intifada in activities such as stone throwing, demonstrating, distributing leaflets, painting graffiti, and enforcing strikes. In other words, this part of the suicides' personal history does not distinguish them from the average Palestinian youngster in the period under consideration. Indeed, 19 of the suicides were described by their families as "very active" during the intifada, and 8 were described as "active." In most cases, therefore, a high level of militancy preceded a personal trauma, although such trauma might later add to the already existing hatred and desire for revenge.

Personality Factors and Psychopathology

In none of the cases did interviews with would-be suicides or parents and siblings' descriptions of their personality and behavior (for complete suicides) suggest the existence of a major psychopathology. No evidence was found for hospitalization in a mental institution or outpatient psychological treatment. Furthermore, the descriptions did not reveal a common personality type for all or most of the suicides (however, relying solely on family descriptions was not a sufficiently sensitive method for characterizing personality types). Still, significantly, no evidence was found for the existence of risk factors for suicide. Three main risk factors are generally recognized in psychiatry and psychology: the existence of affective disorders (especially depression), substance abuse, and a history of suicide attempts (Lester & Lester 1971; Barraclough & Hughes, 1987; Klerman, 1987; World Health Organization, 1993; Jacobs, Brewer, & Klein-Benheim, 1999; Linehan, 1999; Miller & Paulsen, 1999; Moscicki, 1999). None of these was present among the Palestinian suicides of the 1993–1998 period. It is, of course, possible that more sensitive techniques would have revealed more subtle suicidal ideation in at least some of the terrorist suicides.

Furthermore, existing sociological and psychological theories of suicide seem to be inappropriate for explaining suicidal terrorism. A full survey of the compatibility of suicide theories with the phenomenon of terrorist suicide is beyond the scope of this chapter, and I therefore address this issue rather succinctly. Of the sociological theories, the one that comes closest to explaining this phenomenon is Durkheim's concept of altruistic suicide, more specifically, his subcategory of "optional" altruistic suicide (Durkheim, 1951). Optional altruistic suicide comprises cases in which suicide is considered a merit by society but is not obligatory, such as the Japanese Samurai custom of seppuku, or hara-kiri.

However, the suitability of Durkheim's concept to the phenomenon of terrorist suicide is questionable on several grounds. Durkheim used the concept of altruistic suicide to characterize societies, not individuals. He explained the differences in the suicide rates of various societies by the attributes of these societies. He inferred the motivation for committing suicide from the characteristics of the society to which the suicides belonged. Thus, he characterized suicides in the military as "altruistic" because of the characteristics that he attributed to the army, such as obedience and a sense of duty. He perceived altruistic suicide as a stable rather than a situational characteristic of the society in question. Altruistic suicide characterizes societies that are highly "integrated," in Durkheim's terms (i.e., very cohesive) and therefore exert much influence on their members. Hence, to apply Durkheim's concept of altruistic suicide to the phenomenon of terrorist suicide is to attribute these suicides to the traits of the societies in which they occurred—a religious group, an ethnic community, a caste, or a social organization such as the army.

Terrorist suicide, however, has taken place in very diverse societies. In addition to the Lebanese Shi'ites, Lebanese Sunnis, secular Lebanese, Palestinians, Egyptians, Armenians, Marxist Kurds, and Tamil Hindus, suicide for a political cause has also been committed by communist Germans, Catholic Irish, and Protestant Americans (John Wilkes Booth, who assassinated President Lincoln, committed suicide after the murder). It can be argued that the important factor is not the larger social unit—the ethnic group, religious group, or nation—but the microsociety of a terrorist group itself that provides the social milieu amenable to generating self-sacrificial suicide, in accordance with Durkheim's altruistic variety.

Highly cohesive and rigorous, they create rules of conduct and behavior ethics that members are expected to abide and live by. Yet, the great majority of the terrorist groups, regardless of their structure, have not resorted to suicide attacks at all. Furthermore, there is no evidence that terrorist groups, which maintain a particularly strict discipline and a tight structure, have resorted to suicide tactics more than the looser groups. On the contrary: Among the Palestinian groups, the Popular Front for the Liberation of Palestine (PFLP) has a much tighter structure and discipline than Hamas. Yet, the PFLP has generated only a few suicide attacks, whereas Hamas has carried out many.

Psychological theories of suicide cannot readily explain the phenomenon of terrorist suicide either. Psychoanalytic theories view suicide as a result of an "unconscious identification of the self with another person who is both loved and hated.

Thus it becomes possible to treat oneself, or some part of oneself (typically one's disavowed body), as an alien and an enemy" (Maltsberger, 1999, p. 73). While my study did not provide tools for examining the suicides' unconscious processes, no external supportive evidence of this theoretical explanation of suicide was found either. A more specific form of this approach was offered by Zilboorg (1996), who has stressed the importance of identification with an important person who died when the suicide was a child. The data do not support this theory. In the Palestinian sample, for instance, only 6 (out of 34) of the suicides lost a parent prior to carrying out the attack (at ages that ranged from 2 to 10). It is unlikely, although theoretically possible, though, that the suicides lost other psychologically important persons in childhood. But these theories would find it hard to explain the waves of suicide terrorism in the Lebanese, Palestinian, and Sri Lankan cases, as well as the episodes of cluster suicides, such as the September 11, 2001, attacks in the United States, the Irish hunger strikers in 1981, and the cases of Palestinian suicide attacks in duo or trio.

Whereas psychoanalytical theories have basically viewed suicide as aggression (directed internally), other psychological theories emphasize the element of despair. In this view, the wish to commit suicide is almost always caused by intense psychological pain that is generated by frustrated psychological needs. Suicide is committed by those who view it as the best way to stop the pain. The prevailing emotion of suicides is the feeling of hopelessness-helplessness (Shneidman, 1985, 1999). Several other researchers (e.g., Farber, 1968; Beck, Kovacs, & Weissman, 1996) also underscored the role of hopelessness in generating the wish to commit suicide. The greater the feeling of hope, the less the likelihood of suicide. Hope is the perceived ability to influence and to be satisfied by the world. This concept of hope, however, relates to people's expected ability to function within their own social milieu, rather than to a general communal situation, such as being under occupation. Lester and Lester (1971, p. 45) noted in this regard that suicidal people tend to see not only the present but also the future as gloomy, expecting to be socially isolated in the future. With regard to terrorist suicide, however, whereas it can be argued that at least in some cases the suicide attacks are motivated by despair that exists at the national or community level and is associated with frustrated *national* needs, the families' interviews revealed no evidence that those who carried out the suicide attacks suffered from despair at the individual level (although it is possible that the interviews failed to discover more subtle personality characteristics and motivations that would have surfaced in psychological interviews and tests administered to the suicides themselves). It is noteworthy in this respect that, in times of war, when the whole community is under duress, suicide rates tend to go down (Lester & Lester, 1971, pp. 109–110).

The profiles of the terrorist suicides gleaned from the interviews did not resemble typical suicide candidates, as described in the literature. By their family members' accounts, 47% of the 1993–1998 Palestinian suicides occasionally said that they wished to carry out an act of martyrdom, and 44% used to talk about paradise. However, the young people who eventually committed suicide had no record of earlier attempts of self-immolation and were not at odds with their family and friends, and most of them expressed no feelings of being fed up with life. In the suicides' notes and last messages, the act of self-destruction was presented as a form of struggle rather than as an escape. There was no sense of helplessness or hopelessness. On the contrary, the suicide was presented as an act of projecting power rather than expressing weakness. It thus seems that most terrorist suicides in the Palestinian sample were not "suicidal" in the usual psychological sense.

Terrorist Groups as Suicide Production Lines

The preceding sections suggest that neither demographic nor individual psychological characteristics can in themselves explain the phenomenon of terrorist suicide.

An important clue to understanding the phenomenon of terrorist suicide can be found in the hunger strike of 10 Irish Republican Army (IRA) and Irish National Liberation Army (INLA) members in Belfast's Maze Prison in 1981. These Irish nationalists, led by Bobby Sands, starved themselves to death one after the other when their demand to be recognized as political (rather than common criminal) prisoners was rejected by the British government.

Although this event does not qualify as an act of suicidal terrorism because the hunger strikers did not kill anyone but themselves, it was an act of self-destruction for a political cause and, as such, can teach us much about the psychological mechanisms involved in suicide terrorism.

Self-starvation is an extremely demanding way to die, much more difficult than the instantaneous death caused by a self-inflicted explosion. It took the hunger strikers from 50 to more than 70 days to die. During that time mothers, wives, and priests begged at least some of the hunger strikers to stop their self-destruction (Beresford, 1987). The force that led them to continue their strike to the very end, ignoring all pressures, must have been very strong. What was this force that sustained their determination? The assumption that all ten were suicidal persons who happened to be in jail at the same time is rather implausible. It is also unlikely that they were motivated by religious fanaticism and the promise of a place in paradise.

The only way to understand this frightening demonstration of human readiness for self-sacrifice is to look at the group's influence on its individual members. The suicide was a product of a group contract that one could not break. The group pressure in that situation was as strong as the group pressure that led hundreds of thousands of soldiers in World War I to charge against enemy machine gun fire and artillery to almost sure death. And it was even stronger once the first hunger striker died. From that point on, the contract to die could no longer be broken because the person who could release the next person in line from his commitment was already dead.

A more comprehensive picture of the process of making suicide bombers was gained from data collected on Palestinian suicide terrorists, including interviews with trainers for these missions and surviving would-be suicides. The findings of these data are supported by circumstantial evidence from suicide terrorism in other countries. The data suggest that there are three main elements in the preparation of a suicide bomber by an organization, namely, indoctrination, group commitment, and a personal pledge.

Indoctrination

Throughout the preparation for a suicide mission, the candidates are subjected to indoctrination by authoritative members of the group. Although the candidates are presumably convinced from start of the justification of the cause for which they are willing to die, the indoctrination is intended to further strengthen their motivation and to keep it from dwindling. Indoctrination in the religious Palestinian groups (Hamas and PIJ) included nationalist themes (Palestinian humiliation by Israel, stories of Arab glory in the days of Mohammad and the Caliphate, examples of heroic acts during the Islamic wars) and religious themes (the act of self-sacrifice is Allah's will, and the description of the rewards guaranteed a place in paradise for *shahids*—martyrs).

Group Commitment

The mutual commitment of candidates for suicide operations to carry out a self-sacrificial attack is a very powerful motivation to stick to the mission despite hesitations and second thoughts. The chain suicide of the Irish hunger strikers in 1981 is an example of this social contract, which is extremely hard to break (Merari, 1990). A similar situation exists when several members of a terrorist cell prepare together for carrying out suicide attacks, such as the September 11, 2001, attacks in the U.S., the multiple attacks in Morocco on May 16, 2003, and the London suicide attacks of July 7, 2005. Palestinian suicides are usually recruited and prepared individually for their mission. Sometimes, however, two or three youngsters decide jointly to carry out a suicide attack and undergo the preparations together.

In the LTTE, both male and female suicides have been trained in special "Black Tigers" units. Most likely they are also bonded in a social contract to carry out the suicidal mission. In fact, the power of the group commitment and the inability to break it formed the basis of the willingness of the Japanese pilots in World War II to fly on kamikaze missions. The last letters of the kamikazes to their families, written shortly before they took off for their last flight, indicated that, although some of them went on their suicidal attack enthusiastically, others regarded it as a duty that they could not evade (Inoguchi & Nakajima, 1958, pp. 196–208).

Personal Commitment

Many Middle Eastern groups have adopted a routine of releasing a videotape to the media shortly after a suicide attack. In addition, after the operation, the organization usually presents these tapes to the suicide's family as a farewell message. Typically, in this tape the suicide is seen with rifle in hand (and, in Islamic groups, a Koran in the other hand), declaring his intention to go on the suicide mission. This act is not only meant for propaganda. It is primarily a ceremony intended to establish the candidate's irrevocable personal commitment to carry out the suicide attack. This ritual constitutes a point of no return.

Having committed himself in front of a television camera (the candidate is also asked at that time to write farewell letters to his family and friends, which are kept by the group along with the videotape for release after the completion of the mission), the candidate cannot possibly renege on his promise. In fact, in both Hamas and PIJ, from that point on, the candidate is formally referred to as "the living martyr" (*al-shahid al-hai*). This title is often used by the candidates themselves in the opening sentence of the video statement, which routinely starts this way: "I am [the candidate's name], the living martyr." At this stage, the candidate is seemingly in a mental state of a living dead person and has already resigned from life.

Public Support

The magnitude of public support for suicide operations seems to affect both the terrorist group's willingness to use this tactic and the number of volunteers for suicide missions. Most, if not all, terrorist groups that have used suicide attacks are not indifferent to the opinions and attitudes of what they view as their constituency—the population whose interests they claim to serve and from which they recruit their members. In choosing tactics and targets, the groups tend to act within the boundaries of their constituency's approval. During the last 6 months of 1995, for example, Hamas refrained from carrying out suicide attacks because its leadership realized that such actions would not be supported by the Palestinian population at that time and would thus have had an adverse effect on the organization's popularity. In the Palestinian case, public support for terrorist attacks against Israel in general and for suicide attacks in particular has waxed and waned since the Oslo agreement of 1993, ranging from as low as 20% support in May 1996 to more than 70% in

May 2002 (Center for Palestine Research and Studies, 2000; Jerusalem Media and Communication Centre, 2002; Palestinian Center for Policy and Survey Research, 2002).

The great increase in the frequency of suicide attacks during the second intifada, al-Aqsa intifada, reflects the greater willingness of Palestinian youth to volunteer or to be recruited for what the community generally regards as acts of ultimate patriotism and heroism. Songs praising the shahids are the greatest hits, the walls in the streets and alleys of Palestinian towns in the West Bank and the Gaza Strip are covered with graffiti applauding them, and their actions are mimicked in children's games. In this atmosphere, not only do the terrorist groups perceive a public license to continue the suicide attacks, but they also have a constant flow of youngsters ready to become human bombs. The role of the preparation of the suicide candidate is to make sure that the youngsters who, because of social pressure, have said "yes" to an offer to become a shahid (or even an enthusiastic volunteer) would not have second thoughts and change their mind.

The importance of public attitude notwithstanding, it should be emphasized that so far there has not been even a single case of a person who carried out a true terrorist suicide attack for a political cause on an independent, personal whim. In every case it was an organization that decided to use this tactic, chose the target and the time, prepared the explosive charge, and arranged the logistics necessary for getting the human bomb to the target. Evidently, therefore, the terrorist group's decision to use suicide attacks as a tactic and the group's influence on the candidates are the key elements in this phenomenon.

Coping With the Psychological Effects of Suicide Terrorism

Terrorism in general and suicide attacks in particular constitute a major source of stress. This section deals with the ways that potential targets have adopted to deal with this stress. As Israel has faced a continuous series of suicide terrorist attacks since 1993, it is an appropriate case in point. Suicide attacks have exacerbated the Israeli-Palestinian conflict and have had a significant adverse political effect on the peace process. They have also had a deleterious impact on the economy. This final section, however, deals only with their individual psychological effects and the ways that Israel has coped with them.

Terrorist events are known to be a source of psychological trauma. In addition to acute stress disorder, which appears immediately following such an event, a longer-term posttraumatic stress disorder (PTSD) emerges in some of those exposed to the traumatic event. In a review of several studies of PTSD among people in various countries who witnessed a terrorist attack, Gidron (2002) found an average PTSD rate of 28.2%. Symptoms of posttraumatic stress disorder may appear not only among those present at the site of an attack but also among some of those who consider themselves as potential victims or who are exposed to the event through the mass media or personal accounts by relatives and friends. Studies conducted after the 9/11/ attacks in New York found PTSD symptoms among people who had not personally witnessed the attack (Cohen Silver, Holman, McIntosh, Poulin, & Gil-Rivas, 2002; Galea et al., 2002). PTSD rates were higher among people who lived in proximity to the site of the attack and therefore felt a greater direct danger.

Although psychological trauma of civilian victims of terrorism in Israel has been studied since the 1970s, interest in this problem has grown since the 1990s, when suicide attacks became a frequent occurrence. These attacks intensified in the second intifada, which started on September 29, 2000. The nearly 6 years of the intifada (as of this writing) have been marked by suicide attacks, which have been the most deadly form of terrorism by far. Although suicide attacks in this period have constituted only about 0.5% of the total number of terrorist attacks, they have accounted for 59% of the civilian fatalities (Israel Defense Forces, 2003). Suicide attacks are more frightening than other forms of terrorism not only because they generate a larger number of victims but also because these incomprehensible acts of self-sacrifice seem unstoppable. They create a sense of insecurity and lack of control. An explosive charge hidden in an innocent-looking package or a shopping bag can be detected and rendered harmless, but most of the suicides activate their charge upon detection. People avoid public places, such as shopping centers, coffee shops, and buses because these are the targets of suicide attacks.

Surveys conducted in Israel during the recent quarter century have consistently found a very high rate of expressed worry of terrorism. Since 1979, in most of the surveys, more than 70% of representative samples of the adult Israeli population have said that they were "very worried" or "worried" that they or members of their families would be hurt in a terrorist attack. The rate of worry was high even when the intensity of terrorism was much lower than during the second intifada (Merari and Friedland, 1980; Arian, 2003, p. 19).

Nevertheless, this high rate of worry is not necessarily associated with stress disorder. A 2003 survey by Bleich, Gelkopf, and Solomon determined the occurrence of PTSD among Israelis. The survey was conducted in April and May 2002, at a time when Israeli civilians were exposed to frequent suicide attacks. Although more than 60% expressed a low sense of safety for themselves and their relatives, the authors found that only 9.4% met the symptom criteria for PTSD. This low rate is especially surprising because more than 16% of the sample reported that they had been directly exposed to a terrorist attack, and 37.3% had a family member or friend who had been exposed. In comparison, in the United States, various surveys found that 10%–20% suffered from several PTSD symptoms a couple of months after 9/11 (Schlenger et al., 2002; Cohen Silver et al., 2002). The difference may be explained not only by methodological variations (e.g., in the length of time since the exposure to the traumatic event) but also by a habituation process that has taken place in the Israeli population. Another possible explanation is that the Israeli mental health system is more adept at handling the psychological effects of terrorist attacks.

Coping with the psychological effects of terrorism in general and suicide attacks in particular comprises two general categories: (1) preparatory measures, and (2) intervention after the attack. Preparatory measures include the training of organizations and units involved in responding to actual or threatened suicide attacks (police, military units of the homeland command, medical corps, public information, etc.). Public knowledge of the existence of an effective response system and trust in its committed and professional performance reduce anxiety and create some sense of control of a situation that is inherently surprising and uncertain.

Warnings that are based on intelligence information and concern an actual or intended launching of a terrorist attack in a certain area are followed by a massive effort to dissuade or stop the perpetrator by police and military roadblocks and searches. This effort is often successful and helps to reduce the feeling of uncertainty and give the public a sense of control over the situation. The credibility of the warnings is highly important for establishing public trust in the authorities. In the absence of trust, public responses might have resulted in a paralysis of economic and social activities. As the suicide bombers target public places, guards are stationed at the entrances to cafes, shopping malls, theaters, and schools. These guards constitute the last line of defense, and some of them have been killed as they prevented the suicide attacker from getting inside the target building, thus saving the lives of many people.

Intervention after the attack necessitates the coordinated action of many organizations. Police, fire fighters, medical corps, and victim identification teams are the first responders on the scene. Concurrently, hospitals in the area of attack are alerted and get ready with medical and mental health teams to take in a large number of casualties. At the same time, the municipalities activate teams whose task is to inform victims' families and provide psychological and social support. Several studies suggest that social support (by the family or community) is negatively correlated with posttraumatic stress (e.g., Solomon, Mikulincer, & Flum, 1988; Cohen Silver et al., 2002). The activity of social services and volunteer organizations is important mainly in the days and months following the attack.

Persons who suffer acute stress reaction as well as PTSD patients are entitled to social security compensation for their loss of ability to work and to financing for psychological treatment. Following an incident, social security personnel contact psychological patients and invite them to attend support groups that start a week after the incident. Those who suffer long-range psychological incapacitation get a permanent social security allowance commensurate with the degree of incapacitation.

In conclusion, the Israeli experience suggests that even a protracted campaign of suicide terrorism does not necessarily cause widespread psychological trauma. A credible warning system and trust in the authorities' effectiveness reduce anxiety. Mental health and social support services may effectively reduce and limit the psychological trauma associated with direct or indirect exposure to terrorist attacks.

Acknowledgment. I would like to thank Nasra Hassan, who conducted the interviews.

References

Andoni, L. (1997). Searching for answers: Gaza's suicide bombers. *Journal of Palestine Studies, 24*(4), 33–45.

Arian, A. (2003). Israeli public opinion on national security 2003. Memorandum no. 67. Tel Aviv: Tel Aviv University, Jaffee Center for Strategic Studies.

Arzt, D. E. (1997). *Refugees into citizens: Palestinians and the end of the Arab-Israeli conflict.* New York: Council on Foreign Relations.

Atran, S. (2003). Genesis of suicide terrorism. *Science, 299,* 1534–1539.

Barraclough, B., & Hughes, J. (1987). *Suicide: Clinical and epidemiological studies.* London: Croom Helm.

Beck, A. T., Kovacs, M., & Weissman, A. (1996). Hopelessness and suicidal behavior. In J. Maltsberger & M. Goldblatt (Eds.), *Essential papers on suicide* (pp. 331–341). New York: New York University Press.

Beresford, D. (1987). *Ten men dead.* London: Harper-Collins.

Bleich, A., Gelkopf, M., & Solomon, Z. (2003). Exposure to terrorism, stress-related mental health symptoms, and coping behaviors among a nationally representative sample in Israel. *Journal of the American Medical Association, 290*(5), 612–620.

Center for Palestine Research and Studies. (2000). *Public opinion polls 1–48.* Retrieved May 20, 2000, from http://www.cprs-palestine.org

Chandran, S. (2001, October 6). Suicide terrorism. *Hindu Online Edition.* Retrieved July 8, 2003, from http://www.hinduonnet.com/thehindu/2001/10/06/stories/05062524.htm

Cohen Silver, R., Holman, E. A., McIntosh, D. N., Poulin, M., & Gil-Rivas, V. (2002). Nationwide longitudinal study of psychological responses to September 11. *Journal of the American Medical Association, 288,* 1235–1244.

Cronin, A. K. (2003, August 28). Terrorists and suicide attacks. CRS Report for Congress, Congressional Research Service, Library of Congress, order code RL32058.

Durkheim, E. (1951). *Suicide: A study in sociology.* New York: Free Press.

Ergil, D. (2001). Suicide terrorism in Turkey: The Workers' Party of Kurdistan. In *Countering suicide terrorism: An international conference* (pp. 105–128). International Policy Institute for Counter-terrorism at the Interdisciplinary Center, February 20–23, 2000. Herzliya, Israel: International Policy Institute for Counter-terrorism.

Farber, M. L. (1968). *Theory of suicide.* New York: Funk & Wagnalls.

Fisk, R. (2001, August 11). What drives a bomber to kill the innocent child? *Independent* (UK). Retrieved January 20, 2002, from http://www.independent.co.uk/story.jsp?story=88134

Galea, S., Ahern, J., Resnick, H., Kilpatrick, D., Bucuvalas, M., Gold, J., et al. (2002). Psychological sequelae of the September 11 terrorist attacks in New York City. *New England Journal of Medicine, 346*(13), 982–987.

Gidron, Y. (2002). Posttraumatic stress disorder after terrorist attacks: A review. *Journal of Nervous and Mental Disease, 190,* 118–121.

Gunaratna, R. (2000). Suicide terrorism: A global threat. *Jane's Intelligence Review,* October 20, 2002. Retrieved June 1, 2002, from http://www.janes.com/security/international_security/news/usscole/jir001020_1_n.shtml

Hassan, N. (2001, November 19). An arsenal of believers. *New Yorker,* 36–41.

Hoffman, B. (1998). *Inside terrorism.* London: Victor Gollancz.

Holmes, S. (2005). Al-Qaeda, September 11, 2001. In D. Gambetta (Ed.), *Making sense of suicide missions* (131–172). New York: Oxford University Press, 2005.

Hopgood, S. (2005). Tamil Tigers, 1987–2002. In D. Gambetta (Ed.), *Making Sense of Suicide Missions* (pp.43–76). New York: Oxford University Press.

Hudson, R. (1999). The sociology and psychology of terrorism: Who becomes a terrorist and why? Washington, DC: Federal Research Division, U.S. Library of Congress.

Hurwitz, E. (1999). *Hizballah's military echelon: A social portrait.* Tel Aviv: Dayan Center for Middle Eastern Studies, Tel Aviv University.

Inoguchi, R., & Nakajima, T. (1958). *The divine wind: Japan's kamikaze force in World War II.* Annapolis, MD: Naval Institute Press.

Israel Defense Forces. (2003). Casualties since 30.9.00 (Updated November 20, 2003). Retrieved November 22, 2003, from http://www.idf.il/daily_statistics/english/1.doc

Israeli, R. (1997). Islamikaze and their significance. *Terrorism and Political Violence, 9,* 96–121.

Jacobs, D. J., Brewer, M., & Klein-Benheim, M. (1999). Suicide assessment: An overview and recommended protocol. In D. G. Jacobs (Ed.), *The Harvard Medical School guide to suicide assessment and intervention* (pp. 3–39). San Francisco: Jossey-Bass.

Jerusalem Media and Communication Centre (JMCC). (2002). JMCC public opinion polls 1–48. Retrieved June 20, 2003, from http://www.jmcc.org

Joshi, C. L. (2000, June 1). Sri Lanka: Suicide bombers. *Far Eastern Economic Review.* Retrieved June 24, 2002, from http://www.feer.com/_0006_01/p64currents.html

Kimhi, S., & Even, S. (2004). Who are the Palestinian suicide bombers? *Terrorism and Political Violence, 16*(4), 815–840.

Klerman, G. L. (1987). Clinical epidemiology of suicide. *Journal of Clinical Psychiatry, 48*(12, Suppl.), 33–38.

Kramer, M. (1991). Sacrifice and fratricide in Shiite Lebanon. *Terrorism and Political Violence, 3,* 30–47.

Lester, G., & Lester, D. (1971). *Suicide.* Englewood Cliffs, NJ: Prentice Hall.

Linehan, M. M. (1999). Standard protocol for assessing and treating suicidal behaviors for patients in treatment. In D. G. Jacobs (Ed.), *The Harvard Medical School guide to suicide assessment and intervention* (pp. 146–187). San Francisco: Jossey-Bass.

Maltsberger, J. T. (1999). The psychodynamic understanding of suicide. In D. G. Jacobs (Ed.), *The Harvard Medical School guide to suicide assessment and intervention* (pp. 72–82). San Francisco: Jossey-Bass.

Merari, A. (1990). The readiness to kill and die: Suicidal terrorism in the Middle East. In W. Reich (Ed.), *Origins of terrorism: Psychologies, ideologies, theologies, states of mind* (pp. 192–207). New York: Cambridge University Press.

———, & Friedland, N. (1980). Public opinion on terrorism. Memorandum. Tel Aviv: Center for Strategic Studies, Tel Aviv University.

Miller, M. C., & Paulsen, R. H. (1999). Suicide assessment in the primary care setting. In D. G. Jacobs (Ed.), *The Harvard Medical School guide to suicide assessment and intervention* (pp. 520–539). San Francisco: Jossey-Bass.

Moscicki, E. K. (1999). Epidemiology of suicide. In D. G. Jacobs (Ed.), *The Harvard Medical School guide to suicide assessment and intervention* (pp. 40–51). San Francisco: Jossey-Bass.

Palestinian Center for Policy and Survey Research. (2002). Public opinion polls 1–8. Retrieved July 1, 2003, from http://www.pcpsr.org

Palestinian Central Bureau of Statistics. (1997). Summary of final results: Population, housing, and establishment census, 1997. Retrieved July 28, 2003, from http://www.pcbs.org/english/phc_97/popu.htm

———. (2002). Education: Current main indicators. Retrieved July 30, 2003, from http://www.pcbs.org/inside/selcts.htm

Pape, R. (2005). *Dying to win: The strategic logic of suicide terrorism.* New York: Random House.

Post, J. (2001, October 30). Killing in the name of God: Osama bin-Laden and radical Islam. A presentation at the New York Academy of Medicine. Retrieved June 24, 2002, from http://www.theapm.org/cont/Posttext.html.

Ricolfi, L. (2005). Palestinians, 1981–2003. In D. Gambetta (Ed.), *Making sense of suicide missions* (pp. 77–130). New York: Oxford University Press, 2005.

Shavit, U., & Banna, J. (2001, July 6). The Palestinian dream, the Israeli nightmare. *Ha'aretz* (weekly supplement; published in Tel Aviv in Hebrew), 18–28.

Schlenger, W. E., Caddell, J. M., Ebert, L., Jordan, B. K., Rourke, K. M., Wilson, D., et al. (2002). Psychological reactions to terrorist attacks: Findings from the national study of Americans' reactions to September 11. *Journal of the American Medical Association, 288*(5), 581–588.

Schweitzer, Y. (2001). Suicide terrorism: Developments and main characteristics. In *Countering suicide terrorism: An international conference* (pp. 75–85). International Policy Institute for Counter-Terrorism at the Interdisciplinary Center, February 20–23, 2000. Herzliya, Israel: International Policy Institute for Counter-Terrorism.

———, & Shay, S. (2002). *An expected surprise: The September 11th attacks in the USA and their ramifications.* Herzliya, Israel: Mifalot, IDC and ICT Publications.

Shneidman, E. S. (1985). *Definition of suicide.* New York: Wiley.

———. (1999). Perturbation and lethality. In D. G. Jacobs (Ed.), *The Harvard Medical School guide to suicide assessment and intervention* (pp. 83–97). San Francisco: Jossey-Bass.

Solomon, Z., Mikulincer, M., & Flum, H. (1988). Negative life events, coping responses, and combat-related psychopathology: A prospective study. *Journal of Abnormal Psychology, 97,* 302–307.

Sprinzak, E. (2000, September–October). Rational fanatics. *Foreign Policy,* 66–73. Retrieved February 22, 2006, from http://www.foreignpolicy.com/Ning/archive/archive/120/rationalfanatics.pdf.

Taylor, M. (1988). *The terrorist.* London: Brassey's Defence Publishers.

Weinberg, L., Pedahzur, A., & Canetti-Nisim, D. (2003). The social and religious characteristics of suicide bombers and their victims. *Terrorism and Political Violence, 15*(3), 139–153.

World Health Organization. (1993). Guidelines for the primary prevention of mental, neurological, and psychosocial disorders, 4: Suicide. Publication no. WHO/MNH/MND/93.24. Geneva: Author, Division of Mental Health.

Zilboorg, G. (1996). Considerations on suicide, with particular reference to that of the young. In J. T. Maltsberger & M. J. Goldblatt (Eds.), *Essential papers on suicide* (pp. 62–82). New York: New York University Press.

9

The Strategy of Terrorism and the Psychology of Mass-Mediated Fear

James N. Breckenridge
Philip G. Zimbardo

Throughout the history of violent conflict, adversaries have resorted to terrorism when their opponents' superior material and military assets prohibited a direct struggle for strategic goals. Acts of terror, especially suicide terrorism, represent a growing transnational threat due specifically to the psychological advantages terrorism possesses in modern asymmetrical warfare. Modern terrorism derives this tactical advantage from its reliable ability to evoke *disproportionate* fear and to create an enduring, pervasive apprehension of threat. Terrorists appear to have a keen, intuitive appreciation of psychological mechanisms that spread the effects of terror well beyond their primary victims and amplify the perception of risk and vulnerability far out of proportion to reasonable probabilities. Modern terrorism is necessarily mass-mediated political violence, and the media play a critical role in facilitating the psychological processes that intensify the public's fears and apprehensions.

Countering terrorists' intuitive use of the tactics of mass-mediated fear demands an appreciation of the underlying psychology and requires strategies that exploit scientific progress in understanding the nature of emotionally biased judgment and perception. Although scholarly works routinely acknowledge the psychological nature of

terrorist strategy, few discuss the relevant psychological science in any detail. In this chapter we examine the psychological basis of terrorism and the important ways in which public reactions differ from responses to other tragic and disastrous events. People's reactions are more complex than a mere visceral sense of personal danger, and the multifaceted aspects of their fears can strongly influence the public's trust in and support for government policy. Disproportionate reactions to the threat of terrorism, we argue, result from emotionally driven biases associated with appraising risks and making decisions with uncertain prospects. The threat of terrorism is further augmented by a variety of sociopsychological processes, especially the priority that human attention assigns to negative information and the narrative frames with which the mass media surround reports of terrorist actions. Finally, we maintain that the threat of terrorism is made more menacing by stereotypical, dispositional explanations of evildoers, characterizations that are also central to the terrorists' own view of the enemies they seek to harm.

Acts of terrorism can serve many goals from simply injuring an enemy to venting longstanding hostilities and frustration. Inciting widespread fear and vulnerability, however, may represent the terrorists' most important objective.

Fear: The Critical Element of Terrorist Strategy

Although newspaper, magazine, and television accounts have often focused on the potential use of chemical, biological, radiological, or nuclear weapons to inflict mass casualties or severe damage to critical infrastructure, experts have long questioned whether such objectives are essential or perhaps even counterproductive to the strategy of terrorism. A few months prior to September 11 some experts questioned whether objective data supported "media-hyped" concerns about a growing threat of high-casualty terrorism (Johnson, 2001). Despite the enormity of September 11, subsequent dramatic bombings in Madrid and Bali and the increase in terrorist attacks internationally following U.S. wars in Iraq and Afghanistan, the "new terrorism" may yet continue a conservative approach to high-technology weapons of mass destruction (Crenshaw, 2000; Hoffman, 2001a, 2001b; Lesser et al., 1999; Tucker, 2001). It has been argued that terrorists can carry out less costly, more restrained acts of terror that nevertheless "could have disproportionately enormous consequences, generating fear and alarm and thus serving the terrorists' purpose just as well as a larger weapon or more ambitious attack with massive casualties" (Hoffman, 2001a, p. 8).

Terrorists choose terrorist tactics—even suicide terrorism—because historically the underlying logic has realized some success. Suicide terrorist tactics, for instance, apparently produced incremental gains for the terrorists' side in Lebanon in the 1980s and the Gaza Strip and the West Bank in the 1990s; they have also resulted in progress for the position of the Kurds in Turkey and for the Tamils in Sri Lanka (Pape, 2003). These gains, however, have not been a consequence of the number of people harmed or the magnitude of damage to critical infrastructure but resulted from the political impact of public fear and the perception of personal vulnerability multiplied throughout the victimized society.

The critical role fear plays in the terrorist strategy has been acknowledged by leading security experts. The Geneva Declaration on Terrorism (United Nations, 1987) asserts that "the distinguishing feature of terrorism is fear and this fear is stimulated by threats of indiscriminate and horrifying forms of violence directed against ordinary people everywhere." Because terrorists lack the military prowess, political power, and material resources of their adversary, their strategy is critically dependent upon the strategic benefits of inciting a perception of vulnerability that far exceeds realistic dangers, an aim that depends heavily upon mass-media publicity. The threat of terrorism should thus bear "no relation to the actual statistical probability of one's being killed or injured in a terror attack, or even of a terror attack taking place at all," (Ganor, 2004). The strategy of terrorism aims to undermine the public's sense of security, disrupt everyday life, and sway public opinion by "creating an unremitting, paralyzing sensation of fear" (Ganor, 2004). Terrorists strive to provoke a pervasive feeling of threat that comes to assume priority over all other social and political concerns.

A heightened sense of crisis can lead to political disaffection and diminished confidence in government. For example, the terrorist bombings in Madrid just prior to the 2004 elections in Spain appear to have significantly influenced both electoral outcomes and subsequent foreign policy. To maximize discontent and crisis, terrorists typically target civilian noncombatants to heighten the sense of public threat. Reports suggest, for instance, that recent suicide attacks by insurgents in Iraq, hoping to foment a breakdown of social trust and cooperation, have shifted priorities from attacks on military and government targets to high-casualty suicide bombings in civilian settings (Bunker & Sullivan, 2005).

Mass-mediated acts of terror can also strengthen popular support for a more militant counterterrorism policy and for bold restrictions on civil liberty, as well as encourage public acceptance of potentially misplaced priorities. A national survey conducted soon after September 11, 2001, for instance, found that the greater the public's sense of threat, the greater the willingness to place restrictions on civil liberties to increase safety and security (Davis & Silver, 2004). Another post–September 11 New York Times poll found widespread support for military action against terrorism even if "many thousands of innocent people" were killed (Berke & Elder, 2001). A longitudinal review of national polling data found that public support for restricting civil liberties to combat terrorism peaked in the early days following September 11, and although support diminished over the next year, a majority of Americans continued to support restrictions on their civil liberties if personal costs were relatively low (Kuzma, 2004).

Trust in government is a significant, albeit occasionally overstated, moderator of public threat perceptions (Viklund, 2003). Public trust in government and support for counterterrorism policy expenditures increased significantly following September 11, in sharp contrast to a long period of public cynicism regarding government capabilities (Chanley, 2002). However, a year later, public confidence in government was almost evenly divided between optimistic and pessimistic appraisals (Kuzma, 2004). Fear mixed with cynical distrust can also undermine compliance with public safety and other security instructions during a crisis. Several studies have observed a troubling percentage of Americans who report that they would ignore or disobey the recommendations of authorities during a terrorist attack (Boscarino, Figley, & Adams, et al., 2003; Fischhoff, González, Small, & Lerner, et al2003; Lasker, 2004).[1]

Mass-mediated attention to acts of terror can also encourage public acceptance of misguided policy priorities. The public's political attention is highly selective and ultimately emotionally driven. In addition, the consensus among political scientists is that sustained public awareness of the details of current events, politics, and public policy is limited at best. It is no coincidence that government leadership is often eager to focus public attention on decisions and programs that are consistent with opinion polls. If people's perceptions are shaped by mass-mediated accounts of recent acts of terror, public concerns may focus on "yesterday's threat." For example, the public's support for the national airline passenger-screening program may reflect the indelible impact of the (mediated) events of September 11, coupled with limited public knowledge of the deficiencies in the screening of airline cargo. The potential for misplaced threat-related priorities may represent a particularly daunting challenge for the United States, which can anticipate a vast array of possible terrorist targets and methods, but relative to many areas of conflict, it has had little historical experience with terrorist attacks.[2]

It is not surprising that fear and apprehension can have considerable political consequence. The role of emotions in most matters of political interest is powerful and pervasive because emotions bias judgments, frame perceptions, prime supporting memories, and influence agenda setting (Marcus, 2000, 2003). Precisely these psychological constructs also characterize the basis of the media's influence on public opinion. Affective influences on attention, memory, and judgment contribute to the widespread experience of disproportionate vulnerability and looming threat appraisal that make terrorism a more psychologically complex phenomenon than mere "scare tactics."

More Than Personal Fear and Different From Responses to Other Types of Disasters

Reactions to an act of terror and to the threat of future attacks are more complicated than mere visceral experiences of personal danger. Emotions can range from a mix of sadness, fear, anger, and even positive emotions, such as gratitude for lives spared and increased affiliation and social connectedness. A predominantly fearful response can produce an effect on the perception of future terrorist threat that is opposite to what an angry reaction may evoke (Lerner & Keltner, 2001). Fear stimulates a pessimistic estimate of risk, whereas anger is associated with a more optimistic outlook. Fearful versus angry emotional responses can also differentially influence support for public policy. For example, a post–September 11 national study using video stimuli to experimentally manipulate emotional reactions found that angry respondents had more optimistic future risk appraisals but favored more vengeful government actions than did fearful respondents (Lerner, Gonzales, Small, & Fischhoff, 2003).

Individuals' perceptions of fear of harm to themselves do not automatically determine their perceptions of sociotropic fear, that is, their estimation of danger or risk to society. Sociotropic fears following terrorist acts appear more common and more strongly related to public policy views than do perceptions of personal threat. The separation of personal and sociotropic fears is consistent with a widely observed positive bias in self-perceptions. That is, on the average, each of us tends to view our own prospects and circumstances as superior to that of others (Mezulis, Abramson, Hyde, & Hankin, 2004). Personal threats violate ordinary expectations and may be especially likely to promote anxiety and traumatic responses.

This is precisely what was observed in a national survey of reactions in the 6 months following September 11, 2001: Heightened perceptions of personal threat were associated with increased rates of fear, anxiety, and somatic features of affective distress (Huddy, Feldman, Lahav, & Taber, 2003). Personal self-interest (e.g., fear of personal harm) had relatively little relationship, however, to support for government policy or with expectations for risk to the nation. On the contrary, fear for the community and the nation was predictive of stronger support for military intervention and government counterterrorism policy. Similarly, perceptions of *personal* threat were not correlated with participants' predictions of future threats of terrorism in a study of New York residents following September 11 (Huddy et al., 2002). Perceptions of personal and national threat are distinct but clearly related, nevertheless; those who expect little risk to the nation, for example, typically do not anticipate personal risk.

Although well beyond the scope of this chapter, it should also be noted that people vary greatly in terms of their vulnerability to trauma. For a significant portion of the public, especially persons with current or past psychiatric disorders or those who have been exposed to prior trauma, the psychological consequences can include depressive, traumatic, or other mental health disorders (for a review, see Chapter 3 in this volume and Danieli, Engdahl, & Schlenger, 2004). Traumatic consequences can be especially severe for young children and older adults (F. H. Norris, Byrne, & Díaz, 2002). Certain fortunate individuals, however, exhibit an overall positive emotional response to calamities, and, regardless of whatever anger, fear, sadness, and other negative emotions they experience, demonstrate a resistance to traumatic psychological injury and more resilient coping in the aftermath of crisis. For example, a small study of college students begun before September 11 found that students who reported feelings of gratitude and increased social affiliation appeared to have superior resistance to depression in the weeks following the catastrophe (Fredrickson, Tugade, Waugh, & Larkin, 2003).

Fear, especially sociotropic fear, is widespread in the aftermath of terrorist acts, but mass hysteria or panic is rare. Panic is highly situation specific. Studies of natural and technological disasters indicate that only on some occasions, when there is a perception of immediate, severe danger coupled with the appearance of narrowing opportunities for escape, has mass panic been observed (Perry & Lindell, 2003). Even in such circumstances, panic is not inevitable.

Contrasting Terror to Other Catastrophes

How comparable psychologically are natural disasters or unintentional human-made catastrophes to acts of terrorism? Prior experience with natural disasters has much to inform the development of programs to prepare for acts of terrorism, especially with regard to organizing, coordinating, and deploying resources. Can we borrow from disaster management experience as we attempt to understand and counter the terrorist strategy of fear? We believe that natural disasters and accidental human-made catastrophes provide only an incomplete comparison with acts of terror. Just as disasters present problems quite unlike routine emergencies, acts of terror pose unique challenges that differ distinctly from other traumatic catastrophes. In stark contrast to natural disasters, terrorism *intentionally* targets basic social infrastructure in a manner that inspires lingering fear throughout society (Fullerton, Ursano, Norwood, & Holloway, 2003). Public consciousness of the deliberate, intentional nature of acts of terror is a critical emotional distinction. Despite the traumatic impact of natural disasters,

> the resulting psychological fallout is not as devastating because these events are understood to be the result of circumstances beyond human responsibility, and therefore unpreventable. These acts of God or nature or human error are also seen as unusual circumstances not attributable to malevolence. (Ditzler, 2004)

Actions with obvious malevolent intent have much more powerful emotional impact. Thus, in a review of studies of 102 disasters, more than two-thirds of victims of mass violence catastrophes incurred severe impairment as opposed to 34% of those who were subject to natural disasters (F. H. Norris et al., 2002). Paul Slovic, a pioneer in the psychology of risk perception, dubs terrorism a "new species of trouble" because it entails calculated mal-evolent intent (Slovic, Fischhoff, & Lichtenstein, 2000).

Malevolent intent targets a society or a nation. While there are inevitable costs to the nation, nat-ural disasters victimize localities (e.g., hurricanes strike coastal residents, and tornados ravage the Midwest). Most importantly, society recognizes that every citizen is a potential target of future malevolence. It is this perception of lingering threat that best distinguishes terrorism from other calamities. The psychological strategy of terrorism is to ensure that no matter what defensive actions are taken, the next act of terror seems inevitable and likely to occur sooner rather than later, threatening each of us personally.

The temporal boundaries of natural disasters are defined by a return to normality, a pattern of recovery socially constructed in terms of memories of past disasters. Psychologically, normality does not return after an act of terrorism. A "new nor-mality" begins and brings unexpected concerns and new threats (Hills, 2002). While scientists develop uncertain, but comfortably distant, predictions of future natural disasters, security officials worry immediately about copycat responses and hoaxes in the aftermath of terrorism. It is unusual for natural disasters to reoccur soon; thus, survivors of natural calamities such as earthquakes and tsuna-mis do not expect to be victimized again in the near future. In contrast to second-guessing natural dis-asters, intelligence officials are told their greatest failure has been a failure of imagination, a failure to anticipate a new or an unusual form of terrorist attack (Peters, 2004). Yet, there are so many targets, so many citizens, so many methods. If we recognize that we cannot defend ourselves against every possible threat, can we ever feel safe?[3]

The perception of continuing threat is therefore the crucial distinction between terrorism and other traumatic calamities. Lay threat perceptions typically differ dramatically from professional risk appraisals, and this considerable difference favors the terrorist.

Why Do We Feel So Vulnerable? Public Fears Versus Statistical Odds

Expert risk appraisals tend to correlate well with statistical evidence of potential harm, especially mortality rates (Slovic, Finucane, Peters, & Mac-Gregor, 2004). Rationale analyses strive to conform to the laws of probability, using new data to revise expectations in a Bayesian fashion. Classical deci-sion theory comes to conclusions by weighting ex-pectations by some estimate of the utility of each possible factor. Thus, the probability of success and failure are weighted by some quantified valuation of the cost and benefits of each alternative. "Correct" decisions optimize the combination. Most people, however, do not make risky decisions in this way.

Whereas expert risk appraisals are bounded by probabilities, public worries about extreme threats typically dwarf any "rational" or statistical assess-ment of risk. In an opinion piece for the AEI-Brookings Joint Center, Michael Rothschild sum-marizes the paradoxical nature of disproportionate risk appraisals assigned to acts of terror following September 11:

> The odds of dying in an automobile accident each year are about one in 7,000, yet we con-tinue to drive. The odds of dying from heart disease in any given year are one in 400 and of dying from cancer one in 600, yet many of us fail to exercise or maintain a healthy diet. We have learned to live with these common threats to our health. Yet we are afraid to return to malls and the skies. (Rothschild, 2001, p. 1)

Rothschild further calculates that, even if air travel resumed at normal rates and one plane per month were attacked, the odds of flyers encounter-ing terrorists were more than 500,000 to 1. Even more striking, the odds of dying in a terrorist bombing at a shopping mall are approximately 1.5 million to 1, even if it is assumed that terrorists totally destroy one mall per week.

Indeed, the public perceives that these risks pose a much greater threat than Rothschild's ap-praisal indicates they actually present, with enor-mous consequence to U.S. society. The economic costs of avoiding airline travel in the aftermath of September 11 are staggering. The volume of U.S. commercial airline traffic did not return to pre–September 11 levels until February 2005. The economic damage to the national and international airline industry and to tourism—more than $57 billion for the U.S. travel industry alone—has been enormous (Frey, Luechinger, & Stutzer, 2004).

Terrorism is not society's only exaggerated fear. Social scientists have long recognized that many public fears are often grossly inconsistent with objective data. In his popular pre–September 11 book, *The Culture of Fear,* sociologist Barry Glassner (1999) questions why American fear the "wrong" things and are obsessed with apprehensions about crime, drugs, health risks, and other threats that are either unsupported or completely contradicted by empirical evidence. Disproportionate fears of crime, for example, have endured in the face of many years of well-publicized declining crime rates. The public's misplaced worries about crime, however, present an alluring opportunity for media outlets seeking readers or viewers. A longitudinal study of public perceptions of crime in the early 1990s, for example, revealed a dramatic 52% increase in the number of Americans who rated crime as the most important problem facing the country despite widely published FBI statistics to the contrary (Lowry, Nio, & Leitner, 2003). Television news coverage was identified as the primary source of the public's distorted perception of crime. Clearly, disproportionate apprehensions about crime also represent an attractive opportunity for the "politics of fear" (Baer, 1997).[4]

Despite the "irrational" excesses of public risk perceptions, homeland security professionals cannot ignore public opinion. Response and preparedness efforts to counter terrorism will involve large numbers of the lay public, many more than the growing number of trained professionals. It can also be argued that, in a democracy, interventions that address the misguided fears of a majority, or at least a large number of citizens, are legitimate even if only anxiety is reduced and objective threat reduction is negligible (Sunstein, 2003). Parenthetically, such reasoning raises critical questions about the value of government actions such as the Homeland Security Advisory System, which elevates fears with alerts but offers citizens no tangible actions to foster even the illusion of control or preparedness.

The public's perceptions of threat can escalate rapidly, outpacing rational analysis. Because human beings do not weigh negatively and positively valenced information evenly, the perception of terrorist threat, like other public fears, can intensify in the face of compelling empirical disconfirmation and contrary probabilities. Negativity bias impacts a wide range of psychological processes, including attention, memory, decision making, and impression formation. Negativity works in concert with a

set of heuristics—mental shortcuts—that most of use to predict risk and make decisions under uncertainty.

Perceived Risk and Negativity Bias

Judgment and Heuristics

Risk perceptions and many other judgments are guided by heuristics, implicit and intuitive shortcuts, which often contrast dramatically with the logical, probability-based analytical process employed by professional experts. Although the range of processes identified by advances in psychology and cognitive neuroscience is beyond the scope of this brief chapter, two such cognitive biases exert a critical role in the public's evaluation of the threat of terrorism: the availability heuristic and the affect heuristic.

Under conditions of uncertainty, emotionally evocative events are more easily imagined and more readily available for cognitive processing. This enhanced availability—our ability to easily imagine images of the event—influences our judgment about the likelihood of similar events. The *availability heuristic* refers to a widely observed tendency of people to assign a higher perceived probability (or risk) to vivid, easily imagined (available) events (Teversky & Kahneman, 1974). In the aftermath of a terrorist act, powerfully facilitated by mass media reporting, the event is highly available, thus elevating disproportionately the perception that another act is likely. The availability heuristic is exploited strategically by many "availability entrepreneurs" (Kuran & Sunstein, 1999), including terrorists, who capitalize on intense, elevated perceptions of danger by creating and publicizing threatening events.

People also rely upon an *affect heuristic* to make judgments (Finucane, Alhakami, Slovic, & Johnson, 2000), tacitly employing feeling states to facilitate decision making and risk appraisals. Simply put, ordinary people use their feelings to estimate risk. In general, the public's assessment of risk utilizes an intuitive, emotional process that deems highly dreaded, unusual, or uncontrolled events as more probable. Psychometric studies have shown that at least two qualitative characteristics of threats underlie people's risk perceptions (Slovic et al., 2004; Slovic et al., 2000). A diverse array of threats or hazards can be differentiated in terms of perceived "dread," the most important factor, and the degree to which they are viewed as unfamiliar or new. Thus, those threats that are most feared (i.e., evaluated as the most dreadful and unfamiliar) are actually perceived as greater risks. Acts of terror were second only to warfare and the use of nuclear weapons in one psychometric risk perception study (Slovic et al., 2000).

The influence of both heuristics is compounded by the difficulty most people experience in contrasting rare events and comparing quantitative outcomes in different contexts or frames. Studies have demonstrated, for instance, that people will judge interventions to save the same absolute number of lives quite differently if the different outcomes represent different relative proportions. Thus, if one intervention saves 50 people out of a possible 100, it will be seen as much more effective than an intervention that saves 50 out of 1,000. Dubbed "psychophysical numbing," this is a highly ingrained, robust example of our struggles to compare tragic or catastrophic outcomes (Fetherstonhaugh, Slovic, Johnson, & Friedrich, 2000). The dramatic, emotionally charged, and dreadful context that frames terrorist casualties produces a converse effect, belying the relative odds of actual personal threat.

Negativity Bias

Human beings are much more powerfully influenced by negative than by positive information. Judgments concerning *valence*—the positive versus negative evaluative aspect of information—are ubiquitous, automatic, and largely outside conscious awareness (Slovic et al., 2004). The greater emotional force of negatively valenced material results in a *negativity bias* that pervades human perception, impression formation, attention, judgment, and decision making, frequently in ways that appear irrational (Baumeister, Bratslavsky, Finkenauer, & Vole, 2001; Rozin & Royzman, 2001; Skowronski & Carlston, 1989). Negative information tends to be construed as more informative and influential than positive data, and when positive and negative information are both presented together, the emphasis on the negative is greater than would be predicted for an equally weighted, emotionally balanced combination. For example, research suggests that negative messages

indicating the presence of risk are evaluated as more trustworthy than positive messages communicating the absence of risk (Siegrist & Cvetkovich, 2001). Furthermore, with respect to political context, voters lend greater weight to negative information about candidates (Klein, 1991). Similarly, negativity bias can play a powerful role in shaping public trust. Negative events appear to have a greater impact on damaging public trust than positive events have on bolstering trust (Poortinga & Pidgeon, 2004; Slovic, 1993). Slovic (1993) dubs this imbalance the "asymmetry principle" (i.e., that it is easier to destroy than to build public trust in the capacity of government to mitigate risks).

Negativity bias is also associated with observations of prospect theory (Kahneman & Tversky, 1979). For example, people exhibit a pronounced risk aversion when decisions about uncertain outcomes are framed in terms of negative results. Thus, if the risks of a medical procedure are presented to a patient in terms of the odds of death, the patient will respond very differently than if the same risks are presented in terms of the chances of survival. Even though the odds of death and survival are necessarily codetermined, patients are less likely to consent to statistically equivalent risks when framed in terms of the negative outcome. In addition, people tend to overreact to small chances of bad outcomes. Furthermore, they subjectively overestimate the probability of highly undesirable but objectively rare outcomes. When intense negative emotions are involved, as in the case of all terrorist threats, our attention is captured by the dreaded outcome, and we overlook the relatively small chance of the threat actually occurring. Such "probability neglect" (Sunstein, 2003) is an important contributor to sustaining disproportionate fears of terrorism.

Because negativity biases and the emotional basis of risk perception are fundamental aspects of the psychology we all share, perceptions of threat can easily ripple through society. The propensity for social amplification further bolsters terrorist threats.

Social Amplification

These fears and apprehensions that can ripple through society are compounded by *social amplification*. Social amplification is especially common when there is ambiguity, doubt, or misinformation, which promote fear and instigate rumor. Social amplification, for example, deeply exacerbated perceptions of risk and stigmatization of British beef following the identification of "mad cow disease" and contributed to the ultimate long-lasting collapse of the British beef market in 1996. Similarly, technological or product stigmatization (Gregory, Flynn, & Slovic, 1995) is a likely and potentially severely destructive consequence of a biochemical terrorist attack on the agricultural system. Parallel consequences are likely to characterize public reactions to terrorists' use of infectious disease agents or radiological weapons.

The consequences of socially amplified fears are not simply psychological. For example, the mad cow crisis costs to the European Union were at least $2.8 billion and more than 4 billion pounds to the United Kingdom (Powell, 2001). Exaggerated fears destroyed public confidence in British regulatory authorities and forced the creation of a new food standards agency (Food safety: Experiences of four countries in consolidating their food safety systems, 1999). A deliberate attack on the food supply could have similar economic impact in the United States, where one out of every eight people is employed in a food-related occupation (Risk assessment for food terrorism and other food safety concerns, 2003). American travel, tourism, and the airline and dining industries in metropolitan areas following September 11 are estimated to have lost more than one million jobs in 2002 due to public trepidations over the threat of terrorism (Joint Committee on Economics, 2002). Strong public fears represent a powerful disincentive to participate in industries marked by the threat of terrorism, as well as a costly incentive to accelerate the pace of resource diversion to antiterrorist security measures. Disproportionate fears can easily result in proportionate cuts in commerce.

The Role of the Media

A primary strategic goal of terrorism is to communicate its message via violent acts (Hoffman, 2002). Consequently, the mass media have been called the essential "oxygen" of terrorism (Dettmer, 2004). It has been suggested that modern terrorism began only after the first television satellite was launched in the late 1960s (Hoffman, 1998). The terrorists' aim to maximize their audience and commercial journalism's competition for readers and viewers have spawned a symbiotic terrorist-media relationship.

The Geneva Declaration on Terrorism (United Nations, 1987) recognized that the media could play a direct role in terrorism by "uncritically disseminating disinformation" and playing an indirect role through a pattern of selective coverage. Twenty-first-century terrorists are no longer dependent upon formal media outlets to disseminate their message. Most national and international media outlets exercise disciplined restraint with respect to obvious terrorist propaganda and avoid replaying terrorist announcements or communiqués. Unfortunately, terrorists can readily circumvent journalistic censorship. Recorded instructions and coded communications, as well as videos of executions, beheadings, hostage pleadings, and "documentaries" of suicide bombings are now easily distributed over the Internet and nonmainstream sources.

While terrorists are likely to continue to exploit the publicity potential of the Internet, the psychology of risk perception dictates that media coverage, especially television journalism, will continue to play a crucial role in fueling public fears. Vivid, repetitive coverage of acts and threats of terror prime the cognitive and emotional processes that help create a disproportionate sense of risk and vulnerability. Images of terror become more readily available and underscore the sense of emotional dread. Dramatic media accounts of terrorism capture public attention, and the perception of a greater risk of future attacks is heightened by the availability and affect heuristics.

Televised reporting of acts of terror appears to have stronger emotional impact than print news (Cho et al., 2003). Clearly, all of the tools of the modern film industry are available to television journalism, and only professional ethics and convention restrain the exploitation of high-production sound, music, graphics, animation, and video to deliver the maximum emotional impact. Compelling dramatic images of victims and their suffering personalize the implicit threat of terrorism, tacitly conveying a persuasive implication of the viewers' vulnerability: This has happened to people like us; therefore it could happen to us. The importance of television is underscored in studies of reactions to the September 11 terrorist attacks. For instance, greater monitoring of television reports was associated with adverse reactions (Huddy et al., 2003), and increased media reliance before September 11 was associated with greater threat perceptions after the attacks (Lowry et al., 2003). Even in countries with prolonged exposure to terrorism and emotionally hardened populations, media exposure has a significant impact. Prior to the war in Iraq, Israelis represented a major portion of terrorist casualties. A recent Israeli study (Keinan, Sadeh, & Rosen, 2003) has demonstrated that exposure to media coverage of terrorist attacks was correlated with an increase in traumatic symptoms even in this seasoned population.

Contemporary trends in terrorist tactics further call attention to the media's critical role, with ironic, but terrible, consequences for working members of the press. Three developments characterize recent acts of terrorism (Pfefferbaum, 2003). First, there has been a substantial increase in the lethality and brutality of terrorist acts, which may speak to the greater publicity value and inherently terrifying qualities associated with more dramatic violence (Stern, 1999).

In contrast to earlier policies employed by European terrorist groups (e.g., IRA and Basque ETA), which minimized casualties but maximized publicity by alerting police or journalists of planned bombings with sufficient time to allow evacuation, terrorists in Iraq and Afghanistan prepare their own videos documenting the extent of death and damage of their efforts for distribution after attacks to maximize media exposure. The growing technical proficiency of international television journalism creates an expanding market that may have provided such excesses with an unintended encouragement. In addition, the use of Web-based streaming video clips of beheadings and pleading hostages are often described, if not replayed, by professional media outlets. Second, anonymous acts of terrorism have increased but would have limited tactical value without media dissemination. Dramatic, graphic media coverage of anonymous, unattributed acts of terror—such as suicide bombings—nevertheless incites fear and apprehension among the public. Third, there has been an increase in terrorist attacks on journalists, a tragic indicator of the media's indispensable role in the strategy of terrorism.

Negativity bias is a fundamental factor in the media's selection and framing of news events and the public's trust in media analysis and reporting, and studies reveal a powerful bias toward coverage of negative events and outcomes (Niven, 2001). In their recent comprehensive review of the intersection of media, communication, and psychology, Byron Reeves and Clifford Nass (2003) conclude that people relate to mediated events in ways that reflect fundamental psychological processes that underlie human information processing. In particular, they note that human attention and memory—supported by "hardwired" neuropsychophysical processes—assign priority to negatively valenced, high-arousal stimuli. The underlying processes occur automatically and without conscious awareness and are probably the result of evolutionary adaptational advantages accrued from increased vigilance to potential threats. Memory for events following negative and high-arousal stimuli is proactively enhanced, and prior material is retroactively inhibited.

Interestingly, the effects of arousal are cumulative. Reeves and Nass argue, citing substantial supporting evidence, that mediated events are processed psychologically in much the same manner as "real world" events. Thus, it is not surprising that television networks, perpetually engaged in fierce competition for ratings and viewers, would feature reports with qualities that grab people's attention and stick in their memories: those that are negative and arousing. These qualities govern the selection and prominence assigned to stories that ultimately make it to the television screen, as well as shape their "packaging," that is, the editorial emphasis, the images selected, the music, the accompanying graphics, and all the other subtle nuances that set the emotional tone.

Thus, psychological processes give priority to negative, arousing material, and the news media act in accordance with the psychology of their audience. The media create a wider audience of spectators to terrorist acts while intensifying their emotional reactions, which engenders a greater sense of threat. If the availability and affect heuristics contribute to a disproportionate perception of risk and vulnerability, the media—especially television—augment and exacerbate the underlying psychology.

In addition to serving as a source of intense emotional stimuli, the media play a crucial role in profoundly shaping the public's understanding of terrorism. In fact, almost all areas of political interests are influenced by the media's powerful ability to set agendas and frame our understanding of events (Kinder, 1998). The media's influence lies not so much with its potential to persuade or to propagandize but rather with its reliable capacity to determine the facts, data, arguments, explanations, and theories to which its audience attends. The media tend not so much to persuade us but to dictate the facts, choices, or questions we should consider, evaluate, or debate. Risk perceptions are not exclusively emotional. Indeed, risk appraisals also depend on our ability to project future implications on the basis of our understanding of present circumstances. With respect to terrorism, our understanding of present circumstances is heavily dependent upon the news media's determination of what to report and how to report it, and this determination begins with how reports are framed.

Framing is a potent, yet inescapable, influence on the interpretation of reported events (Scheufele, 1999). In its simplest form, framing refers to the central organizing story. The frame simplifies the report and cues the audience to the report's "place" in a familiar, shared social construction of everyday reality. Tacitly, the frame signals another instance of a familiar theme (e.g., another report of wasteful government spending, another example of political corruption, another instance of gang violence). Sometimes a single image establishes the frame. For instance, the images of Muhammed Dura, a Palestinian boy supposedly killed in his father's arms, "clinches the 'larger narrative'" linking the event to "a chain of iconic images which (rightly or wrongly) signify historical events in public memory" (Liebes & First, 2003, p. 59). Why one frame rather than another is chosen remains an object of intense debate and study (P. Norris, Kern, & Just, 2003). Clearly, the process is immune to neither political partisanship (Niven, 2001) nor the influence of social power or material sponsorship (Carragee & Roefs, 2004).

Studies suggest that news coverage of terrorism, after the initial focus on the details of the act and the government's early response during the aftermath, rapidly (often in only a few weeks) restricts consideration of alternative explanations and motives for the attack. One study of terrorist reporting in a prominent national newspaper, for instance, found that, while the volume of coverage

devoted to the September 11 attack continued for many months, the number of alternative reasons, explanations, or motives considered diminished dramatically within just a few weeks (Traugott & Brader, 2003). Another study of editorials for the ten largest U.S. newspapers during the year after September 11 concluded that editors quickly— within the first month—arrived at a consistent, consensus narrative frame of the "war on terrorism" with little disagreement or dissent (Ryan, 2004).

Even the decision to characterize an act of political violence as "terrorism" is subject to implicit editorial biases. For instance, many studies indicate that regional media tend to report incidents of political violence against their own citizens as acts of terror but use other terms for similar acts against foreigners elsewhere (Nacos, 2002). Subtle variations in the use of descriptive terms can have very different psychological and political implications. Our own preliminary results in an ongoing study of terrorist media coverage reveal interesting variations in reports of a suicide bombing attack after a recent truce agreement with the new Palestinian government. While most countries explicitly described the attack as a suicide bombing, most Israeli sources consistently omitted the term "suicide," perhaps choosing to stress the damage to civilians over terms that convey the sense of martyrdom the terrorists seek to emphasize. In addition, we found considerable variation among the framing of this event among U.S. newspapers. We observed that front-page headlines describing the incident were split between those framing it as a major threat to a fragile truce and those emphasizing the act of suicide bombing. Nearly a third of the newspapers chose not to put the story on the front page, implicitly framing the incident below front-page priority and importance.

As discussed earlier, people often experience great difficulty in estimating risks using probabilities and percentages and instead fall back on psychological shortcuts or heuristics. The media must make parallel choices between reporting base rate data and statistical analyses or relying primarily on illustrative examples or case histories. Although news reports commonly employ examples of "typical cases," which are frequently chosen for their sensational qualities, base rate data are often omitted. If examples are exaggerated, they can be perceived as more broadly representative than actually borne out by facts. For example, in an experimental study (Gibson & Zillmann, 1994) that manipulated levels of exemplar distortion, readers of news reports featuring highly exaggerated examples of carjacking considered carjacking to be a much more serious national problem than readers of reports with less distorted exemplars. This effect was not mitigated by the presentation of accurate base rate data, a result consistent with the consensus of literature in this area, which concludes that base rate information "fails to exert a strong effect on news consumers' perceptions" (Gibson & Zillman, 1994, p. 608). Thus, the implied threat of terrorism is likely to be magnified by vivid, evocative examples of terrorist attacks despite efforts to balance conclusions by including precise statistical data about objective relative risk.

Although threats to public welfare are more likely to capture the attention of mass media than less negative and arousing events, not all risks become headline news. In an analysis of risk reporting for three very different well-publicized events in Great Britain, the authors conclude that risks will be reported when "there are decisive scientific statements, major disasters, fresh human interest stories, official reactions and/or when major organizations or governments come into conflict over the extent of the danger" (Kitzinger & Reilly, 1997, p. 344). They further conclude, however, that the media are poorly equipped to sustain "high level coverage for long-term threats" beyond the immediate controversies of the day.

Not only can mass media's preference for controversy over scientific subtleties and careful exposition of risks elevate the public's sense of danger and vulnerability, but it can also limit the public's understanding of the enemy. This is clear with respect to an understanding of the mind of the terrorist, a distortion that has potential to further exacerbate public fears.

Dispositional Stereotypes Versus Situational Explanations of Terrorists

Popular characterizations in many countries and political contexts typically portray terrorists as mentally deranged, homicidal madmen who are driven by severe psychopathology and antisocial personalities (Ruby, 2002). Early psychological

theories of terrorism offered hypothetical support for dispositional explanations, attributing the choice of the terrorist path to narcissistic rage, "hostile neuroses," paranoia, and other intrapsychic factors (Hudson, 1999).

In fact, however, comprehensive reviews of both classified and unclassified data regarding psychological features of known terrorists consistently conclude that the distribution of psychopathology among terrorist groups is similar to that of other groups (Atran, 2003; Crenshaw, 2000; Hoffman, 2002; Horgan, 2003; Hudson, 1999; Silke, 2003; Victoroff, 2005). In contrast to popular dispositional accounts, much current research and analysis emphasizes the powerful influence of situational factors in explaining the origins and motivations of terrorists. For example, situationally based explanations have greater validity in explorations of the development and influence of terrorist networks (Sageman, 2004), the influence of the decision-making process under clandestine circumstances (McCormick, 2003), the effects of social relationships and religious factors (Strenski, 2003), and the social and psychological processes that facilitate the recruitment and moral disengagement of those who choose the terrorist path (Moghaddam, 2005). Why, then, do dispositional characterizations of mentally deranged terrorists persist and in fact flourish in popular and professional accounts?

The *fundamental attribution error* (Ross, 1977), that is, the tendency of people to explain behavior in terms of internal, dispositional causes and to overlook or ignore situational factors clearly underlies the intuitive appeal of the deranged terrorists portrayed as victims of pathology or character flaws (Atran, 2003). Moreover, in stark contrast to dispositional explanations of "bad" actions, social psychologists have demonstrated that even among otherwise "good" people, evil can readily arise from situational factors (Zimbardo, 1995, 2004). The influence of social factors such as obedience to authority (Milgram, 1974) and the structure of social roles (Haney, Banks, & Zimbardo, 1973) can interact with ordinary psychological processes common to most people to disengage or diffuse their natural moral restraints (Bandura, 1999). Situational factors may have explanatory application to understanding evil ranging from petty crimes to horrendous atrocities, yet the fundamental attribution error regularly obscures the situationist perspective. It is not surprising, then, to witness a popular but misplaced focus on the "mind" of the terrorist.

Attributional errors can have important and destructive consequences. Political psychologists have observed that attributional bias can lead to flawed threat assessments in international politics because adversaries are understood in dispositional terms, while behavior on the part of one's own country is explained by situational factors (Levy, 2003). Thus, because situational factors, including threatening policies and actions of one's own country, are often discounted in favor of a focus on the adversary's perceived hostile intentions, the adversary is seen as more dangerous and malevolent. Actions on the part of one's own country are viewed as forced by situational factors (perceived threats). Thus, "if we take security measures because we have no choice, presumably others recognize this and understand that we are no threat to them, so that if they buy arms or mobilize forces it must be because they have hostile intentions" (Levy, 2003, p. 266). The cycle of attributing malevolent intent to the adversary and overlooking the provocative interpretation of our own well-intentioned reactions can spiral out of control.

Parallel patterns can occur with popular perceptions of terrorists. Certainly, the terrorists' intention is indeed hostile and malevolent, but a focus on disposition can both increase the sense of threat and obscure appropriate counterresponses. Portrayals of terrorists as madmen fit well with the psychological processes we have argued create a disproportionate sense of threat and, to that extent, may further the terrorists' agenda. "Deranged, crazed terrorists" are simultaneously *unfamiliar* and *dreadful*—extreme on both psychometric dimensions associated with elevated risk perceptions. Negativity bias furthers bolsters the intuitive appeal of dispositional characterizations of evildoers because, as we noted earlier, negative descriptors are perceived as more credible and more trait informative. The primarily dispositional portrayal of terrorists is quite compatible with the media's bias toward negatively valenced and high-arousal content, while exploration of situational factors challenges the media's reluctance to take on complex stories that unfold only after sustained analysis. Furthermore, terrorism is always understood within a political context. The dispositional portrayal is

more easily utilized politically because it avoids the complicated examination of situational factors, some of which may include policies and behaviors on both sides of the conflict.

Therefore, although terrorists are clearly evil, it is important to recognize all of the systemic factors that support and facilitate terrorism. Despite the power of situational explanations, they are sometimes mistaken as excuses: "Social circumstances compelled terrorists' violent, evil actions." The validity of situational contributions does not exonerate terrorists, who remain culpable for their crimes in any case. Situational explanations of terrorist behavior do not imply situational ethics. In his discussion of the origins of the Rwandan genocide, Diamond (2005) reminds us that explanations of misconduct can be misconstrued as excuses, but

> whether we arrive at an over-simplified one-factor explanation or an excessively complex 71-factor explanation for genocide doesn't alter the personal responsibility of the perpetrators . . . for their actions. This is a misunderstanding that arises regularly in discussion of the origins of evil; people recoil at any explanation, because they confuse explanation with excuses. But it *is* important that we understand the origins of Rwandan genocide—not so that we can exonerate the killers, but so that we can use that knowledge to decrease the risk of such things happening again in Rwanda or elsewhere. (pp. 326–327)

A preoccupation with intrapsychic, dispositional factors not only helps make terrorists more frightening, which is to their strategic advantage, but can also result in a failure to fully scrutinize the recruitment processes, group decision-making structures, and various societal influences that support the evil of terrorism (see Chapter 8 in this volume). The same cognitive and emotional processes that facilitate the disproportionate sense of danger and vulnerability, however, present a serious challenge to the public's appreciation of situational explanations.

Recommendations

It is essential that government leadership make every effort to "take the terror out of terrorism" by deploying programs to address the psychosocial processes that underlie public perceptions before, during, and after a terrorist emergency. Fear management programs are unlikely to achieve success without strong executive leadership. Because public reactions are complex, they cut across the province of medical, law enforcement, and other disaster-response stakeholders and entail sensitive attention to the priorities and concerns of diverse ethnic, cultural, and religious segments within states. Moreover, the economic, political, and social consequences of failure are so substantial that the intricacies of managing public fear in an era of terrorism must not be ignored.

Several factors are key to successfully responding to human-made attempts to exploit the psychology of fear:

Provide Full Information That Speaks to Local Concerns. Fear management efforts must recognize that psychological reactions to acts of terror are actually composed of a diverse, complex array of emotions and perceptions that can have very different effects on traumatic outcomes, public trust, and support for government policy. The public must have ready access to accurate information concerning threat assessment and preparedness, as well as to developments and protective governmental responses, following acts of terror. Risk alerts or warnings should stress realistic probabilities rather than dramatize catastrophic possibilities. In addition, neither federal government public affairs efforts nor national media communications are likely to adequately address public concerns at state and local levels. Fears of tainted or contaminated products following an act or threat of agroterrorism, for instance, present different concerns and challenges for food production than for recipient communities. Governments should consider investing in the development and field testing of risk communications tailored specifically to local concerns, priorities, and cultural norms and attitudes. Of course, materials and information should be made available in languages other than English where appropriate.

Plan for Realistic Psychological Reactions. Fear management programs must avoid focusing on the relatively unlikely probability of public panic and hysteria. Fear management plans should emphasize more probable scenarios, for example, the mass convergence of spectators, volunteers, and media on

the vicinity of Ground Zero or the strain on public health resources caused by a flood of "worried well" urgently seeking medical evaluations.

Stress Preparation and Training. Preevent organized activities can have enormous impact on public trust, and perceptions of trust can mitigate the impact of negativity bias and heightened feelings of fear and vulnerability. Simulations and exercises to educate the public, practice responding, enlist the cooperation of civic organizations, and disseminate accurate and authoritative information regarding best practices in response to various terrorist actions are absolutely essential. Simulations and other exercises can contribute to public perceptions of government competence and bolster public trust. Such activities may also help develop valuable relations with media representatives. Public and government leaders should insist upon adequate support for state programs, as well as advocate for comprehensive integration with nongovernmental organizations, including private medical facilities, the American Red Cross, charitable organizations, and healthcare professional organizations that provide voluntary disaster relief services.

Regular preevent simulations and exercises are valuable opportunities to ensure the optimal use of influential social networks within the structure of a state's communities. Preparedness efforts should ensure that fear managers capitalize on opportunities to integrate resources well in advance of terrorist threats rather than relegate integration to belated attempts to introduce leadership and "trade business cards" at the site of the disaster. Finally, preevent training provides opportunities for leadership to rehearse its decision-making process governing the release of information. Within reasonable bounds, full public disclosure is critical to rebutting rumor, misinformation, and distrust. Homeland security leadership should exploit every opportunity, including preevent simulations, to develop, practice, and evaluate policy and methods for determining the reasonable boundaries on information management.

Use Scientifically Credible Risk Communication. Risk communication about acts of terror should be informed by social scientists who are familiar with the psychological challenges that characterize public response. Effective fear management requires a well-considered, practiced media strategy. Public relations specialists can make an important contribution. Public trust in the sincerity and competence of government, however, is critical and will be undermined by any appearance of political spin or misguided efforts to calm public reactions by obscuring or strategically reframing information. Preparedness and response programs should encourage media access and build local media relationships with the clear recognition, however, that media coverage during a crisis will likely be dominated by out-of-state, national outlets whose priorities will often trump local relationships and media guidelines.

Unmask the Anonymous Perpetrator. The unknown is inherently more frightening than the known. Even if data are limited, providing the public with information about specific terrorists, especially information that highlights their fallibility and pedestrian qualities, is preferable to inviting the public to project an unwarranted sense of capability onto the absence of information.

Exercise Particular Care With Warnings. Given the power of negative information to aggravate public fear and vulnerability, public alerts or warnings of potential terrorist threats should be reconsidered if available information is vague and no specific public actions can be recommended. All warnings should stress the low magnitude of relative risk, perhaps by comparison with ordinary familiar hazards, such as car accidents, lightning strikes, and so on. Official warnings should be coupled with detailed information regarding government preparedness actions, preferably including a clearly prescribed role for concerned citizens. (It should be noted that research, albeit limited, on warnings and response allocation suggests that scant political cover is likely to be provided by vague, seemingly gratuitous warnings that happen to precede actual attacks.)

Anticipate the Needs of Special Populations. Fear management plans should strive to identify in advance populations with particular vulnerability to the traumatic impact of terrorists' actions (e.g., children) and also anticipate ethnic or cultural groups at risk for retribution or backlash following actions apparently linked to particular cultural or religious origins. Homeland security leadership should encourage school systems to develop disaster plans and implement routine age-appropriate training and drills. Preparatory efforts that target students may have a productive impact on otherwise apathetic parents, who might fail to

develop an emergency plan for themselves but will respond to their children's interest. Governors should also actively recruit cultural, ethnic, and religious leaders to serve as advisors and consultants in building and implementing fear management programs, as well as to serve as communication facilitators and spokespersons within diverse communities during crises.

Take Advantage of Technological Communication Resources. Internet-based information resources can effectively supplement fear management efforts. Web-based resources to rebut urban legends and potentially destructive product misinformation and rumor may serve as useful examples (Kimmel, 2004).

It is the quintessential nature of terrorism that perceptions of vulnerability, fear, and apprehension, however exaggerated or unrealistic, will inevitably represent the shared concerns of a large majority of citizens. Therefore, during an era of terrorism a democratic society has every right to expect the highest standards in fear management. Despite much progress, extensive research and development is needed to optimally mitigate our enemies' efforts to promote public terror.

Public policy for managing responses to terrorism should be guided by attention to three factors: education, resource integration, and scientific credibility. Government must invest in executive education that is designed specifically for homeland security leaders and managers. Executive education should include a comprehensive but pragmatic review of risk perception and communication, as well as the psychology of fear management. Leadership and their staff must be well trained in practical psychological principles and effective communication and media strategies.

Resource integration is critical, and people are a critical human capital resource. Effective fear management depends upon well-managed collaboration among many government and nongovernmental constituencies. Government leadership should advocate and fund state-tailored programs to reach out to government and community leaders, to provide continuous training, and to monitor progress and revise programs. The aim should be to develop an integrated community of stakeholders that can provide a valuable forum for discussion and public education.

The range of possible terrorist threats is daunting. In the long run, the most important advances in fear management will result from a better-educated (and hardened) public. Government should lead a continuing dialogue—one that is carefully and repeatedly presented in the mass media—about realistic limitations on our true capacities to protect against any threat.

Finally, in too many ways, fear management threatens to become a cottage industry fueled by the economics of fear. Many popular fear management interventions have not stood up to rigorous evaluation. It is essential that fear management programs be scientifically validated. Expert opinion is simply no substitute for empirical evidence. A large body of scientific work exists to inform future program development, and the safety of citizens should rest upon a scientifically credible foundation.

In summary, terrorists exercise their intuitive appreciation of the psychology of fear to promote widespread, disproportionate fear and vulnerability among the public. Their strategy is critically dependent upon the mass media but highly consistent with ingrained, fundamental psychological processes that guide the attention of the media's audience. Surely an effective response to terrorism will capitalize on a comprehensive understanding of the relevant psychology.

Notes

1. The apparent relationship between willingness to restrict civil liberties and the perceived risk of terrorism may depend on how "risk" is quantified. In a 2002 survey of Harvard Law School students, for instance, although respondents were willing to trade off civil liberties under certain conditions, their willingness was not associated with their perceptions of risk expressed in terms of the number of lives that might be lost in future attacks (Viscusi & Zeckhauser, 2003).

2. For example, since 1970 there have been only eight terrorist attacks on airplanes that resulted in the deaths of U.S. citizens. This tally includes the September 11 hijackings. (Compare Flynn, 2004.)

3. Despite exaggerated fears of crime, soon after 9/11 surveys indicated that the threat of terrorism surpassed perceptions of the risk of crime (see Gallup Crime Survey, 2001).

4. It has been argued that violent action and some limitations on civil liberties—lesser "evils" in the opinion of liberal democracies—can be a justified and necessary response to the greater evil of terrorism (Ignatieff, 2004). It seems especially important, therefore, to get the complexities of evil right and not settle for emotionally biased and perhaps politically expedient simplifications. This concern is elevated to even greater importance if recent assertions that the use of fear as a political justification has become a more favored pragmatic political method in democracies as faith in political principles fades (Robin, 2004).

References

Atran, S. (2003). Genesis of suicide terrorism. *Science, 299*(5612), 1534–1539.

Baer, J. (1997). Generating fear: The politics of crime reporting. *Crime, Law, and Social Change: An Interdisciplinary Journal, 27*(2), 87–107.

Bandura, A. (1999). Moral disengagement in the perpetration of inhumanties. *Personality and Social Psychological Review, 3,* 193–209.

Baumeister, R. F., Bratslavsky, E., Finkenauer, C., & Vole, K. D. (2001). Bad is stronger than good. *Review of General Psychology, 3*(4), 323–370.

Berke, R., & Elder, J. (2001, September 16). Poll finds strong support for U.S. use of military force. *New York Times,* p. 6.

Boscarino, J. A., Figley, C. R., & Adams, R. E. (2003). Fear of terrorism in New York after the September 11 terrorist attacks: Implications for emergency mental health and preparedness. *Journal of Emergency Mental Health, 5*(4), 199–203.

Bunker, R. J., & Sullivan, J. P. (2005, January–February). Suicide bombing operations in Operation Iraqi Freedom. *Military Review,* 69–82.

Carragee, K. M., & Roefs, W. (2004). The neglect of power in recent framing research. *Journal of Communication,* 214–233.

Chanley, V. A. (2002). Trust in government in the aftermath of 9/11: Determinants and consequences. *Political Psychology, 23*(3), 469–483.

Cho, J., Boyle, M. P., Keum, H., Shevy, M. D., McLeod, D. M., Shah, D. V., et al. (2003). Media, terrorism, and emotionality: Emotional differences in media content and public reactions to September 11 terrorist attacks. *Journal of Broadcasting and Electronic Media, 47*(3), 309–327.

Crenshaw, M. (2000). The psychology of terrorism: An agenda for the 21st century. *Political Psychology, 21*(2), 405–420.

Danieli, Y., Engdahl, B., & Schlenger, W. E. (2004). The psychosocial aftermath of terrorism. In F. M. Moghaddam & A. J. Marsella (Eds.), *Understanding terrorism: Psychosocial roots, consequences, and interventions* (pp. 223–246). Washington, DC: American Psychological Association.

Davis, D. W., & Silver, B. D. (2004, January). Civil liberties vs. security: Public opinion in the context of the terrorist attacks on America. *American Journal of Political Science, 48*(1), 28–46.

Dettmer, J. (2004). Supplying terrorists the "oxygen of publicity." In T. J. Badey (Ed.), *Annual editions: Violence and terrorism, 2004/2005* (pp. 136–137). Guilford, CT: McGraw-Hill/Dushkin.

Diamond, J. (2005). *Collapse: How societies choose to fail or succeed.* New York: Viking.

Ditzler, T. F. (2004). Malevolent minds: The teleology of terrorism. In F. M. Moghaddam & A. J. Marsella (Eds.), *Understanding terrorism: Psychosocial roots, consequences, and interventions* (pp. 187–207). Washington, DC: American Psychological Association.

Fetherstonhaugh, D., Slovic, P., Johnson, S. M., & Friedrich, J. (2000). Insensitivity to the value of human life: A study of psychophysical numbing. In P. Slovic (Ed.), *The perception of risk* (pp. 372–389). London: Earthscan.

Finucane, P. L., Alhakami, A., Slovic, P., & Johnson, S. M. (2000). The affect heuristic in judgments of risks and benefits. In P. Slovic (Ed.), *The perception of risk* (pp. 413–429). London: Earthscan.

Fischhoff, B., González, R. M., Small, D. A., and Lerner, J. S. (2003). Evaluating the success of terror risk communication. *Biosecurity and Bioterrorism: Biodefense Strategy, Practice, and Science, 1*(43), 255–258.

Flynn, S. (2004). *America the vulnerable: How our government is failing to protect us from terrorism.* New York: HarperCollins.

Food safety: Experiences of four countries in consolidating their food safety systems. (1999). GAO/RECED-99–80, pp. 5–6. Washington, DC: U.S. General Accounting Office.

Fredrickson, B. L., Tugade, M. M., Waugh, C. E., & Larkin, G. R. (2003). What good are positive emotions? A prospective study of resilience and emotions following the terrorist attacks on the United States on September 11, 2001. *Journal of Personality and Social Psychology, 84*(2), 365–376.

Frey, B. S., Luechinger, S., & Stutzer, A. (2004). Calculating tragedy: Assessing the costs of terrorism. Unpublished manuscript.

Fullerton, C. S., Ursano, R. J., Norwood, A. E., & Holloway, H. H. (2003). Trauma, terrorism, and disaster. In R. J. Ursano, C. S. Fullerton, & A. E. Norwood (Eds.), *Terrorism and disaster: Individual and community mental health interventions* (pp. 1–22). New York: Cambridge University Press.

Ganor, B. (2004). Terror as a strategy of psychological warfare. In T. J. Badey (Ed.), *Annual editions: Violence and terrorism 2004–2205* (pp. 5–8). Guilford, CT: McGraw-Hill/Dushkin.

Gibson, R., & Zillmann, D. (1994). Exaggerated versus representative exemplification in news reports: Perception of issues and personal consequences. *Communications Research, 21*(5), 603–624.

Glassner, B. (1999). *The culture of fear: Why Americans are afraid of the wrong things.* New York: Basic Books.

Gregory, R., Flynn, J., & Slovic, P. (1995). Technological stigma. *American Scientist, 83,* 220–223.

Haney, C., Banks, C., & Zimbardo, P. (1973). Interpersonal dynamics in a simulated prison. *International Journal of Criminology Penology, 1,* 69–97.

Hills, A. (2002). Responding to catastrophic terrorism. *Studies in Conflict and Terrorism, 25,* 245–261.

Hoffman, B. (1998). *Inside terrorism.* New York: Columbia University Press.

———. (2001a). Change and continuity in terrorism. *Studies in Conflict and Terrorism, 24,* 417–428.

———. (2001b, September 26). Re-thinking terrorism in light of a war on terrorism. Testimony presented by Hoffman (vice president, External Affairs, and director, RAND, Washington office) to the Subcommittee on Terrorism and Homeland Security, House Permanent Select Committee on Intelligence, U.S. House of Representatives, pp. 1–10.

———. (2002). The mind of the terrorist: Perspectives from social psychology. In H. W. Kushner (Ed.), *Essential readings on political terrorism: Analyses of problems and prospects for the 21st century* (pp. 62–69). Lincoln: University of Nebraska Press/Gordon Knot Books.

Horgan, J. (2003). The search for the terrorist personality. In A. Silke (Ed.), *Terrorists, victims, and society: Psychological perspectives on terrorism and its consequences* (pp. 3–28). New York: Wiley.

Huddy, L., Feldman, S., Lahav, G., & Taber, C. (2003). Fear and terrorism: Psychological reactions to 9/11. In P. Norris, M. Kern, & M. Just (Eds.), *Framing terrorism: The news media, the government, and the public* (pp. 255–278). New York: Routledge.

Huddy, L., Friedman, S., Capelos, T., & Provost, C. (2002). The consequences of terrorism: Disentangling the effects of personal and national threat. *Political Psychology, 23*(3), 485–509.

Hudson, R. A. (1999). *The sociology and psychology of terrorism: Who becomes a terrorist and why?* Washington, DC: Federal Research Division, Library of Congress.

Ignatieff, M. (2004). *The lesser evil: Political ethics in the age of terrorism*. Princeton, NJ: Princeton University Press.

Johnson, L. C. (2001). The future of terrorism. *American Behavioral Scientist, 44*(6), 894–913.

Joint Committee on Economics. (2002, May). *The economic costs of terrorism*. U.S. Congress, Washington, DC.

Kahneman, D., & Tversky, A. (1979). Prospect theory: An analysis of decisions under risk. *Econometrica, 47*, 263–291.

Keinan, G., Sadeh, A., & Rosen, S. (2003). Attitudes and reactions to media coverage of terrorist acts. *Journal of Community Psychology, 31*(2), 149–165.

Kimmel, A. J. (2004). *Rumors and rumor control: A manager's guide to understanding and combating rumors*. Mahwah, NJ: Erlbaum.

Kinder, D. R. (1998). Communication and opinion. *Annual Review of Political Science, 1*, 167–197.

Kitzinger, J., & Reilly, J. (1997). The rise and fall of risk reporting. *European Journal of Communication, 12*(3), 319–350.

Klein, J. G. (1991). Negativity effects in impression formation: A test in the political arena. *Personality and Social Psychological Review, 17*, 412–418.

Kuran, T., & Sunstein, C. R. (1999). Availability cascades and risk regulation. *Stanford Law Review, 51*, 683–768.

Kuzma, L. M. (2004). Security versus liberty: 9/11 and the American public. In W. Crotty (Ed.), *The politics of terror: The U.S. Response to 9/11* (pp. 160–190). Boston: Northeastern University Press.

Lasker, R. D. (2004). *Redefining readiness: Terrorism planning through the eyes of the public*. New York: New York Academy of Medicine.

Lerner, J. S., Gonzales, R. M., Small, D. A., & Fischhoff, B. (2003). Effects of fear and anger on perceived risks of terrorism: A national field experiment. *Psychological Science, 14*(2), 144–150.

Lerner, J. S., & Keltner, D. (2001). Fear, anger, and risk. *Journal of Personality and Social Psychology, 81*(1), 146–159.

Lesser, I. O., Hoffman, B., Arquilla, J., Ronfeldt, D. F., Zanini, M., & Jenkins, B. M. (1999). *Countering the new terrorism*. Santa Monica: RAND.

Levy, J. S. (2003). Political psychology and foreign policy. In D. O. Sears, L. Huddy, & R. Jervis (Eds.), *Oxford handbook of political psychology* (pp. 253–284). New York: Oxford University Press.

Liebes, T., & First, A. (2003). Framing the Palestinian-Israeli conflict. In P. Norris, M. Kern, & M. Just (Eds.), *Framing terrorism: The news media, the government, and the public* (pp. 59–74). New York: Routledge.

Lowry, D. T., Nio, T. C. J., & Leitner, D. W. (2003, March). Setting the public fear agenda: A longitudinal analysis of network TV crime reporting, public perceptions of crime, and FBI crime statistics. *Journal of Communication, 53*, 61–73.

Marcus, G. E. (2000). Emotions in politics. *Annual Review of Political Science, 3*, 221–250.

———. (2003). The psychology of emotion and politics. In D. O. Sears, L. Huddy, & R. Jervis (Eds.), *Oxford handbook of political psychology* (pp. 182–221). New York: Oxford University Press.

McCormick, G. H. (2003). Terrorist decision making. *Annual Review of Political Science, 6*, 473–507.

Mezulis, A. H., Abramson, L. Y., Hyde, J. S., & Hankin, B. L. (2004). Is there a universal positivity bias in attributions? A meta-analytic review of individual, developmental, and cultural differences in the self-serving attributional bias. *Psychological Bulletin, 130*(5), 711–747.

Milgram, S. (1974). *Obedience to authority*. New York: Harper & Row.

Moghaddam, F. M. (2005). The staircase to terrorism: A psychological explanation. *American Psychologist, 60*(2), 161–169.

———, & Marsella, A. J. (Eds.). (2003). *Understanding terrorism: Psychosocial roots, consequences, and interventions* (pp. 323–246). Washington, DC: American Psychological Association.

Nacos, B. L. (2002). *Mass-mediated terrorism: The central role of the media in terrorism and counter-terrorism*. Lanham, MD: Rowman & Littlefield.

Niven, D. (2001). Bias in the news: Partisanship and negativity in media coverage of presidents George Bush and Bill Clinton. *Harvard International Journal of Press/Politics, 6*, 31–46.

Norris, F. H., Byrne, C. M., & Díaz, E. (2002). 60,000 disaster victims speak, part 1: An empirical review of the empirical literature, 1981–2001. *Psychiatry, 65*, 207–239.

Norris, P., Kern, M., & Just, M. (2003). Framing terrorism. In P. Norris, M. Kern, & M. Just (Eds.), *Framing terrorism: The news media, the government, and the public* (pp. 3–23). New York: Routledge.

Pape, R. A. (2003). The strategic logic of suicide terrorism. *American Political Science Review, 97*(3), 21–43.

Perry, R. W., & Lindell, M. K. (2003). Understanding citizen response to disasters with implications for terrorism. *Journal of Contingencies and Crisis Management, 11*(2), 49–60.

Peters, B. G. (2004). Are we safer today? Organizational responses to terrorism. In W. Crotty (Ed.), *The politics of terror: The U.S. response to 9/11* (pp. 235–251). Boston: Northeastern University Press.

Pfefferbaum, B. (2003). Victims of terrorism and the media. In A. Silke (Ed.), *Terrorists, victims, and society* (pp. 175–187). Hoboken, NJ: Wiley.

Poortinga, W., & Pidgeon, N. F. (2004). Trust, the asymmetry principle, and the role of prior beliefs. *Risk Analysis, 24*(6), 1475–1486.

Powell, D. (2001). Mad cow disease and the stigmatization of British beef. In J. Flynn, P. Slovic, & H. Kunreuther (Eds.), *Risk, media, and stigma* (pp. 219–228). London: Earthscan.

Reeves, B., & Nass, C. (2003). *The media equation: How people treat computers, television, and new media like real people and places.* Palo Alto: CLSI Publications, Stanford University.

Risk assessment for food terrorism and other food safety concerns. (2003, October 7). Department of Health and Human Services, U.S. Food and Drug Administration, Center for Food Safety and Applied Nutrition/Office of Regulations and Policy. Retrieved January 12, 2006, from http://www.cfsan.fda.gov/~dms/rabtact.html

Robin, C. (2004). *Fear: The history of a political idea.* New York: Oxford University Press.

Ross, L. (1977). The intuitive psychologist and his shortcomings: Distortions in the attributional process. In L. Berkowitz (Ed.), *Advances in experimental social psychology: Vol. 10* (pp. 173–220). New York: Academic Press.

Rothschild, M. L. (2001). Terrorism and you: The real odds. *AEI-Brookings Joint Center: Policy Matters, 1*(31), 1–2.

Rozin, P., & Royzman, E. B. (2001). Negativity bias, negativity dominance, and contagion. *Personality and Social Psychological Review, 5*(4), 296–320.

Ruby, C. L. (2002). Are terrorists mentally deranged? *Analyses of Social Issues and Public Policy, 2*(1), 15–26.

Ryan, M. (2004). Framing the war against terrorism: U.S. newspaper editorials and military action in Afghanistan. *Gazette: International Journal for Communication Studies, 66*(5), 363–382.

Sageman, M. (2004). *Understanding terror networks.* Philadelphia: University of Pennsylvania Press.

Scheufele, D. A. (1999, Winter). Framing as a theory of media effects. *Journal of Communication,* 103–122.

Siegrist, M., & Cvetkovich, G. (2001). Better negative than positive? Evidence of a bias for negative information about possible health dangers. *Risk Analysis, 21,* 199–206.

Silke, A. (2003). Becoming a terrorist. In A. Silke (Ed.), *Terrorists, victims, and society: Psychological perspectives on terrorism and its consequences* (pp. 29–53). Hoboken, NJ: Wiley.

Skowronski, J. J., & Carlston, D. E. (1989). Negativity and extremity biases in impression formation: A review of explanations. *Psychological Bulletin, 105*(1), 131–142.

Slovic, P. (1993). Perceived risk, trust, and democracy. *Risk Analysis, 13*(6), 675–682.

———, Finucane, M. L., Peters, E., & MacGregor, D. C. (2004). Risk as analysis and risk as feelings: Some thoughts about affect, risk, and rationality. *Risk Analysis, 24,* 311–322.

Slovic, P., Fischhoff, B., & Lichtenstein, S. (2000). Facts and fears: Understanding perceived risk. In P. Slovic (Ed.), *The perception of risk* (pp. 137–153). London: Earthscan.

Stern, J. (1999). *The ultimate terrorist.* Cambridge: Harvard University Press.

Strenski, I. (2003). Sacrifice, gift, and the social logic of Muslim "human bombers." *Terrorism and Political Violence, 15*(3), 1–34.

Sunstein, C. R. (2003). Terrorism and probability neglect. *Journal of Risk and Uncertainty, 26*(2/3), 121–136.

Traugott, M. W., & Brader, T. (2003). Explaining 9/11. In P. Norris, M. Kern, & M. Just (Eds.), *Framing terrorism: The news media, the government, and the public* (pp. 183–202). New York: Routledge.

Tucker, D. (2001, Autumn). What's new about the new terrorism and how dangerous is it? *Terrorism and Political Violence, 13,* 1–14.

Tversky, A., & Kahneman, D. (1974). Judgment under uncertainty: Heuristics and bias. *Science, 185,* 1124–1131.

United Nations. (1987, May 29). Geneva declaration on terrorism. Paper presented at the United Nations General Assembly, Geneva, Switzerland.

Victoroff, J. (2005). The mind of the terrorist: A review and critique of psychological approaches. *Journal of Conflict Resolution, 49*(1), 3–42.

Viklund, M. J. (2003). Trust and risk perception in Western Europe: A cross-national study. *Risk Analysis, 23*(4), 727–738.

Viscusi, W. K., & Zeckhauser, R. J. (2003). Sacrificing civil liberties to reduce terrorism risks. *Journal of Risk and Uncertainty, 26*(2/3), 99–120.

Zimbardo, P. G. (1995). The psychology of evil: A situationist perspective on recruiting good people to engage in anti-social acts. *Japanese Journal of Social Psychology, 11*(2), 125–133.

———. (2004). A situationist perspective on the psychology of evil: Understanding how good people are transformed into perpetrators. In A. Miller (Ed.), *The social psychology of good and evil: Understanding our capacity for kindness and cruelty.* New York: Guilford.

III

Consequences of Terrorism

10

The Role of Religion, Spirituality, and Faith-Based Community in Coping With Acts of Terrorism

Timothy A. Kelly

On September 11, 2001, the world changed, and, like it or not, civilization is now enduring an age of terrorism. On that clear Fall morning, the world watched in horror as the Twin Towers collapsed, and thousands of innocent lives were lost. The television footage was horrendous, showing some plunging to their death from the flames, others fleeing monstrous clouds of dust in panic, and still others exhausted and covered in ghastly soot from top to toe. On average, adults watched more than 8 hours of coverage that day (Schuster et al., 2001), enough to see the towers come down dozens of times, enough to traumatize the hapless viewer. Acts of terrorism are of course designed to do just that—to traumatize a population into submission (Linley, Joseph, Cooper, Harris, & Meyer, 2003). The United States has not submitted, but it has been traumatized by the terror of 9/11.

Where do people turn in times of trauma? Where is help to be found when the very infrastructure of society collapses as it did in New York City? A RAND survey conducted less than a week after 9/11 discovered that people relied primarily on two resources—one another and their understanding of God. As the survey authors state, "most turned to religion, and also to one another for social support" (Schuster et al., 2001, p. 1511). In fact, a full 90% reported turning to prayer, religion, or spiritual feelings. That is slightly more than the 85% of Americans who report that religion is "fairly or very important" in their lives (Gallup, 2003). In a similar vein, survivors of the Oklahoma City bombing were found to consistently use "positive religious coping strategies" as a means of working through the trauma of that attack (Harrison, Koenig, Hays, Eme-Akwari, & Pargament, 2001, p. 88).

Shortly after 9/11, the Department of Justice distributed the Office for Victims of Crime Handbook for Coping after Terrorism (U.S. Department of Justice, 2001). The handbook refers several times to the fact that victims of terrorism may need to consider "professional or spiritual" counseling, meaning help from a counselor or minister.[1] Recognizing this fact, the city of New York generously provided for the thousands of workers charged with the grisly task of sorting through the rubble of the Twin Towers. Dozens of mental health professionals and clergy were brought in to make themselves available for the workers as needed. To whom does one turn when you have just recovered a coworker's body or perhaps the arm of a child from the wreckage? Mental health professionals can help rescue workers process their thoughts and feelings in a manner that is certainly helpful in many instances. But for many trauma victims, clergy can offer more: a level of comfort, a means of grace, a touch of the divine in the midst of the struggle to cope with incomprehensible tragedy. So it has been found that, in times of cataclysmic trauma, people turn first to clergy for emotional support and only later, if at all, to mental health workers (Everly, 2003).

On the other hand, religiously oriented persons experiencing a life trauma may find that their religious beliefs do not necessarily help. They may struggle endlessly with the age-old question of theodicy—how to reconcile the reality of evil with the concept of an all-powerful and all-good God. This is most poignantly expressed as a syllogism:

- A good and omnipotent God must be willing and able to prevent evil.
- Evil exists.
- Therefore, God is either not omnipotent or not good.

For example, a study of Vietnam veterans suffering from posttraumatic stress disorder (PTSD) found that 74% have difficulty reconciling their religious beliefs with the trauma they experienced in Vietnam. Slightly more than half (51%) stated that they abandoned their religious faith in Vietnam (Drescher & Foy, 1995). For these veterans, religion and spirituality did not help them to cope with the horror of warfare.

What is to be made of the fact that those who were traumatized by a terrorist attack turned in large numbers to religion and spirituality, yet many Vietnam veterans abandoned their faith? Do religion and spirituality provide a critical resource in times of national trauma, or is this a false hope? If it is indeed an important resource, precisely what aspect of religion or spirituality helps one to cope in times of trauma? This chapter addresses these and related questions as they pertain to individual and community preparedness for terrorist attack. Since there is some confusion as to the definitions of basic concepts such as "religion" and"spirituality," the chapter begins by introducing and defining key terms: spirituality, religion, faith-based community, posttraumatic stress disorder, posttraumatic depression, and posttraumatic growth. Next current research on trauma care and on the role of religion and spirituality in coping with trauma is reviewed. The chapter closes with a discussion of practical recommendations for emergency mental health professionals, individuals, and faith-based communities in drawing on spirituality and religion to help those affected cope with the trauma of a terrorist attack.

Key Concepts and Terms

Religion, Spirituality, and Faith-Based Community

Wars have long been fought (and are still being fought) over which concept of God and which definition of religion will stand. In fact, the terrorism the world faces today—primarily that of militant Islam—is often justified by the perpetrators as necessary in order to protect and expand a way of life based on strict religious beliefs. It is both ironic and tragic to note that militant Islamic terrorists kill in the name of God, while at the same time many victims of their attacks turn to God in order to cope with the inflicted trauma. It is not surprising, then, that no precise definition of religion can be offered with which all theologians and policymakers would agree. Instead, this chapter offers a dictionary definition that is generic enough to reflect a pluralistic approach, yet specific enough to be meaningful:

> Religion: belief in a divine power to be worshipped and obeyed as the creator and ruler of the universe, expressed in conduct and ritual. (Webster, 1979)

"Spirituality," too, is a word with variable usage and meanings. Currently in postmodern America the term is frequently used to refer to a more personal, subjective, psychological, and less formalized type of religious orientation. Thus, a person can be spiritual without necessarily being religious. To some, it is more authentic to be spiritual in one's own way than to be religious by following the directives of an organization such as a church, synagogue, or mosque. However, this dichotomized view of religion and spirituality is problematic. After all, many traditionally religious people place a high value on spirituality as well and hold that these are not mutually exclusive concepts. Perhaps it is more helpful to suggest that spirituality and religion are overlapping concepts with a difference in focus. Spirituality focuses more on individual and psychological expression, whereas religion focuses more on corporate and sociological expression. It is possible to experience one without the other, but many would say that they function best as two sides of one coin. A religious person who lacks spirituality may be seen as superficial, and an antireligious spiritual person may be seen as simply self-indulgent. In contrast, a person who is both spiritual and religious can be seen as demonstrating a credible maturity of faith and practice.

Consider, for example, notable religious leaders such as Mother Teresa and Inamullah Khan, Christian and Muslim recipients of the Templeton Prize, or Lord Jakobovits, former chief rabbi of Great Britain. Each of these remarkable people can be said to have demonstrated a life that was both religious and spiritual. Acknowledging, then, that these concepts are distinct yet complementary, we may define spirituality as follows:

> Spirituality: the individual's personal, subjective expression of their search for transcendent meaning and purpose, which may or may not involve organized religion.

With these definitions in mind, it is possible to state with some clarity what "faith-based community" means. Since religious beliefs are not subject to empirical verification and concepts of the divine are not subject to standard scientific tests, faith is a prominent component in both religion and spirituality. (Of course, even the hardest science requires faith in the empirical method and scientific interpretation, but that is another discussion.) Thus, religiously or spiritually oriented people are often described as "people of faith," and many consider themselves part of a community of those who believe as they do (though some are more individualistic and idiosyncratic in their faith and do not associate with any religious organization). The faith community typically revolves around a parish, church, synagogue, mosque, or some other anchor point for like-minded believers:

> Faith-based community: that group of like-minded believers with whom the individual participates and identifies regarding religious/ spiritual beliefs and practices. It is to such communities that survivors of terrorist attacks invariably turn for help.

Posttraumatic Stress Disorder

The concept of psychological trauma following in the wake of physical trauma is generally well accepted by professionals and the general public alike. The central idea, as presented in Chapter 13, is that people who have experienced an overwhelming trauma may find afterward that they are simply unable to cope well with life's stressors. Instead, they experience debilitating symptoms that may continue unabated unless treated. During and after the world wars of the twentieth century, for example, many servicemen were found to suffer from shell shock and to need hospitalization. The need for treatment for postcombat servicemen helped drive the expansion of Veterans Administration hospitals and sped the growth of clinical psychology.

Not until after the Vietnam War was the term "posttraumatic stress disorder" (PTSD) coined as a way to capture the disabling experiences that many combat veterans endured. PTSD is defined for mental health professionals in the *Diagnostic and Statistical Manual of Mental Disorders* (American Psychiatric Association, 2000). The condition can occur after exposure to a life-threatening stressor that induces fear, helplessness, and/or horror (e.g., combat, sexual assault, torture, terrorist attack). Exposure may involve being present at and experiencing a direct threat of death or injury, as was the case for those in the Twin Towers on 9/11, or it may involve witnessing such an event either close at hand or via media coverage (Linley et al., 2003). The result is an array of difficult symptoms such as feelings of extreme anxiety or panic, recurrent nightmares or flashbacks, a mental and emotional reliving of the event, ceaseless hyperactivity, and significant dysfunction at home or work.

Results of a national survey in the mid-1990s showed that PTSD was fairly widespread in the United States even before 9/11 (Kessler, Sonnega, Bromet, Hughes, & Nelson, 1996), and rates appear to rise after major disasters. For instance, nations that have experienced extreme conflict show extremely high rates of this disorder: Algeria (37%), Cambodia (28%), and Gaza (18%) (de Jong et al., 2001).

In sum, PTSD is a well-recognized emotional disorder, triggered by a traumatic event, that seriously impairs one's quality of life. If untreated, PTSD can result in permanent mental disability involving intense psychological suffering, social alienation, disorganization, decreased productivity in the workplace, and ongoing medical and legal expenses. Since a terrorist attack is by definition a potentially overwhelming traumatic event, survivors of such attacks are at high risk for PTSD. This is confirmed by research that was completed 6 months after 9/11 in New York City, which found that 36.7% of those who were in the World Trade Center met the criteria for PTSD (Galea et al., 2003).

Posttraumatic Depression and Other Disorders

Survivors of a terrorist attack are clearly at risk for PTSD. They are also at risk for other emotional disorders that may be either related to PTSD or totally distinct but triggered by the same trauma (Flannery, 1999). For instance, posttraumatic depression can occur as a survivor finds that, following a trauma, a profound sense of hopelessness and sadness becomes overwhelming and debilitating. Such depression may include loss of sleep and appetite, loss of motivation and energy, feelings of guilt or anxiety, and suicidal thoughts. Unless treated, posttraumatic depression may become chronic and even lead to suicide attempts.

Other emotional disorders may also be triggered by trauma, though PTSD and posttraumatic depression are the most common. Trauma survivors may experience panic attacks, agoraphobia (fear of leaving the safety of one's home), or psychosomatic pains such as stomach cramps or headaches. Survivors may also find that, for the first time, they struggle with drug and alcohol abuse or other high-risk behaviors. After 9/11, surveys found that the trauma of terrorist attack led large numbers of Americans to seek help for substance abuse (National Center of Addiction and Substance Abuse, 2001). It is not known why the same trauma evokes different disorders in different people, but it is clear that these disorders call for timely and effective help. If no help is available, these disorders may result in intense psychological pain, an increase in accidents or illness, lost productivity in the workplace, permanent disability, or suicide (Flannery, 1999).

Posttraumatic Growth

Whereas the fairly common experience of PTSD and related emotional disorders is well studied and well accepted, clinicians and researchers have more recently identified another possible aftereffect of trauma that is only beginning to be understood—posttraumatic growth. Actually, the possibility of positive change resulting from negative events has been recognized through the ages in philosophy, literature, and religion. Consider, for example, the mythological story of the Egyptian phoenix—a great bird that was destroyed, only to rise again from the ashes. Or consider the actual story of Lance Armstrong, multiple winner of the Tour de France after surviving cancer. In his autobiography Armstrong discusses how the trauma of cancer and chemotherapy led to his resolve to become a world champion: "[The] truth is that cancer is the best thing that ever happened to me" (Armstrong, 2001, p. 4). Of course, this does not mean that Armstrong welcomed the scourge of cancer; rather, it means that even the worst experience can lead to remarkable benefit. Thus the concept of new birth or growth resulting from trauma and suffering is not new.

For the past 10 years a growing number of researchers have been studying this intriguing concept. Although various terms are used, the concept is the same—long-term positive outcome following crisis (e.g., "stress-related growth," "adversarial growth"). As a result, a growing body of literature has found that a significant number of those who have been victimized by trauma experience posttraumatic growth (Affleck & Tennen, 1996; Arnold, Calhoun, Tedeschi, & Cann, 2005; Calhoun & Tedeshi, 2006; Linley & Joseph, 2004; McMillen, 1999; Tedeschi & Calhoun, 1995; Tedeschi, Park, & Calhoun, 1998; Woodward & Joseph, 2003).

It is possible to experience growth after illness, bereavement, and other major life stressors. It is also possible to experience growth after the severe trauma of a terrorist attack. But just what does posttraumatic growth mean, and how is it best understood? Most researchers suggest that it consists of positive changes in interpersonal relationships, positive changes in life philosophy, and/or a sense of peace and optimism in the face of adversity. As a result, the posttraumatic individual ends up at a significantly higher level of functioning at home, at work, and with others. This positive change is labeled "posttraumatic growth."

It is important to note that posttraumatic growth is not the same thing as resilience or recovery (e.g., Bonanno, 2004, 2005), topics that are addressed in Chapters 12 and 21. It is certainly true that many people are able to recover from even a disastrous trauma and carry on, especially with the support of friends and family. These are emotionally strong people who have the ability to return to normal functioning with little help and who will likely not experience PTSD. However, posttraumatic growth means more than just recovering one's normal state of functioning, as important as that is. It also means that the trauma victims actually end up surpassing their pretrauma state of functioning and report being significantly better off for having suffered the event. This does not at all suggest that the trauma is therefore welcomed or trivialized, nor does it mean that there is no negative impact from the trauma. It is possible for a survivor to go through periods of severe anxiety and grief on the way to posttraumatic growth. Nevertheless, it does mean that the final outcome is actually superior to the starting point.

In sum, there are three possible outcomes to trauma: PTSD, recovery, and posttraumatic growth. Not only do these outcomes yield different experiences for the victims of trauma, but they also require different treatment responses, as trauma care researchers are now recognizing.

Trauma Care and the Role of Religion and Spirituality

Critical Incident Stress Management: A Trauma Care Standard

Every major metropolitan area across the United States has designated resources for meeting a community's needs after a disaster, whether that involves food and housing, physical healthcare, or mental healthcare. Emergency mental health (EMH) services are designed to meet the mental health needs of individuals and communities after a major disaster such as a terrorist attack (Flannery, 1999). These services are typically coordinated from a central crisis-response center and involve those who have been selected and trained to serve the community as EMH professionals in times of crisis. Thus in any given area there should be a team of psychiatrists, psychologists, social workers, and/or other mental health practitioners who are ready to serve when called upon. What guides the services that EMH professionals offer?

The most widely recognized treatment approach is known as critical incident stress management (CISM; Everly & Mitchell, 1999), which provides a paradigm for postcrisis care. CISM is designed to reduce the acute psychological distress suffered by victims of a trauma such as a terrorist attack and to reduce the incidence of emotional disorders such as PTSD that may be triggered by that trauma.

CISM necessarily requires planning and preparation on the part of emergency care agencies, such as selecting and training EMH professionals and developing area strategies. Once these are implemented, there are four primary treatment components that can be helpful both for the residents of an affected area and for disaster workers attending them:

- Individual acute crisis counseling, consisting of one-on-one sessions, with or without medications. This is typically offered as soon as possible to those who are severely traumatized and who may have difficulty with daily life functioning.
- Brief small-group debriefings. These discussions are designed to reduce acute symptoms such as high anxiety levels and grief by working through such feelings. The goal is to offer this service early on so as to defuse what could otherwise become debilitating emotional trauma.
- Longer-term small-group discussions known as critical incident stress debriefing (Mitchell & Everly, 1996). The goal of long-term debriefing is to work through traumatic events and achieve a sense of closure so that victims can move on with their lives without difficulty. This may take weeks or months of focused effort, especially for those who have difficulty expressing negative thoughts and feelings.
- Family crisis intervention procedures. Living with traumatized individuals can be hard on a family unit or on others who live or work closely with the victim. In this intervention, EMH professionals go into the neighborhoods and homes of trauma victims and offer family therapy and other supportive and problem-solving services that may be called for.

The goal of these interventions is to reduce pathological symptoms, build caring networks of friends and family for ongoing support, and restore a sense of mastery and purpose in life. If the interventions do not adequately meet the needs of those impacted by the trauma, CISM calls for referrals for psychological assessment and treatment on an as-needed basis. CISM is supported by empirical evidence (Everly, Flannery, & Mitchell, 2000; Everly & Mitchell, 1999) and is considered by many as an international standard of trauma care for mental health needs (Mitchell & Everly, 2000). For this reason it was widely offered as a standard "blanket" intervention after 9/11 for those who were exposed to the trauma of the World Trade Center attack (Miller, 2002).

Research on the Effectiveness of Trauma Care

Until recently CISM and related approaches were assumed to constitute state-of-the-art effective treatment for all trauma victims. The assumption was that all those who were exposed to life-threatening stressors would benefit from the described services. After all, common sense suggests that it is helpful to work through grief and anxiety following trauma and loss and that the alternative is to deny emotions at one's own risk. Surprisingly, a growing literature demonstrates that that is not the case (e.g., Bonanno & Kaltman, 1999; Stroebe & Stroebe, 1991; Wortman & Silver, 1989). As it turns out, not only is CISM sometimes ineffective, but in some cases it may actually be harmful. One review of grief therapies, which overlap considerably with CISM strategies, found that 38% of those who received treatment actually got worse (Niemeyer, 2000). CISM is most likely helpful for some trauma victims who are spiraling downward emotionally and need help to process their negative feelings and thoughts, but it is not necessarily appropriate for those who have a different experience in reaction to trauma (Bonanno, 2004).

Thus, it seems increasingly clear that there are differential treatment needs among survivors of a terrorist attack. Some may benefit from CISM and related approaches, as detailed in Chapter 16. However, according to George Everly, who heads up the International Critical Incident Stress Foundation, many people need what might be called "pastoral crisis intervention." Everly defines this as "the use of traditional pastoral interventions applied within a context of sound emergency mental health skills." He states that pastoral crisis intervention is "nowhere . . . more useful than in response to real or threatened terrorism" (Everly, 2003, p. 1). Thus a well-recognized proponent of CISM acknowledges the limitations of that approach to posttraumatic treatment, as well as the unique relevance of spiritual and religious resources.

The Role of Religion and Spirituality in Coping With Trauma

Terrorism demoralizes a population with fear, anger, paranoia, and grief. Those who have lost loved ones are devastated, and witnesses (even via media) are horrified. Trust in one's community and government may fail, and the very fabric of society may seem to be crumbling. Saathoff and Everly point out that these feelings have the potential to spread by contagion, in that the population inadvertently spreads the intended impact of a terrorist attack by losing perspective and resolve (Saathoff & Everly, 2002). We thus further terrorize ourselves. If CISM is not capable of neutralizing such trauma sequelae for all victims, what recourse is there?

One recourse is to draw on the near-universal human experience of faith, spirituality, and religion. These resources have been historically neglected by the field of psychology for various reasons, yet are now recognized as strongly related to mental health (Hill & Pargament, 2003; Kelly & Strupp, 1992; Miller & Thoresen, 2003). Perhaps one could add that this rediscovery is coming in the nick of time, as the United States faces an enemy capable of destruction on the order of a nuclear war, yet without the predictability of the cold war. Thankfully, because of the rediscovery of the role of spirituality in mental health, there is a growing literature on the topic of spirituality and trauma—sometimes referred to as "religious coping." Researchers have found that positive religious coping is associated with lower rates of depression and with fewer symptoms of psychological distress such as those found in PTSD (e.g., Calhoun, Cann, Tedeschi, & McMillan, 2000; Drescher & Foy, 1995; Everly, 2003; Harrison et al., 2001; Meisenhelder, 2002; Overcash, Calhoun, Cann, & Tedeschi, 1996; Pargament, Tarkeshwar, Ellison, & Wulff, 2001; Pargament et al., 1990; Sowell et al., 2000). More specifically, research points toward three key resources that religion and spirituality provide for victims coping with the trauma of a terrorist attack: openness to religious growth, engagement in spiritual reflection, and involvement in a faith-based community.

Openness to Religious Growth

In earthquake-prone California, much has been learned about the type of building construction that can withstand a major earthquake. Standard building practices produce rigid structures that are unable to flex or sway in response to a tremor, and these buildings are much more likely to suffer damage or even collapse. Earthquake-resistant structures are built with flexibility so that they may give and sway during a quake. Although the swaying can be unnerving for those inside, it protects them from harm. In like manner, those who experience a major trauma are going to discover whether their faith and spirituality are rigid or flexible.

A rigid approach to religion means that simplistic concepts are maintained at all costs, such as "a faithful person will not suffer tragedy." Those with this (or a similar) rigidly held religious belief are left with only three options after experiencing a major trauma. They may attempt to deny that the trauma was as bad as it seems, thus maintaining their belief that they are not subject to life's tragedies despite evidence to the contrary. They may draw the depressogenic conclusion that the tragedy proves they lack faith. Or they may abandon their religious beliefs altogether since the trauma experience was not consistent with their unrealistic and rigid theology. Needless to say, none of these options are desirable. Neither a life in denial nor depression nor a life shorn of faith will help a victim cope with the trauma of a terrorist attack.

The alternative is to be flexible in response to the trauma and open to change and growth as a person of faith. This means holding onto one's core religious beliefs even while searching for answers, and turning to one's understanding of God in a heartfelt manner for help and direction. Where better to turn in time of overwhelming trauma? After the 9/11 terrorist attacks, 90% of New York City residents turned to prayer, religion, or spiritual feelings (Gallup, 2003). In short, they turned to God as a source of comfort, strength, and understanding. For a person of faith, only in God can ultimate meaning and purpose be found—especially in the face of death and terror. This means trusting that God exists and is greater than all traumas and being open to spiritual growth and change even in the midst of pain and suffering.

Empirical evidence suggests that openness to religious growth is not only helpful in coping with trauma but is also related to posttraumatic growth. Calhoun et al. (2000) tested 54 students who had experienced a major traumatic event within the past 3 years. They measured posttraumatic growth with the Posttraumatic Growth Inventory (Tedeschi & Calhoun, 1996) and openness with the Quest Scale (Batson, Schoenrade, & Ventis, 1993), which includes a subscale on openness to religious change (e.g., "there are many religious issues on which my views are still changing"). Five other variables thought to be related to posttraumatic growth were also measured, including "early event rumination." When they ran a simultaneous multiple regression equation, with posttraumatic growth as the dependent measure, only two of the variables were significantly predictive of growth—openness to change and early event rumination. Thus, openness to religious change is found to be an important factor in the very desirable outcome of posttraumatic growth. This suggests that a willingness to learn and grow, coupled with a focus on one's understanding of God, function together as a powerful coping mechanism after a trauma-inducing event.

The research therefore seems to suggest that there are two possible responses to trauma relevant to personal growth. One response focuses inward on self, holds rigidly to grievances, and increases the misery of posttraumatic stress. The other focuses outward on one's understanding of God, is open to learning new things in the midst of suffering, and leads to posttraumatic growth. For some the latter may be very difficult, for a variety of reasons. Thus it is never appropriate to blame trauma victims for the anguish of their posttraumatic stress. The only correct response is compassion. At the same time, it is important that trauma victims be made aware of the potential benefits of openness to religious growth. In that way, those who are so inclined will be encouraged to access this important resource and experience its benefits.

Engagement in Spiritual Reflection

If being open to religious growth is a significant help when coping with trauma, by what mechanism does that help occur? After all, "openness" is a fairly static concept, seemingly more attitudinal than behavioral. Just what does a person do who is turning to God and open to posttraumatic growth? Among other things, they think carefully about what happened and all that it means for them. An appropriate visual metaphor would perhaps be Rodin's Thinker, sitting with elbow on knee and chin on fist while contemplating. After experiencing a traumatic event such as a terrorist attack, numerous questions inevitably press in on the mind. What should I conclude from this terrifying experience? How do I make sense of it? Why did it happen? Where was God? What must I do now to be safe? These and related questions flow through the victim's consciousness, and it is easy to become preoccupied with the search for answers. If such thinking leads nowhere and no answers are found, discouragement follows and adds to the weight of posttraumatic distress. But if reflection leads to new realizations and conclusions that help explain not only the event but also deeper questions regarding life's ultimate meanings, that is another matter. Productive, positive spiritual reflection is a significant help for victims struggling to cope with trauma.

It should not be surprising that constructive cognitive processes constitute a significant coping mechanism for dealing with trauma. Since the rise of cognitive therapy in the 1970s and 1980s (e.g., Beck, 1976; Ellis, 1987; Meichenbaum, 1977), it has been clear that negative cognitive processes are related to many forms of psychopathology. Changing those negative cognitions thus leads to improvement. In fact, in the long run, cognitive therapy and related cognitive-behavior therapy, which target specific negative cognitions, have been found to be more effective than medication in treating anxiety disorders (Gould, Otto, Pollack, & Yap, 1997). Additionally, most therapists currently declare themselves to be cognitive-behavioral in orientation (Craighead, 1990; Prochaska & Norcross, 2003).

Although the focus has traditionally been on diminishing negative thought processes in order to relieve pathology, ongoing work by Martin Seligman adds a complementary positive point of view. Seligman points out that psychology as a field has tended toward a negative focus on psychopathology and argues for a more positive and optimistic mental health focus to include concepts such as a person's strengths, values, and life goals (Seligman, 1990). For spiritual reflection, it is this broader view of the importance of cognitive processes—including both positive and negative cognitions—that is most relevant. Spiritual reflection thus draws on concepts found in cognitive psychotherapy but incorporates a positive focus such as Seligman's work discusses.

Here too, empirical evidence suggests that spiritual reflection is not only helpful in coping with trauma but also related to posttraumatic growth. Calhoun and colleagues used a "rumination" scale, defined as "recurrent [event-related] thinking, including making sense, problem solving, reminiscence, and anticipation" (Calhoun et al., 2000, p. 522). The scale covers the following items:

- deliberately thinking about the event to try to understand it
- deliberately trying to make something good come out of the struggle with the event
- deliberately trying to see benefits in the event
- thinking about the meaning or purpose of life (p. 524)

Using a multiple regression equation, the researchers found that early event-related rumination was related not just to coping with trauma but also to posttraumatic growth. Calhoun et al. note that there is a negative, intrusive, unabated type of rumination (negative cognitive process) that is unhelpful. Thus, simply obsessing over worries in a circular manner does not help. However, constructive reflection does help and contributes significantly to posttraumatic growth. This means that the trauma victim takes the time to reflect on the event (what to make of it, what it really means, etc.) in a positive manner that leads at least in part to satisfactory answers.

In this way spiritual reflection, functioning as a mechanism for openness to change, leads to positive outcomes in trauma victims. According to the research, it needs to occur early on, and it must lead at least in part to satisfactory conclusions that help the victim make sense of the trauma. A critical discrimination is between positive spiritual reflection (which is productive) and pointless rumination (which continues endlessly without conclusion). The latter simply adds to the agony of the trauma, but the former constitutes a powerful tool for coping with it. Moreover, it adds to the likelihood that the victim will experience posttraumatic growth.

Involvement in a Faith-Based Community

A trauma victim engaging in spiritual reflection and open to religious growth is more likely to cope well with posttraumatic stress and to experience posttraumatic growth. Nevertheless, an individual's efforts can go only so far, and most victims turn to family and friends as well—a healthy instinct given the universal need for community and support. For those who are already part of a local faith community, that community constitutes a third resource that is not to be overlooked. A mosque, church, or synagogue can play a unique role in coping with trauma since it can provide both social support and a shared belief system that together offer effective help. This social support reminds victims they are not alone and encourages them to rely on others who are struggling to work through similar trauma. The shared belief system provides a meaningful theological and philosophical framework for thinking through what has occurred and helps the victim to avoid extreme and counterproductive conclusions. This is not so, however, if the religious culture is one of rigidity, punishment, and harsh theological teachings (such as "God is punishing you because of your lack of faith [or your disobedience]"). A punitive faith community only adds to the burden of posttraumatic stress, but one that offers love and acceptance, as well as a reasoned and wholesome theology, constitutes a critical resource for the victim of trauma.

There is a growing literature that recognizes the importance of local faith-based organizations in times of personal or community trauma. Harrison et al. have found that, although punitive religious reframing is counterproductive, "it appears that seeking congregational support and reframing the event in benevolent terms have positive health benefits" (2001, p. 86). Meisenhelder states that "attending religious services brings people together in a supportive environment, where pain can be acknowledged and comforted. The shared belief system in itself decreases the sense of isolation accompanying crisis or trauma. . . . People who use positive religious coping see their life as part of a larger spiritual force and try to find the lesson for them in the crisis" (2002, p. 775). That lesson may refer to, for example, a new appreciation for the sanctity and beauty of life, and the importance of being more other-oriented. These researchers seem to support what is generally well recognized—that participation in a local faith-based community can be good for body and soul, especially in times of crisis.

Each of these three responses to trauma is helpful for coping with the enormous stressors a victim experiences. Even more than that, the three together constitute a comprehensive strategy for survival and growth that is hard to match with standard treatment plans. Trauma victims do well to adopt an attitude of openness to religious growth, to think through concerns in constructive spiritual reflection, and to link up with their faith-based community. Such a strategy provides powerful help in coping with trauma and increases the likelihood of eventually experiencing posttraumatic growth rather than PTSD. Perhaps this is why almost half of Americans surveyed after 9/11 reported that their faith was actually stronger after the terrorist attack (Wagner, 2001).

Recommendations and Next Steps

It is clear that spirituality, religion, and faith-based communities can play a key role in coping with the trauma of a terrorist attack. Although the mental health profession has historically neglected these resources, the recognition of their importance for mental health services is growing (Kelly, 2003; Miller & Thoresen, 2003). In fact, this is precisely where many turn in times of crisis. More importantly, research shows that the help that trauma victims find there sometimes surpasses what is available via standard mental health care. Such comfort not only provides a resource for coping with trauma but also increases a victim's likelihood of experiencing posttraumatic growth. A nation locked in combat with terrorism cannot afford to overlook such a resource.

Practically speaking, what does this mean for the emergency mental health professionals, individuals, and faith-based communities? What steps can they take in preparation for and in response to terrorist attack? Furthermore, what additional research is needed in order to better understand this important resource?

For Emergency Mental Health Professionals

The standard protocol for emergency mental health care—critical incident stress management—needs major modification. CISM is likely helpful for some trauma victims who are spiraling downward emotionally and need help to process their negative thoughts and feelings but not for others who react differently to trauma. Emergency mental health professionals must be trained to differentiate between those who might benefit from CISM and those who might not, especially since the misapplication of CISM can be harmful. Differentiation may involve using an assessment instrument capable of clearly identifying appropriate candidates for CISM versus other treatments or strategies. Those in need of treatment but not likely to respond well to CISM could be referred to other modalities such as cognitive-behavioral therapy or exposure therapy. Those not in need of treatment should be encouraged to turn to other sources of help such as family, friends, or spiritual/religious resources.

Since the field is advancing so rapidly, EMH professionals must not rely on traditional, outdated protocols for emergency mental health care. Instead, it is critical to keep up with the literature, conferences, and training opportunities. Increasingly, researchers are turning their attention to developing strategies for working with survivors of terrorism (e.g., Gil-Rivas, Holman, & Silver, 2004; Kelly, 2004, 2005). One of the findings is that some members of a community are predictably more at risk than others for being negatively impacted by trauma. For instance, a recent study found that adolescents with a history of mental illness or learning difficulties were more at risk for difficulties following 9/11 than the general population (Gil-Rivas, Holman, & Silver, 2004). Accordingly, EMH professionals should be trained to assess for these and other risk factors among the target population before prescribing care. They can then tailor services and supports to meet individual needs rather than automatically offering them to all comers.

It is important to note that a person of faith (one for whom spiritual and/or religious matters are very important) may benefit from CISM or other treatment modalities as well as from faith-based resources. It is not an either-or scenario, so whether or not a person of faith receives professional care, they should also be encouraged to access the full spectrum of spiritual/religious resources available to them. For this reason, EMH professionals need to be trained to understand the importance of spirituality and religion as coping resources in times of trauma. In sum, they must be ready to provide CISM when clearly indicated, refer to cognitive-behavioral or other treatment modalities as needed, encourage all victims to turn to family and friends, and encourage people of faith to draw on their spiritual and religious resources, including their faith-based community.

For the Individual

According to the Department of Homeland Security there are several ways that an individual can prepare for times of crisis, including purchasing needed items (emergency food, radio, flashlight; duct tape and plastic for creating a "safe room," etc.) and developing plans for meeting and communicating with loved ones. But how is one to prepare to draw on spiritual and religious resources at these times? Here are recommendations for individuals who are preparing for and possibly responding to trauma such as a terrorist attack:

Preparation for Crisis

1. Do not be satisfied with religious or spiritual beliefs that are rigid and unrealistic and that cannot flexibly respond to your needs during a crisis. For example, if your belief system leads you to expect that no harm can come to you or your loved ones (as long as you are faithful, obedient, etc.), you are less likely to cope well with trauma. It may be helpful to expand your theological understanding so that it can assimilate the reality of tragedies that sometimes afflict good and faithful people. At that point you will be better prepared to weather a crisis.

2. Regularly practice productive spiritual reflection as a natural part of life during times of peace so that, when crisis comes, this resource will not be foreign to you. This may involve prayer and meditation, the study of religious writings, keeping a spiritual journal, or discussing key theological issues with others. Such practices prepare you for crisis by familiarizing you with positive spiritual reflection and making it less likely that you will fall into fruitless rumination in the aftermath of a trauma.

3. Align yourself with a faith-based community that is capable of providing interpersonal support during times of crisis. The faith community must have a belief system you are

comfortable with and that can account for life's tragedies in a realistic and meaningful manner. A faith-based community built primarily upon superficial interactions, whose members are smiling and friendly but seldom wrestle with life's difficulties, will not do. Only a community whose members support one another in meaningful ways and who share a wholesome and realistic theology will be a helpful resource during a tragedy.

Posttraumatic Response

1. Remember the importance of your faith, your spirituality, and your religion because these resources can make all the difference as you struggle to cope with tragedy and loss. Remember who you are spiritually and where to turn for help.

2. Be open to religious change and deliberately avoid rigid attitudes and unrealistic expectations. Instead of focusing inward on yourself, focus outward on your understanding of God and on seeking God. Expect that some of your assumptions will be challenged, and be willing to let them be modified or expanded. Expect that managing the trauma may change your spiritual and religious understanding in significant and helpful ways, and be open to that. Expect that posttraumatic suffering will hurt but that it will also create new things in your life that will come to have deep and satisfying spiritual significance.

3. Embrace spiritual reflection early on as a key resource for handling crises. This does not mean to engage in pointless rumination but to invest time and energy into productive prayer and meditation, discussion, and so on, as you search for answers. Remember that it is appropriate and necessary to do so and that consequently you may not be as focused as usual on life's daily tasks for some time. Record your thoughts and prayers in a journal, and share them with loved ones and members of your faith community. Do not be afraid to draw conclusions that might have seemed quite foreign to you before the trauma (e.g., "There is a struggle in this broken world between good and evil, with real consequences and innocent casualties. Therefore it is best to actively support the good and to live life to the fullest in a godly manner."). It is a time for growth.

4. Become fully engaged with your faith-based community, whether synagogue, church, mosque, or other organization. Remember that this will not help if that group is rigid and harsh, perhaps with a focus on punishment. However, if it is a community of compassion and sound shared beliefs, it will serve as a tremendous resource for all of its members. Attend functions, volunteer for programs and activities, and become as involved as possible. This will not only provide needed support for you, but it will also allow your support to be given to others, which is healing for both parties. Moreover, it will allow for discussion of core existential and theological questions that are the natural sequelae to major trauma events.

5. Expect not only that these resources will help you to cope with posttraumatic stress but that you may also experience posttraumatic growth.

6. Do not hesitate to access standard mental health resources as needed—such as mainline psychotherapy and medication or CISM—for emotional needs that persist. To do so does not negate the value of your spirituality, religion, or faith, as it is not an either-or matter.

For the Faith-Based Community

Unfortunately, not all faith-based communities rise to the occasion when crisis hits. It was reported that in Manhattan, after 9/11, some of the local church pastors immediately left to stay with family and friends in other areas (A. D. Hart, personal communication, Oct. 3, 2003). This seems akin to dereliction of duty, as the faith-based community has a critical role to play in times of disaster. Following are several recommendations for faith-based communities that desire to prepare for crises and to be ready to help their members in an effective and compassionate manner.

Preparation for Crisis

1. The governing body of a faith-based organization, especially those located in large metropolitan areas or near high-value terrorist targets, should recognize the importance of preparation for terrorist attack. This should

include discussion among the membership, as well as with national representatives (if applicable). Making an effort to be prepared for potential disaster is consistent with most theological traditions and is one example of caring for the faith community. A clear decision should be made to allocate the time and resources necessary for planning and preparation.

2. Once the decision to move ahead with planning and preparation has been made, the governing body (or those tasked) should locate and appropriate any and all available resources. There are at least three sources to consider:

   a. Faith-based communities with a national leadership organization should look to that group for help with plans and resources. If such help is not yet available, the national organization should be strongly encouraged to move in that direction. There is no excuse for any national faith-based organization to ignore critical current issues, and this one is of primary import.

   b. Local government disaster relief agencies should be contacted so that their emergency plans may be coordinated with those of the faith community in a mutually helpful manner. It may be helpful for a representative of the faith community to begin attending emergency preparation meetings, which are generally open to the public. Such interest and help would likely be welcomed by the relief agency.

   c. Federal government agency websites should be accessed so that available plans and resources there may be had. There are many government-sponsored websites filled with relevant and helpful information for individuals and communities wanting to prepare for terrorist attack (e.g., Centers for Disease Control and Prevention, Department of Homeland Security, Federal Emergency Management Agency, National Institute on Mental Health, and the Substance Abuse and Mental Health Services Agency). One or more faith community members could be tasked with downloading relevant information and presenting it to the governing body (see websites listed in Chapter 27).

3. Utilizing these resources, the faith-based organization needs to put in place a plan of action to be followed in times of crisis. This may involve stipulating which staff or members cover which function, how members will be contacted and communication maintained, what resources (housing, emotional support, etc.) will be offered, how to liaison with local emergency services, and so on. In this way, the faith-based community becomes prepared to take a major role in time of posttraumatic recovery. This will of course dramatically benefit the faith-based community's members, and it also positions the organization to be of help to the wider community.

Posttraumatic Response

1. Remember the critical importance of the "faith" part of your faith-based community and where your help ultimately comes from.

2. Make sure that all organizational staff and representatives stay local, remain engaged, and make themselves available as necessary.

3. Implement the faith-based community's plan of emergency action with courage and compassion, knowing that to do so is to provide a tremendous resource both to members and to the wider community.

4. To the extent possible, ensure that all community members are accounted for and that they feel accepted, supported, and encouraged throughout the posttrauma period.

5. Focus on the importance of talking through all that has occurred in the context of the faith community's shared beliefs. Make sure that multiple, ongoing opportunities are provided for such discussion and that all questions are taken seriously.

6. Encourage members to help one another to cope with the extreme stress of a terrorist attack, to be open to religious growth, to engage in productive spiritual reflection, and to participate in as many faith-community activities and programs as possible. Encourage them to expect that they will find strength for coping and to be open to posttraumatic growth.

7. Be ready to refer members with ongoing emotional needs to standard mental health resources such as mainline psychotherapy,

medication, and CISM. This must not be seen as a sign of failure any more than would visiting a doctor for penicillin to treat an infection.

8. Expect the unexpected, and be ready to improvise or change the plan of action quickly, creatively, and as often as needed.

Research Recommendations

Although much is known about the importance of the three spiritual and religious resources discussed earlier in responding to trauma, the research literature is still nascent on these and related topics. There is a pressing need, made more so by the threat of terrorist attack, to push ahead with comprehensive and programmatic research to build on the foundation that has been laid. Here are some of the areas that warrant priority attention:

1. Emergency mental health professionals must be able to accurately differentiate between those trauma victims who would benefit from CISM and those who would not. Reliable and valid assessment instruments and protocols must be developed for this purpose. For instance, a brief, psychometrically sound survey with high discriminant validity (few false positives regarding the need for CISM) would be of tremendous help.

2. In a similar fashion, emergency mental health professionals must be able to clearly identify those who are likely to benefit from their personal spiritual and religious resources in a posttrauma period. A brief survey or interview protocol addressing this topic would be of great help in identifying people of faith or others who would want to be referred to those resources and would benefit from them (e.g., the Religious Commitment Inventory developed by Worthington et al., 2003).

3. The concept and clinical reality of posttraumatic growth is clearly relevant to trauma care. Several psychometrically sound measures of posttraumatic growth are now available (e.g., the Posttraumatic Growth Inventory developed by Tedeschi & Calhoun, 1996). Research that applies these measures to different populations in different trauma scenarios and with sufficiently large numbers of participants to gen-

erate firm conclusions statistically would add to the growing literature on this important topic. Especially significant would be research that addresses the facilitation of posttraumatic growth and explores its course and clinical importance.

4. The three spiritual and religious resources so far identified in trauma research are of critical importance. Openness to religious growth, engagement in spiritual reflection, and involvement in a faith-based community all have very practical and clinically significant applications for victims of trauma such as a terrorist attack. Additional research that replicates these findings and also identifies other spiritual and religious resources would help expand our current understanding, as well as our present strategies for coping with disaster. Eventually, an array of evidence-supported spiritual resources and strategies could be identified and incorporated in EMH trauma care protocol.

Conclusion

The world changed on 9/11, and for a long time to come, life in the United States is not likely to be as secure as it once was. We cannot ignore the ever-present threat of a suicidal/homicidal religious terrorist breaking through the nation's security apparatus. It is only prudent, therefore, for the nation to begin preparing for the next 9/11, even as we fervently hope it will never occur and do all that can be done to prevent it. Furthermore, the next 9/11 may be significantly worse than the first, especially if it involves biochemical or radioactive weapons designed to kill large numbers of unsuspecting citizens.

In such a scenario society would by necessity turn to binding up the wounds of the survivors and rebuilding what was destroyed. Since some of the most grievous wounds are psychological rather than physical, attending to psychological posttrauma needs becomes a top priority. This chapter has explored a topic that policymakers and mental health professionals alike have historically overlooked—spiritual and religious resources that can help in times of crisis. As we have seen, these resources can be as healing as standard mental health services and, in many cases, are more readily desired by trauma victims. Such resources cannot be ignored in this time of potential peril. It is of utmost importance that federal, state, and local agencies charged with emergency preparedness and care (including but not limited to the newly created Department of Homeland Security) take note. The once-neglected spiritual factor must be included in policy deliberation, research priorities, and treatment considerations. Why? Because survivors almost universally perceive it as having the utmost importance as a help in times of need.

On a more philosophical and theological note, one cannot reflect on the importance of spirituality and religion in times of crisis without coming face to face with some of the most enduring and perplexing questions ever to face humankind. Does God exist? If so, how do we know? Either way, how do we explain the reality of what appears at times to be a very broken world filled with unwarranted tragedies? How can it be that life is at times wonderful beyond words and at other times hellish beyond belief? In light of that, just what is the purpose of life?

These questions may seem irrelevant to public policy and crisis care, but they are not, for people's ability to productively address such questions determines to some extent how well they will be able to cope with the trauma of a terrorist attack. It would of course be inappropriate in a pluralistic society for any government agency to promote a given set of answers to these fundamental life-questions. The strength of a free and democratic society is that it allows citizens to reach their own religious and philosophical conclusions and pursue their own destiny as they see fit, as long as they respect social and legal norms. This is in marked contrast with cultures that demand allegiance to a given set of philosophical or theological propositions, such as is the case with militant Islam. In fact, were militant Islam to spread, one of the first rights to be lost would be that of religious freedom.

However, it is not inappropriate for the pluralistic agencies of the U. S. government to recognize the importance of spiritual and religious resources to most citizens, especially during times of crisis, and to promote access to those resources as desired by the survivors. To continue to neglect this topic would be to deprive trauma victims of a powerful coping resource after the next 9/11. Thus policymakers at all levels of governance would do well to attend to the content of this chapter. In so doing, all

of us are perhaps recognizing that the effort to create a "naked public square" (Neuhaus, 1984) devoid of all things religious and spiritual was in large measure mistaken. In a pluralistic society that champions freedom of religion (among other basic rights), what is needed is not a naked public square but simply an open public square where all ideas—theological, philosophical, governmental, policy related, and so on—are welcomed in the marketplace of public opinion and debate. Let individuals, not governmental or religious authorities, decide which ideas to adopt.

This chapter exemplifies an open public square approach in that it recognizes the importance of religion, spirituality, and faith in response to the disaster of a terrorist attack. When crisis strikes, when the next 9/11 occurs, give surviving victims permission to draw on their own spiritual and religious resources, and help them to do so by following these recommendations. This will help a stricken community to find strength and prevail even in the face of terror.

Acknowledgments. The author deeply appreciates the contribution made by research assistants Elizabeth A. Secrist and Sherry M. Walling to this chapter.

Note

1. Here the term "minister" is used broadly to indicate "one who ministers to others in the name of a given religious or spiritual perspective." Thus, the term would apply to pastors, priests, rabbis, imams, and others who represent faith traditions.

References

Affleck, G., & Tennen, H. (1996). Construing benefits from adversity: Adaptational significance and dispositional underpinnings. *Journal of Personality, 64,* 899–922.

American Psychiatric Association. (2000). *Diagnostic and statistical manual of mental disorders* (4th ed.). Washington, DC: Author.

Armstrong, L. (2001). *It's not about the bike.* New York: Penguin.

Arnold, D., Calhoun, L. G., Tedeschi, R., & Cann, A. (2005). Vicarious posttraumatic growth in psychotherapy. *Journal of Humanistic Psychology, 45,* 239–263.

Batson, T. W., Schoenrade, P., & Ventis, W. L. (1993). *Religion and the individual: A social-psychological perspective.* New York: Oxford University Press.

Beck, A. T. (1976). *Cognitive therapy and the emotional disorders.* New York: International Universities Press.

Bonanno, G. A. (2004). Loss, trauma, and human resilience. *American Psychologist, 59,* 20–28.

———. (2005). Clarifying and extending the construct of adult resilience. *American Psychologist, 60,* 265–267.

———, & Kaltman, S. (1999). Toward an integrated perspective on bereavement. *Psychological Bulletin, 125,* 760–776.

Calhoun, L. G., Cann, A., Tedeschi, R. G., & McMillan, J. (2000). A correlational test of the relationship between posttraumatic growth, religion, and cognitive processing. *Journal of Traumatic Stress, 13,* 521–527.

Calhoun, L. G., & Tedeshi, R. G. (Eds.). (2006). *Handbook of Posttraumatic Growth.* Mahwah, NJ: Lawrence Earlbaum Associates, Inc.

Craighead, W. E. (1990). There's a place for us, all of us. *Behavior Therapy, 21,* 3–23.

De Jong, J., Komproe, T. V. M., Ivan, H., von Ommeren, M., El Masri, M., Araya, M., et al. (2001). Lifetime events and posttraumatic stress disorder in four postconflict settings. *Journal of the American Medical Association, 286,* 555–562.

Drescher, K. D., & Foy, D. W. (1995). Spirituality and trauma treatment: Suggestions for including spirituality as a coping resource. *National Center for PTSD Clinical Quarterly, 5,* 4–5.

Ellis, A. (1987). Rational-emotive therapy: Current appraisal and future directions. *Journal of Cognitive Therapy, 1,* 73–86.

Everly, G. S., Jr. (2003). Pastoral crisis intervention in response to terrorism. *International Journal of Emergency Mental Health, 5,* 1–2.

———, Flannery, R. B., Jr., & Mitchell, J. T. (2000). Critical Incident Stress Management (CISM): A methodological review. *Aggression and Violent Behavior: A Review Journal, 5,* 23–40.

Everly, G. S., Jr. & Mitchell, J. T. (1999). *Critical Incident Stress Management (CISM): A new era and standard of care in crisis intervention* (2d ed.). Ellicott City, MD: Chevron.

Flannery, R. B., Jr., (1999). Psychological trauma and posttraumatic stress disorder: A review. *International Journal of Emergency Mental Health, 2,* 135–140.

Galea, S., Vlahov, D., Resnick, H., Ahern, J., Susser, E., Gold, J., et al. (2003). Trends of probable posttraumatic stress disorder in New York City and the September 11 terrorist attacks.

American Journal of Epidemiology, 158, 514–524.

Gallup, G., Jr. (2003). *The Gallup poll: Public opinion 2003.* Lanham, MD: Rowman & Littlefield.

Gil-Rivas, V., Holman, E. A., & Silver, R. C. (2004). Adolescent vulnerability following the September 11th terrorist attacks: A study of parents and their children. *Applied Developmental Science, 8,* 130–142.

Gould, R. A., Otto, M. W., Pollack, M. H., & Yap, L. (1997). Cognitive behavior and pharmacological treatment of generalized anxiety disorder: A preliminary meta-analysis. *Behavior Therapy, 28,* 285–305.

Harrison, M. O., Koenig, H. G., Hays, J. C., Eme-Akwari, A. G., & Pargament, K. I. (2001). The epidemiology of religious coping: A review of recent literature. *International Review of Psychiatry, 13,* 86–93.

Hill, P. C., & Pargament, K. I. (2003). Advances in the conceptualization and measurement of religion and spirituality. *American Psychologist, 58,* 64–74.

Kelly, T. A. (2003, August). Transforming the mental health system: Principles and recommendations. Paper presented at the annual meeting of the American Psychological Association, Toronto.

———. (2004, July). Strategies for working with survivors of terrorism and diminishing fear. Symposium on the psychology of terrorism and fear management: what leaders need to know. Panel presentation at the annual meeting of the American Psychological Association, Honolulu.

———. (2005, April). Media management for emergency mental health professionals: how to get the right message out after a terrorist attack. Presentation for the Pasadena Emergency Preparedness Partnership Mental Health Subcommittee meeting, Pasadena.

———, & Strupp, H. H. (1992). Patient and therapist values in psychotherapy: Perceived changes, assimilation, similarity, and outcome. *Journal of Consulting and Clinical Psychology, 60,* 34–40.

Kessler, R. C., Sonnega, A., Bromet, E., Hughes, M., & Nelson, C. B. (1996). Posttraumatic Stress Disorder in the National Comorbidity Survey. *Archives of General Psychiatry, 52,* 1048–1060.

Linley, P. A., & Joseph, S. (2004). Positive change following trauma and adversity: A review. *Journal of Traumatic Stress, 17,* 11–21.

———, Cooper, R., Harris, S., & Meyer, C. (2003). Positive and negative changes following vicarious exposure to the September 11 terrorist attacks. *Journal of Traumatic Stress, 16,* 481–485.

McMillen, J. C. (1999). Better for it: How people benefit from adversity. *Social Work, 44,* 455–468.

Meichenbaum, D. (1977). *Cognitive-behavior modification.* New York: Plenum.

Meisenhelder, J. B. (2002). Terrorism, posttraumatic stress, and religious coping. *Issues in Mental Health Nursing, 23,* 771–782.

Miller, J. (2002). Affirming flames: Debriefing survivors of the World Trade Center attack. *Brief Treatment and Crisis Intervention, 21,* 85–94.

Miller, W. R., & Thoresen, C. E. (2003). Spirituality, religion, and health. *American Psychologist, 58,* 24–35.

Mitchell, J. T., & Everly, G. S., Jr. (1996). *Critical incident stress debriefing (CISD): An operations manual for the prevention of traumatic stress among emergency services and disaster workers* (2d ed.). Ellicott City, MD: Chevron.

———. (2000). Critical incident stress management and critical incident stress debriefing: Evolutions, effects, and outcomes. In B. Raphael & J. P. Wilson (Eds.), *Psychological debriefing: Theory, practice, and evidence* (pp. 71–90). New York: Cambridge University Press.

National Center of Addiction and Substance Abuse at Columbia University. (2001). Results of post–September 11th survey of substance use in America. Retrieved December 5, 2001, from http:www.yahoo.com.

Niemeyer, R. A. (2000). Searching for the meaning of meaning: Grief therapy and the process of reconstruction. *Death Studies, 24,* 541–558.

Neuhaus, R. J. (1984). *The naked public square: Religion and democracy in America.* Grand Rapids, MI: William B. Eerdmans.

Overcash, W. S., Calhoun, L. G., Cann, A., & Tedeschi, R. G. (1996). Coping with crises: An examination of the impact of traumatic events on religious beliefs. *Journal of Genetic Psychology, 157,* 455–464.

Pargament, K. I. (1997). *The psychology of religion and coping: Theory, research, practice.* New York: Guilford.

———, Smith, B. W., Koenig, H. G., & Pérez, L. (1998). Patterns of positive and negative religious coping with major life stressors. *Journal for the Scientific Study of Religion, 37,* 710–724.

Pargament, K. I., Ensing, D. S., Falgout, K. Olsen, H., Reilly, B., Van Haitsma, K., & Warren, R. (1990). God help me (I): Religious coping efforts as predictors of the outcome to significant negative life events. *American Journal of Community Psychology, 18,* 793–824.

Pargament, K. I., Tarakeshwar, N., Ellison, C. G., & Wulff, K. M. (2001). The relationship between religious coping and well-being in a national sample of Presbyterian clergy, elders, and members. Journal for the Scientific Study of Religion, 40, 497–513.

Prochaska, J., & Norcross, J. (2003). Systems of psychotherapy: A transtheoretical analysis. (5th ed.). Pacific Grove, CA: Brooks/Cole.

Saathoff, G., & Everly, G. S., Jr. (2002). Psychological contagion. *International Journal of Emergency Mental Health, 4,* 245–252.

Schuster, M. A., Stein, B. D., Jaycox, L. H., Collins, R. L., Marshall, G. N., Elliot, M. N., et al. (2001). A national survey of stress reactions after the September 11, 2001, terrorist attacks. *New England Journal of Medicine, 345,* 1507–1512.

Seligman, M. E. P. (1990). *Learned optimism.* New York: Knopf.

Sowell, R., Moneyham, L., Hennessy, M., Guillory, J., Demi, A., & Seals, B. (2000). Spiritual activities as a resistance resource for women with human immunodeficiency virus. *Nursing Research, 49,* 73–82.

Stroebe, M. S., & Stroebe W. (1991). Does "grief work" work? *Journal of Consulting and Clinical Psychology, 59,* 479–482.

Tedeschi, R. G., & Calhoun, L. G. (1995). *Trauma and transformation: Growing in the aftermath of suffering.* Thousand Oaks, CA: Sage.

———. (1996). The posttraumatic growth inventory: Measuring the positive legacy of trauma. *Journal of Traumatic Stress, 9,* 455–471.

Tedeschi, R. G., Park, C. L., & Calhoun, L. G. (Eds.). (1998). *Posttraumatic growth: Positive changes in the aftermath of crisis.* Mahwah, NJ: Erlbaum.

U.S. Department of Justice. (2001). Office for victims of crime handbook for coping after terrorism. Publication no. NCJ 190249. Washington, DC: U.S. Government Printing Office.

Wagner, A. (2001, October 31). Coping. *National Journal, 41,* 3206.

Webster, A. M. (1979). *Webster's New Collegiate Dictionary.* Springfield, MA: G & C Merriam Company.

Woodward, C., & Joseph, S. (2003). Positive change processes and posttraumatic growth in people who have experienced childhood abuse: Understanding vehicles of change. *Psychology and Psychotherapy: Theory, Research and Practice, 76,* 267–283.

Worthington, E. L., Wade, N. G., Hight, J. S., Ripley, M. E., McCullough, M. E., Berry, J. W., et al. (2003). The religious commitment inventory 10: Development, refinement, and validation of a brief scale for research and counseling. *Journal of Counseling Psychology, 50,* 84–96.

Wortman, C. B., & Silver, R. C. (1989). The myths of coping with loss. *Journal of Consulting and Clinical Psychology, 57,* 349–357.

11

Psychological Consequences of Actual or Threatened CBRNE Terrorism

Glenn R. Sullivan
Bruce Bongar

The acquisition of chemical, biological, radiological, nuclear, and high-yield explosive (CBRNE) weapons remains a priority of several terrorist organizations, including al-Qaeda. The extreme lethality and disruptive effect of CBRNE weapons make them highly attractive to these groups, who conceive that their use will help them to achieve their strategic goals. CBRNE weapons could be said to be true "terror weapons" because their psychological impact usually exceeds the extent of their physical destructiveness, however massive.

Terrorism is psychological warfare, and the civilian population is the primary target. Terrorist groups do not, and will never, possess the means to limit or even reduce the strategic capabilities of a nation such as the United States. Their only hope is to inflict sufficient psychological trauma on civilians, who will in turn pressure their governments to effect policy changes that favor the terrorists' interests. Promoting psychological resilience and minimizing psychological trauma in the wake of terrorist attacks has therefore become a matter not only of individual health but also of national security.

This chapter presents several historical models that illustrate critical psychological aspects of this threat. In addition to the psychological reactions to the 9/11 attacks, we examine gas exposure in World War I, ballistic missile attacks on Tehran and Israel, a radiological accident in Brazil, an outbreak of plague in India, and a chemical attack on the Tokyo subway. We describe the potential psychological impact of various CBRNE weapons and present evidence that argues against the likelihood of mass panic in the aftermath of a CBRNE attack. We discuss the phenomenon of mass psychogenic illness and offer recommendations for treatment and planning.

The majority of victims of CBRNE terrorism will be psychological, not physical, casualties. In the aftermath of a CBRNE attack, public health authorities should expect that for every person actually exposed to radiation or chemical or biological agents, many (perhaps hundreds) more will seek medical screening. A significant percentage of nonexposed individuals seeking screening will present with psychosomatic symptoms that mimic those of victims who were actually exposed. Enormous numbers of people will present with symptoms of fear that will need to be managed by overtaxed medical personnel.

The threat of chemical attack or an outbreak of a highly contagious and lethal disease could result in a mass exodus of civilians from population centers. This demonstrated loss of faith in the government's ability to protect its citizens can compel a nation's leaders to effect drastic policy changes. The economic losses following such an event could be catastrophic. Effective preparation and official communication are critical to preventing unplanned evacuations.

Fortunately, a reasonably well-prepared civilian population can withstand prolonged terrorist campaigns, even those marked by the realistic threat of CBRNE attack. The rate of psychological casualties will decline precipitously as people habituate to the attacks, which they tend to do rapidly. Understanding these nightmarish weapons as instruments of psychological warfare and not as weapons of mass (physical) destruction is critical to planning and executing an effective response.

The Psychological Impact of CBRNE Weapons

This modality of terrorism is exceptionally well suited to the apparent objectives of contemporary terrorist organizations. CBRNE attacks spread fear, foster uncertainty, and undermine confidence in government and leadership. They elicit irrational and repressive countermeasures, including, potentially, a nuclear response demanded by an incensed American public. They have the potential to rend "the fabric of trust that bonds society" (Hoffman, 2002, p. 313). Potential individual psychological reactions to CBRNE terrorism include numbness; anxiety and fear; horror and disgust; anger and scapegoating; paranoia; loss of trust; demoralization, hopelessness, and helplessness; and survivor guilt (Holloway, Norwood, Fullerton, Engel, & Ursano, 1997).

Survivors of mass violence (e.g., terrorism or shooting rampage) are more likely to suffer subsequent psychiatric illness than are survivors of natural or technological disasters (Norris et al., 2002). One reason for this is that intentional attacks "might happen again at any moment," whereas respites are expected after natural disasters. Further, mass violence reveals a degree of human malevolence that most people cannot integrate into their worldview.

The very nature of chemical, biological, and radiological agents inspires terror. People are unable to see or feel the agent and in most cases are unable to smell or taste it. Because of this intangibility, direct exposure is impossible to detect

without specialized equipment or medical tests (at least during the physiologically asymptomatic stage of exposure). The possibility of person-to-person transmission magnifies our natural fear of contagion. When people fear infection from others or infecting those close to them, social support networks disintegrate. CBRNE events evoke the primal human fear of being permanently disfigured or disabled. Years after an attack, there will be residual fears of subsequent birth defects or the delayed appearance of cancers, and so on.

External factors also serve as "terror multipliers" during CBRNE events. Inconsistent or incomplete information from the media and authorities can heighten anxiety and deplete trust. Perceived contradictions regarding preventative measures, prognosis, and treatment effectiveness among public health officials and kibitzers appearing on 24-hour news channels can contribute to anxiety. Stress and anxiety are compounded when treatments (e.g., Cipro) are identified but availability is perceived to be limited. Witnessing large numbers of dead or injured people can demoralize or shock even those not directly exposed to the attack. This effect is maximized when images of dead or injured children are broadcast.

The novelty of CBRNE weapons is perhaps their most potent aspect: Human beings dread most that with which they are unfamiliar. Fortunately, habituation to frightening stimuli occurs rapidly (Rachman, 1990). The first offensive use of gas in World War I produced panic among the defenders, but subsequent attacks did not (Moscrop, 2001). Similarly, all other factors remaining constant, if an airliner were flown into the Empire State Building tomorrow, the psychological reaction would be less intense than the reactions observed on September 11, 2001.

Credibility of the Threat

In 1975 terrorism analyst Brian Jenkins said famously, "Terrorists want a lot of people watching and a lot of people listening and not a lot of people dead" (p. 15). Over the ensuing 30 years, a new paradigm has emerged, which Jenkins (1999) himself has acknowledged:

> A number of America's foes and potential foes are actively conducting research on chemical,

biological, or nuclear weapons. As motives change and their self-imposed constraints erode, today's terrorists seem more interested in running up high body counts than in advancing a political agenda.

CBRNE terrorism is a low-probability/high-consequence event. To date, the airliner attacks of September 11, 2001, remain the sole example of mass casualty CBRNE terrorism on U.S. soil.[1] The best evidence that terrorist groups do not yet possess the biologic, chemical, or nuclear means to inflict hundreds of thousands of civilian casualties is that there have been no such attacks to date. Security concerns, particularly the fear of interception before delivery, would compel any terrorist organization committed to megacasualty operations to launch such attacks almost immediately upon acquiring the means to do so (Friedman, 2004).

The desire of terrorist masterminds to commit murder on an apocalyptic scale is well documented. Jessica Stern (1999) observed that religious militants conceive of weapons of mass destruction (WMD) as the perfect means to "conjure a sense of divine retribution" (p. 8).[2] Osama bin Laden has proclaimed the acquisition of WMD a "religious duty" and has diligently curried clerical support in order to justify future mass killings (Scheuer, 2005). It should be remembered that the intention of Ramzi Yousef, architect of the 1993 World Trade Center bombing, was to topple one of the Twin Towers into the next, sending both crashing lengthwise onto lower Manhattan, killing perhaps 250,000 people (Friedman, 1999).

The technical challenges involved in developing CBRNE weapons remain formidable (Steinhausler, 2003). Even Aum Shinrikyō, an apocalyptic cult with vast economic and intellectual resources, failed in its extensive efforts to develop effective CBRNE weapons. However, concerns persist regarding both the security of nuclear materials in the former Soviet states and the willingness of some scientists (e.g., Pakistan's A. Q. Khan) to share their expertise with terrorist groups or states that support terror. Due to technical obstacles, it is more likely that terrorists will obtain CBRNE weapons by indirect means.

It is especially worrying that the "calculus of deterrence" that helped prevent a nuclear exchange between the Cold War superpowers does not apply to nonstate actors.[3] Groups such as al-Qaeda already know that the United States is committed to its absolute destruction; therefore, they do not fear additional retaliation. Indeed, al-Qaeda's strategic intent has been described as deliberately provocative of massive retaliation (McCauley, 2002). Jihadist terror organizations do not feel an ethical obligation to limit civilian casualties. Moreover, they do not fear alienating anyone with the nature of their outrages because (unlike the IRA) their funding and manpower do not rely on broad-based public support.

Former chief U.S. weapons inspector David Kay (2001) has noted that even nation-states may be tempted to engage in CBRNE terrorism because they perceive no alternatives to U.S. ascendancy. Kay has stated that, as the power of the United States increases, the probability that its strategic competitors will employ CBRNE weapons through indirect means (or proxies) will increase as well:

> Nations will seek courses of action that will allow them operational freedom from U.S. conventional attack or, at least, the ability to inflict significant losses on the United States if it does attempt to frustrate their ambitions with military actions. Terrorism, and particularly mass casualty terrorism, is a logical counter for such states. Chemical, biological, and radiological terrorism offers tremendous difficulties of attribution—that is, proving who really carried out an attack. Biological terrorism even has the added difficulty of determining or proving that one is really under attack and not simply seeing a natural disease outbreak.

On the individual level, people who ascribe to apocalyptic ideologies or religious fanaticism may be more likely to engage in CBRNE terrorism because they may be less concerned about the need for self-protection while handling deadly agents in preparation for an attack (Moores, 2002). A commonly cited bioterrorism scenario involves martyrdom teams infecting themselves with smallpox and then boarding as many commercial airline flights as possible before they are overcome.

Mass Panic

Mass panic is defined as an "acute fear reaction marked by loss of self-control which is followed by nonsocial and nonrational flight" (Quarantelli, 1954, p. 265). It is important to differentiate mass panic from "mass anxiety," a classic example of which is the public's reaction to Orson Welles's "War of the Worlds" broadcast. Those who were listening to their radios on Halloween night 1938 may have been nervous and uncertain, but they were not running for their lives. An example of mass panic is the 1942 Cocoanut Grove nightclub fire in Boston. A total of 492 people died in 15 minutes in large part because panic prevented the crowd from using the revolving doors at the main entrance or other exits in a socially appropriate manner (Thomas, 1992).

It is a commonly held opinion among emergency planners that the public responds to disaster with either passivity or panic (Perry & Lindell, 2003). However, public responses to a variety of actual disasters do not support this view. Mass panic, in particular, appears to be quite rare in the historical record. Panicked flight did not occur during the bombings of British, German, or Japanese cities during World War II. Mass panic did not break out in the wake of the 1995 Tokyo subway sarin attack, despite the horrifying invisibility of the debilitating agent and the fears of contamination and mutation that have affected Japanese society since the 1945 atomic bombings. The repeated Scud missile raids on Israel during the Gulf War did not provoke a mass exodus from the cities, despite a rational expectation of chemical attack. There was no mass panic by civilians after the Oklahoma City Federal Building bombing, although the circumstances of the attack were highly ambiguous and no one could be sure that other office buildings would not be next.

Perhaps the most compelling example of non-panic in response to disaster is that of the 1993 and 2001 World Trade Center attacks. Orderly evacuations were executed after both incidents. Former New York mayor Rudolph Giuliani estimated that 20,000 people were safely evacuated before the Twin Towers collapsed on September 11, 2001 (Giuliani, 2004). Giuliani attributes this remarkable feat to both the courage of first responders and to the calmness of the civilians: "People exited this building carefully, they exited this building quickly, they exited this building without harming or hurting each other" (p. 15).

Some of the evacuees on 9/11 had walked down those same stairwells after the 1993 bomb-

ing, but the "practice effect" of that experience and of half-hearted fire drills during the intervening years is dubious. Far more important is that people tended to make the long descent among friends and coworkers after the decision to evacuate was made by individual office groups. This familiarity not only provided social support but also enforced socially appropriate behavior.

Individual heroism played a large role as well. The head of security for Morgan Stanley's Individual Investor Group, Silver Star–decorated Vietnam veteran Rick Rescorla, is credited with saving the lives of almost 2,700 of that company's employees (Stewart, 2003). During the evacuation, he sang patriotic songs through a bullhorn in order to calm people's nerves. He was last seen walking back up the stairs, searching for stragglers, shortly before the towers collapsed.

Multiple factors may contribute to an outbreak of panic behavior: (1) perceiving oneself at high risk of illness or injury; (2) limited availability of resources that are apportioned on a first-come, first-served basis; (3) perceived lack of effective management of the catastrophe; and (4) loss of credibility by the authorities (Hall et al., 2003). Perhaps most relevant to the situation in the upper stories of the burning Twin Towers is this combination of contributing factors: any situation in which a mortal threat is present and there are limited escape routes (Pastel, 2001).

Mass Psychogenic Illness

The phenomenon of *mass psychogenic illness*, in other times and contexts, has gone by other names, including epidemic hysteria, conversion hysteria, mass sociogenic illness, mass hysteria, somatization, and, most recently, outbreaks of medically unexplained physical symptoms (MUPS). Mass psychogenic illness (MPI) has been defined as "a constellation of symptoms suggestive of organic illness, with no identifiable cause and little clinical or laboratory evidence of disease, which occurs among persons who share beliefs regarding their symptoms" (Jones, 2000, p. 2650).

Ironically, vigorous emergency response to suspected or actual CBRNE terrorism (and consequent intense media attention) may facilitate the emergence of mass psychogenic illness. The emergence, maintenance, and resolution of physical symptoms occurs completely outside the bounds of conscious awareness; people suffering from MPI are not consciously malingering or feigning illness. CBRNE attacks will likely trigger epic outbreaks of mass psychogenic illness that could easily overwhelm medical and government institutions and threaten civil order (DiGiovanni, 1999).

Direct exposure to an agent is not required to develop somatic symptoms (in fact, no *agent* is required at all). The literature contains countless examples of people in schools, military bases, churches, and so on falling ill due to a purported gas leak or toxic exposure, and upon investigation no such exposure was found (e.g., Jones et al., 2000). If medical care is perceived to be a scarce resource, more people will develop symptoms of exposure, and somatic symptoms will become more severe. Rumor, irresponsible media coverage, or inconsistent official announcements could increase the prevalence of psychogenic cases. Within the context of a CBRNE event, it is highly probable that large numbers of unaffected persons will inaccurately attribute physical stress reactions (headache, shortness of breath, diaphoresis, etc.) to lethal agents (Alexander & Klein, 2003).

The most commonly presented symptoms of MPI are headache; dizziness or lightheadedness; nausea; abdominal cramps or pain; cough; fatigue; drowsiness or weakness; sore or burning throat; hyperventilation or breathing difficulties; and watery or irritated eyes (Jones, 2000). Causal factors may include hyperventilation or syncope (Jones, 2000). "Symptom sharing" and "line-of-sight" transmission (in which an individual becomes ill upon witnessing others becoming ill is common (Jones, 2000).

Drawing from the experience of military medical personnel charged with treating psychiatric casualties and the work of contemporary researchers in the field (e.g., Engel, 2001; Holloway, Norwood, Fullerton, Engel, & Ursano, 1997; Jones, 2000), we offer the following treatment recommendations and guidelines:

1. Keep suspected MPI patients separate from patients with known exposure.
2. Off-site treatment is preferable, whenever possible.
3. Identify and manage symptoms of hyperarousal.
4. Encourage patients to hydrate, eat, and sleep.

5. Do not label MPI patients as psychiatrically ill or identify members of the treatment team as psychiatrists or psychologists.
6. As soon as possible, have patients engage in useful work.
7. Quickly return patients to their social network.
8. Remember that a "skeptical attitude may induce efforts by patients to *prove* their symptoms are *real*" (Engel, 2001, p. 47).
9. Remember that nonphysical origin does not rule out real distress.
10. Remember that psychological distress is often comorbid with physical exposure.

Individual differences may determine a person's susceptibility to MPI. These differences include preexisting anxiety levels, suggestibility, personal belief systems, and connection to social networks (Bartholomew & Victor, 2004). MPI may disproportionately affect more females than males and frequently involves adolescents and children (Jones, 2000). MPI is more common among patients suffering from preexisting psychological disorders, severe stress, or perceived lack of social support (Jones, 2000).

Post-9/11 Incidence of Mass Psychogenic Illness

The anthrax mailings of October 2001 were a prime opportunity for a widespread outbreak of mass psychogenic illness. Letters containing the weaponized form of this bacteriological agent were mailed to prominent media and government figures. In all, 5 people died, and 22 became ill, many of them postal workers who handled the letters. Moreover, "[m]illions of people were made anxious and the routine act of opening the mail became dangerous" (Hall et al., 2003, p. 139). The publicized symptoms of anthrax exposure were dismayingly similar to those of influenza or a severe cold: fever, chills, chest pain, cough, nausea, vomiting, and labored breathing. In describing the effects of the anthrax attacks, Bruce Hoffman (2002) has noted that "[t]errorists do not have to kill 3,000 people to create panic and foment fear and insecurity: five persons dying in mysterious circumstances is quite effective at unnerving an entire nation" (p. 313).

Nevertheless, no reports have been published of medical facilities being overwhelmed or overly burdened by a sudden influx of people who were concerned that they had been exposed to the anthrax bacillus. Perhaps those who were worried about possible exposure sought assistance from their primary care providers and not from local emergency departments. If there was a large-scale outbreak of MPI directly related to the 2001 anthrax attacks, it has escaped our review of the research literature.

A handful of localized, small-scale, bioterrorism-related MPI scares did occur in the immediate aftermath of 9/11 (for a review, see Wessely, Hyams, & Bartholomew, 2001). However, MPI events occur with regularity, especially in schools and other regimented social contexts such as military training posts. There is no evidence that the events of September 11, 2001, prompted an increase in these events.

Radiation Hysteria: Goiania, Brazil, 1987

The detonation of a radiological dispersion device (RDD)—or "dirty bomb"—could immediately kill dozens to hundreds of victims, sicken thousands of others, and make a large section of a major city uninhabitable for many years. Clean-up costs from a single RDD have been estimated at more than $100 billion (Stern, 1999). Yet the primary impact of a dirty bomb lies not so much in its lethality or economic cost but in the psychological terror it could engender.

Although we have been living in the "nuclear age" for more than 60 years, the general public remains both ignorant and highly fearful of radiation (Slovic, Fischhoff, & Lichtenstein, 1980). The regular outpouring of concerns regarding the potentially harmful effects of radiation (e.g., the agricultural irradiation of apples) often bears striking resemblance to mass hysteria. The psychological effects of the Chernobyl nuclear disaster (depression, anxiety, and stress reactions) are far more prevalent and range farther from the focal point of the incident than the physical effects (e.g., increased risk of developing thyroid cancer). Reports from Chernobyl suggest that some people who thought they might have been exposed to fallout committed suicide rather than face the terror of death by radiation sickness (Salter, 2001). For months after the Chernobyl accident, many people

in neighboring regions refused to go outside or eat anything but canned food (Salter, 2001).

The 1987 radiation accident in Goiania, Brazil, serves as a useful model for public response to a dirty bomb attack. A radiotherapy machine was stolen from an abandoned medical clinic and sold for scrap metal. When the machine was dismantled, a curious powder that glowed in the dark was discovered inside. This powder (the radioactive isotope cesium 137) was played with and shared among the family and friends of the machine's appropriators. Soon after, many people who were directly exposed to the radioactive powder developed flulike symptoms (e.g., anorexia, nausea, vomiting, and diarrhea).

The extent of the exposure—and the cause—eventually came to the attention of local public health authorities. Any residents who thought they might have been exposed to the stolen radioactive substance were invited to come to the city's soccer stadium for a free radiological screening. More than 10% of Goiania's 1.2 million residents presented themselves for screening (Pastel, 2001). The actual number of people who were found to have been contaminated with radiation was 249; of these, 20 required hospitalization, and 4 eventually died from their exposure (Pastel, 2001). Therefore, the ratio of "concerned" to "contaminated" people in this event was greater than 500 to 1.

A significant portion of Goiania's citizens demonstrated their apprehension by traveling to a central location and standing in long lines for many hours before undergoing screening with Geiger-type radiation detectors. Undoubtedly, many more residents were *passively* concerned or anxious about possible exposure, but other factors (the need to work, inability to travel, or fear of medical authorities) kept them away from the screening center.

Of the 125,800 people screened at Goiania, 8.3% presented with psychosomatic reactions that mimicked the symptoms of radiation exposure (Pettersen, 1988). People fainted and vomited while they waited to be screened; many complained of diarrhea, and most were visibly fearful (Pastel, 2001). Using the experience of Goiania as a guide, we might reasonably expect that for every person actually exposed to radiation in the aftermath of a dirty bomb attack, more than 500 will seek medical screening for possible contamination, and more than 40 will exhibit fear-related physical symptoms that mimic the symptoms of radiation exposure.

Plague: Surat, India, 1994

A potential analogue to a widespread bioterrorism attack is the 1994 outbreak of pneumonic plague in Surat, India. A total of 5,150 suspected cases of plague were identified by health officials; 49 residents eventually died of the disease (Ramalingaswami, 2001). Fear of contagion was so great that approximately 600,000 people (almost 33% of the city's population) fled the city by any means at their disposal—and on foot if necessary (Ramalingaswami, 2001). Even medical doctors fled the city and left their patients unattended. In Calcutta—more than 1,500 kilometers away—people stayed indoors and off the streets. Tetracycline and other drugs were hoarded and quickly became unavailable.

This medical crisis is estimated to have cost billions of dollars. The tourism industry for the entire subcontinent virtually shut down for a time. There were widespread cancellations of existing orders for Indian exports. Economic activity in the affected areas dropped to nearly nothing.

The government's mishandling of this emergency contributed to its magnitude. Initially, the Indian government attempted to minimize the scale of the outbreak and play down the risk of contagion (Ramalingaswami, 2001). Official communications were dilatory, often inaccurate, conflicting, and sometimes intentionally misleading (Ramalingaswami, 2001). Government attempts to obfuscate or minimize the disease outbreak and the flight of health care personnel from the affected area were major factors in the unplanned evacuation.

The "War of the Cities," 1987–1988

Toward the end of the brutal and protracted war between Iran and Iraq (1980–1988), both nations attempted to break civilian morale and end popular support for the opposing regime by targeting the public at large with intermediate-range ballistic missiles. In 1987 Saddam Hussein ordered 150 Scud missiles fired at Tehran, but these attacks achieved little strategic or tactical effect. One year later, rumors began to circulate in Tehran that

Saddam was planning a major chemical attack on the capital city (Findley, 1991). This threat was not unfounded, as Iraq had employed chemical weapons on the frontlines beginning in 1984.

Between February 29 and April 20, 1988, in response to missile attacks against Baghdad, Iraq launched 190 conventional Scud-B missiles at Tehran and other major Iranian cities (Findley, 1991). No chemical weapons were deployed (perhaps only because Saddam did not possess the capability to deploy such weapons in that manner at that time). Nevertheless, in the wake of this 6-week-long aerial assault, at least 100,000 civilians fled Tehran (some estimates put the figure as high as 1.5 million—25% of the city's population) (Martin, 2002).

An estimated 2,000 people were killed during these attacks, and an additional 6,000 were wounded (Martin, 2002). In terms of the amount of destruction inflicted as a ratio of ordnance expended, the ballistic missile attacks during the so-called War of the Cities were roughly equivalent to the V1 and V2 rocket attacks on London during World War II (Fetter, Lewis, & Gronlund, 1993). However, the Nazi rocket attacks did not prompt a mass exodus of the civilian population from the targeted capital city.

The variable of interest here is the *realistic threat* of chemical warfare, which multiplied the psychological impact of the attacks many times. Indeed, the threat of chemical warheads delivered via ballistic missile not only depopulated Tehran and weakened support for the revolutionary regime but also pushed Iran's leaders to accept a disadvantageous UN peace resolution.

Scud Missile Attacks on Israel, 1991

The psychological impact of ballistic missile attacks on Israeli civilians during the 1990–1991 Gulf War did not nearly approach the regime-threatening magnitude of the War of the Cities. From January 17 to February 25, 1991, 39 Scud missiles were launched at Israeli cities in 18 separate attacks (Bleich, Dycian, Koslowsky, Solomon, & Weiner, 1992). As during the Iran-Iraq War, expectations of chemical attack were high among both civilians and government officials. Saddam Hussein's prior use of chemical weapons and his strategic interest in drawing Israeli forces into hostilities heightened the fear of impending chemical attack. Memories of the Holocaust, in which poison gas was used to kill millions of Jews, maximized the psychological impact.

A total of eight people were killed as a result of the missile attacks. Only two of those deaths were directly caused by missile-related injuries. Six deaths were attributed to suffocation resulting from the improper use of gas masks (Bleich et al., 1992). Even though they were choking, these people refused to remove their masks because they were convinced that poison gas was filling the room (Bleich et al., 1992). It can be fairly said that these people died of fear.

A total of 773 war casualties were hospitalized during this 4-week period. Nearly 30% of the hospitalizations were due to missile-related physical injuries (Bleich et al., 1992). These were broadly defined to include falls taken while running to shelter, injuries sustained in car accidents that occurred during air raids, and so on. A majority of the hospitalizations were for either psychological stress reactions (43%) or unjustified atropine reactions (27%) (Bleich et al., 1992). The unjustified atropine injections are a symptom of anxiety, specifically the unfounded belief that poison gas is present in the environment and must be counteracted.

As civilians became habituated to the air raids, the number of stress-related hospital admissions fell. Ambulance crews adapted to the raids as well and became less likely to transport psychological casualties to the hospital (Bleich et al., 1992). No mass exodus from Tel Aviv or any other Israeli city was reported. The resilience of the Israeli people to air attack may have been bolstered by the government's policy of outfitting all of its citizens with modern gas masks. (Israeli citizens who do not maintain their masks in good working order are subject to fines.) In addition, universal military training may increase this population's confidence that they "know what to do in case of an emergency." In addition, public trust in the government and the media was very high.

Sarin Gas Attack in Tokyo Subway, 1995

On March 20, 1995, members of the apocalyptic religious cult Aum Shinrikyō dispersed deadly sarin gas within the confines of the Tokyo subway system. The cult had been under increasing pressure and scrutiny from Japanese security forces, which fed their leader's already paranoid worldview (Lifton, 2000). One of the reasons for the increased scrutiny was the group's suspected involvement in a sarin gas attack the previous year in Matsumoto that killed seven people. In Shoko Asahara's rush to "strike first," his followers produced and disseminated a relatively low-lethality version of the deadly chemical (Lifton, 2000). While much has been made of Aum Shinrikyō's vast financial and intellectual resources, the members who dispersed the cult's chemical weapons were not trained microbiologists but rather "gifted amateurs" with professional experience in chemistry or medicine.

On the chaotic day of the attack, more than 5,000 civilians and first responders were rushed to Tokyo emergency rooms for treatment of suspected exposure to the deadly nerve agent (Pangi, 2002). Almost all of these people displayed signs of psychological reactions to the event, including severe anxiety or shock (Hall et al., 2003). Nearly 80% of those who were brought to emergency rooms that day were examined and discharged. Of the 5,081 people who received medical attention in the aftermath of the attack, 19% were hospitalized for sarin exposure ($n = 984$), 1.2% were severely injured ($n = 62$), and 12 died (Asukai & Maekawa, 2002).

Many researchers (Ohbu et al., 1997; Asukai & Maekawa, 2002; Pangi, 2002) have suggested that an unknown but significant percentage of the people examined and discharged on the day of the sarin attack had never actually been exposed to the gas. On the patients' initial arrival at an emergency room, the combination of shock, emotional distress, and fear-related physical symptoms (e.g., shortness of breath, nausea, rapid heartbeat) would make those who have actually experienced low-level exposure to a nerve agent virtually indistinguishable from those who merely believe they were exposed. However, it is important to emphasize that patients suffering from *actual exposure* to nerve agents are also likely to exhibit signs of intense fear, anxiety, and emotional distress.

Gas Mania in World War I

Modern understanding of mass psychogenic illness in the context of actual or threatened exposure to chemical weapons began during World War I. Exposure to gas, whether to blister agents such as mustard gas or choking agents such as phosgene or chlorine, had a relatively low mortality rate. About 2% of soldiers exposed to gas died (Shepard, 2001). Therefore, chemical warfare during World War I was primarily concerned with disrupting enemy operations, denying territory to the enemy, and disabling (usually temporarily) enemy personnel. Chemical weapons were not employed simply in order to kill swathes upon swathes of enemy soldiers.

For each soldier who was exposed to gas on the Western Front, 2 applied for medical care, without any evidence of exposure (Pastel, 2001). Put another way, 2 out of 3 soldiers seeking medical care for gas exposure during World War I had not actually been exposed to gas. Soldiers commonly presented with symptoms that mimicked exposure to gas (e.g., fatigue, chest pain, difficulty breathing, coughing, tingling or burning in the throat, watery or itchy eyes, blurred vision). In a famous incident, 500 soldiers of the U.S. 3rd Division became disabled with symptoms of gas exposure even though their unit was *not in an area in which gas had been deployed* by either side (Pastel, 2001).

This phenomenon became known as "gas mania," and victims were treated much like other psychological casualties during that conflict. Soldiers were treated as close to the front as possible, usually "within the sound of the guns." They were fed and encouraged to sleep. The expectation of a rapid return to one's fighting unit was emphasized. Simple treatment approaches (e.g., proximity, immediacy, expectancy) minimized the disruption caused by fear of chemical attack.

Summary and Recommendations

In the Age of Terrorism, civilians are both the targets of direct violence and the intended audience for violent outrages. The strategic intent of terrorist groups is to inflict psychological trauma on civilian populations and thereby undermine popular support for the current policies of democratic governments. Seen through this strategic prism, civilians are not merely the potential victims or indirect agents of terrorists but also combatants in the war against terrorism. Mental health professionals have an important duty to help citizens

marshal their personal resources in order to arm themselves against the psychological onslaught of terrorism. We offer the following guidelines and recommendations to inform terrorism response planning and preparation:

1. In any CBRNE attack, psychological casualties will exceed physical casualties. For every physical injury, expect 10–100 times as many psychological casualties. All simulations, tabletop or real life, should include a realistic number of psychological casualties.

2. When planning, assume higher than normal absenteeism among first responders and hospital staff. Healthcare and emergency workers will fear contamination and also feel compelled to help their families first.

3. The symptoms of anxiety prompted by a CBRNE attack can easily mimic the effects of exposure to chemical, biological, or radiological weapons.

4. Large numbers of trained people will be required to perform initial assessment and triage. Develop a simple charting system to handle large numbers of patients. If possible, screen for "actual exposure versus MPI" off-site (in churches, schools, etc.) to prevent hospitals from being overwhelmed. Automated telephone or web-based screening tools may reduce the number of nonexposed individuals seeking medical care.

5. Create a informative, nonsensational, easy-to-understand public education campaign about terrorist use of CBRNE weapons. Officials can reduce fear by providing the public with specific, relevant information regarding the scope and nature of threatening situations. The perception that information is being withheld or that necessary actions are not being taken will only increase the public's anxiety.

6. People will take steps to protect themselves from threat, so officials should provide the public with clear instructions regarding the most effective actions to take and the reasons for those actions. Should necessary responses go beyond the scope of individual action, then governments should explain what protective actions are being carried out and why (Perry & Lindell, 2003).

7. Civilian resilience has been chronically underestimated by government planners and

public health officials. Fear and anxiety are normal human reactions to threat and should not be confused with psychiatric illness. During World War II, mental health experts in Britain before the blitz predicted that *three to four million* cases of "acute panic, hysteria and other neurotic conditions" would require psychiatric care during the first 6 months of air raids (Shepard, 2001, p. 175). The actual number of psychiatric casualties during the blitz was "astonishingly small" (p. 178).

8. A significant minority of the affected population will suffer long-term psychological consequences that require professional care. At highest risk are those with preexisting psychiatric illnesses or poor social support systems. Also at increased risk are those who suffered physical injuries, lost family in the event, directly witnessed the deaths of others, handled dead bodies, or experienced significant loss of property or economic reversal.

Notes

1. The high-yield explosive employed was the hijacked airliners' aviation fuel. Examples of high-yield explosive attacks include those on Oklahoma City's federal building (April 19, 1995); Russian and Dagestani apartment buildings (August–September, 1999); and the World Trade Center and Pentagon (September 11, 2001).

2. The terms "WMD" and "CBRNE" are used here interchangeably.

3. Hitler did not use chemical weapons against the Allies during World War II because he believed that the United States possessed a more deadly stockpile than Germany's. Saddam Hussein refrained from using WMD in Gulf War I because he feared nuclear retaliation by the United States.

References

Alexander, D., & Klein, S. (2003). Biochemical terrorism: Too awful to contemplate, too serious to ignore. *British Journal of Psychiatry, 183,* 491–497.

Asukai, N., & Maekawa, K. (2002). Psychological and physical health effects of the 1995 sarin attack in the Tokyo subway system. In J. Havenaar & J. Cwikel (Eds.), *Toxic turmoil: Psychological and societal consequences of ecological disasters* (pp. 149–162). New York: Kluwer Academic/Plenum.

Bartholomew, R., & Victor, J. (2004). A social-psychological theory of collective anxiety attacks: The "Mad Gasser" reexamined. *Sociological Quarterly, 45*(2), 229–248.

Bleich, A., Dycian, A., Koslowsky, M., Solomon, Z., & Weiner, M. (1992). Psychiatric implications of missile attacks on a civilian population: Israeli lessons from the Persian Gulf War. *Journal of the American Medical Association, 268*(5), 613–615.

DiGiovanni, C. (1999). Domestic terrorism with chemical and biological agents: Psychiatric aspects. *American Journal of Psychiatry, 156,* 1500–1505.

Engel, C. C. (2001). Outbreaks of medically unexplained symptoms after military action, terrorist threat, or technological disaster. *Military Medicine, 166*(12), 47–48.

Fetter, S., Lewis, G. N., & Gronlund, L. (1993). Why were casualties so low? *Nature, 361,* 293–296.

Findley, T. (1991). Chemical weapons and missile proliferation. Boulder: Lynee Rienner.

Friedman, G. (2004). *America's secret war: Inside the hidden worldwide struggle between America and its enemies.* New York: Doubleday.

Friedman, T. L. (1999). *The Lexus and the olive tree.* New York: Farrar, Straus, & Giroux.

Giuliani, R. (2004). *Testimony before the National Commission on Terrorist Attacks upon the United States.* Retrieved March 15, 2005, from http://www.9-11commission.gov/archive/hearing11/9-11Commission_Hearing_2004-05-19.pdf

Hall, M. J., Norwood, A. E., Ursano, R. J., & Fullerton, C. S. (2003). The psychological impacts of bioterrorism. *Biosecurity and Bioterrorism: Biodefense Strategy, Practice, and Science, 1*(2), 139–144.

———, & Levinson, C. J. (2002). Psychological and behavioral impacts of bioterrorism. *PTSD Research Quarterly, 13*(4), 1–7.

Hoffman, B. (2000). *Change and continuity in terrorism.* Address delivered at the conference on "Terrorism and Beyond: The Twenty-first Century," Oklahoma City, OK, April 17. Retrieved March 15, 2005, from http://www.mipt.org/hoffman-ctb.asp

———. (2002). Rethinking terrorism and counterterrorism since 9/11. *Studies in Conflict and Terrorism, 25,* 303–316.

Holloway, H. C., Norwood, A. E., Fullerton, C. S., Engel, C. C., & Ursano, R. J. (1997). The threat of biological weapons: Prophylaxis and mitigation of psychological and social consequences. *Journal of the American Medical Association, 278*(5), 425–427.

Jenkins, B. M. (1975). International terrorism: A new mode of conflict. In D. Carlton & C. Schaef (Eds.), *International terrorism and world security* (pp. 13–49). New York: Wiley.

———. (1999, October 20). Testimony delivered to the House Committee on Government Reform.

Jones, T. (2000). Mass psychogenic illness: Role of the individual physician. *American Family Physician, 62,* 2649–2653, 2655–2656.

———, Craig, A., Hoy, D., Gunter, E., Ashley, D., Barr, D., et al. (2000). Mass psychogenic illness attributed to toxic exposure at a high school. *New England Journal of Medicine, 342*(2), 96–100.

Kay, D. A. (2001). WMD terrorism: Hype or reality? In J. M. Smith & W. C. Thomas (Eds.), *The terrorism threat and U.S. government response: Operational and organizational factors.* Retrieved March 15, 2005, from http://atlas.usafa.af.mil/inss/terrorism.htm

Lifton, R. J. (2000). *Destroying the world to save it: Aum Shinrikyō, apocalyptic violence, and the new global terrorism.* New York: Owl Books.

Martin, E. S. (2002). Missiles of terror: Hitler's and Hussein's use of ballistic missiles. Master's thesis, Louisiana State University.

McCauley, C. R. (2002). Psychological issues in understanding terrorism and the response to terrorism. In C. Stout (Ed.), *The psychology of terrorism, Vol. 3: Theoretical understandings and perspectives* (pp. 3–30). Westport, CT: Praeger.

Moores, L. E. (2002). Threat credibility and weapons of mass destruction. *Neurosurgery Focus, 12,* 1–3.

Moscrop, A. (2001). Mass hysteria is seen as main threat from bioweapons. *British Medical Journal, 323,* p. 1023.

Norris, F. H., Friedman, M. J., Watson, P. J., Byrne, C. M., Díaz, E., & Kaniasty, K. (2002). 60,000 disaster victims speak: Part 1: An empirical review of the empirical literature, 1981–2001. *Psychiatry, 65*(3), 207–239.

Ohbu, S., Yamashina, A., Takasu, N., Yamaguchi, T., Murai, T., Nakano, K., et al. (1997). Sarin poisoning on the Tokyo subway. *Southern Medical Journal, 90,* 587–593.

Pangi, R. (2002). Consequence management in the 1995 sarin attacks on the Japanese subway system. BCSIA Discussion Paper 2002–2004. John F. Kennedy School of Government, Harvard University.

Pastel, R. (2001). Collective behaviors: Mass panic and outbreaks of multiple unexplained symptoms. *Military Medicine, 166*(12), 44–47.

Perry, R. W., & Lindell, M. K. (2003). Understanding citizen response to disasters with implications for terrorism. *Journal of Contingencies and Crisis Management, 11*(2), 49–60.

Pettersen, J. S. (1988). Perception versus reality of radiological impact: The Goiania model. *Nuclear News, 31,* 84–90.

Quarantelli, E. L. (1954). The nature and conditions of panic. *American Journal of Sociology, 60,* 265–275.

Rachman, S. J. (1990). *Fear and courage* (2d ed.). New York: Freeman.

Ramalingaswami, V. (2001). Psychosocial effects of the 1994 plague outbreak in Surat, India. *Military Medicine, 166*(12), 29–30.

Salter, C. A. (2001). Psychological effects of nuclear and radiological warfare. *Military Medicine, 166*(12), 17–18.

Scheuer, M. (2005). Al-Qaeda's completed warning cycle: Ready to attack? *Terrorism Focus, 2*(5), 4–5.

Shepard, B. (2001). *A war of nerves: Soldiers and psychiatrists in the twentieth century.* Cambridge, MA: Harvard University Press.

Slovic, P., Fischhoff, B., & Lichtenstein, S. (1980). Facts and fears: Understanding perceived risk. In R. Schwing & W. A. Albers Jr. (Eds.), *Societal risk assessment: How safe is safe enough?* (pp. 181–214). New York: Plenum.

Steinhausler, F. (2003). What it takes to become a nuclear terrorist. *American Behavioral Scientist, 46*(6), 782–795.

Stern, J. (1999). *The ultimate terrorists.* Cambridge, MA: Harvard University Press.

Stewart, J. B. (2003). *Heart of a soldier.* New York: Simon & Schuster.

Thomas, J. (1992, November 22). The Cocoanut Grove inferno. *Boston Globe,* p. 1.

Wessely, S., Hyams, K. C., & Bartholomew, R. (2001). Psychological implications of chemical and biological weapons. *British Medical Journal, 323,* 878–879.

12

Psychological Weapons of Mass Disruption Through Vicarious Classical Conditioning

Dennis D. Embry

Danger requires response. When a hurricane nears the U.S. shore, all manner of warnings and preparations follow, depending on the magnitude and path of the threat. Similarly, when meteorologists spot a tornado, warnings sirens signal the depth of the emergency, and broadcast media immediately inform those who should seek shelter.

Dangers differ. For some, people have advance knowledge, but others, like earthquakes, strike suddenly and without warning. Some are chronic dangers and some are acute, and they vary in the type of response they require. Tobacco, alcohol, and other drugs have a chronic, adverse impact on safety and health. Health promotion psychology has tested any number of strategies to reduce or prevent the hazard they pose. In the past few decades exposure to violent offenses such as rape, assaults, and homicides have caused a rush of other strategies that utilize community policing, prevention, and security systems.

Terrorism is a newly acknowledged danger in the United States, although its threats have been apparent for some time, and it has substantial history in many other parts of the world. The attacks of September 11, the anthrax letters, shoe bombs, other actions, and *threats* of action by terrorists have raised the specter of sustained vigilance and made apparent the need for planned responses by government (at all levels), law enforcement, health professionals, the private sector, and private citizens. It is equally clear the military's defeat of the Taliban and al-Qaeda or the capture of leading terrorists will not end future risk.

The greatest danger of terrorism is not to be found in the typical territorial acquisition, body counts, or target destruction of historical wars. The essential danger—and objective—of terrorism is the creation of terror—a state of mind and its resultant behavioral responses. Terrorism applies the science and practice of psychology for political purposes in much the same way that thermonuclear weapons apply the science of physics for military purposes. More powerful, plentiful, technologically sophisticated weapons and military strategies are the common response to promote security in the face of conventional warfare threats. An essential policy, strategic, and tactical question now is, how might we achieve those same levels of safety and security when the threat is psychological?

Multiple areas of psychological research offer guidance to help shape policy and practice for homeland security. Failure to make use of lessons from these sources could seriously increase real risks for future acts of terrorism or slow recovery from such events. Effective use of psychological research and technology could substantially improve the competence, resilience, and protection of U.S. citizens. This chapter explores several approaches for using psychology in the defense of the United States.

The New Type of War Using the Psychology of Mind and Behavior

In the United States, we are equipped and trained to fight large conventional wars. We make more tanks, more ships, more airplanes, and more of everything to overwhelm an enemy. Regardless of who the enemy is, they are matched tank for tank, plane for plane, or weapon for weapon. Military strategists call this a symmetric war, and the United States has excelled in symmetric wars. They have typically worked well and ensured security for the country and its citizens.

Some wars in recent history, such as the Gulf War, have been disymmetric: Iraq was a weak force facing a strong force. Iraq fought conventionally against an immensely stronger opponent.

The current situation, however, is asymmetric, not disymmetric like Iraq. Presently, the United States has unquestioned hegemony in world affairs and conventional warfare. It is the remaining world superpower. Asymmetric war dictates that any opponent of the United States, representing the superior force, needs to avoid the strengths of the United States and concentrate on its vulnerabilities. U.S. military strategies have for some time warned that the United States is (as the 911 attacks and the anthrax letters demonstrably proved) vulnerable to asymmetric strategies of warfare.

Asymmetry is about the qualitative difference in the means, values, and styles of the new enemies. Once a power like the United States achieves military superiority and singular influence in world affairs, its disadvantaged enemies resort to unconventional asymmetrical means to fight it, avoiding its strengths and concentrating on its vulnerabilities. The greatest vulnerability is the mind of its citizens, who use perceived safety as the behavioral foundation to maintaining the very fabric of the U.S. productivity system and the global economy.

Asymmetric Strategy One: Condition Fear and Anxiety

Terrorism aims not just at any fear. Terrorism works best from a strategic perspective if the very symbols of everyday life become classically conditioned fear and anxiety stimuli, which then render your stronger opponent (if you are the weaker player in the asymmetric war) strategically wounded.

Classical conditioning especially affects either aversive- or approach-type behaviors and specifically emotionally laden behaviors or thoughts (e.g., Carlson, 1994). Here I am concerned with aversive or emotional conditioning. The mechanism is fundamental in behavioral sciences and has been well studied for nearly a hundred years. Classical conditioning is a form of learning in which a previously unimportant stimulus (visual, auditory, tactical, or internal body event) acquires the property of an important stimulus. For example, your new baby sees a balloon for the first time. Another child pops the balloon, and the baby is startled by the loud noise (important, unconditioned stimulus) and cries from the fright (unconditioned response to fear in babies). Thereafter, balloons evoke fear in the baby. The conditioning often becomes much more complicated. For example, what if exposure to the balloons were paired with birthday paraphernalia such as signs, hats, and noisemakers? Subsequently, sheer exposure to any of those stimuli might trigger the fear or anxious response—especially if the fearful events were relatively singular or potent. A simple map of classical conditioning is shown in Figure 12.1.

The power of classical conditioning in creating fear and anxiety was obviously not lost in the planning of the terrorist attacks of 9/11. The entire event resembled a large-scale Pavlovian conditioning experiment:

1. Strong iconic symbols were chosen with matched visual and auditory cues—the Twin Towers, the Pentagon, and perhaps the White House or Capitol, had the fourth plane found its target. This alone increased the chances of conditioned fear and anxiety. The image of the Twin Towers and the words describing that image are the same, which is also true of the Pentagon.

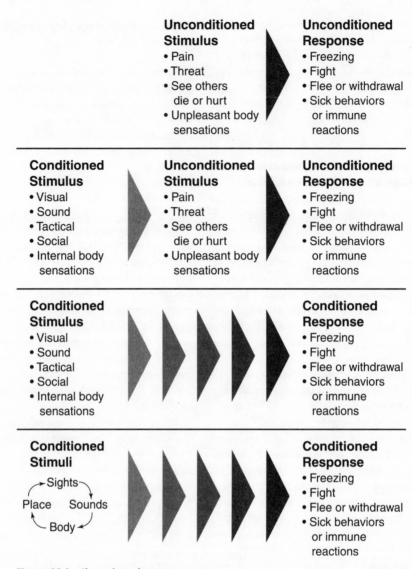

Figure 12.1. Classical conditioning sequence.

2. The instruments of violence or trauma were verbally associated with the country's name—*United* and *American* Airlines. This would mean that the very words and colors associated with the United States could have fear-evoking properties.

3. The attacks injured or destroyed symbols that were associated with high efficacy and power—Wall Street (in fact, world capitalism), the largest dollar exporter and symbol of U.S. technology (Boeing), and the U.S. Defense Department, representing the strongest military forces in the world. Had the White House or Capitol building been hit, the prime symbols of our form of government would have been destroyed.

4. The timing ensured that live news coverage would show the attacks, guaranteeing that almost every citizen would watch the scenes over and over and over again, which further guaranteed that news networks and the acronyms (CNN, NBC, CBS, etc.) associated with them would become paired with fear and anxiety.

5. Facial expressions of fear or terror, weeping from loss, fleeing from danger, and probably raging fire are unconditioned stimuli in humans—evoking visceral reactions of fear and anxiety.

All of these items contain the basic components of the classic conditioned fear and anxiety paradigm, yet this author could find no references in any popular commentary to this fact. The responses by the public were rather predictable. These also meet the requirements of stimulus equivalence based on relational frame theory (Barnes, 1994; Hall, 1996; Hayes & Wilson, 1993, 1995; Peoples, Tierney, Bracken, & McKay, 1998).

Consider the evidence for classical conditioning responses. First, the popular media have universally reported visceral responses such as "I felt sick," "My head hurt," or "I couldn't concentrate." Second, "freezing" and withdrawal responses quickly followed. People stayed put in settings they deemed historically safe, and many adults whisked their children out of school. Other multiple conditioned responses then tended to emerge. For the most part, these responses were all across the United States, only mediated by watching TV or listening to the radio.

Military objectives for conditioned fear in an asymmetric war are quite potent. A major aim is to disrupt normal business and economic transactions that sustain the infrastructure of the enemy. The attacks of 9/11 did that brilliantly. While one would have forecast attacks against people of Middle Eastern descent or appearance in the aftermath, the real secondary shock wave of the attack was near universal fear and avoidance of travel (or anything remotely connected with travel symbolically), big buildings, consumer spending, and impaired stock trading for anything related to Wall Street and the "center of world finance."

These fear and anxiety responses hurt the country greatly. Because uncertainty strengthens the fear conditioning toward U.S. icons, the military objectives of the attacks were further served by al-Qaeda's *not* taking credit for the attacks; taking credit would have diluted the psychological factors. A cardinal precept of asymmetric war is to maximize fear and anxiety conditioning, not necessarily to maximize loss of life or property—a very big difference from symmetric warfare.

Whereas conventional warfare may seek to cause surrender by shock and awe, asymmetric war seeks to cause fear, freezing, and withdrawal.

Classically conditioned fear serves the strategist well in an asymmetric war. First, it undermines the authority of the government of the stronger party. By choosing to attack the very symbols of the United States, this fear made leaders look weak, further enhancing fear conditioning in many segments of the population. Second, conditioned fear severely weakens the productive capacity of the stronger party. Fear and anxiety are well documented to cause significant reductions in task performance—even in less vulnerable, highly trained groups. This can translate into major losses of productivity or market performance.

Few would conceive of simple classical conditioning as a "weapon of mass disruption." Indeed, when teaching the principles of classical conditioning to students, educators, business leaders, or policy makers, many will say, "Oh, that applies only to lower animals—certainly not to humans." Those who understand the role of classical conditioning in modern society are presently two groups outside of researchers on human behavior: (1) Advertising and marketing companies routinely pair unimportant stimuli (a new product) with an important stimulus (e.g., sex appeal) to evoke desired behaviors toward their product; (2) terrorists have proven the immense power of classical conditioning of fear and anxiety as a weapon. The loss of business in the financial markets and travel industry in the few months after the attacks is estimated to have exceeded hundreds of billions of dollars, which is primarily the result of classically conditioned fear and anxiety.

Asymmetric Strategy Two: Increase Long-Term Prevalence Rates of Fear, Anxiety, and Mental Depression

Depression is epidemic in Western culture. The U.S. National Comorbidity Survey (e.g., Kessler, Berglund et al. 2005) reveals a striking rise in the lifetime prevalence of depression (Figure 12.2). A similar pairing can be seen in the increased number of prescriptions for depression paid for by Medicaid and private insurance companies, shown in the related graph. Both of these sets of data have implications for homeland security.

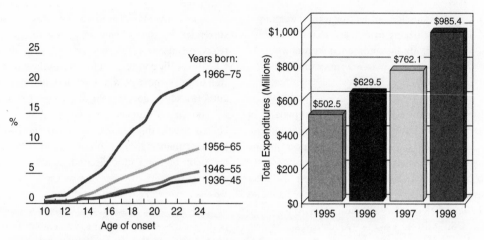

Figure 12.2. Depression prevalence data and Medicaid expenditures.
Source: The Lewin Group analysis of HCFA Medicaid Drug Rebate Program data, 1995–1998. 46
states reporting, 1995–1997, 45 states reporting, 1998.

At first blush, depression would seem to have nothing to do with an asymmetric war against the United States. If your purpose is, however, to wreck havoc in a country by capitalizing on its vulnerabilities, then increasing the prevalence rates of depression or the severity of the condition suits the purpose well as a target of opportunity for terrorism. Active depression has a number of notable symptoms:

• lowered cognitive function and diminished performance on tasks
• decreased energy and motivation
• increased physical illnesses, irritability, and pessimistic ruminations

In clinical psychology, these symptoms are seen in the context of an individual, not in their broader social impact. However, hundreds of thousands of people with depressive symptoms can have a major adverse impact on the larger society, with corresponding economic and political reverberations. Increased prevalence of depression can have manifold adverse societal-level effects, the most prevalent of which are the following:

• decreased consumer confidence and spending
• decreased work productivity and satisfaction
• decreased participation in everyday life, which in turn is associated with
• increased social isolation and withdrawal
• increased rates of domestic violence and instability

What some pundits may not appreciate is the huge impact of all of these aggregate outcomes on state and local budgets. An increased prevalence of depression will substantially drive up health costs, unemployment benefits, and family service costs in the United States during a time in which the nation's governors report that a majority of states will experience at least a 10% shortfall in revenue (Associated Press, 2002). The current vulnerability to depression in Western society has thus been used as a "weapon of mass destruction."

Further, a seminal study by Zullow (1991) has demonstrated, quite amazingly, that national economic trends are predicted by pessimistic ruminations and/or headlines in popular music or news magazines. One need only pick up these publications to grasp the frequency of negative ruminations after September 11. The abstract of Zullow's study foreshadows current events:

Content analyzed lyrics of the top 40 US songs of each year from 1955 to 1989 for 2 depressive psychological traits: rumination about bad events and pessimistic explanatory style. Cover story captions of *Time* magazine for those years were also analyzed for rumination. Increased pessimistic ruminations (PRs) in popular music predicted: (1) changes in the American media and public's view of real world events with a 1- to 2-yr lead-time, (2) increased rumination about bad events in *Time* magazine, and (3) increased pessimism about the economy in nationwide consumer surveys. PR in songs and rumination in *Time* predicted changes in consumer optimism, which in turn predicted personal consumption expenditures and GNP growth. Although PR in songs was an indirect predictor of GNP growth, it may provide early warning of recessions, since its 2-yr moving average correlated highly with the moving average of GNP change in the subsequent two years. (p. 501)

Asymmetric Strategy Three: Stimulate the Prevalence of Substance Abuse and Misuse

According to a wide variety of research reports (e.g., Kosten, Rounsaville, & Kleber, 1986), perceived stress (e.g., danger, fear, worry, depression, anxiety) among humans increases the rate of substance abuse. Increased substance abuse or misuse is an obvious likely outcome from psychological, physiological, and sociological events such as terrorist attacks. Such information is freely available. For example, in testimony in 1991, I reported that alcohol sales at U.S. military base exchanges in Germany stayed the same in the month of January 1991 even though some 100,000 troops had been deployed from these bases while their dependents remained and were exposed—via television—to threats of terrorism and potential casualties.

For most people, the pain of terrorism is vicarious classical conditioning, and substantial research shows that a whole array of substances short-circuit the felt pain from classical conditioning (e.g., Davis, 1992). For example, opiates, benzodiazepines, marijuana, and alcohol can affect the potency of classical conditioning, although the mechanism may differ by type of drug. For example, opiates and benzodiazepines directly affect the learning of the pairing of stimulus and response. Alcohol may increase perceived safety through serotonergic and opiate receptor mechanisms, yet still affect conditioned fear responses (e.g., Chung, Yoon, & Park, 1998; Stromberg, 1992). Further, the pain- or fear-reduction properties, however, are typically achieved only if the substance use state is maintained. Noyes and Baram (1974) report that cannabis may work as a mild analgesic, which would be potentially desirable for those who experience perceived pain as a result of terrorism.

Why would the creators of terrorist strategy even think about increasing substance abuse or misuse among their enemies? There are several reasons that have military significance. First, substance abuse or misuse has obvious adverse consequences on productivity, health, law enforcement, and government operations. These harmful consequences are extremely well documented by a variety of reports such as *Shoveling Up! The Cost of Substance to States* (Center on Substance Abuse and Addictions, 2001). Second, zealots need cash: The illegal drug trade has been linked to the funding of terrorism—even the funding of likely al-Qaeda activities in the United States (Wannenburg, 2003). Third, the illegal drug trade provides a powerful cover to overwhelm the mechanisms that detect the smuggling of items or people who might be used in a terrorist attack—even though early surveillance of drug smuggling might increase, as happened at both Mexican and Canadian border crossings (Kelleher, 2001).

Thus, organized terrorism of the kind that occurs in an asymmetric conflict has many solid strategic reasons to seek to increase substance abuse and misuse among the population of its enemy. Is there any evidence of increased substance abuse yet? I am not aware of any organized studies, but there are already some indices and evidence of the awareness of the strategy's utility and emerging outcomes in the wake of September 11:

- The *New York Times* has variously reported (e.g., Mcfadden, & Moynihan, 2005) that al-Qaeda had elaborate plans to produce and sell a very high-grade heroin for export to the United States and Western Europe. The Speaker of the U.S. House of Representatives formed a special committee to investigate the way in which the illegal drug trade is being used to fund terrorism (Associated Press, 2001a).
- Bar sales of alcohol have increased substantially in airports, despite fewer fliers (Reel, 2001).
- States are substantially cutting treatment dollars for substance abuse and related disorders in the aftermath of September 11 (*Alcoholism and Drug Abuse Weekly,* 2002), which further enhances the military goals of the terrorist attacks.
- The illegal drug trade increased by 25% in the Caribbean area following the terrorist attacks in the United States (Associated Press, 2001b).

- A survey of all states showed an increase in treatment seeking in 23 in the wake of the attacks (The COMPA Bulletin, 2002).

Increasing substance abuse and misuse is a powerful strategy that organized terrorist groups utilize to harm a more powerful opponent and an equally potent strategy for funding those attacks. The principles for increasing likely substance abuse or misuse are available to anyone who can use the Internet (e.g., http://www.nida.nih.gov/) and understands basic psychological research.

Asymmetric Strategy Four: Increase Errors in Detecting Threats

Successful terrorist attacks depend on normal citizens not noticing things—losing the ability to process potential threats or increasing responses to "false positives" for the sake of disruption. Noticing potential threats requires sustained vigilance. Vigilance is a well-studied cognitive skill in psychology, going back to research on radar operators in World War II. Homeland security involves vigilance by average citizens and by paid employees at airports, immigration offices, and other locations vulnerable to acts of terrorism.

Vigilance by Private Citizens

Increasing the vigilance of private citizens poses a paradox. Pressure to maintain or increase vigilance can have an adverse consequence on the behavior of citizens in the market place, increasing the chance that the economy will suffer, thus creating a military victory in the context of an asymmetric war. Maintaining vigilance, however, is potentially aversive for citizens, who are likely to have heightened fear or anxiety as a result of constant cajoling to pay increased attention to potential threats. Under such conditions, psychologists predict several outcomes: (1) Some people will make many errors in failing to distinguish real threat from the mere pressure to perform; (2) some will detect too many perceived threats that are not real; and (3) some people will opt not to engage in sustained attention because they may perceive it as too aversive—creating an incentive for avoidance (e.g., Krohne, 1993). Perceived control also interacts with vigilance accuracy in that lower perceived control reduces accuracy (e.g., Lawler & Schmied, 1987). All of these errors provide some military

advantage to the weaker force in an asymmetric war. Poor detection or nondetection aids actual terrorist attacks, and false positives undermine appeals for homeland security.

Mass appeals to increase vigilance to potential threat may also have some serious, unintended consequences for mortality and morbidity from various diseases. For example, sustained attention to potential threat increases the risk of cardiovascular disease (e.g., Gump & Matthews, 1998; Winters, McCabe, Green, & Schneiderman, 2000). It is possible that more people could die from sustained vigilance than from terrorist attacks. For the theoreticians of asymmetric war, this is simply a bonus from a military strategy perspective.

Vigilance by Security Personnel

Homeland security involves thousands of persons hired to engage in vigilant behavior—airport personnel, law enforcement officers, immigration officials, post office employees, military personnel, intelligence officers, and many more. Part of the military strategy of terrorists is to increase the failure of such personnel, both to create opportunity for attacks and to disrupt government. The mechanisms for both are easy to manipulate with a modicum of knowledge from psychological research that is easily available.

The first tactic is to foster all sorts of stress and anxiety among those who are doing the screening. Too much stress and anxiety reduces the accuracy of their vigilance tasks. It is easy to make such stress and anxiety happen. For example, mass media reports regularly chastise airports and airlines for failures, and the jobs of security personnel have regularly been challenged as a way to "shape up behavior." This type of pressure to be more vigilant as a result of threats to job security (e.g., "If you don't find more security violations, you'll get fired") has already been shown to decrease vigilance (e.g., Singh and Singh, 1985). Emotional distress alone is sufficient to impair the performance of even the most highly trained people (e.g., Simonov, Frolov, & Ivanov, 1980). Vigilance can be sustained with accuracy for only a short period of time without significant training, positive reinforcement, and support.

Decision making in emergency situations has been studied and is relevant here. For example, Janis and Mann (1977) detailed how defensive avoidance or hypervigilance can become dominant in some disaster detection settings, which generally leads to maladaptive actions. For example, many people may become nonsensitive to cues while others become oversensitive, meaning too many false positives or false negatives in the detection of threats. Empirical evidence (e.g., Trivizas & Smith, 1997) indicates that the attack strategies of terrorists seem well primed to evoke maladaptive behaviors by supervisors and line personnel associated with homeland security, with only short-lived effects of actual events on both employees and the general public.

Asymmetric Strategy Five: Foster Piggyback Events

An old saying exists in war: "An enemy of your enemy is your friend." Terrorism strategy seeks therefore to increase the likelihood that others will commit copycat or piggyback attacks. The rationale ought to be obvious. The more copycats or piggyback actions there are, the greater the impact will be of vicarious classical conditioning because of perceived helplessness and lack of control. Further, the threat will be perceived as even more diffuse and unpredictable. It would seem quite likely that any well-educated person involved in planning terrorist attacks that are grounded in psychological research would be likely to know of the probability of imitation following highly visible crimes. There are several reasons to believe this theoretically:

1. Suicidal behavior is clearly more likely to follow a high-profile suicide or suicidally motivated homicide, especially when accompanied by extended media coverage in an apparent dose-response relationship (Etzersdorfer, Voracek, & Sonneck, 2001; Phillips & Hensley, 1984; Sonneck, Etzersdorfer, & Nagel-Kuess, 1994; Stack, 2000).
2. Retributive violence may be copied more as a function of ensuing military action (Bebber, 1994; Diefenbach & West, 2001).

The piggyback events, whether using the same targets as the original terrorists, are not material to the impact on affected communities. In 1978 a dozen children in Holland and West Germany were hospitalized after terrorists deliberately contaminated citrus fruit from Israel with mercury. This ploy was then copied by others—with devastating effects on the Israeli economy (Khan, Swerdlow, & Juranek, 2001).

Asymmetric Strategy Six: Undermine Perceived Authority by Role Rigidity

In a classic study, Haney, Banks, and Zimbardo (1973) had college students pretend to be inmates or guards in the basement of the psychology department of Stanford University. Soon the "guards" began to evidence the behaviors that typically lead to the excesses often documented in prison settings. The "inmates" complied for the most part, subject to their roles. Few people aside from research psychologists and military force-management personnel know how much people assume the behaviors of their structured role. Thus, it would be reasonable to predict that many of those who "don the uniform" of homeland security might come to engage in overzealous behaviors in the name of reducing terrorism. This would increase as a function of perceived job stress and the pressure to be vigilant against the nefarious plots of terrorists. In the famous Stanford experiment, it took only days for these behaviors to unfold.

Role stereotypy and role "freezing" naturally create an adverse reaction to the behavior of those in authority by others who are not part of the uniform "script" or context. To some extent this effect is clearly an outcome of the Arab-Israeli conflict, wherein public support for the Israeli position has eroded in many countries—precisely the goal of many of the Arab tacticians who fought against the overwhelming military power of Israel. This dissatisfaction has even been voiced by academics and scholars within Israel (Shalhoub-Kevorkian, 2004). To the extent that others come to see the exercise of authority as illegal or immoral, terrorist strategies begin to work.

Using Psychological Theory to Guide the Prediction of Targets of Mass Disruption

As I reflected on the attacks of September 11, it became more and more clear that the targets, methods, and processes were very carefully thought out from a psychological perspective, just as they were considered from a structural and logistical point of view. When I have voiced this opinion, some people have seemed angry that one could give the terrorists credit for being intelligent or knowledgeable. To ignore their intelligence risks grave danger and disruption. One rule exists in the military and intelligence operations: If *you* can think of it, your enemy already has.

Can psychological theory be used to predict likely targets of terrorism in the United States or other countries? I believe so, and I suggest the following hypotheses:

Hypothesis 1

Targets or conditioned stimuli that have high visual and iconic salience with related auditory cues will be preferentially selected for attack. For example, the Twin Towers are a better vicarious classical conditioning stimulus for fear than a building like the Sears Tower or the Empire State Building. The visual image and verbal labels are not as strong in the latter cases, and this assertion could be tested in rather simple classical conditioning experiments in which the stimulus is embedded in brief presentations associated with unconditioned stimuli.

Hypothesis 2

Targets or conditioned stimuli that are associated with projections of power, potency, and universality in the United States will be preferentially selected for attack. Thus, terrorist operations would be far more likely to involve Federal Express, United Parcel Service, or the dollar currency than U-Haul trucks, DHL, or bank checks. United and American Airlines are far more likely to be selected as a delivery mechanism than Delta or Southwest Airlines.

Hypothesis 3

Targets or conditioned stimuli that convey everyday connotations of safety, happiness, productivity, and/or pleasure are more likely to be selected. Thus, something like Coca-Cola, fire trucks, or school buses would be a better vehicle for the delivery of terrorism than a bottled water company, a regular truck, or a tour bus.

Vicarious classical conditioning is testable by rather simple laboratory experiments that were first pioneered more than 50 years ago. A computer or slide projector could be used to present the visual stimuli, and either one could easily be yoked to an audio source. The sheer simplicity of vicarious classical conditioning and the strong relationship of classical conditioning to issues of consumer behavior, addictive behaviors, mental disorders, and cognitive competence under stress make classical conditioning one of the most powerful and low-cost strategies of an asymmetric war. Vicarious classical conditioning, as in the case of September 11, caused a crippling blow to the United States. The question is, can we learn to design a preventative strategy short of engaging the very purposes of strategists of terrorism?

Author's Postscript

At the time of final editing, the Dubai Ports controversy had just surfaced, and the deal was scuttled before sending back the final manuscript. Arabic nationality, terrorism risk, and serious threat had become so conditioned in the public mind that a political firestorm emerged, resulting in a cancellation of the deal. While the merits of the issue can be debated in honest ways, the vicarious classical conditioning effect set in motion on September 11th continued to achieve rippling asymmetric military effects, as predicted. That is, perceived prejudice multiplied between the United States and Arabic peoples, setting fertile ground for terrorism recruitment; public trust in leaders (e.g., the President and its backers) was further eroded as witnessed by spot polls and pundits; and economic commerce is set back now with threats of commercial boycotts of United States products by key Arabic trading partners. While the specifics could not be predicted theoretically, the general trajectory of a culture of posttraumatic conditioning could.

References

Alcoholism and Drug Abuse Weekly (2002, January 7). *Treatment Dollars Cut After 9/11.*

Armfield, J. M., & Mattiske, J. K. (1996). Vulnerability representation: The role of perceived dangerousness, uncontrollability, unpredictability, and disgustingness in spider fear. *Behaviour Research and Therapy,* 34(11–12), 899–909.

Associated Press. (2001a, September 21). "Hastert forms task force on drugs."

Associated Press. (2001b, October 17). "Caribbean Drug Trade Increases After 911."

Bandura, A., & Rosenthal, T. L. (1966). Vicarious classical conditioning as a function of arousal level. *Journal of Personality and Social Psychology, 3*(1), 54–62.

Barnes, D. (1994). Stimulus equivalence and relational frame theory. *Psychological Record, 44*(1), p. 91.

Bebber, C. C. (1994). Increases in U.S. violent crime during the 1980s following four American military actions. *Journal of Interpersonal Violence, 9*(1), 109.

Carlson, N. R. (1994.) Physiology of behavior, 5th edition. Boston: Allyn and Bacon.

Chung, B. K., Yoon, B. S., & Park, S. K. (1998). Effects of alcohol and diazepam on fear of acquisition and extinction in rats. [Korean]. *Korean Journal of Biological and Physiological Psychology, 10*(1), 1–17.

Davis, M. (1992). The role of the amygdala in fear-potentiated startle: implications for animal models of anxiety. *Trends in Pharmacological Science, 13,* 35–41.

Diefenbach, D. L., & West, M. D. (2001). Violent crime and Poisson regression: A measure and a method for cultivation analysis. *Journal of Broadcasting and Electronic Media, 45*(3), 432.

Etzersdorfer, E., Voracek, M., & Sonneck, G. (2001). A dose-response relationship of imitational suicides with newspaper distribution. *Australian and New Zealand Journal of Psychiatry, 35*(2), 251.

Gump, B. B., & Matthews, K. A. (1998). Vigilance and cardiovascular reactivity to subsequent stressors in men: A preliminary study. *Health Psychology, 17*(1), 93–96.

Hall, G. (1996). Learning about associatively activated stimulus representations: Implications for acquired equivalence and perceptual learning. *Animal Learning and Behavior, 24*(3), 233.

Haney, C., Banks, C., & Zimbardo, P. (1973). Interpersonal dynamics in a simulated prison. *International Journal of Criminology and Penology, 1*(1), 69.

Hayes, S. C., & Wilson, K. G. (1993). Some applied implications of a contemporary behavior-analytic account of verbal events. *Behavior Analyst, 16*(2), 283.
———. (1995). The role of cognition in complex human behavior: A contextualistic perspective. *Journal of Behavior Therapy and Experimental Psychiatry, 26*(3), 241.Increased demand for alcohol and drug treatment. (2002, June 15). *The COMPA Bulletin, 2*(4), n.p.

Janis, I., & Mann, L. (1977) *Decision making: A psychological analysis of conflict, choice and commitment.* New York: Free Press

Keller, P. A. (1999). Converting the unconverted: The effect of inclination and opportunity to discount health-related fear appeals. *Journal of Applied Psychology, 84*(3), 403–415.

Kelleher, S. (2001, October 28). Big hole in nation's defense: Our ports. *The Seattle Times,* n.p.

Kessler, R. C., Berglund, P., Demler, O., Jin, R., Merikangas, K. R., & Walters, E. E. (2005). Lifetime prevalence and age-of-onset distributions of *DSM-IV* disorders in the National Comorbidity Survey Replication.[see comment][erratum appears in *Arch Gen Psychiatry.* 2005, July;62(7):768 Note: Merikangas, Kathleen R [added]]. *Archives of General Psychiatry, 62*(6), 593–602.

Khan, A. S., Swerdlow, D. L., & Juranek, D. D. (2001). Precautions against biological and chemical terrorism directed at food and water supplies. *Public Health Reports, 116*(1), 3–14.

Kosten, T. R., Rounsaville, B. J., & Kleber, H. D. (1986). A 2.5-year follow-up of depressions, life crises, and treatment effects on abstinence among opioid addicts. *Archives of General Psychiatry, 43,* 733–739.

Krohne, H. W. (Ed.). (1993). *Attention and avoidance: Strategies in coping with aversiveness.* Kirkland, WA: Hogrefe & Huber.

Lawler, K. A., & Schmied, L. A. (1987). The relationship of stress, Type A behavior, and powerlessness to physiological responses in female clerical workers. *Journal of Psychosomatic Research, 31*(5), 555–566.

Lver, A. I., & Greco, T. S. (1975). A comparison of the effects of vicariously instigated classical conditioning and direct classical conditioning procedures. *Pavlovian Journal of Biological Science, 10*(4), 216–225.

Mcfadden, R.D. & Moynihan, C. (2005, October 25). Drug suspect in afghan ring is sent to U.S. *New York Times,* section b, page 1, column 5.

McCabe, P. M., Schneiderman, N., Field, T., & Wellens, A. R. (Eds.). (2000). *Stress, coping, and cardiovascular disease.* Mahwah, NJ: Erlbaum.

Noyes, R., & Baram, D. A. (1974). Cannabis analgesia. *Comprehensive Psychiatry, 15*(6), 531–535.

Ogston, K. M., & Davidson, P. O. (1972). The effects of cognitive expectancies on vicarious conditioning. *British Journal of Social and Clinical Psychology, 11*(2), 126–134.

Peoples, M., Tierney, K. J., Bracken, M., & McKay, C. (1998). Prior learning and equivalence class formation. *Psychological Record, 48*(1), 111.

Phillips, D. P., & Hensley, J. E. (1984). When violence is rewarded or punished: The impact of mass media stories on homicide. *Journal of Communication, 34*(3), 101.

Rachman, S. (1991). Neo-conditioning and the classical theory of fear acquisition. *Clinical Psychology Review, 11*(2), 155–173.

Reed, P. (1994). Learning theory: The determinants of conditioned responding. In T. Digby & M. Birchwood (Eds.), *Seminars in psychology and the social sciences* (pp. 22–41). College seminars series. Washington, DC: American Psychiatric Press.

Reel, M. (2001, December 8). Stranded in airports, fliers turning to bars: Alcohol sales soar at airport lounges. *Washington Post.*

Reiss, D. (1972). Vicarious conditioned acceleration: Successful observational learning of an aversive Pavlovian stimulus contingency. *Journal of the Experimental Analysis of Behavior, 18*(1), 181–186.

Shalhoub-Kevorkian, N. (2004). Racism, militarization, and policing: Police reactions to violence against Palestinian women in Israel. *Social Identities: Journal for the Study of Race, Nation, and Culture, 10*(2), 171.

Silver, A. I., & Greco, T. S. (1975). A comparison of the effects of vicariously instigated classical conditioning and direct classical conditioning procedures. *Pavlovian Journal of Biological Science, 10*(4), 216–225.

Simonov, P. V., Frolov, M. V., & Ivanov, E. A. (1980). Psychophysiological monitoring of operator's emotional stress in aviation and astronautics. *Aviation Space and Environmental Medicine, 51*(1), 46–50.

Singh, I. L., & Singh, S. P. (1985). Job anxiety and vigilance performance. *Perceptual and Motor Skills, 61*(3, pt. 2), 1030.

Sonneck, G., Etzersdorfer, E., & Nagel-Kuess, S. (1994). Imitative suicide on the Viennese subway. *Social Science and Medicine, 38*(3), 453.

Stack, S. (2000). Media impacts on suicide: A quantitative review of 293 findings. *Social Science Quarterly, 81*(4), 957.

Stromberg, M. F. (1992). The effects of ethanol on conditioned freezing: Support for the endorphin compensation hypothesis of ethanol abuse. *Dissertation Abstracts International, 53*(5-B), 2569.

Trivizas, E., & Smith, P. T. (1997). The deterrent effect of terrorist incidents on the rates of luggage theft in railway and underground stations. *British Journal of Criminology, 37*(1), 63–74.

Wannenburg, G. (2003) Links between organised crime and Al-Qaeda. *South African Journal of International Affairs, 10* (2), 1–14.

Winters, R. W., McCabe, P. M., Green, E. J., & Schneiderman, N. (2000). Stress responses, coping, and cardiovascular neurobiology: Central nervous system circuitry underlying learned and unlearned affective responses to stressful stimuli. In McCabe, Schneiderman, Field, & Wellens (Eds.), *Stress, coping, and cardiovascular disease* (pp. 1–49). Mahwah, NJ: Erlbaum.

Witte, K., & Allen, M. (2000). A meta-analysis of fear appeals: Implications for effective public health campaigns. *Health Education and Behavior, 27*(5), 591–615.

Zullow, H. M. (1991). Pessimistic rumination in popular songs and news magazines predict economic recession via decreased consumer optimism and spending. *Journal of Economic Psychology, 12,* 501–526.

13

Near- and Long-Term Psychological Effects of Exposure to Terrorist Attacks

Susan E. Brandon
Andrew P. Silke

Newspapers mentioned that a recent survey showed that seven out of every ten Americans suffer psychological problems following the attacks on New York and Washington.

Osama bin Laden to Mullah Omar, quoted in Cullison (2004)

Humans show an extraordinary capacity to survive in adverse situations. Although there are tragic instances of people who are permanently scarred by trauma, these are relatively few; the majority of those who are involved in violent or life-threatening events do not exhibit long-term symptoms of distress. On the whole, they recover and may even exhibit resilience (Bonanno, 2004). When terrorists strike neighborhoods, what people most often do is wash the blood off the streets and continue on. How and when such recovery occurs is the theme of this chapter.

Here we consider the possibility that the survival, recovery, and occasional resilience seen after terrorist incidents or other disasters reflect processes of dissipation, adaptation, habituation, and sensitization that are ubiquitous to biological organisms. We also consider that many instances of human survival—including thriving—are the result of broad cognitive and affective reappraisal processes that mediate the impacts of our interactions with the world and of normative tendencies to seek out others under conditions of stress.

We describe the near- and long-term psychological effects of exposure to terrorist attacks and the threats of terrorist attacks here, largely ignoring important differences in location, type of strife,

and local and national histories, not because these are not important but because we want to consider the most frequently occurring behaviors and the most general behavioral trends. While there is relatively little empirical analysis of terrorism or terrorists' behaviors (Silke, 2003, 2004)—despite the plethora of materials published since 9/11—there is a significant body of scientific investigation on how people respond to trauma. It is that domain of science that we draw on to understand and predict how people are most likely to respond to terrorist attacks.

Powerful Forces for Normalcy

Dissipation, Adaptation and Habituation, and Sensitization

Common patterns of responses to single or repeated aversive events have been well documented in the psychological literature. However, the apparent robustness and ubiquity of these responses across many organisms and circumstances suggest that a typology of such responses may help us to understand what kinds of behaviors are likely to ensue when an organism confronts a potentially

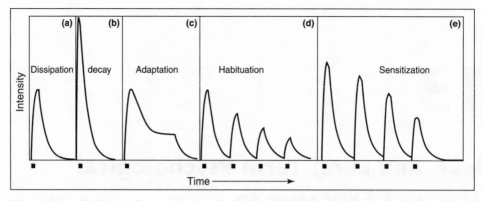

Figure 13.1. A likely immediate reaction to a threatening or harmful event. The Y-axis represents the intensity of the response, and the X-axis represents the passage of time. Discrete traumatic events are represented by the black squares below the X-axis. (a) A single response to a single event. (b) A more salient event evokes a stronger response. (c) Adaptation, observed following longer-term exposure to a single event. (d) Habituation, observed as a decreasing response to a traumatic event that occurs repeatedly across time in an otherwise stable context. (e) Sensitization, observed as an invigorated response elicited when the organism is in a heightened state of anxiety, fear, or vigilance.

harmful event. How well these patterns predict responses to events as complex as natural or technological disasters is an empirical issue. We offer the patterns here to serve as a heuristic and to help organize the discussion.

A single exposure to a threatening or harmful event is likely to provide an immediate reaction (see Figure 13.1).[1] The y-axis represents the intensity of the response, and the x-axis represents the passage of time. Discrete traumatic events are represented by the black squares below the x-axis. A single response to a single event, shown in (a), reaches its peak quickly and then dissipates. For purposes of explanation, we might assume that the aversive event is a spider crawling up the arm of a spiderphobic person. The response, which might be fear, could be assessed by measuring an increase in heart rate or respiration, by recording how vigorously the person shakes his arm to get rid of the spider, or by asking this person how afraid he feels. In the absence of repeated or continued exposure to the event (if the spider is removed), psychological and biological systems typically show the simple return to baseline shown in (a). The simplest explanation for the return to baseline is the decay or *dissipation* of these "high alert" response systems.

If the event is more salient—more frightening, more intense, more catastrophic (a huge tarantula)— the response is stronger, as shown in (b). With longer-term exposure to an event (if the spider sits on the person's arm), adaptation is the likely outcome, illustrated in (c). Although some decay occurs after the initial response, the system does not return to baseline but settles at some intermediate level, above baseline. This adaptation to the change in status quo occurs via the expenditure of the psychological, neural, neuroendocrine, and neuroimmune systems' protective mechanisms. This expenditure, however, is likely to result in the depletion of the ability to respond to further assault or need (McEwen, 1998; McEwen & Mendelson, 1993).

When a traumatic event occurs repeatedly in an otherwise stable context, as shown in (d), the response to the event decreases in vigor, a phenomenon called *habituation* (Thompson & Spencer, 1966). Thus, if a person is repeatedly exposed to a spider crawling up his arm, even the phobic will begin to show a decreased fear response. Habituation has three characteristics that are relevant here. First, it is relatively specific to the eliciting event: Habituation to a spider is not likely to transfer to another fearful insect or event (e.g., a snake) and even less to a fear of elevators or public speaking. Second, habituation itself may dissipate under conditions in which the aversive event does not reoccur for a significant period of time. Third, habituation is sensitive to the context in which it occurs, where the term *context* refers to the external physical environment and internal psychological and physical states of the organism. The ability of most habituated responses to generalize across contexts—to be elicited within a different context—is fickle, and habituation that occurs or is acquired in one context does not often transfer to a novel context. Thus, acquiring a robust habituated response to a spider in the doctor's office may not be of much use when the spider is found at home in bed.

What appears in some ways to work against habituation is sensitization. Many response systems show increased vigor when they are elicited while the organism is in a heightened state of anxiety, fear, or vigilance, a phenomenon referred to as *sensitization* (Borszcz, Cranney, & Leaton, 1989; Cacioppo et al., 2002; Connolly & Firth, 1978; Davis, 1972; Hammond, 1967). Imagine walking alone in a dark forest, fearful of what is all around: A spider landing ever so lightly on one's arm is likely, in this context, to elicit an especially fearful response. This pattern of invigorated responding is illustrated in a comparison of Figure 13.1(d) with Figure 13.1(e). As can be seen, habituation is in effect attenuated.

The temporal characteristics of these processes appear to be a function of the intensity of the initial, impacting event: Very strong events provoke a stronger initial response and a slower return to baseline in the absence of further stimulation. These responses are also modified by experience—that is, they involve significant learning—so that how someone reacts changes across time: People are likely to vary in the intensity and duration of these various responses as a result of their own unique life experiences.

Baseline: Normal Levels of Emotion and Stress

Epidemiological studies within the past decade have found that the risk for exposure to a significant aversive event or trauma in the general population of the United States is as high as 50%–60% (Breslau, Davis, Andreski, & Peterson, 1991; McFarlane, 1986; Norris, 1992; Ozer & Weiss, 2004), but the large majority of victims of trauma do not develop chronic posttraumatic mental health problems (Breslau et al., 1991; Kessler, Sonnega, Bromet, & Hughes, 1995; Ozer & Weiss, 2004). The degree of vulnerability correlates with the magnitude and severity of the trauma as well as

the history of psychiatric problems and the availability of helping resources (Breslau et al., 1991; Norris et al., 2001a, 2001b; North et al., 1999; Shalev, Peri, Canetti, & Schreiber, 1996).

Currently, the most common measure of psychological impairment following trauma such as a car accident, rape, victimization in a violent crime, or exposure to terrorist attack and other technological or natural disasters is the assessment of a relatively complex cluster of factors that, when they occur together, provide a diagnosis of posttraumatic stress disorder (PTSD). PTSD describes the condition of someone who has been exposed to a traumatic event; experiences at least one recurrent symptom related to the event (such as intrusive, repeated recollections or dreams of the incident); persistently avoids people, activities, or places associated with the event; and cannot recall important aspects of the trauma. This person also shows disinterest in the usual daily activities and a restricted range of affect or a sense of foreboding about the future to the extent that they no longer expect to have a normal life. These symptoms, in conjunction with hyperarousal (difficulty in falling or staying asleep, outbursts of anger, hypervigilance, inability to concentrate, or exaggerated startle responses), may lead to significant impairment in social, occupational, or other important areas of the person's life. To the extent that such dysfunction is present, the individual exhibits PTSD (American Psychiatric Association, 1996). It has been estimated that baseline rates of PTSD among Americans is about 3%–4% (National Institute of Mental Health, 2004).

Exposure to psychological trauma has consequences for physical as well as psychological health. To the extent that such trauma disrupts home, family, and community life, as well as the ability to work and play, it will have profound effects on everyday behavior—including those everyday social and individual behaviors that are related to half of all causes of morbidity and mortality in the United States (National Center for Health Statistics, 2003). Psychosocial variables have also been shown to be significant risk factors for chronic disease risk and recovery (Barefoot et al., 2000; Leserman et al., 1999). For example, stress may contribute directly to heart disease by narrowing the blood vessels, leading to atherosclerosis (Rutledge et al., 2003). Blascovich and

Tomaka (1996) report that extreme levels of arousal, such as terror, rage, lust, and ecstasy, are likely to play a role in stress and stress management, and dysfunctional arousal plays a role in coronary heart disease (Blascovich & Katkin, 1993) and immunosuppression (O'Leary, 1990). Negative emotions have been linked to enhanced susceptibility to infection (Herbert & Cohen, 1993), poorer response to an influenza vaccine (Kiecolt-Glaser, Glaser, Gravenstein, Malarkey, & Sheridan, 1996; Rosenkranz et al., 2003), and impaired wound healing (Kiecolt-Glaser et al., 1996). Alternatively, positive emotions are correlated with good health: A longitudinal study of Catholic nuns found that those who expressed the most positive emotions when they were young lived up to 10 years longer than those who had expressed less positive emotions earlier (Danner, Snowdon, & Friesen, 2001).

It is important to recognize that expectations and perceptions mediate the impact of many stressors and that an event has a stressful impact to the extent that it is appraised as taxing or exceeding one's resources and endangering a person's well-being (Lazarus & Folkman, 1986; McEwen & Mendelson, 1993). Antonovsky (1985) has argued that stress can be health enhancing when stressful situations are perceived as challenges and when these challenges are subsequently perceived as being met; that is, he argued for the salutogenic, as well as the pathogenic, effects of stress (Durkheim, 1951; Selye, 1991; Suedfeld, 1997).

Coping With Large-Scale Single Events

A Lexis/Nexus search of all major English newspapers and TV news in the last week of August 2001 showed approximately 50 news stories [that] were devoted to public health scares or crises. During the week of October 23–30 (the height of the anthrax events in the U.S. in the Fall of 2001), there were 558. About 1 month later, the rate dropped to approximately 120.

Osterholm (2001)

Dissipation

The attacks of September 11, 2001, on New York and Washington, DC, produced widespread reactions among residents of those cities, as well as across the country and the world. Three to five days after the attacks, about 90% of the residents of New York City and Washington reported feeling

upset, being bothered by disturbing memories, or having difficulty concentrating or falling asleep (Schuster et al., 2001). The impacts of the attacks were even felt far beyond New York and Washington: Almost 20% of Americans across the country reported symptoms of distress (Silver, Holman, McIntosh, Poulin, & Gil-Rivas, 2002).

As might be expected, the degree of exposure to an attack mediates responses to it. People who are close to the site experience more salient events; furthermore, they are subsequently reminded of the attack more often by seeing, hearing, and smelling disaster-related cues. Disaster relief workers, firefighters, police, and emergency personnel show the highest rates of PTSD, particularly when the disaster is of human origin (North et al., 2002). Data collected after 9/11 show that 10% of adults who lived south of 110th Street in Manhattan (roughly the bottom two-thirds of the island) reported symptoms consistent with a diagnosis of current PTSD after the attacks, while south of Canal Street, only blocks from the site of the devastation, the incidence was 20% (Galea et al., 2002; Galea et al., 2003). In general, the prevalence of probable PTSD was higher in New York City (11%) than in Washington, DC (3%), and the rest of the country (4%). People in the New York City metropolitan region were about three times more likely to have a probable case of PTSD than those who were elsewhere that day (Schlenger et al., 2002). Similar data were reported following the 1995 Oklahoma City bombing of the Murrah Building: Seven weeks after the violence, a clinical needs assessment of more than 3,000 sixth-through twelfth-grade students in Oklahoma City showed posttraumatic stress symptoms (15% reported that they did not feel safe, and 34% said that they worried about themselves and their families) (Pfefferbaum et al., 1999). These symptoms were the highest among those who had experienced a personal loss. Two hundred fifty-five survivors of the direct blast showed a high incidence of postdisaster stress (45%) and PTSD (34%) 6 months after the bombing (North et al., 1999). (The fatality rate inside the Murrah Building was 46%, and 93% of those in the building were injured [North et al., 1999].)

The effective intensity and the temporal characteristics of such attacks are also mediated by victim characteristics that, in some instances, may override proximity effects (Galea et al., in press).

After the Oklahoma City bombing, women reported about twice the rate of PTSD symptoms of men, and more than half of the victims with bombing-related PTSD had a predisaster lifetime history of psychiatric illness (North et al., 1999). In New York City after 9/11, Hispanics, African Americans, and those with poor general health, less education, and lower income were more stressed than others (Galea et al., 2003; Rasinski, Berktold, Smith, & Albertson, 2002).

For most people, the distress produced by exposure to a single incident does not persist for very long. With some exceptions, responses to the attacks on 9/11 dissipated with the simple passage of time and the absence of any additional attacks on U.S. soil. Surveys of adults in New York City 1 month, 4 months, and 6 months after the attacks showed that the prevalence of probable PTSD related to the violence in Manhattan had declined to 9.5% after 1 month, to 1.7% after 4 months and to 0.6% after 6 months (Galea et al., 2003). The distress was transitory for the rest of the United States as well (Schlenger et al., 2002); a nationwide probability sample indicated that distress symptoms fell from 17% after 2 months to 6% after 6 months (Silver et al., 2002).

Adaptive Behavior: Seeking Others

Stress and uncertainty produce social behaviors: People seek out others, perhaps to enhance social support (Cohen & Willis, 1985; Mehl & Pennebaker, 2003) or to help to affirm their cultural view of the world and the threat (Pyszczynski, Solomon, & Greenberg, 2002). Almost 100% of Americans surveyed after 9/11 reported that what they did that day was to talk with others about the attacks (Schuster et al., 2001). Passengers on Flight 93, which crashed in the Pennsylvania countryside, and as many as 353 workers in the World Trade Center towers, called family and friends when they realized that what was happening around them was likely to be catastrophic (Glanz, 2002). The calls were to say good-bye, send love, and, in at least one instance, to confirm their location so that their family would know of their certain death and not wonder what had happened (9/11 Commission Report, 2004). Almost 30% of Americans polled said that they had called or emailed a friend or relative in New York or Washington on 9/11, and 75% of Americans checked on the safety of close family members,

making such actions the most common coping behavior (Schuster et al., 2001). In retrospect, civilian and emergency response personnel report that, when under attack, their most urgent need is to find out whether their family and friends are all right. The most frequent coping activities among Israelis, after more than 2 years of exposure to repeated violence directed at civilians, was to check on the location and safety of friends and family after an attack; the second most common was to seek social support (Bleich, Gelkopf, & Solomon, 2003).[2]

The most frequently reported emotional responses among Americans to the attacks on 9/11 were anger, sadness, and disbelief (NBC News/*Wall Street Journal*, September 12, 2001). Sadness was the most frequent reaction among New Yorkers, followed by anxiety and fear (Felton, 2002). Sixty percent of Americans said that they cried, 50% that they were tense or nervous, and more than 45% reported feeling "sort of dazed and numb." This pattern of responses is similar to that found among Americans after the Kennedy assassination in 1963 (Rasinski et al., 2002).

Sadness fosters reflection, resignation, and acceptance and evokes sympathy and helping responses in others (Izard, 1992, 1993). Preliminary data on the initial reaction to 9/11 among some 90,000 service recipients of New York City's Project Liberty (a consortium of New York State Office of Mental Health, county and New York City mental health departments) showed that people did many things in response to the attacks, but what they did *not* do was withdraw from others (Felton, 2002). Donations of bottled water, food, clothing, and dog food for the animals helping in the search around the World Trade Center swamped the capabilities of food banks and local Salvation Army posts so that some of it had to be shipped to warehouses 90 miles from New York City (Dwyer, 2001). A national survey found 36% of Americans making donations to relief services (Schuster et al., 2001). A large-scale survey of more than 50,000 people in various disaster situations found that social continuity and access to substantial personal and community resources mitigate impact. Disasters with more dire effects, such as Hurricane Andrew in 1992 and the 1989 Exxon *Valdez* oil spill in Alaska, involved not only destruction and threat to life but also prolonged social and financial disruption and loss of resources (Norris, Watson, Hamblen, & Pfeffer-baum, 2003).

Adaptation: Compensatory Responses and Positive Emotions

The *New York Times* series "Portraits of Grief," which ran from September 2001 to December 31, 2002, offered a small photo and paragraph about each of some 1,800 of the 2,937 people who died in the World Trade Center on 9/11. Unlike the usual obituary, these "portraits" offered joyful and humorous anecdotes that family and friends remembered about those who died that day. Lazarus, Kanner, and Folkman (1980) have suggested that positive emotions serve as breathers (temporarily freeing a person from the stress of an experience and allowing pleasurable diversions), as sustainers (fostering the persistence of coping efforts), and as restorers (replenishing damaged or depleted resources or fostering the development of new resources). Nonpathological grief, which occurs in the majority of instances of loss, is known to involve the recognition of positive outcomes, such as happy thoughts, beliefs, and appraisals, positive emotion, and laughter (Bonanno, 2004).

Two weeks after the 9/11 attacks, almost 70% of Americans reported positive emotions, such as being excited about and interested in life; feeling proud, pleased, or accomplished; and "on top of the world" and as if "things were going their way." Less than 35% reported negative emotions, such as feeling restless, lonely, bored, depressed, or upset. By the end of 2003, 70% of Americans claimed that the threat of terrorism had had a positive impact on their lives, either by making them evaluate what is important in their lives or by making them stronger and more resilient. At the same time, the number of Americans who thought that others were helpful was higher than it had been since the 1970s, a view that remained consistent in the subsequent year (Rasinski et al., 2002). Similarly positive outcomes were reported among Americans after the Cuban missile crisis in 1962 (Smith, 2002).

Positive emotions appear to have a "broadening" effect (Frederickson, 1998, 2001), which is to produce flexible, creative, and open-minded thinking (Frederickson & Branigan, 2001; Frederickson, Tugade, Waugh, & Larken, 2003), an outcome that may be correlated with an increase in circulating brain dopamine, which is also associated with rewarding events (Ashby, Isen, & Turken, 1999). It has been suggested that positive emotions are part of resilient individuals' reactions to adversity (Bonanno, Papa, & O'Neill, 2002; Keltner & Bonanno, 1997). Positive emotions can help reduce distress both by distracting from and undoing the effects of negative emotions (Frederickson & Levinson, 1998; Keltner & Bonanno, 1997). Importantly, positive emotions may work by increasing contact with a social support network. To the extent that groups or communities lose loved ones and members, remedial social processes and social bonding are likely to counteract the devastating effects of loss due to violence. An interesting possibility is that the human tendency to seek out and engage in social behaviors that are elicited and exacerbated by the threat of an attack is sufficient not only to help people to cope with that immediate challenge but serves a broader healing function as well (Curran, 1988). The supportive role of others has been shown to buffer cardiovascular reactivity to psychological stress (Uchino, Cacioppo, & Kielcolt-Glaser, 1996).

Social psychologists have discovered a peculiar human tendency to recover better and faster to major trauma than to minor trauma. This pattern may be part of what Gilbert, Lieberman, Morewedge, and Wilson (2003) call the *region-beta paradox*, where the time to recovery from a minor insult is longer than the time to recovery from a major one. The notion is that, in the instance of a major assault, psychological attenuation processes are more likely to come into play (cf. Aronson & Mills, 1958; Zimbardo, 1966). Wilson and Cairns (1992) reported that residents of Enniskillen, Northern Ireland, where a bomb killed 11 people and injured 60 others, exhibited more active and fewer passive coping behaviors than residents of communities less under attack. Rather than engaging in denial or distancing mechanisms, the residents of Enniskillen accurately recalled the violent event and actively sought social support, often via church attendance and religiosity. Similarly, among Americans who knew someone hurt or killed in the 9/11 attacks, the high levels of stress reported immediately after the attacks had returned to normal within less than a year, and those who knew someone hurt or killed in the attacks had some of the highest levels of recovery of any subgroup, reporting nearly three fewer symptoms (Rasinski et al., 2002).

Adaptation: Compensatory Responses and Affective Reappraisal

An event is stressful to the extent that it is appraised as taxing or exceeding one's resources and endangering one's well-being (Lazarus & Folkman, 1986). What appears to matter most is what we expect about the world. These expectations shape our perceptions, and our perceptions shape our emotional, cognitive, and physiological reactions to stressful events. Wilson and Cairns (1992) found that residents of Northern Ireland who were living in towns with a greater incidence of civil violence were more likely to exhibit psychological disorders only if they perceived a high level of violence; those who perceived little or no violence exhibited no more psychological distress than did residents of towns with a lower incidence of civil violence.

In the instance of both the Japanese attack on Pearl Harbor on December 7, 1941, and the attacks on New York and Washington on September 11, 2001, the events were unanticipated by the American public. The immediate response to 9/11 was comparable to or greater than that to Pearl Harbor in terms of surprise and dismay (CBS news poll, September 12, 2001; NBC News/Wall Street Journal poll, September 12, 2001). In one national poll, more than 85% thought that the attacks on 9/11 comprised "the most tragic news" in their lifetime (CNN/USA Today/Gallup poll, September 11, 2001). Moreover, although the attackers targeted Washington, DC, and New York City, the events were viewed as attacks on the nation at large, and people across the country reported intense emotional responses. Decreased heart rate variability—a characteristic associated with increased cardiovascular and sudden death in patients with and without heart disease—was reported for the week following 9/11 among 12 patients in the Yale New Haven Hospital, located some 90 miles northeast of New York City (Lampert, Baron, Craig, McPherson & Lee, 2002). Because the more unexpected an event, the greater the emotion it provokes (Kamin, 1968; Ortony, 1988), the robust emotional responses to the attacks on 9/11 were in many respects predictable.

Once an unexpected event occurs and people have an intense emotional response to it, they are able and likely to make sense of the event quickly, even without realizing that they are doing so (Heider, 1958; Piaget, 1952). Post hoc analysis of an event makes it understandable, and to the extent that this is so, people will think less about it, and the intensity of the emotional response is likely to decrease (Wilson & Gilbert, 2003). Within 1–2 days, Americans went from thinking such an attack would not happen on domestic soil to expecting another assault. On September 13, 2001, a Time/CNN Poll found that 64% of their national sample had thought that an attack as serious as those that had occurred would never happen; an NBC News/Wall Street Journal poll at the same time found that 66% of respondents thought that another attack in Washington and New York was likely. A Gallup poll on September 11, 2001, found that the assaults were interpreted as "an act of war" by 86% of their sample, and 78% identified Osama bin Laden as "very likely" to have been personally involved in the violence; another poll 2 days later showed that 83% of the sample blamed bin Laden (Pew research survey, September 13–17, 2001), and a majority interpreted the attacks as a result of U.S. foreign policy in the Middle East (Pew, 2001).

One might wonder why Americans were so surprised. Terrorism was not new to the United States. However, previous attacks could be described as not only distant but also increasing gradually in intensity, allowing for habituation and adaptive processes to mute reactions. Until the 1960s, international terrorism focused on individuals and occurred primarily via assassination; random attacks and the killing of innocent bystanders began in the late 1960s. Hostage taking and airplane hijacking began in the early 1970s, and embassy attacks began in the late 1970s. Casualties began to number in the hundreds by the 1980s, with car bombs among military personnel and civilians and the downing—rather than hijacking—of airplanes. In the United States, the first successful attack by international terrorists was the 1993 bombing of the World Trade Center, which killed 6 (and wounded more than 1,000). The 1995 bombing of the Murrah Building in Oklahoma City, which killed 167, was not characterized as an attack by an organized, international terrorist network but as the behavior of one or two individuals, which probably marginalized its significance as a threat for most Americans (Hoffman, 1998; Stern, 1999). In some respects, this pattern of gradual increases in the ferocity of the attacks, with a concomitant rise in the number of deaths, made it highly likely that the next terrorist assault would go largely unnoticed by the American and perhaps the Western European public, unless the perception of the attacks was that they were significantly beyond accommodation ranges.

Adaptation: Compensatory Responses and Cognitive Reappraisal

Stressful life events are more likely to cause long-term difficulties if they shatter a person's view of the world (Davis & Nolen-Hoeksema, 2001; Parkes, 1971). Religion is known to foster recovery during bereavement, perhaps by affording a way of understanding how the loss is consistent within a larger, stable belief system and by providing social support from a religious community (McIntosh, Cohen Silver, & Wortman, 1993; Stroebe & Stroebe, 1993). Finding meaning and an acceptable worldview is a core component of the grieving process (Davis & Nolen-Hoeksema, 2001; Parkes, 1971). People under stress often exhibit more religious behaviors than they do when not under stress: The Centers for Disease Control's ongoing Behavioral Risk Factor Surveillance System found that about 50% of the residents of Connecticut, New Jersey, and New York had participated in religious or community memorial services within 1–2 months after 9/11, and more than 10% had attended a funeral or memorial service for an acquaintance, relative, or community member (Morbidity and Mortality Weekly Report, 2002). A nationwide survey found that 90% of Americans had religious thoughts or engaged in religions actions and that 60% had participated in memorial or commemorative group activities (Schuster et al., 2001).

Coping With Instances of Repeated Attacks

An early anecdotal report of civilian behavior during the air raids in England recalled that reactions to the air raids seemed to be a function of how much experience the populace had with them: Early in the war, "the mere sounding of sirens was enough to send large numbers to shelters. ... Their gruesome wail readily frightened people, and, at nights, the noises of automobile or tramcar gears were continually mistaken for warnings. Before the end of 1940, Londoners were general taking no notice of sirens at all ... unless accompanied by the noise of planes, gunfire, or bombs. ... In some areas [it] is a social faux pas to mention the fact that they have sounded. They provoke irritation and boredom."

Vernon (1941, p. 459)

State and local responders in Israel, where suicide bombers have killed more than 300 Israelis and injured more than 3900 others since the 2000 start of the al-Aqsa intifada, have developed an impact-mitigation strategy by removing as much evidence of the attack as quickly as possible. After immediate medical aid, teams come to pick up body parts and wash off blood from the streets and buildings where a blast occurred, and structural damage to those streets and buildings is repaired as quickly as possible.

Hoffman (2004)

Habituation and Sensitization

In the past 10 years, more than 210,000 Americans have been the victims of criminal murder, more than 300,000 people have taken their own lives in suicide, 420,000 people have been killed in car accidents, 5,400,000 have died of cancer, and nearly 7,500,000 have died as a result of heart disease (Anderson, 2001; Fox & Zawitz, 2001). In the same 10 years, some 3,300 Americans have lost their lives as a result of terrorism. Relatively few Americans know someone who was directly affected by a terrorist attack, whereas many of us know people who have died as a result of murder, suicide, car accidents, cancer, or heart disease. We might consider that part of what makes terrorism so frightening is that it is unfamiliar.

More than 30 years of violence in Northern Ireland have offered an opportunity to study the effects of long-term exposure to civil violence and terrorist attacks. The violence, which began in the late 1960s, peaked in 1972 with more than 10,500 shooting incidents in that year alone (Curran, 1988). Records from more than 1,500 bomb victims seen in emergency departments between 1969 and 1972 indicate that about 50% showed psychological disturbances. A study of civilians injured between 1979 and 1984 found more than 20% with diagnosable PSTD, primarily overarousal (startle and sleep disturbances) (Loughrey, Bell, Kee, Roddy, & Curran, 1988). These people exhibited varying symptom thresholds—the longer they were exposed to the violence, the more likely they were to exhibit the PTSD symptoms initially—but there was some apparent habituation as well because only half of the victims had emotional reactions lasting longer than 3 months (Kee, Bell, Loughrey, Roddy, & Curran, 1987; see Bleich, Dycian, Koslowsky, Solomon, & Wiener, 1992, for evidence of apparent habituation during the First Persian Gulf war [1991]). An in-depth analysis of psychiatric morbidity in Derry, which has a social deprivation among the worst in Northern Ireland as well as a 30-year history of civil conflict, found 1-month and 1-year prevalences of psychiatric disorder not different from those of a deprived inner-city section of London (McConnell, Bebbington, McClelland, Gillespie, & Houghton, 2002).

In Israel, since the 2000 start of the al-Aqsa intifada, suicide bombers have killed more than 300 people and injured more than 3,900 others. In 2002, a nationally representative sample of about 500 Israelis queried by a telephone survey after 19 months of attacks that had occurred with increasing frequency showed that about 10% exhibited symptom criteria for PTSD, 77% reported at least one traumatic stress–related symptom, and 59% reported feeling depressed (Bleich, Gelkopf, & Solomon, 2003). A significant portion of the respondents in this survey had experienced earlier traumatic attacks such as previous wars, terrorist attacks, or the Holocaust. Despite these histories and the fact that almost half of the participants in the sample had been exposed to civilian violence either personally or through a friend or family member (with 60% reporting that they felt their lives were in danger), the emotional impact appeared to be moderate. The rate of PTSD found among Israelis after 19 months of repeated attacks was lower than the rates reported for people in the immediate vicinity of the World Trade Center towers 2 months after 9/11, which might be interpreted as habituation among Israelis to the repeated attacks.

There is evidence that habituation and resilience processes might be different among children and that they need to be assessed differently. Children who are exposed to civil violence sometimes exhibit exaggerated levels of antisocial behavior, although this is complicated by the fact that the same civil violence is likely to result in other disadvantages for these children, especially as they enter adulthood, such as educational disruptions and a shortage of jobs (Cairns, 1987; Thabet, Abed, & Vostanis, 2002). High rates of PSTD were found among Kuwaiti and Kurdish children after the 1991 Gulf War, as well as among children in Croatia and Bosnia, especially if they were displaced from their homes and communities (Thabet, Abed & Vostanis, 2002; see also Freud & Burlingham, 1943, for similar observations about children who experienced the bombings of London in World War II). Thabet & Vostanis reported in 1999 that more than 40% of Palestinian children showed moderate to severe PTSD reactions, and more than 20% showed high rates of anxiety and behavioral problems, presumably as a function of the longstanding, armed intifada conflict between 1987 and 1993. These compared with an overall prevalence of 1%–15% for emotional and behavioral disorders of children in the population as a whole. As the conflict subsided, evidence of children's PTSD decreased to about 10% (a 1-year follow-up; Thabet & Vostanis, 1999), although the rate of general emotional and behavioral disorders was as high as 20%, as rated by parents.

There is some evidence of sensitization effects (heightened arousal after repeated exposure to trauma) among children who are exposed to repeated threats of violence. The more recent al-Aqsa intifada in Palestine has been characterized not only by civil violence and armed conflict but also by bombardment and home demolition. Thabet, Abed, and Vostanis (2002) found severe to very severe PSTD among children who had lost their homes. These rates were significantly higher than among children who had also lived in the Gaza Strip but had not been directly bombarded or lost their homes (although they had likely been exposed to bombardment by helicopters, mutilated bodies on TV, and media coverage of the conflict). The most frequent symptoms were difficulty concentrating, sleep disturbances, and avoidance of reminders; these children also had higher total fear scores than did the comparison children. However, a reverse trend—perhaps an instance of the region-beta paradox referred to earlier (Wilson & Gilbert, 2003)—was observed for anxiety problems: These were higher in the group not directly bombarded than in the group that was. This same trend was observed among children involved in the Bosnian conflicts (Smith, Perrin, Yule, & Rabe-Hesketh, 2001). As the authors noted, this divergence may also have occurred because the more severe PTSD masked the anxiety in the exposed children.

Adaptation: Compensatory Responses Lead to Resilience

It has been suggested that, in England during World War II, there was a "Britain can take it mood" for much of the period from 1940 to 1941, and prewar hysteria about mass casualties was replaced by a new myth of universal resilience. Investigators were unable to describe a significant increase in "neurotic disturbances," even though there was an apparent increase in functional somatic disorders (headache, fatigue, dyspepsia, joint and muscle pain, indigestion) (Jones, Woolven, Durodie, & Wessely, 2004, 2006).

A telephone survey of Israeli residents conducted in 2002, some 2 years after the beginning of the al-Aqsa intifada in Israel—and after the deaths of 318 Israeli civilians by knife or gun attacks, drive-by shootings, or suicide bombings—showed that although symptom criteria for PTSD were met by 9.4% of the sample, the majority of the participants felt optimistic about their personal future (82%) and the future of Israel (66%) (Bleich, Gelkopf, & Solomon, 2003). The construct of resilience was developed on the basis of observations of people who not only survive but also thrive in situations of extreme adversity. The notion comes from early investigations of atypical schizophrenic patients who had premorbid histories of relative competence at work, good social relations, marriage, and capacity to fulfill responsibilities (Garmezy, 1991). It was posited that such disordered patients, who had the least severe course of illness, were less dysfunctional because of these relatively resilient trajectories.

Similarly, children of schizophrenic mothers sometimes have thrived despite their high-risk status, which has led to a characterization of the children as resilient (Garmezy & Masten, 1991): It was thought that attributes of the children themselves, their families, and their wider social environments were critical to this resilience (Masten, Best, & Garmezy, 1990). (There is evidence that, for children, resilience may be inconsistent: Although some at-risk children excel at a particular point in time, they may falter subsequently [Luthar, Cecchetti, & Becker, 2000].) Notably, resilience is more than recovery: Recovery is a return

to normal functioning, which had ceased temporarily. Functioning returns to preevent levels, whereas resilience is viewed as the ability to *maintain* equilibrium (Bonanno, 2004). In addition, resilience is more than the absence of psychopathology; resilient people may show transient perturbations in functioning (for several weeks) but demonstrate a stable trajectory of healthy functioning over time and "the capacity for generative experiences and positive emotions" (Bonanno, 2004, p. 2).

On the individual level, resilience differs from optimism in that resilient people recognize the effects of stressful situations, yet still experience positive outcomes (Masten, 2001; Tugade & Frederickson, 2002). These people are likely to elicit positive emotions though humor, relaxation, and optimistic thinking. Factors related to resilience include hardiness (Kobasa, Maddi, & Kahn, 1982), which is defined as the capability of finding meaningful purpose in life, the belief that one can influence one's surroundings and the outcome of events, and the belief that one can learn from both positive and negative experiences; a kind of self-enhancement (Greenwald, 1980). Bonanno et al. (2005) found that "self-enhancing" individuals who were in or near the World Trade Center at the time of the 9/11 attacks reported better adjustment and more active social networks and were rated more positively by their friends. Physiological assessments of resilient people indicate that they experience less stress as indicated via salivary cortisol measures (Brindley & Rolland, 1989). These people apparently regulate their emotions more effectively (Lazarus, 1993; Masten, 2001; Rutter, 1987), perhaps via repressive coping (Weinberger & Davidson, 1979), which is the tendency to repress or avoid unpleasant thoughts, emotions, and memories (Weinberger & Schwartz, 1990).

Adaptation: Compensatory Responses Enable Victims to Thrive

Civil unrest and violence do not always result in a damaged populace. Sometimes just the opposite appears to occur, where such strife is accompanied by a suspension or decrease in the use and perhaps need for psychological and physical remediation. One of the outcomes of civil violence may be improved psychological health (Fogelson, 1970; Greenley, Gillespie, & Lindenthal, 1975; Mira,

1939), perhaps because of the increased social cohesion shown in response to a common threat or enemy (Durkheim, 1951). Lyons (1972) observed that, in areas closely associated with violence, male depression and suicide rates drop, whereas in areas less directly exposed, the reverse is true. In England and Wales, the number of suicides reported in the month of September 2001 was significantly lower than in other months for every September of the previous 27 years (Salib, 2003). During and after the 1975–1976 civil war in Lebanon, admissions to psychiatric hospitals decreased, and outpatient treatment fell more than what might have been expected on the basis of transportation or communication disruptions. When the hostilities ceased, outpatient treatment appeared to rebound (Nasr, Racy, & Flaherty, 1983).

Curran (1988) points to data from racial rioting in U.S. cities in 1968 and in Kuala Lumpur in 1969, as well as to earlier data from the Algerian civil war, the Spanish civil war, and World War II, as showing no increase in demand for psychiatric services and, in some cases, decreased demands for such services during the period when the violence was ongoing, with some evidence of a rebound effect after the violence had peaked. Bleich et al. (1992) reported that, during the Scud missile attacks on Israel in 1991, there was an inverse relationship between the number of physical casualties and the number of psychological stress casualties reporting to hospitals. As Curran (1988) noted, there may be multiple reasons for such outcomes, including the failures of people to report distress and seek help, the migration out of the area of those who are most distressed, the fact that people are distracted by the more immediate demands of external stressors (Ierodiakonous, 1970), or the tendency of people to engage in active denial or reappraisal (Gross, 1998).

What to Expect for the Future

Although one must carefully qualify such a statement, what we have observed for most people in instances of terrorist attacks in the United States, Northern Ireland, and Israel is the dissipation of the effects of isolated attacks and habituated and adaptive behaviors to repeated attacks. Dissipation, habituation, and adaptation are behaviors that can be predicted on the premise that behavior is, in

large part, principled. This view begs the question, what should we expect for the future?

Habituation Versus Sensitization of Emotional Reactions

We should expect, at least for the majority of people, adaptation and accommodation to living with terrorist attacks and with the threats of terrorist attacks. This has already been noted for communities in Northern Ireland, Israel, and Palestine. Similar habituation could be claimed for the public in the United States before 9/11, which was affected by terrorist attacks only incrementally until 2001.

The attacks on 9/11 killed 3,063 people. Although there were multiple sites, similar methods were used: Each involved airplanes and suicide terrorists. From what we know about habituation and adaptation, we might expect one of the following scenarios: (1) For a subsequent attack to significantly increase public perceptions of vulnerability, fear, and stress, it will likely have to be of larger perceived intensity than those that occurred on 9/11, unless a significant period of time elapses before the next attack; or (2) in the near term, repeated, similar attacks will generate less disruption due to habituation and adaptation effects. However, (3) a series of smaller attacks that vary in location, method, and target—that is, that do not entail habituation or adaptation because of the variance in the nature of the attacks, such as the bombing of shopping malls, schools, and hospitals—can be expected to be as effective (or more so) than a single, large-scale attack, even in the near term.

It may be instructive to consider the impact of the Washington, DC, sniper attacks in 2002 in view of this notion that Americans might "habituate to terrorist attacks." Few systematic data are yet available about the impacts of these incidents (although studies are in progress). Public perception is that, rather than exhibit habituation or adaptation as a function of the previous exposure to the attacks on the Pentagon on 9/11 and the anthrax events the following fall, residents in the greater Washington metropolitan area showed a sensitization effect: They exhibited hypervigilance, that is, behavior that could be described as inappropriate given the statistically low level of being a victim, which actually put people in positions of greater likelihood of injury from other sources. (Examples of such behavior were driving long distances in order to avoid neighborhood gas stations or shopping malls, keeping school children indoors during recess and after school, and canceling sporting events in numerous schools for many weeks.)

One way to understand this pattern of behavior is to grasp the fact that habituation is context and event specific and occurs with repeated exposure to a traumatic event under otherwise stable conditions; thus the event can be anticipated on the basis of the context in which it occurs. Habituation does not generalize to different contexts or to a substantial change in the nature of the fearful event. When events change over time—such as planes smashing into buildings, then anthrax being sent in the mail, and finally, snipers cropping up at shopping malls—the outcome is the opposite of habituation or sensitization—the increase, rather than decrease, in anxiety or fear as a function of repeated exposure to fearful events. This leads to the expectation that, should the public be exposed to a series of different types of attacks (the third scenario just listed), sensitization may exaggerate the effects of any one of the attacks, even though any one as a single instance would have had a small effect.

Cognitive and Affective Reappraisal

The American public has been encouraged to believe that it is vulnerable to future terrorist attacks. Affective and cognitive reappraisals can be expected to occur in the context of such expectations because we try to make sense of the world around us. It is likely that this psychological preparation will depend, to some extent, on our assessment of the likelihood of such an assault. When people expect an event to occur in a future over which they perceive themselves as having little or no control, they tend to engage in anticipatory reconstrual, that is, they get a head start on interpreting its meaning. Wilson and his colleagues found that, when events that had either positive or negative connotations were probable but not certain, people engaged in little anticipatory reconstrual (e.g., Wilson, Wheatley, Kurtz, Dunn, & Gilbert, 2004). Instead, they adopted a "wait and see" strategy, postponing their interpretation of the meaning of an event until after it occurred. However, when events were perceived as highly likely or even certain, people engaged in more anticipatory reconstrual, making sense of the event ahead of time. To the extent, then, that a population perceives a terrorist attack to be an inevitable part of its future, it is more likely to adjust its understanding of an attack ahead of time on the basis of its current knowledge and understanding of such an event. These views and attitudes are likely to be difficult to change, even in the face of additional information or contradictory evidence.

On the basis of what is known about affective forecasting—our abilities to predict how we will feel about an event that will happen in the future—we can surmise that we expect we will be more distressed about future attacks than we actually will be (e.g., Read & Loewenstein, 1995). We will also misconstrue and misremember important aspects of the event in hindsight (e.g., Kaplan, 1978), especially the intensity and frequency of our emotions about it (Christianson & Safer, 1996). Further, our initial understanding of an attack will largely determine our long-term understanding of it, even when provided with subsequent information to correct for errors (Tversky & Kahneman, 1974). In short, we will work hard to transform the meanings of the attacks so as to mitigate their negative impacts, all the while remaining curiously unaware of this tendency (Loewenstein & Adler, 1995). This kind of "misforecasting," while probably resulting in more positive emotions than would otherwise accrue, will nonetheless make people vulnerable to decision errors because people act in accordance with how they expect to feel about that action. To the extent that our affective forecasting is inaccurate, these decisions will be unsound.

Preparation Strategies

How might we take advantage of these guesses about the future to inform response and recovery preparations? There are several implications, all of which are extrapolations from assumptions about basic mechanisms but need empirical validation. We offer them here as food for thought. First, a preparedness strategy that focuses on fear is likely to produce either habituation to alerts and threats or adaptation and a chronic state of anxiety that depletes individual and community resources. A strategy that highlights our strengths and capacity for recovery would not only save resources but may even help create them (Durodie, 2002, 2004). Public participation in dealing with community disasters has repeatedly been shown to bolster public morale and ameliorate psychological stress—from the bombings in London during World War II (Jones et al., in press) to the modern-day Israeli/Palestinian conflict (Bleich et al., 2003).

Second, if we try to "expect the unexpected" and then incorporate the unexpected within the context of normal as much as possible, we will react less vigorously to a novel attack event. Our expectations are based on what we have experienced and already know, and we are most likely to be disrupted by what we do not expect. It is likely that Americans expect future attacks, should they occur, to involve airlines, large buildings, suicide terrorists, and New York or Washington. These expectations are probably encouraged by the most obvious change—greatly enhanced airport security. There is remarkably little national dialogue about alternatives to that scenario. A national discussion of alternative attacks would not only allow for realistic and detailed descriptions of what might happen but also engage the public so that the views and practices of communities and their possible responses could inform response and recovery strategies (cf. Lasker, 2004), as well as education and preparedness strategies (Vineburgh, 2004). To the extent that Americans begin to view terrorist attacks in other countries as occurring, in some sense, also to ourselves, our expectations should begin to change so that even the unimaginable, such as a school bombing, is perceived as "experienced," if only vicariously. One might argue that such anticipatory preparation is appropriate to the fact that the current threats come from loosely organized, international networks of terrorists, which are likely to employ a variety of methods against a variety of targets (Burke, 2003).

Such a discussion would also engage some degree of adaptation to the fear responses that might be provoked; obviously, such dialogue would be of most benefit if it were conducted in the context of understanding what people fear, what they would be likely to do in such scenarios, and how we might adapt risk communications and recovery strategies to those behaviors (Fischhoff, 2002; Fischhoff, Gonzales, Small, & Lerner, 2003). This sort of discussion might also help to put particularly unexpected scenarios into a more familiar context, which would lessen anxiety and increase response capacity. For example, chemical toxins could be described within the context of advice about which protective and palliative behaviors are likely to be useful. If the similarity between the chemical weapons of terrorists and the chemicals that sit under our own kitchen sinks is pointed out, we might take advantage of the habituated emotional response we have already learned to paint thinners and drain cleaners and of the knowledge we already have about what to do when exposed to harm from such agents.

Finally, we reflect, talk, and listen so that we can understand the world around us, especially when feeling threatened or experiencing loss. Might anxiety be alleviated, strengths encouraged, and wisdom engendered to the extent that the nation engages in learning about the people and ideas that motivate the terrorists that attack us (Ilardi, 2004; McNamara & Blight, 2003)? This, too, is an empirical issue worth pursuing (Fischhoff, personal communication, June 29, 2004).

Conclusion

The quote at the beginning of this chapter reflects a common belief that Americans and other victims of terrorism remain vulnerable to the trauma that terrorist attacks evoke. It implies that fear and anxiety, once aroused, do not dissipate, adapt, or habituate. But humans, like all animal organisms, have evolved to deal with changing environments, especially those that threaten us. Perhaps what we know about how we respond can be used to protect us.

Notes

1. This graph is from a real-time, computational theory of conditioning that describes the modulation of learned and unlearned behaviors by fear (Wagner & Brandon, 1989; Brandon & Wagner, 1998). This theory assumes that the nature and strength of responses to discrete events are predictable, based on the learning history of the responding organism and the nature of the eliciting event. Most of the data upon which this theory is based come from reduced or simple learning preparations with nonhuman animals. However, the theoretical processes are known to map onto many aspects of the biological systems that the

theory embraces and may well be ubiquitous to the fundamental processes of learning and emotion in all vertebrate systems. The SOP model is used here, however, because it offers a straightforward, albeit theoretical, picture of these fundamental processes, which we believe can be used to describe the behaviors of humans in both mundane and extraordinary circumstances.

2. As noted by Wessely (in press), the implications of such findings are that, given that communication is a vital coping mechanism, ensuring that cell phone systems are maintained after a terrorist attack is important not only to emergency responders but to the public as well and will serve to significantly mitigate the impacts of an attack.

References

9/11 Commission report: Final report of the National Commission on Terrorist Attacks Upon the United States. (2004). New York: Norton.

American Psychiatric Association. (1987). *Diagnostic and statistical manual of mental disorders IV* (3d ed.). Washington, DC: Author.

Anderson, R. (2001). Deaths: Leading causes for 1999. *National Vital Statistics Reports 49*(1). Hyattsville, MD: Department of Health and Human Services, National Center for Health Statistics, Leading Causes of Death, 1900–1998. Retrieved January 16, 2006, from http://www.cdc.gov/nchs/data/lead1900_98.pdf

Antonovsky, A. (1985). The life cycle, mental health, and the sense of coherence. *Israel Journal of Psychiatry and Related Sciences, 22*(4), 273–280.

Aronson, E., & Mills, J. (1958). The effect of severity of initiation on liking for a group. *Journal of Abnormal and Social Psychology, 59,* 177–181.

Ashby, F. G., Isen, A. M., & Turken, U. (1999). A neuropsychological theory of positive affect and its influence on cognition. *Psychological Review, 106*(3), 529–550.

Barefoot, J. C., Brummett, B. H., Helms, M. J., Mark, D. B., Siegler, I. C., & Williams, R. B. (2000). Depressive symptoms and survival of patients with coronary artery disease. *Psychosomatic Medicine, 62*(6), 790–795.

Blascovich, J., & Katkin, E. S. (1993). *Cardiovascular reactivity to psychological stress and disease.* Washington, DC: American Psychological Association.

Blascovich, J., & Tomaka, J. (1996). The biopsychosocial model of arousal regulation. *Journal of Experimental Social Psychology, 28,* 1–51.

Bleich, A., Dycian, A., Koslowsky, M., Solomon, A., & Wiener, M. (1992). Psychiatric implications of missile attacks on a civilian population. *Journal of the American Medical Association, 268,* 613–615.

Bleich, A., Gelkopf, M., & Solomon, A. (2003). Exposure to terrorism, stress-related mental health symptoms, and coping behaviors among a nationally representative sample in Israel. *Journal of the American Medical Association, 290,* 612–619.

Bonanno, G. A. (2004). Loss, trauma, and human resilience: Have we underestimated our capacity to thrive after extremely aversive events? *American Psychologist, 59*(1), 20–28.

———, Rennicke,, C., & Dekel, S. (2005). Self-enhancement among high-exposure survivors of the September 11th terrorist attack: Resilience of social maladjustment? *Personality Processes and Individual Differences, 88,* 984–998.

Borszcz, G. S., Cranney, J., & Leaton, R. N. (1989). Influence of long-term sensitization on long-term habituation of the acoustic startle response in rats: Central gray lesions, preexposure, and extinction. *Journal of Experimental Psychology: Animal Behavior Processes, 15,* 54–64.

Brandon, S. E., & Wagner, A. R. (1998). Occasion setting: Influences of conditioned emotional responses and configural cues. In N. Schmajuk & P. Holland (Eds.), *Occasion setting: Associative learning and cognition in animals* (pp. 343–382). Washington, DC: American Psychological Association.

Breslau, N., Davis, G. C., Andreski, P., & Peterson, E. (1991). Traumatic events and posttraumatic stress disorder in an urban population of young adults. *Archives of General Psychiatry, 48*(3), 216–222.

Brindley, D., & Rolland, Y. (1989). Possible connections between stress, diabetes, obesity, hypertension, and altered lipoprotein metabolism that may result in atherosclerosis. *Clinical Science, 77,* 453–461.

Burke, J. (2003). *Al-Qaeda: Casting a shadow of terror.* New York: I. B. Taurus.

Cacioppo, J. T., Gardner, W. L., Berntson, G. G., Rogers, R. D., Owen, A. M., Middleton, H. S., et al. (2002). Social applications: Motivation and emotion. In J. T. Cacioppo & G. G. Berntson (Eds.), *Foundations in social neuroscience* (pp. 493–572). Social Neuroscience Series. Cambridge, MA: MIT Press.

Cairns, E. (1987). *Caught in crossfire: Children and the Northern Ireland conflict.* New York: Syracuse University Press.

———, & Wilson, R. (1991). Northern Ireland: Political violence and self-reported physical symptoms in a community sample. *Journal of Psychosomatic Research, 35*(6), 707–711.

Christianson, S. A., & Safer, M. A. (1996). Emotional events and emotions in autobiographical memory. In D. Rubin (Ed.), *Remembering our past: Studies in autobiographical memory* (pp. 218–243). New York: Cambridge University Press.

Cohen, S., & Willis, T. A. (1985). Stress, social support, and the buffering hypothesis. *Psychological Bulletin, 98,* 310–357.

Connolly, J. F., & Firth, C. D. (1978). Effects of a varying stimulus context on habituation and sensitization of the OR. *Physiology and Behavior, 21,* 511–514.

Cullison, A. (2004, September). Inside al-Qaeda's hard drive. *Atlantic Monthly,* 55–70.

Curran, P. S. (1988). Psychiatric aspects of terrorist violence: Northern Ireland 1969–1987. *British Journal of Psychiatry, 153,* 470–475.

Danner, D. D., Snowdon, D. A., & Friesen, W. V. (2001). Positive emotions in early life and longevity: Findings from the nun study. *Journal of Social and Personality Psychology, 80,* 804–813.

Davis, C. G., & Nolen–Hoeksema, S. (2001). Loss and meaning: How do people make sense of loss? *American Behavioral Scientist, 44,* 736–741.

Davis, M. (1972). Differential retention of sensitization and habituation of the startle response in the rat. *Journal of Comparative and Physiological Psychology, 78,* 260–267.

Durkheim, E. (1951). *Suicide: A study in sociology* (J. A. Spaulding & G. Simpson, Trans.). Glencoe, IL: Free Press of Glencoe.

Durodie, B. (2002). Perception and threat: Why vulnerability-led responses will fail. *Security Monitor, 1,* 16–18.

———. (2004). Facing the possibility of bioterrorism. *Current Opinion in Biotechnology, 15,* 1–5.

Dwyer, J. (2001, September 16). Donated goods deluge the city and sit unused. *New York Times,* p. 1.

Felton, C. J. (2002). Project Liberty: A public health response to New Yorkers' mental health needs arising from the World Trade Center terrorist attacks. *Journal of Urban Health: Bulletin of New York Academy of Medicine, 79,* 429–433.

Fischhoff, B. (2002). Assessing and communicating the risks of terrorism. In T. Nelson & L. Washington (Eds.), *Science and technology in a vulnerable world* (pp. 51–64). Washington, DC: American Association for the Advancement of Science.

———, Gonzales, R., Small, D., & Lerner, J. (2003). Evaluating the success of terror risk communications. *Biosecurity Bioterrorism, 1,* 255–258.

Fogelson, R. M. (1970). Violence and grievances: Reflections on the 1960s' riots. *Journal of Social Issues, 26,* 141–163.

Fox, J., & Zawitz, M. (2001). Homicide trends in the United States. Retrieved January 16, 2006, from http://www.ojp.usdoj.gov/bjs/homicide/homtrnd.htm

Frederickson, B. L. (1998). What good are positive emotions? *Review of General Psychology, 2,* 300–319.

———. (2001). The role of positive emotions in positive psychology. *American Psychologist, 56,* 218–236.

———. (2003). The value of positive emotions. *American Scientist, 91,* 330–335.

———, & Branigan, C. (2001). Positive emotions. In T. J. Mayne & G. A. Bonanno (Eds.), *Emotions: Current issues and future directions* (pp. 123–151). New York: Guilford.

Frederickson, B. L., & Levinson, R. W. (1998). Positive emotions speed recovery from the cardiovascular sequelae of negative emotions. *Cognition and Emotion, 12,* 191–220.

Frederickson, B. L., Tugade, M. M., Waugh, C. E., & Larkin, G. R. (2003). What good are positive emotions in crises? *Journal of Personality and Social Psychology, 84,* 365–376.

Freud, A., & Burlingham, D. (1943). *War and children.* New York: Medical War Books.

Galea, S., Ahern, J., Resnick, H., Kilpatrick, D., Bucuvalas, M., Gold, J., et al. (2002). Psychological sequelae of the September 11 terrorist attacks in New York City. *New England Journal of Medicine, 346,* 982–987.

Galea, S., Ahern, J., Resnick, H., & Vlahov, D. (in press). Post-traumatic stress symptoms in the general population after a disaster: Implications for public health. In N. Y. Gross, R. Gross, R. Marshall, & E. Susser (Eds.), *Mental health in the wake of a terrorist attack.* New York: Cambridge University Press.

Galea, S., Vlahov, D., Resnick, H., Ahern, J., Susser, E., Gold, J., et al. (2003). Trends of probable post-traumatic stress disorder in New York City after the September 11 terrorist attacks. *American Journal of Epidemiology, 158,* 514–524.

Garmezy, N. (1991). Resiliency and vulnerability to adverse developmental outcomes associated with poverty. *American Behavioral Scientist, 34,* 416–430.

———, & Masten, A. S. (1991). The protective role of competence indicators in children at risk. In E. M. Cummings & A. L. Greene (Eds.), *Life-span developmental psychology: Perspectives on stress and coping* (pp. 151–174). Hillsdale, NJ: Erlbaum.

Gilbert, D. T., Lieberman, M. D., Morewedge, C. K., & Wilson, T. D. (2003). The peculiar longevity of things not so bad. *Psychological Science, 15,* 14–19.

Glanz, J. (2002, June 2). The haunting final words: "It doesn't look good, babe." *New York Times*, p. 1.

Greenley, J. R., Gillespie, D. P., & Lindenthal, J. J. (1975). A race riot's effects on psychological symptoms. *Archives of General Psychiatry, 32,* 1189–1195.

Greenwald, A. G. (1980). The totalitarian ego: Fabrication and revision of personal history. *American Psychologist, 35,* 603–618.

Gross, J. J. (1998). Antecedent- and response-focused emotion regulation: Divergent consequences for experience, expression, and physiology. *Journal of Personality and Social Psychology, 74,* 224–237.

Hammond, L. J. (1967). Human GSR pseudoconditioning as a function of change in basal skin resistance and CS-US similarity. *Journal of Experimental Psychology, 73*(1), 125–129.

Heider, F. (1958). *The psychology of interpersonal relations.* New York: Wiley.

Herbert, T. B., & Cohen, S. (1993). Depression and immunity: A meta-analytic review. *Psychological Bulletin, 113,* 472–486.

Hoffman, B. (1998). *Inside terrorism.* New York: Columbia University Press.

———. (2004, Vol. 293(1), January/February). Aftermath. *Atlantic Monthly* online. Retrieved March 15, 2006, from http://www.theatlantic.com/doc/200401/hoffman.

Ierodiakonous, C. S. (1970). The effect of a threat of war on neurotic patients in psychotherapy. *American Journal of Psychotherapy, 24,* 643–651.

Ilardi, G. J. (2004). Redefining the issues: The future of terrorism research and the search for empathy. In A. Silke (Ed.), Research on terrorism: Trends, achievements, and failures (pp.214–228). London: Frank Cass.

Izard, C. E. (1992). Basic emotions, relations among emotions, and emotion-cognition relations. *Psychological Review, 99,* 561–565.

———. (1993). Four systems for emotion activation: Cognitive and noncognitive processes. *Psychological Review, 100*(1), 68–90.

Jones, E., Woolven, R., Durodie, W., & Wessely, S. (2004). Civilian morale during the Second World War: Responses to air raids re-examined. *Social History of Medicine, 17,* 463–479.

Jones, E., Woolven, R., Durodie, W., & Wessely, S. (2006). Public panic and morale: Second World War civilian responses re-examined in the light of the current anti-terrorist campaign. *Journal of Risk Research, 9,* 57–73.

Kamin, L. (1968). Attention-like processes in classical conditioning. In M. R. Jones (Ed.), *Miami symposium on the prediction of behavior: Aversive stimulation* (pp. 9–32). Coral Gables: University of Florida Press.

Kaplan, H. R. (1978). *Lottery winners: How they won and how winning changed their lives.* New York: Harper and Row.

Kee, M., Bell, P., Loughrey, G. C., Roddy, R. J., & Curran, P. S. (1987). Victims of violence: A demographic and clinical study. *Medicine, Science, and the Law, 27,* 241–247.

Keltner, D., & Bonanno, G. A. (1997). A study of laughter and dissociation: Distinct correlates of laughter and smiling during bereavement. *Journal of Personality and Social Psychology, 73*(4), 687–702.

Kessler, R. C., Sonnega, A., Bromet, E., & Hughes, M. (1995). Posttraumatic stress disorder in the National Comorbidity Survey. *Archives of General Psychiatry, 52*(12), 1048–1060.

Kiecolt-Glaser, J. K., Glaser, R., Gravenstein, S., Malarkey, W. B., & Sheridan, J. (1996). Chronic stress alters the immune response to influenza virus vaccine in older adults. *Proceedings of the National Academy of Sciences USA, 93,* 3043–3047.

Kobasa, S. C., Maddi, S. R., & Kahn, S. (1982). Hardiness and health: A prospective study. *Journal of Personality and Social Psychology, 42,* 168–177.

Lampert, R., Baron, S. J., Craig A., McPherson, C. A., &. Lee, F. A. (2002). Heart rate variability during the week of September 11, 2001. *Journal of the American Medical Association, 288,* p. 575.

Lasker, R. (2004). *Redefining readiness: Terrorism planning through the eyes of the public.* New York: New York Academy of Medicine, Center for the Advancement of Collaborative Strategies in Health.

Lazarus, R. S. (1993). Coping theory and research: Past, present, and future. *Psychosomatic Medicine, 55*(3), 234–247.

———, & Folkman, S. (1986). Cognitive theories of stress and the issue of circularity. In M. H. Appley & R. Trumbull (Eds.), *Dynamics of stress: Physiological, psychological, and social perspectives* (pp. 63–80). Plenum Series on Stress and Coping. New York: Plenum.

———, Kanner, A. D., & Folkman, S. (1980). Emotions: A cognitive-phenomenological analysis. In R. Plutchik & H. Kellerman (Eds.), *Theories of emotion* (pp. 189–217). New York: Academic Press.

Leserman, J., Jackson, E. D., Petitto, J. M., Golden, R. N., Silva, S. G., Perkins, D. O., et al. (1999). Progression to AIDS: The effects of stress, depressive symptoms, and social support. *Psychosomatic Medicine, 61*(3), 397–406.

Loewenstein, G., & Adler, D. (1995). A bias in the prediction of tastes. *Economic Journal, 105,* 929–937.

Loughrey, G. C., Bell, P., Kee, M., Roddy, R. J., and Curran, P. S. (1988). Post-traumatic stress disorder and civil violence in Northern Ireland. *British Journal of Psychiatry, 153,* 554–560.

Luthar, S. S., Cecchetti, D., & Becker, B. (2000). The construct of resilience: A critical evaluation and guidelines for future work. *Child Development, 71,* 543–562.

Lyons, H. A. (1972). Depressive illness and aggression in Belfast. *British Medical Journal, 1,* 342–345.

Masten, A. S. (2001). Ordinary magic: Resilience processes in development. *American Psychologist, 56,* 227–238.

———, Best, K., & Garmezy, N. (1990). Resilience and development: Contributions from the study of children who overcome adversity. *Development and Psychopathology, 2,* 425–444.

McConnell, P., Bebbington, P., McClelland, R., Gillespie, K., & Houghton, S. (2002). Prevalence of psychiatric disorder and the need for psychiatric care in Northern Ireland. *British Journal of Psychiatry, 181,* 214–219.

McEwen, B. S. (1998, May 1). Stress, adaptation, and disease: Allostasis and allostatic load. In S. M. McCann, E. M. Sternberg, J. M. Lipton, et al. (Eds.), *Neuroimmunomodulation: Molecular aspects, integrative systems, and clinical advances (Annals of the New York Academy of Sciences, Vol. 840* (pp. 33–44). New York: New York Academy of Sciences.

———, & Mendelson, S. (1993). Effects of stress on the neurochemistry and morphology of the brain: Counterregulation versus damage. In L. Goldberger & S. Breznitz (Eds.), *Handbook of stress: Theoretical and clinical aspects* (2d ed.) (pp. 101–126). New York: Maxwell Macmillan International.

McFarlane, A. C. (1986). Posttraumatic morbidity of a disaster: A study of cases presenting for psychiatric treatment. *Journal of Nervous Mental Disorders, 147,* 4–13.

McIntosh, D. N., Cohen Silver, R., & Wortman, C. B. (1993, October). Religion's role in adjustment to a negative life event: Coping with the loss of a child. *Journal of Personality and Social Psychology, 65(4),* 812–821.

McNamara, R. S., & Blight, J. G. (2003). *Wilson's ghost: Reducing the risk of conflict, killing, and catastrophe in the 21st century.* New York: Perseus Books.

Mehl, M. R., & Pennebaker, J. W. (2003). The social dynamics of a cultural upheaval: Social interactions surrounding September 11, 2001. *Psychological Science, 14,* 579–585.

Mira, E. (1939). Psychological work during the Spanish War. *Occupational Psychology 13,* 166–177.

Morbidity and Mortality Weekly Report (MMWR). (2002, September 6). Psychological and emotional effects of the September 11 attacks on the World Trade Center: Connecticut, New Jersey, and New York, 2001. *CDC Weekly, 51(35),* 784–786.

Nasr, S., Racy, J., & Flaherty, J. S. (1983). Psychiatric effects of the civil war in Lebanon. *Psychiatric Journal of the University of Ottawa, 8,* 208–232.

National Center for Health Statistics. (2003). Accessed January 16, 2006, http://www.cdc.gov/nchs/icd9.htm

National Institute of Mental Health (2004). Facts about posttraumatic stress disorder. Retrieved January 16, 2006, from http://www.nimh.nih.gov/publicat/ptsdfacts.cfm

Norris, F. H. (1992). Epidemiology of trauma: Frequency and impact of different potentially traumatic events on different demographic groups. *Journal of Consulting and Clinical Psychology, 60(3),* 409–418.

Norris, F. H., Byrne, C. M., Díaz, E., & Kaniasty, K. (2001a). Psychosocial resources in the aftermath of natural and human-caused disasters: A review of the empirical literature, with implications for intervention. Online at http://www.ncptsd.org/facts/disasters/fs_resources.html

———. (2001b). Risk factors for adverse outcomes in natural and human-caused disasters: A review of the empirical literature. Retrieved February 7, 2006, from http://www.ncptsd.org/facts/disasters/fs_riskfactors.html

Norris, F. H., Watson, P. J., Hamblen, J. L., & Pfefferbaum, B. J. (2003). Provider perspectives on disaster mental health services in Oklahoma City. In Y. Danieli, D. Brom, & J. B. Sills (Eds.), *The trauma of terror: Sharing knowledge and shared care* (pp. 649–662). Binghamton, NY: Haworth.

North, C. S., Nixon, S. J., Shariat, W., Mallonee, S., McMillen, J. C., Spitznagel, E. L., et al. (1999). Psychiatric disorders among survivors of the Oklahoma City bombing. *Journal of the American Medical Association, 282,* 755–762.

North, C. S., Tivis, L., McMillen, J. C., Pfefferbaum, B., Cox, J., Spitznagel, E. L., et al. (2002). Coping, functioning, and adjustment of rescue workers after the Oklahoma City bombing. *Journal of Traumatic Stress, 15,* 171–175.

O'Leary, A. (1990). Stress, emotion, and human immune function. *Psychological Bulletin, 108,* 363–382.

Ortony, A. (1988). Subjective importance and computational models of emotion. In V. Hamilton, G. H. Bower, & N. H. Frijda (Eds.), *Cognitive perspectives on emotion and motivation* (pp. 321–333). NATO ASI series D. Boston: Kluwer.

Osterholm, M. T. (2001, November). Framing the debate: Applying the lessons learned. Biological threats and terrorism: Assessing the science and response capabilities. Based on a workshop of the Institute of Medicine. Washington, DC: National Academy Press.

Ozer, E. J., & Weiss, D. S. (2004). Who develops posttraumatic stress disorder? *Current Directions in Psychological Science, 13,* 169–172.

Parkes, C. M. (1971). Psycho-social transitions: A field for study. *Social Science and Medicine, 3,* 101–115.

Pfefferbaum, B., Nixon, S. J., Krug, R. S., Tivis, R. D., Moore, V. L., Brown, et al. (1999). Clinical Needs Assessment of Middle and High School Students Following the 1995 Oklahoma City Bombing. *Am J Psychiatry, 156,* 1069–1074.

Piaget, J. (1952). *The origins of intelligence in children.* New York: International Universities Press.

Pyszczynski, T. A., Solomon, S., & Greenberg, J. (2002). Black Tuesday: The psychological impact of 9/11. In T. Pyszczynski, S. Solomon, et al. (Eds.), *In the wake of 9/11: The psychology of terror* (pp. 93–113). Washington, DC: American Psychological Association.

Rasinski, K. A., Berktold, J., Smith, T. W., & Albertson, B. L. (2002). America recovers: A follow-up to a national study of public responses to the September 11 terrorist attacks. Report by the National Opinion Research Center, University of Chicago, Chicago.

Read, D., & Loewenstein, G. (1995). Diversification bias: Explaining the discrepancy in variety seeking between combined and separated choices. *Journal of Experimental Psychology: Applied, 1*(1), 34–49.

Rosenkranz, M. A., Jackson, D. C., Dalton, K. M., Kolski, I., Ryff, C. D., Singer, B. H., et al. (2003). Affective style and in vivo immune response: Neurobehavioral mechanisms. *Proceedings of the National Academy of Sciences, 100,* 11148–11152.

Rutledge, T., Reis, S. E., Olson, M., Owens, J., Kelsey, S. F., Pepine, C. J., et al. (2003). Socioeconomic status variables predict cardiovascular disease risk factors and prospective mortality risk among women with chest pain: The WISE study. *Behavior Modification, 27*(1), 54–67.

Rutter, M. (1987). Psychosocial resilience and protective mechanisms. *American Journal of Orthopsychiatry, 57,* 316–331.

Salib, E. (2003). Effect of 11 September 2001 on suicide and homicide in England and Wales. *British Journal of Psychiatry, 183,* 207–212.

Schlenger, W. E., Caddell, J. M., Ebert, L., Jordan, K. B., Rourke, K. M., Wilson, D., et al. (2002). Psychological reactions to terrorist attacks: Findings from the National Study of Americans' Reactions to September 11. *Journal of the American Medical Association, 288,* 581–588.

Schuster, M. A., Bradley, D. S., Jaycox, L. H., Collins, R. L., Marshall, G. N., Elliott, M. N., et al. (2001). A national survey of stress reactions after the September 11, 2001, terrorist attacks. *New England Journal of Medicine, 345,* 1507–1512.

Selye, H. (1991). History and present status of the stress concept. In A. Monat & R. S. Lazarus (Eds.), *Stress and coping: An anthology* (3d ed.) (pp. 21–35). New York: Columbia University Press.

Shalev, A. Y., Peri, T., Canetti, L., & Schreiber, S. (1996). Predictors of PTSD in injured trauma survivors: A prospective study. *American Journal of Psychiatry, 153*(2), 219–225.

Silke, A. (2003). *Terrorists, victims, and society: Psychological perspectives on terrorism and its consequences.* Hoboken, NJ: Wiley.

———. (2004). *Research on terrorism: Trends, achievements, and failures.* London: Frank Cass.

Silver, R. C., Holman, E. A., McIntosh, D. N., Poulin, M., & Gil-Rivas, V. (2002). Nationwide longitudinal study of psychological responses to September 11. *Journal of the American Medical Association, 288,* 1235–1244.

Smith, P., Perrin, S., Yule, W., & Rabe-Hesketh, S. (2001). War exposure and maternal reactions in the psychosocial adjustment of children from Bosnia-Herzegovina. *Journal of Child Psychology and Psychiatry, 42,* 395–404.

Smith, T. W. (2002). The impact of the Cuban missile crisis on American public opinion. Report by the National Opinion Research Center, University of Chicago, Chicago.

Stern, J. (1999). *The ultimate terrorists.* Cambridge, MA: Harvard University Press.

Stroebe, W., & Stroebe, M. S. (1993). Determinants of adjustment to bereavement in younger widows and widowers. In M. S. Stroebe, W. Stroebe, & R. O. Hansson (Eds.), *Handbook of bereavement* (pp. 208–226). New York: Cambridge University Press.

Suedfeld, P. (1997). Homo invictus: The indomitable species. *Canadian Psychology, 38,* 164–173.

Thabet, A. A., Abed, Y., & Vostanis, P. (2002). Emotional problems in Palestinian children living in a war zone: A cross-sectional study. *Lancet, 359,* 1801–1804.

Thabet, A. A., & Vostanis, P. (1999). Posttraumatic stress reactions in children of war. *Journal of Child Psychiatry, 40,* 385–391.

Thompson, R. F., & Spencer, W. A. (1966). Habituation: A model phenomenon for the study of neuronal substrates of behavior. *Psychological Review, 73*(1), 16–43.

Tugade, M. M., & Frederickson, B. L. (2002). Positive emotions and emotional intelligence. In L. F. Barrett & P. Salovey (Eds.), *The wisdom in feeling: Psychological processes in emotional intelligence* (pp. 319–340). New York: Guilford Press.

Tversky, A., & Kahneman, D. (1974). Judgment under uncertainty: Heuristics and biases. *Science, 185,* 1124–1131.

Uchino, B. N., Cacioppo, J. T., & Kiecolt-Glaser, J. K. (1996). The relationship between social support and physiological processes: A review with emphasis on underlying mechanisms and implications for health. *Psychological Bulletin, 119*(3), 488–531.

Vernon, P. E. (1941). Psychological effects of air raids. *Journal of Abnormal and Social Psychology, 36,* 457–476.

Vineburgh, N. T. (2004). The power of the pink ribbon: Raising awareness of the mental health implications of terrorism. *Psychiatry, 67,* 137–146.

Wagner, A. R., & Brandon, S. E. (1989). Evolution of a structured connectionist model of Pavlovian conditioning (ÆSOP). In S. B. Klein & R. R. Mowrer (Eds.), *Contemporary learning theories: Pavlovian conditioning and the status of traditional learning theory* (pp. 149–190). Hillsdale, NJ: Erlbaum.

Weinberger, D. A., & Schwartz, G. E. (1990). Distress and restraint as superordinate dimensions of self-reported adjustment: A typological perspective. *Journal of Personality, 58*(2), 381–417.

———, & Davidson, R. J. (1979). Low-anxious, high-anxious, and repressive coping styles. *Journal of Abnormal Psychology, 88,* 369–380.

Wessely, S. (in press). What mental health professionals should and should not do. In N. Y. Gross, R. Gross, R. Marshall, & E. Susser (Eds.), *Mental health in the wake of a terrorist attack.* New York: Cambridge University Press.

Wilson, R., & Cairns, E. (1992). Trouble, stress, and psychological disorder in Northern Ireland. *Psychologist, 5,* p. 347–350.

Wilson, T. D., & Gilbert, D. T. (2003). Affective forecasting. In M. Zanna (Ed.), *Advances in experimental social psychology, Vol. 35* (pp. 345–411). New York: Elsevier.

Wilson, T. D., Wheatley, T. P., Kurtz, J. L., Dunn, E. W., & Gilbert, D. T. (2004). When to fire: Anticipatory versus postevent reconstrual of uncontrollable events. *Personality and Social Psychology Bulletin, 30*(3), 340–351.

Zimbardo, P. G. (1966). Control of pain motivation by cognitive dissonance. *Science, 151,* 217–219.

14

The Response of Relief Organizations to Terrorist Attacks

An Overview of How the Red Cross and Other Relief Organizations Work in Conjunction With Other Agencies

John A. Clizbe
Susan Hamilton

Ironically, on September 10–11, 2001, emergency management leaders from around the country were meeting in Montana. Their agenda was to discuss ways in which they could work together when faced with terrorist events. Included in the group were senior leaders from the American Red Cross and emergency managers from many of the areas directly impacted by the terror of September 11.

While everyone obviously felt an urgent need to return home, in retrospect there were some short-term unforeseen advantages to being stranded together in Montana. It was possible, for example, to work through some of the issues requiring coordination that would have been impossible to do back home, given the chaos within the communication systems. For example, a quick face-to-face meeting between a Red Cross leader and the emergency management group from the Commonwealth of Virginia resolved some challenges with Red Cross access to the Pentagon. Everyone agreed it would have been extremely difficult to track each other down through the turmoil on the eastern seaboard.

A longer-term implication and lesson emerged from this experience as well. Over the subsequent months, problem solving and communication clarification occurred best when key people could meet face to face to talk it out. This was true among the not-for-profits, government agencies, businesses, and just about everyone who was working to respond to the disaster. When these interactions happened, problems were solved. Frequently the problems, challenges, and misunderstandings persisted, however, when the communication was indirect or through the media or other sources.

Context

Although the acts of terror on September 11 were generally unexpected and unpredicted, they happened in the context of decades of relationship building in the emergency management and nonprofit community. At the local, state, and national levels, a number of organizations had been meeting, planning, and working together in a variety of situations. The participants at these events included not only the relief organizations themselves but also a number of partner agencies in government and business (American Red Cross, 2002).

Some of the leaders from the nonprofit organizations also had long-standing relationships with other agencies through their participation in the National Emergency Management Agency, the

National Hurricane Conference, the Natural Hazards Institute, and other organizations. As the association officially responsible for Emergency Support Function #8 in the Federal Emergency Response Plan, the American Red Cross was a regular attendee at planning meetings involving all of the federal agencies involved in emergency preparation and response.

The National Voluntary Organizations Active in Disaster (NVOAD) is, as the name suggests, a consortium of nonprofit organizations who participate in disaster relief nationally and often locally. At annual meetings and smaller gatherings, members of the organization had been reviewing ways in which they could work together more effectively in a wide range of potential emergencies, including acts of terrorism. Most of the member groups and their representatives had been working with each other for a number of years. They had also been discussing the niches each group preferred to fill—often in a deliberately complementary fashion. Included in almost all of their events had been representatives from the Federal Emergency Management Agency and other government organizations.

At the local level, American Red Cross chapters had also spent a number of years planning and responding with their colleagues in NVOAD, other nonprofit organizations, and government agencies. In New York City and Washington, DC—as well as locations in Massachusetts, Rhode Island, Connecticut, New York State, New Jersey, Pennsylvania, Maryland, Virginia, and elsewhere around the country—Red Cross chapters had solidly established relationships, often based on formal statements or memoranda of understanding. These declarations typically spelled out the general terms of the working relationship as well as specific details applicable to exactly how and when the organizations would work together.

Several voluntary relief organizations had also initiated, well before 9/11, new programs in anticipation of possible weapons of mass destruction or terrorist events. Starting in 1998, for example, the Red Cross established a special task force to address ways in which that organization and its partners could prepare for and respond to these kinds of events. Various subgroups were set up, ranging from training to community education to logistics, and they all included members from throughout emergency management and relief organizations. By the year 2000, the Clara Barton Center for Domestic Preparedness Training had been established in Pine Bluff, Arkansas, and trainers and trainees again included representatives from a range of organizations.

At the national, state, and local levels, often working in conjunction with emergency management, voluntary relief organizations participated in a variety of planning and training sessions and exercises. They were, for example, involved in all of these phases with the federally sponsored, multistate TOPOFF 1 (named for the involvement of top officials), which was intended to test the abilities of the entire disaster system to handle serious simultaneous disasters across the country. Red Cross chapters in New York City, Washington, DC, and elsewhere participated with other organizations in similar experiences (American Red Cross, 2002).

An additional context predating 9/11 was the strong emphasis placed on an "all hazards" approach by the entire emergency management community. It became quite clear that the experiences relief organizations had in working together and with other agencies on natural disasters were directly applicable in both preparation and potential responses to acts of terrorism. Many of the same services would need to be delivered, the same working relationships would function, and the same stresses and strains would occur. Thus, discussion in NVOAD and other settings explored ways in which these experiences might translate into situations involving terrorism.

There were, of course, some clear differences between acts of terrorism and natural disasters. The fact that an act of terrorism was a crime meant that law enforcement would be more directly involved in the planning and response. Research seemed to suggest that acts of terrorism would have different psychological and sociological impacts than natural disasters. The scale and scope of the impact was likely to be greater, expanding far beyond the place where the event took place. These and other differences proved to be especially problematic for relief organizations as the days following 9/11 unfolded.

The events of September 11, 2001, did not, then, occur in a vacuum. Advance planning, thinking, relationship building, and theorizing had all taken place. Some of it proved to be well founded, and some of it erroneous. Some new players entered the field with different perspectives. Several organizations with experience in natural disasters struggled to find their niche in this new environment. Some of those with no previous disaster-related experiences found ways in which they could substantially contribute. The established background and context was sometimes helpful but sometimes constraining.

The Need

As the horror of September 11 developed, two different sets of needs quickly emerged. Most important, of course, were those of the survivors, but the definition of just who was a "survivor" expanded exponentially. For example, survivors came to be viewed as not just those who physically walked away from the specific disaster sites but also colleagues and extended family members and residents in the affected communities. Ultimately, people across the country came to view themselves as attempting to "survive" the disasters. A second set of needs related to the institutions attempting to help the survivors and the institutions also became a rapidly expanding pool.

The Survivors

For the survivors, however they were defined, a number of needs were apparent. This was true whether they were people who physically survived at the point of devastation, family members related to those who had been injured or had lost their lives, rescue workers or relief organization workers, or those who were located physically far from the site of impact but were nevertheless profoundly affected.

The Need for Support

One such need was the requirement for quick support. The exact nature of the support was sometimes obvious and sometimes not to either the seeker or the provider, but a wide range of people clearly felt they had to have *some kind* of help.

For the families of those who lost their lives, the required support was often quite complex. It was assumed (not always correctly) that emotional help was crucial, but other kinds of support were often expressed both directly and indirectly. Some families had an immediate need for financial as-sistance, which was not always in direct proportion to the resources available to them. Some required help from their often far-flung families. Many needed someone to simply listen as they talked about what they had experienced; others were looking for someone to tell them what to do, if that was at all possible. Some had to have physical support near the site of the disaster, whereas others needed to move away from the site. In a number of respects, the hierarchy of requirements espoused by Abraham Maslow often seemed to reflect the ways in which people looked for assistance, with safety, survival, and a sense of security taking clear precedence over more "actualizing" needs. Much of this complexity was consistent with the findings published in a National Institute of Mental Health (2002) report on mental health and mass violence.

For many, support was a direct reflection of their personal circumstances. Elderly people who were stranded in high rises needed physical assistance and sustenance. Those with pets required care for their animals. Those in dust-contaminated apartments lacked a place to stay and a way to clean up. Injured people sought physical care and emotional support. Those who were primarily impacted economically were faced with earning a living, finding a new job, or surviving while their employers regrouped. Employers themselves searched for ways to aid their employees.

Perhaps especially striking was the degree to which people throughout the country and around the world were affected—and called for support. The tens of thousands of requests the American Red Cross call-in center received underscored these needs: A mother in Iowa wondered how to deal with her anxious 6-year-old. A couple in Houston struggled to cope with a layoff attributed to 9/11. Korean tourists were stranded in the Midwest without hard-to-find prescribed medication. Thousands of people felt driven to do something to help all those who were expressing a need for some kind of support.

The Need for Linkages

The relief agencies also quickly realized the need for linkages between family and community. First, of course, were those who were desperate to find a loved one they feared was lost in the disasters. If they lived together, the hour-by-hour trauma of trying to make contact was profound. Many tried to reach the physical site in hopes of establishing contact. Others stayed by the phone. Still others had strong reason to believe their loved one had not survived.

Agencies seeking to help faced the huge challenge of trying to reestablish these contacts, often in the face of sparse and inaccurate information. Some of the initial estimates of lives lost approached 50,000, then paused for weeks at around 6,000, and ultimately reached about 3,000. This meant that, for a while, it was not possible to account for tens of thousands of people—almost all of whom had someone hoping to reestablish contact with them.

As time dragged on, those who seemed to have lost loved ones needed linkages with other family members and friends in the community. These connections, which often had to be arranged, provided some of the most important senses of support for those directly impacted. Family members who lived around the country also searched for connection. As many as twenty or thirty family members from a single family often came to New York, Washington, or Pennsylvania to be together with family members living in those areas.

People in the broader community sought comparable linkages. Preestablished, newly formed, and spontaneous community groups provided their members with these connections. A wealth of reports filtered into the Red Cross, for example, describing special church services and meetings at established organizations that focused on the events of September 11, newly formed citizen discussion and action groups, and neighbors bonding in ways they never had before.

The Need for Information

Information often became the most important kind of support. Both people who were located in the impacted areas and others around the world demanded in-depth news of the events. First, they wanted to know about the situation "on the ground" and looked to the relief organizations and their contacts in government to provide it. What had happened? How had it happened? How many people were injured or killed? Who were the victims? What was being done, and what else could be done? A myriad of smaller questions followed. What streets and building were impacted? What

transportation routes were available? How can I get there (or how can I get away from there)?

Second, people required information about available services, which they often sought before the services were established. Who will help me find out about a loved one? Who can tell me what I should do now? Who can get food to the emergency responders? Who can help me financially right now? What kind of services do you offer?

A third kind of information was education about what was going to happen next. Who can help me find a job? Who can tell me how to talk with my children? Who can offer child care services? Who will bring my family together? Who will help with burials? Who offers counseling? Who will help me find another place to live? Who can help look after my long-term financial concerns?

In a related vein, people asked questions about how to prepare for another attack or for some comparable emergency. What kind of planning should families do? What should be stockpiled in a family survival kit? What kind of preventative health care actions should I take? What can communities do to be better prepared?

Others sought information about how they could help. Thousands of spontaneous volunteers arrived at or near the disaster sites wanting to help. Hundred of thousands of others wanted to know how their financial contributions would be put to use. Teachers sought information about how to talk to their students. Children were unsure of how to talk to each other. Agencies were often overwhelmed with people who wanted to be of assistance. All of these requests reflected a need for another kind of information—how to help others.

People also required information on how to cope. Should I go back to work immediately? Should my children go back to school? Should I sell our home and move? Should I go to the banker or the lawyer first? How do I get my life back together? Workers in relief agencies listed hundreds of such questions they were asked.

Survivors, at a minimum, needed multiple kinds of support—help in establishing connections with family and friends and lots of information. The relief organizations had to address these challenges quickly because the needs were pressing. Doing so would require extensive collaboration with each other and with other agencies.

The Institutions

The institutions quickly discovered the needs they themselves faced if they wished to serve and in fact survive. No organization was truly prepared for an event of this nature. People were in desperate straits, but the relief organization often did not have the capacity to immediately deliver the required services. They thus had to balance the difficulty of quickly serving people with the simultaneous challenge of providing those sought-after services.

The Need for Assessment

While challenged to quickly provide assistance, the relief organizations also had to attempt to understand and assess what was happening, what was needed, what would happen next, and what would be needed in a rapidly changing environment. If they were to be able to go beyond simply reacting to the latest piece of accurate or inaccurate information, they had to find ways to understand the full nature of the situation. If they were to plan for and predict demands for services and resources, they had to be able to undertake a broad-ranging assessment.

This assessment was actually twofold. Much like the survivors, the institutions needed an assessment of the situation. How many people had been directly affected? Were there many people in the impacted buildings who were able to walk away? How many were injured? Were the directly affected people from the immediate area or from somewhere else? Who was already delivering what services? They also had to undertake a healthy self-assessment. What was their capacity? What kinds of human and financial resources did they have and still need?

The perplexing nature of the situation on the ground presented an immediate test to the relief organizations. If there were 6,000 victims, they needed to be ready at one level; if there were 3,000, a different level of response was required. Thousands versus hundreds of injuries carried different implications.

Who were the immediate clients? Who would or should be secondary clients? If the primary needs were those of people who had lost loved ones, then the focus had to be in that direction. However, if hundreds or thousands were ulti-mately to be impacted economically, a different clientele would emerge. Should the relief services be provided only in the localities directly impacted, or did the data suggest a wider need? What would be the pattern of the emerging needs—emotional? financial? educational?

The institutions also needed to assess themselves. How did their strengths fit with present needs? How would their shortcomings be exacerbated by the existing situation? In order to evaluate both their current capacity and their capacity for growth, they had to determine their staffs' strengths and capabilities This self-assessment also needed to include an appraisal of the network of potential services and service deliverers. How did their capabilities fit with the community's other resources? What programs would be available through governmental agencies? Did they need to invent a new program, or would they be reinventing the proverbial wheel?

The Need for Coordination

If they did not wish to reinvent the wheel, the relief organizations would have to coordinate with one another and with other agencies. On the one hand, they presumably did not want to duplicate services. On the other hand, they also did not want people's needs to go unmet because of gaps in service. These objectives were not always successfully met. Sometimes services were duplicated, and sometimes gaps in services meant that needs were left unfulfilled. To minimize these possibilities, extra coordination was going to be required.

As the situation evolved, it became even clearer that coordination was key. Government officials and those who were directly impacted were outspoken in their criticism of the lack of coordination. At times this was easier to point out than to resolve. Not only was it necessary for people in the organizations to talk, but their *systems* also had to work together. This called for an entirely new level of coordination.

The Need to Share Information

The events surrounding 9/11 raised the question of whether relief organizations should share information they had traditionally seen as only their own. This issue was not simply a matter of proprietary self-interest; it also involved assumptions (and sometimes promises) made concerning client confidentiality—for example, could such information be passed from one organization to another? Various groups had different information available to them that could potentially lead to better and more efficient service delivery. They might know, for example, that a new walk-in clinic had been established in a particular neighborhood. One organization might learn of a pocket of unmet needs, while another might develop a new service (financial planning, for example) that would be of interest and use to many. Examples occurred of one relief group saying that another organization would provide a specific service when that was not, in fact, what was planned.

Coordination of Communication

The relief organizations also found they had to coordinate their communications to the public. Sometimes inconsistent and even conflicting information was disseminated by different parties. The confusing nature of the available information was, of course, one of the contributing factors, but when various organizations or people were publicizing conflicting information, the confusion was only heightened. At the same time, the prospect of coordinating public statements was, for many groups, a new and challenging concept.

While it did not usually appear necessary for the organizations to speak with only one voice, they had to at least be aware of what their colleagues had said or were going to say. Two different organizations might spend time and resources developing similar communication vehicles (brochures for identical audiences, for example). Organizations working virtually side by side might announce different hours of operation.

Sometimes a single voice was called for. For example, the issue of confidentiality of records was relevant to almost all of the organizations, as was advocacy and appreciation of the work being done by the relief groups. In these instances the relief organizations had to stand together in their messaging.

Communicating in a high risk environment is an acknowledged art and science. As Joshua Gotbaum, former chief executive officer of the September 11 Fund, said, "When in the spotlight, use it—or else" (Gotbaum, 2003). The relief organizations needed to clearly appreciate the complexity of the communication challenges.

The Need to Work With and Strengthen Local Resources

It was immediately clear to many inside observers that New York City and the Pentagon, for example, had some outstanding resource specialists in place. They knew their community and the people in it. They knew local needs and neighborhood assets. Furthermore, they were very likely to be there when others would be long gone. The relief organizations thus had to quickly identify, work with, and strengthen those local, on-the-ground authorities.

The requirement was twofold. The larger organizations responding to September 11 needed to strengthen both their own local affiliates and the other existing local service agencies. In fact, it appeared that many services could be effectively delivered and sustained only if the local resources were primary. Obviously, those local assets were often overwhelmed and welcomed the arrival of help. Yet the long-term need had to be for all of them to be reinforced rather than weakened, taken over, or supplanted.

Smaller organizations moving into the areas found a somewhat different challenge. Lacking existing local affiliates, these new arrivals had to find local resources they could help to shore up. Some called it the "swoop-in factor"—the temptation for organizations outside the impacted area to step in and save the day by delivering services. Clearly, for all, the fundamental principle was the long-term enhancement of existing resources.

Risk Management

The need for risk management also emerges in a crisis environment. Virtually every relief organization had to confront the risks they were taking with their services and their members. While many of them were accustomed to this challenge in natural disasters, certain dimensions of September 11 were different. For example, there was the early temptation for some relief organization workers and volunteers to rush to the disaster site, which was still laden with physical risk. There was also the danger of possible follow-up acts of terrorism and the question of just where it was safe to be. Moreover, it was unclear whether acts of terrorism were covered by the same policies that covered workers in natural disasters.

With the wealth of spontaneous volunteers and the demands of many workers, additional risks included the degree to which traditional standards and credentials needed to be maintained. For example, the Red Cross had a long-standing policy of using only mental health professionals whose credentials had been closely examined in advance. Could and should these same standards be maintained? Could the standards be better maintained by changing the on-the-job requirements—for example, requiring workers to work for shorter lengths of time compared with more typical disasters, thereby making it possible for more people with appropriate credentials to work? Did we even know for certain what kinds of interventions were the most appropriate in this catastrophic event?

Because of the intense demand for services, it was sometimes necessary to balance a desire to do what seemed like the right thing with the risks of actually doing it—perhaps ineffectively. For example, should workers reach out and solicit an opportunity to help by going door-to-door looking for "victims"? Was this professionally appropriate, and did it place the organization at risk? Importantly, the Red Cross center was receiving phone calls that indicated that people wanted help but were unable to come to Red Cross supervised sites.

The Response

The events of September 11 brought to the forefront a multitude of organizations. Some were well established, while others were newly formed. Almost all of them genuinely sought to help; a few were purely opportunistic. Given the extensive needs that were immediately apparent and emerging, both traditional and new methods of response needed to be implemented by the relief organizations.

The American Red Cross had a unique position and set of obligations. Its congressional charter mandates that it provide relief to disaster victims and help people prevent, prepare for, and respond to emergencies. It is the agency selected by the National Transportation and Safety Board (NTSB) to provide assistance at aviation, transportation, and mass casualty incidents—obviously applicable on September 11. The Red Cross is also

the sole nonprofit agency that has been assigned specific responsibilities in the Federal Response Plan (FRP), which describes federal assistance in any federally declared major disaster or emergency. Under the Robert T. Stafford Disaster Relief and Emergency Assistance Act, the Red Cross was required to provide emergency shelter, food, emergency first aid, disaster welfare information, and the bulk distribution of emergency relief items and to support information dissemination, planning, health and medical services, and the bulk acquisition of food.

Previously established relationships and formal statements of understanding and letters of agreement were very quickly activated by the nonprofit organizations and the federal, state, and county agencies. Because these agreements were established in advance and described the parameters and method of cooperation, it was much easier to immediately set up liaisons, working relationships, and information sharing. This cooperation helped bring some order to the complex and chaotic circumstances occurring in New York, Washington, and Pennsylvania.

As one example of multiagency activation, at Boston Logan International Airport, the Logan Massport Authority officials activated their aviation response plan while the Red Cross Mass Bay chapter set up a family assistance center at the Logan Hilton for approximately 78 Massachusetts families directly impacted by the crashes. Among the other responding agencies were the state police, FBI, Massachusetts Corps of Fire Chaplains, the Massachusetts Department of Health, the Trauma Center, the American Psychological Association Disaster Response Network, the American Psychiatric Association Disaster Network, area hospitals, and the Department of Veterans Affairs.

Part of the success of the response in Boston was due to the Logan Airport aviation incident planning initiative and drill exercise sponsored the previous year by Massport. Ten Red Cross chapters had taken part in the exercise, nurturing relationships with state agencies and private-sector professional groups and providing an operational context for mobilizing almost immediately. These relationships also facilitated the necessary flexibility to make changes as needed.

Well-established connections were expanded, and new ones were created, ranging from the National Organization for Victims of Crime and the New York Port Authority to long-term agreements between the Red Cross and the Southern Baptist and Church of the Brethren response networks. Early in the development of Red Cross mental health services, the national mental health associations had developed statements of understanding with the organization and had set up networks whose members were able to be alerted to respond to Red Cross requests for mental health volunteers.

The 9/11 United Services Group (USG) originally consisted of a consortium of 13 New York City human services organizations working on the front lines of the recovery efforts. On December 14, 2001, they came together to oversee assistance to the victims. Their joint mission was to ensure that everyone needing assistance received it in an effective, timely, and supportive manner, while at the same time ensuring accountability and strengthening confidence in the delivery of charitable aid and social services. They formed and maintained a comprehensive tracking service using data provided by the participating groups. In this way they were able to identify service gaps and potential duplication of services.

Integrated services through the USG included financial assistance, training, and help with case management. A case manager was assigned to all those who received assistance, helping them negotiate the system. The USG also served as a liaison to the community-at-large by providing requested reports that would inform the public on how services were provided and how clients were helped. A hotline was developed that operated 24 hours a day, 7 days a week for people with questions or requesting a service coordinator. Immediate crisis counseling was available, and referrals could be made to mental health or substance abuse practitioners or programs. Within a year, 67,000 people had received aid, and the number of participating agencies had grown considerably.

The agencies were also required to rapidly adapt their usual responses to the exceptional needs of the moment. Two cities were experiencing mass casualties on the ground, a plane had crashed in rural Pennsylvania, and bereft families and travelers were stranded by grounded planes around the country. Shelters had to be opened throughout the country for travelers. Family assistance centers were being established at the planes' points of origin (Boston Logan Airport and Dulles Airport in Washington, DC) and destinations (Los Angeles and San Francisco).

Family Assistance Centers

Within 72 hours of the time the planes hit the World Trade Center, New York Mayor Rudolph Giuliani authorized the opening of a family assistance center (FAC). The objective was to establish a center where families and individuals who had lost loved ones or whose loved ones were hospitalized (or if they themselves had been hospitalized) could meet with the relief agencies. It was to be an accessible, one-stop location where multiple agencies could meet multiple needs. The first FAC opened at the Lexington Avenue Armory. Four weeks later it was relocated to Pier 94, a 20,000-foot warehouse that remained open until March 22, 2002. Buses transported families to and from three locations: the Armory, Penn Station, and Chambers Street.

Initially, the FAC served as a place where people could file missing-person reports, obtain information, and bring DNA samples for later identification. It later expanded to assist those who had lost their jobs and homes. Because of the high security and the facilities and services it provided, the FAC evolved into a safe haven for families and friends and provided waiting rooms, child care, telephones, Internet access, and meals. The center was open 7 days a week from 8:00 A.M. until midnight. Areas were set aside for emotional support and spiritual care, for the Federal Emergency Management Agency (FEMA), representatives from the mayor's office, insurance companies, the New York State Crime Victims Board/Safe Horizon, the New York Police Department Command Center, Department of Veterans Affairs, labor leaders, the FBI Crime Victims Assistance, foreign governments, the American Red Cross, the Salvation Army, and other community resources. A separate dining area served meals to the center staff and to workers returning from Ground Zero.

Additional centers were later set up at Liberty State Park in Jersey City, New Jersey, and at the Crystal City Sheraton in Arlington, Virginia, for the families affected by the Pentagon tragedy. As the days progressed and the needs became clearer, more and more services were provided. In Virginia, for example, trained dogs were brought into the center to help create an emotionally supportive climate. Family assistance centers became the vital ingredient in service delivery.

Respite Centers

The purpose of the three respite centers near Ground Zero was to provide support services for rescue personnel and recovery animals working at the site. Their aim was to reduce the psychological and physical stress caused by the demanding work of rescue and recovery. These centers became multifunctional sites in partnership with agencies providing specialized services. The key collaborating agencies in New York were the Office of Emergency Management, the Red Cross, the Salvation Army, the food banks, the New York Health Department, the Hotel and Restaurant Association, local clergy, and veterinary services for the care of the search-and-rescue dogs. The centers provided meals, a place to sleep and relax, clothes, work gear, articles for personal hygiene, emotional and spiritual support, and physical health care. When the three centers downsized to a "big white tent," the Salvation Army assumed overall direction, while the Red Cross provided mental health services.

Service Centers and Cross-Training

The Red Cross established three service centers in Manhattan and several outside the Manhattan area to provide direct financial assistance to displaced families and others. Originally designed as a place for the delivery of Red Cross services, they ultimately housed a number of agencies that worked together cooperatively. As the casework increased, the Red Cross, the Salvation Army, and Safe Horizon cross-trained their volunteer workers at these centers. This not only helped use staff members more efficiently but also enabled clients to receive services from multiple agencies and the agencies to coordinate some of their service delivery.

Unmet Needs Groups

By November 2001, the September 11 Fund stopped soliciting donations and in January 2002 asked the public to stop sending contributions. In much less than a year, well in excess of a billion dollars had been donated to the charities. Surveys indicated that as many as two-thirds of U.S. households had donated money to the charitable organizations.

Yet, despite all of the available dollars and all of the effort, the needs of some groups of people remained unmet. The difficulty was not a lack of money but uncertainty about how to best channel those resources. Focused, special kinds of needs (e.g., for financial planning) emerged. In addition, particular groups (e.g., undocumented workers, people whose livelihood was disrupted, those living outside a designated area) still required assistance. As had usually been the case with natural disasters, it was important to establish mechanisms for addressing these unfulfilled needs.

It became apparent that some people whose family members had died on September 11 would not receive compensation or assistance from some programs either because they were ineligible or because they simply fell through the cracks. For example, in New York City, a Spanish family was unable to claim government assistance because the business that had employed the victim would not confirm the person's employment since it was "off the record." Michelle Archer, a program coordinator for the 9/11 fund at the New Jersey Immigration and Policy Network, disclosed the fact that a number of people who worked at the World Trade Center had held H-I visas (legal work permits), but their spouses and children were undocumented, which made the task of seeking aid daunting. Archer, with other relief groups in New Jersey, set up immigrant centers where translators, attorneys, and interpreters assisted these immigrants and informed other service providers of their needs. Church World Services (CWS) funded Tepeyac, a New York–based group that helped families of immigrants who died.

Specific ethnic groups were also struggling. New Life Center was created to assist the Fujianese, an ethnic group from the Fujian province of China, who did not qualify for assistance because they lived beyond the strict geographical guidelines that many agencies used but whose homes and workplaces were impacted. Their problem was confounded because most of the 9/11 language assistance was available only in Cantonese and other major Chinese languages.

Emerging psychological needs also stimulated additional programs and support. At the time of the tragedies, many national mental health and humanitarian organizations quickly published information for the public. The American Psychological Association, the National Center for Victims of Crime, the Institute of Mental Health, the National Mental Health Association, the New York University Child Study Center, and the Red Cross all published material to help people cope and recover. The National Center on Post Traumatic Stress Disorder published "Dealing with the Aftermath of Terror" and "Facts about PTSD." The Red Cross had its materials translated into many languages and posted them on its website.

Others were victims of secondary economic effects. In April 2002 the United Methodist Committee on Relief (UMCOR) allotted monies for a 3-year program that focused on secondary victims in New York. John Scibilia, director of the September 11 response for Lutheran Disaster Relief in the New York area told the Board of Global Ministries that there was a major shortfall in meeting the needs of the impacted. Some people who lost their jobs because of the terrorist attacks soon exhausted their savings and other funds and began to use their retirement funds. Members of the New Jersey Interfaith Partnership for Disaster Recovery set up an "unmet needs table" to address this problem and help clients with expenses, encouraging them to become self-supporting through retraining and significant changes in lifestyle.

On July 17, 2002, the New York Regional Associations of Grantmakers, the Twenty-first Century Foundation, and the Rockefeller Foundation had decided to cosponsor a program called Unmet Needs: A Special Post-9/11 Session. In February 2003 caseworkers from UMCOR and other major agencies, including the Salvation Army, Catholic Charities, and El Centro, were continuing to bring cases to the New Jersey unmet needs table. Their clients had grown to include laid-off airline personnel and people with delayed psychological reactions. CWS also funded a number of interfaith programs to assist people who were still hurting. These included the New York Disaster Recovery Interfaith, the New Jersey Partnership for Disaster Recovery, the Long Island Council of Churches Disaster Taskforce, and the New York City September 11 Unmet Needs Roundtable.

Despite all of these efforts, some people continued to need assistance after the initial programs were discontinued. Not all of the economic effects of September 11 were felt immediately, and some people came forward only when they absolutely had to, which, unfortunately, was occasionally after other resources had lapsed. Eligibility for the federal program of financial assistance continued for an extended time as families struggled to choose between receiving a cash grant or pursuing legal action against the airlines and others.

Some professionals projected that unmet needs might well emerge over a period of years, rather than just months. A number of organizations, such as the American Red Cross, with the substantial donations it received, expect to continue with assistance for a number of years. While some of those needs are predictable from previous experiences (such as long-term mental health requirements for some rescue workers), others may yet arise.

The Challenges

As the relief organizations worked in conjunction with other agencies to develop methods of responding to communities' needs, new and more effective means of collaboration and service delivery emerged. A great deal was done right, and a great deal of assistance was delivered. However, although the background of pre-9/11 cooperative efforts certainly helped, challenges persisted. Many of those remain as important considerations for whatever future difficulties these organizations may confront.

Making It Easier for Those Who Were Affected

An extraordinary number of relief organizations responded at an unprecedented level, especially in the large metropolitan area in and around New York City and, to a slightly lesser extent, Washington, D.C. Families who lost loved ones lived around the country and world, although most lived in the suburbs of New York, New Jersey, and Connecticut. For those families who sought face-to-face contact with the relief organizations, the logistics were a challenge at best.

Often those who sought assistance from several organizations had to negotiate their way between multiple sites. Once there, they frequently had to fill out different forms asking for much of the same information again and again. These were issues not unique to the nonprofit community; they certainly also included government programs.

A range of possible solutions began to appear. Some were never fully actualized, however, and some are still under discussion. Barriers included simply a lack of time and staff, the need to work through risk and liability issues, problems of physical logistics, special requirements by some organizations to be consistent with their standard practices, and sometimes cultural resistance within associations. Constructively, some groups began to merge their sites—initially at large centers and then at smaller drop-in locations. Staff from different organizations were even cross-trained in each other's forms and procedures so that clients could do "one-stop-shopping." Still under intense discussion (and strongly advocated by some government officials and clients) are the ways in which the relief organizations can use common forms, thereby allowing clients to fill out only one form and eliminate duplication of effort.

Other challenges include the application of technology to allow people to be assisted without physically coming to a site. The Red Cross, for example, established a massive call-in center for just such a purpose. The relief organizations must also deal with the problem of getting their technology systems to interface. Some of them have already found ways in which they can link up with national, state, or local government databases and programs.

Determining the Nature of the Assistance

September 11 changed the ways many organizations thought about the nature of the assistance they offer. Most have historically worked on a clearly defined needs-based approach. The definition of "needs," however, altered on 9/11. For some organizations this not only presented significant challenges internally but also impacted the collaboration among organizations. If one used strict financial criteria and another applied a more liberal interpretation of need, confusion could reign and misunderstanding increase. It was not immediately clear what criteria government programs would use in the future.

Most of the relief groups ultimately chose to use their own criteria, although a few attempted to agree on some common definitions. If similar events happen in the future, this challenge will

have to be faced. A model of institutional triage may need to be developed and implemented.

Sharing Information

There was increasing pressure both to share and not share information. Much of this debate proved to be a forerunner of current concerns about patient/client privacy. As questions about eligibility for assistance escalated, so did the topic of whether organizations should and could share the information they had. Sometimes this was an issue between governmental and nongovernmental agencies, with the clients of the latter expressing concern about their personal information (for example, residency and immigration status) being given to the government. On other occasions, it was a matter for discussion even between nongovernmental agencies.

Aggressive efforts were made to develop a system of sharing appropriate information using outside database consultants in hopes of protecting some kinds of confidential data. Other organizations went through extensive processes of obtaining release-of-information permission. This area is a major challenge confronting the relief community and does not lend itself to quick and easy solutions. Virtually all of the organizations recognized the need for at least some basic sharing of information. Perhaps a starting point would be the determination of what is confidential and what is not. At the very least, relief groups will need to adopt strategies to address this problem.

Understanding Those Who Wanted to Help

There were at least three categories of people who expressed a desire to help: donors of time, donors of goods, and donors of money. All three represented significant challenges, and although this has historically been the case, the challenges became even greater on 9/11. The very nature of the event stimulated new donors, new expectations, and new frustrations.

Tens of thousands of people arrived at various locations volunteering to help. This required a massive process of volunteer management. Here, too, was an area where information sharing could be helpful. Were some organizations looking for people with certain kinds of skills? Were there places where people could be utilized later?

Unfortunately, some potential volunteers left angry because they were not given an opportunity to help. The relief organizations will have to address this challenge of volunteers (including how to credential them), and this may require a higher level of collaboration.

Those who donated goods also posed an unparalleled challenge. Countless truckloads of unsolicited goods arrived hourly. The simple logistics of where to unload them became a daunting task. The process of sorting, organizing, distributing, and/or destroying unusable materials occupied numerous hours. Although the emergency management community has tried in the past to communicate the disadvantages of these kinds of donations, the message still needs to be delivered more effectively.

September 11 was an event that triggered an enormous outpouring of financial support from around the country and the world. What distinguished this outpouring from that after other disasters (in addition to the sheer number of dollars donated) was perhaps the quantity of comparatively small spontaneous donations made in a wide variety of settings—retail establishments, street-corner collections, at-home coffee hours, and so on. These donors in particular, perhaps donating for the first time, had very strong feelings about how their dollars should be used—almost always a direct and full pass through to victims' families. Most notably the Red Cross, but other organizations as well, faced a major challenge in understanding these donors' intentions and determining how best to respond. How to handle similar situations in the future remains an issue to be resolved. A related challenge for the relief community is to find ways of communicating the legitimacy of associated expenses, the need for infamous "infrastructure," and the costs of readiness. We hope that the relief organizations will be able to do this without embarrassment.

Improving Selection and Training

The enormous complexity of the events surrounding September 11 highlight the critical need for training people—whether paid or volunteer. Fortunately, many relief organizations had already invested significantly in training—some of it even focused on terrorism. Yet very few were adequately trained for what they experienced. The training

gaps were not so much in technical know-how but more in the decision making and flexibility.

Arguably, some of these concerns cannot be addressed only with training, and good selection is therefore essential. The relief organizations realized the necessity of doing more advance work in identifying those who are best suited for these kinds of disasters and providing them with the training and systems that enable them to do their jobs.

Safety and Security Issues

One common problem faced by most of the relief organizations was the safety and security of their members. Particularly with the influx of so many groups and volunteers, the task became substantial. It was also a challenge for the law enforcement community to understand and meet these needs of the nonprofits.

One issue was identification. Many sites necessarily had restricted access. Identifying who should have admittance was difficult. Identification badges were forged, and uniforms were mimicked. Most of the traditional identification processes used by the nonprofits were unsophisticated. The relief organizations, working with the law enforcement community, must find ways of effectively and efficiently identifying their people.

Sometimes the safety of staff and clients was also a challenge at the relief sites. Even issues such as protecting lines of clients from inclement weather became difficult. Most of the nonprofit organizations have not felt it necessary to have security experts on their staffs, but the challenges related to September 11 predict that such expertise will be required in similar events in the future.

Handling Turf

Issues of turf arise despite the best of intentions. Relief organizations, like all other groups, take pride in their special skills and mission. Understandably, most of them believe they are very good at what they do. Although not often acknowledged, competition sometimes arises between relief associations just as it does elsewhere.

The task for relief organizations is to keep this phenomenon from detracting from the ultimate good of the people they are seeking to serve. Some lessons have emerged in the wake of 9/11. First, it is important to respect the need of each association to fulfill its fundamental mission. Most groups with a history have evolved a clear sense of their mission. The challenge, while collaborating, is to let them—even help them—do it.

Second, the relief organizations needed to stick to their strengths. When these groups begin to move away from what they are good at doing, then they experience both internal and external problems. Relief organizations must respect each other's turf and also manage their own with respect for their compatriots.

Supporting One Another

The task of supporting one another derives from the challenge of turf management. Joshua Gotbaum, in the commentary cited earlier, noted in particular the failure of much of the nonprofit community (unlike the business community, he says) to pull together when some parts of it were under siege (Gotbaum, 2003). When specific relief organizations were criticized for certain practices, very few members of the broader community of relief groups came to their defense—even though the practices were often common to many of them. As a result, the image of the entire relief community suffered to some extent.

As Gotbaum suggests, the nonprofit community has traditionally failed to see itself as a unified group, instead leaving each organization to fend for itself. Many groups may even have preferred this model. Recent history suggests, however, that these associations have a stake in each other's success and face the job of finding ways to appropriately support each other.

Political Pressures

Relief organizations may find one of the best opportunities to support each other in the political arena. Granted the concerns about lobbying (an issue that is often misunderstood by nonprofits), there are often political issues of common concern to many nonprofits. With September 11, some of these issues (such as sharing information) arose. These provided the organizations with the challenge and the opportunity to discover common purposes and needs and to perhaps work together in the political sphere.

Conclusion

The relief organizations that responded to the events of September 11, 2001, did an amazing job. More people were served faster with more direct assistance than at perhaps any other time in history. In addition, this occurred in a high-stress, first-time-ever climate with substantial ambiguity, confusion, and escalating expectations.

Before 9/11, relationships within the relief organization community and between the community and other agencies certainly facilitated these efforts. The fact that these groups had numerous formal and informal agreements and experiences provided a context in which they could work together. The needs they attempted to serve in some ways paralleled earlier experiences but in other ways were very different. Whole new ways of thinking about the needs of clients, donors, and communities emerged. A wealth of new programs and services evolved. New kinds of controversies arose. Demands for effective collaboration escalated.

The lessons learned from these experiences are also still coming to light as more and more retrospective analyses are published. There seem to be, however, some clear challenges—mostly quite manageable—requiring the attention of relief organizations both independently and collectively. These require new ways of thinking about the "industry," new ways of working with each other and other agencies, and even new ways of envisioning who is to be served and how they are to be aided.

References

American Red Cross. (2002). September 11, 2001: Unprecedented events, unprecedented response. Internal document.

Gotbaum, J. (2003, February 6,). Lessons learned after September 11. *Chronicle of Philanthropy, 15*(8), 37–39.

National Institute of Mental Health. (2002). Mental health and mass violence: Evidence-based early psychological interventions for victims/survivors of mass violence. A workshop to reach consensus. NIH Publication no. 02–5138, Washington, DC.: U.S. Government Printing Office.

15

Understanding How Organizational Bias Influenced First Responders at the World Trade Center

Joseph W. Pfeifer

At 9:59 A.M, the South Tower collapsed. What the world saw on television, we could not see. Our world in the lobby of the North Tower went black. In darkness, I radioed to the firefighters above. "Command to all units in Tower 1, evacuate the building!" While many of the firefighters assisting people heard the message, they were already dozens of floors above ground level. Little did we know that time was running out.

Author's recollection of 9/11

To fully understand the 9/11 response, this chapter will examine how organizational bias influenced the evacuation of first responders from the World Trade Center. Regardless of any prior history of power struggles among first responders, it is inconceivable that any commander on 9/11 would ever deliberately withhold vital information that could potentially save lives. Then why did organizations not think to share critical reports about the signs of collapse of World Trade Center towers? The answer lies in years of organizational bias within the emergency response community, where organizations generally act independently of each other.

One would expect that these organizational biases would be abandoned during times of crises; however, the events of 9/11 in New York illustrate a strong systematic bias towards group self-interest. The analysis of the World Trade Center response illustrates the negative effect organizational bias has on commanding complex incidents. These organizational biases are seen under three command conditions: (1) resistance to a single incident commander, (2) development of blind spots in command capacity, and (3) a diffusion of personal command responsibility. Most importantly,

this chapter provides a unified command model for overcoming organizational bias—something vital for effective Homeland Security and the command of complex incidents of terrorism.

In trying to understand critical aspects of the response of New York City agencies to the crisis at the World Trade Center (WTC) on September 11, 2001, many observers overlook the effects of years of interagency fighting for sole command power. The following analysis explores the impact that social group behavior has on information sharing under conditions of stress and uncertainty.

The action aim of this chapter is to demonstrate that the likelihood of sharing vital information at critical times during complex incidents becomes greater when groups that ordinarily are competing or acting independently are organized to act as an integrated group under a unified command, where all members are equally responsible for command-coordinated action. However, to achieve this level of integration, organizational biases need to be overcome.

Social identity that promotes the power of one organization over another produces two social outcomes during complex incidents. First, it creates a positive in-group bias toward those who are part of the same group and a negative out-group bias against those who are part of an alternate group (Deaux, 1996; Zimbardo, 2004). When providing information across groups, people are prone to give more information to members of their own group and less to members outside it. Second, when under stress, people feel little obligation to share valuable information with those outside their group since the responsibility for acting is diffused within their in-group. This phenomenon excludes the out-group from receiving information that may be vital to their operation.

To fully understand the power of organizational (systematic) bias, one must examine how information sharing within and outside groups influenced the evacuation of first responders from the North Tower of the World Trade Center. This chapter illustrates that the most accurate and timely information reported by police aviation produced a rapid evacuation with a sense of urgency. However, the majority of the first responders, including firefighters within the North Tower, did not receive the same situational-awareness report. That information-transmission failure was responsible for an unhurried evacuation without any apparent sense of urgency.

Comparing these two cases demonstrates the severe consequences of keeping critical information within an organization. This lack of information sharing is referred to as "stovepipe situational awareness." Analogous to a stovepipe, information travels only within a single organization. As a result, one agency had superior situational awareness regarding the fire on the upper floors of the towers, while the fire department had little or no information. This inequity greatly affected the decision-making capacity of emergency responders. It also raises the more important question regarding the reason commanders did not communicate this vital information to each other.

Escape From the North Tower

This case study compares two separate situational-awareness pictures given to first responders. The analysis looks at the radio transmissions on 9/11 between the time the South Tower collapsed at 9:59 A.M. and the collapse of the North Tower at 10:28 A.M. Messages transmitted during those 29 minutes were given by radio to emergency re-

sponders according to each organization's intra-agency protocol. No messages were transmitted by radio, computer, or face-to-face contact between the two primary response agencies. This created a stovepipe situational awareness that resulted in separate and divergent operational pictures of the fires on the upper floors,

NYPD Rapid Evacuation

When the South Tower of the World Trade Center collapsed, the Emergency Service Unit (ESU) teams of the New York Police Department (NYPD) in the North Tower, like the firefighters, had no idea what had just occurred. After witnessing this collapse from the air, the NYPD aviation units immediately radioed a report, and the ESU dispatcher made five emergency transmissions, ordering all of the emergency service officers to get out of the North Tower (Dwyer & Flynn, 2005, p. 214).

At 10:01 A.M., an ESU detective at the NYPD command post on Church and Vesey streets saw the South Tower fall and ordered the evacuation of all ESU units from the WTC complex (9/11 Commission Report, 2004, p. 309). An ESU officer inside the North Tower clearly heard the message but could not comprehend how a 110-story building could collapse, so he asked for the message to be repeated. It was then explained that the South Tower was gone and that the North Tower building, which they were in, was in imminent danger of also coming down (9/11 Commission Staff Report #13, 2004, pp. 24–25). That message was an alarm for all of the ESU units to immediately begin their evacuation.

These officers now understood why they needed to leave rapidly. But it was the additional helicopter radio transmissions of observed fire conditions and building instability that made it more apparent that they were not simply to evacuate the building but to leave rapidly in order to escape its inevitable collapse. The transmissions from the police helicopter were made on an NYPD Special Operation Division (SOD) frequency that was monitored by ESU officers inside and outside the North Tower.[1]

10:00 A.M.   "A member of the NYPD aviation unit radioed that the South Tower had collapsed immediately after it happened and further advised that all people in the WTC complex and nearby area should be evacuated." (9/11 Commission Report, 2004, p. 309).

10:07 A.M.   The pilot of Aviation 14 radioed: "Advise everyone to evacuate the area in vicinity of Battery Park City. . . . About fifteen floors down from the top, it looks like it's glowing red. It's inevitable" (Dwyer & Flynn, 2005, p. 223)."To be certain that the message was delivered, the dispatcher repeated it, practically word by word, so that all the police officers on the air heard the warning. 'All right, he said from the 15th floor down, it looked like the building was going to collapse and we need to evacuate everyone'" (Dwyer & Flynn, 2005, p. 223).

10:08 A.M.   A moment later, the pilot of Aviation 6 reported, "I don't think this has too much longer to go, I would evacuate all people within the area of the second building" (Dwyer and Flynn, 2005, p. 223; supported by 9/11 Commission Report, 2004, p.309 and 9/11 Commission Staff Report #13, 2004, p. 25).

10:20 A.M.   "NYPD aviation unit reports that the top of the tower might be leaning" (National Institute of Standards and Technology [NIST], 2005, p. 37).

10:21 A.M.   "NYPD aviation unit reports that the North Tower is buckling on the southwest corner and leaning to the south" (NIST, 2005, p. 37)."NYPD officer advises that all personnel close to the building pull back three blocks in every direction" (NIST, 2005, p. 37).

10:27 A.M.   "NYPD aviation unit reports that the roof is going to come down very shortly" (NIST, 2005, p. 37).

These reports make it clear that NYPD officers had a comprehensive situational awareness not only of the collapse of the South Tower but also the imminent danger of collapse to the building they were occupying. The McKinsey Report states that NYPD Aviation warned the police department "that WTC 1 collapse is likely and advises immediate evacuation" (2002, p. 50). The officers who received these messages were able to correctly interpret the information they received and quickly leave the building. Each subsequent message had a cumulative effect of added urgency, plus multiple validations of the original report.

Eyewitness reports indicate that ESU officers did not remain and, at one point, were jumping from landing to landing by sliding down the stair banisters. These reports confirm the importance of the helicopter messages for understanding that the building was about to buckle and that the officers

needed to rapidly leave the building. For these officers, the situational-awareness reports they received from NYPD Aviation and fellow officers outside the building were critical to their escape from the North Tower and most likely saved their lives.

FDNY Unhurried Evacuation

The situational-awareness picture for the Fire Department of the City of New York (FDNY) was vastly different from that of the police department. When the South Tower came down at 9:59 A.M., rescuers on the upper floors of the North Tower felt the building shake, similar to what is felt when a small earthquake occurs. Simultaneously, operational commanders in the lobby had debris dust fill their location, forcing them to move to a passageway between the North Tower and 6 World Trade Center (the adjacent building). As the South Tower disintegrated in front of them, the Chief of Department and his command staff, located on the far side of West Street, abandoned their command post and took shelter in a parking garage under the World Financial Center. Throughout the incident, there was an absence of any NYPD commanders at both the incident command post and the operations section. These facts set the stage for operational stovepipe situational awareness and the looming disaster.

10:00 A.M.   "The South Tower total collapse was immediately communicated on the Manhattan dispatch channel by an FDNY [fire] boat . . . but no one at the site received this information, because every FDNY command post had been abandoned" (9/11 Commission Report, 2004, p. 306)."Despite the lack of knowledge of what had happened to the South Tower, a chief in the process of evacuating the North Tower lobby sent out an order within a minute of the collapse: 'Command to all units in Tower 1, evacuate the building'" (9/11 Commission Report, 2004, p. 306). Within minutes, some of the firefighters heard the evacuation order. "At least two battalion chiefs on the upper floors of the North Tower . . . heard the evacuation instruction . . . and repeated it to everyone they came across" (9/11 Commission Report, 2004, p. 307).

10:10 A.M.   Another chief (after moving from the lobby of the North Tower to the North Bridge) "soon followed with an additional evacuation order" (9/11 Commission Report, 2004, p. 306).

10:15 A.M.   The Chief of Department issued a radio
order for all units to evacuate the North
Tower (9/11 Commission Report, 2004,
p. 308).

Of the 100 interviews conducted by the 9/11
Commission and its review of 500 internal oral
histories from members of the FDNY, only three
firefighters mentioned hearing any possibility of
"imminent collapse" (2004, p. 550). Indeed, most
of the firefighters in the North Tower had little
idea that the South Tower had fallen and did not
receive warning messages from police aviation
predicting the collapse of the North Tower (9/11
Commission Report, 2004, p. 554). The FDNY, as
well as the Port Authority police, were never provided with the critical information that the NYPD
possessed.

The Importance of Sharing Information

Although the 9/11 Commission shied away from
using the term *stovepipe situational awareness* to
describe interagency communication, it did recognize that critical information was not shared
among agencies and that FDNY chiefs would have
benefited greatly had they been able to receive the
same situational-awareness picture as the NYPD
(2004, p. 321). The situational-awareness picture
for the fire department members inside the North
Tower was limited to a rumbling sound and orders
to evacuate the building. The fire department received no updates about the spreading fire or the
deterioration of the building. They were given no
warnings from the helicopters of the building's
possible collapse, which would have reinforced the
absolute necessity for a rapid mass departure.

Essential to situational awareness is the need
to make sense of the information one receives.
Organizational psychologist Karl Weick has described the basic human process of "sensemaking"
as a "search for context within which small details
fit together and make sense" (1995, p. 133). The
more detailed the information, the better the
sense-making capability of the receiver.

The NYPD and FDNY case studies dramatically portray how emergency responders reacted to
different levels of situational awareness. Informa-

tion about the collapse of the South Tower, the
spread of the fire, and the potential collapse of the
North Tower provided the police department with
enough data to precipitate a rapid escape, while
the lack of similar information for the fire department translated into an unhurried evacuation—and
its lethal consequences. These facts illustrate how
information sharing—and the lack of it—affected
the emergency responders' interpretation of the
evacuation orders.

The strongest statement about the dangers of
stovepipe situational awareness comes from an
investigation conducted by the National Institute
of Standards and Technology (NIST). The study
concludes that "a preponderance of evidence indicates that emergency responder lives were likely
lost at the WTC resulting from the lack of timely
information-sharing and inadequate communication capabilities" (2005, p. 174). This is further
clarified by the 9/11 Commission Report that any
radio failure, while important, "was not the primary cause of many firefighters' deaths in the
North Tower" (2004, p. 323). The reason so many
firefighters died in the North Tower was that commanders who received vital messages from their
helicopters never shared that information with the
FDNY, resulting in an uneven distribution of critical information.

An unhurried evacuation made perfect sense
to those who lacked situational awareness in the
North Tower. A rapid evacuation made equally
perfect sense to those police officers who heard the
repeated warnings of the North Tower's possible
collapse. "If events are noticed, people make sense
of them, and if events are not noticed, they are not
available for sensemaking" (Starbuck & Milliken,
1988, p. 60). Those emergency responders who
had the power of situational awareness were able
to avoid being trapped in the collapse of the North
Tower; those without it did not stand a chance.

Effective incident command is dependant
upon strengthening information sharing to maintain common situational awareness. When an organization possesses critical information, it must
be immediately shared with other commanders and
all emergency responders operating at an incident.
Only then can emergency responders make sense
of and react quickly to new messages. *The single
most important safety lesson learned by emergency
responders on 9/11 is simply to share information.*

Understanding Organizational Bias

These case studies reveal the vital role that information sharing or lack of it played in the decisions that were made at the World Trade Center. It is shocking to think that critical information was not shared among the first responders from these New York City agencies. Some observers would like to conclude that a technological problem with portable radios was to blame, but the 9/11 Commission Report confirms that the evacuation messages were indeed heard (2004, p. 554). Furthermore, the NIST investigation concludes that the WTC repeater (a system to boost radio signals) was incapable of working after the South Tower collapsed and would not have assisted in the evacuation of firefighters from the North Tower (2005, p. 138).

Inadequate radio interoperability is another theory that may help to account for the communication gap among the agencies. However, agencies, commanders, and personnel were within a short distance of each other (NIST, 2005, p. 162). Regardless of any history of infighting between the police and the fire department, it is inconceivable that any commander would ever deliberately withhold vital information that could save the lives of personnel from other organizations. With that in mind, a critical question arises: Why did police commanders—over the course of 29 minutes—remove their members from the vicinity of the towers and fail to inform the fire department of the dangers observed by police aviation? One answer lies in years of organizational biases within the first responder community, whose organizations are generally autonomous. This is not a conscious bias but rather a long-standing bias on a systematic level.

Organizational bias stems from the desire to belong to an omnipotent group that is capable of excluding those who are not part of the group. In government, it is usually demonstrated through command power and the authority to control information. The turf battles between the NYPD and the FDNY mirror those of CIA and the FBI, which was made public during the 9/11 Commission investigation (Staff Report #9, 2004). In both instances, the key to understanding the failure to share information for command of incidents or operations is ultimately a quest for the superiority of one agency over the other.

This intergroup competition is illustrated by an absence of cooperation, duplication of effort, and strict control of information that might benefit other groups. One frequently wishes to exclude the others from an operation or is not forthcoming with information simply to demonstrate its perceived power. This bias not only gives one group an advantage over another but also systematically conditions groups to think only of themselves.

One would expect that these social biases would be abandoned during times of crises; however, the WTC case studies illustrate a stronger partiality for an individual group's self-interest, which in this case proved to be a fatal flaw for the first responders. Even with thousands of police officers and firefighters at the scene and many only a few feet from each other, reports from the police helicopter never reached any of the fire chiefs. During the 9/11 World Trade Center attack, the first responders were unable to overcome their organizational biases, thus causing a fragmented command structure. One can observe the ramification of these biases under three different command conditions:

- resistance to a single incident commander
- development of blind spots in command capacity
- diffusion of personal command responsibility

The first command condition is the failure of the preincident planners to recognize that, at terrorism incidents with multiple agencies present, social biases cause organizations to resist the control wielded by a single incident commander. The WTC response depicted a refusal by certain agencies to operate under the authority of the fire department's incident commander. Even though both WTC Towers were on fire, "there is no record that the ICP [Incident Command Post] had any senior NYPD personnel assigned to it to provide liaison or assist with operations" (NIST, 2005, pp.161–162). Agencies implicitly think of themselves as being the most important, and, as a group, their natural tendency is to resist deferring to another organization. This is especially true for police and fire departments whose organizational development reinforces a sense of belonging to an important group. These organizations call themselves the "Finest" and "Bravest," and each one has significant roles to play during a terrorist incident.

During large, complex incidents, agencies must change this perception by viewing themselves as part of a unified command, whose members are equally important and necessary to the operation. Doing so will eliminate the tendency to withhold information in the quest for retaining or acquiring power. Organizational social biases will engender considerable resistance to accepting the authority of a single incident commander who is not "one of their own" when the group believes its right to command is equally important to the outcome of the incident.

The second command condition is the development of blind spots in command capacity. These develop as part of a group prejudice toward members of the same group and against those who do not belong to the group. This was evident in the case studies of instances in which information was provided within one group but not shared across groups. It has also been found that, as the stress and complexity of a crisis increase, people tend to narrow their focus on aspects judged most important to them (Weick, 1995, p. 102).

As the intensity of the WTC crisis mounted, commanders became so focused on central organizational tasks that they neglected to perform the critical task of sharing information. Their command capacity became so myopic that they failed to recognize the fact that the reports from helicopters would be of crucial importance to the fire department. Critical messages were never passed from the police to the firefighters or their commanders, nor did the fire commanders ever request information from the police on conditions as seen from the helicopters. Both organizations were so preoccupied with performing their own operations that they developed blind spots that reduced their own command capacity. These agencies never crossed group boundaries to consider the welfare of the other, nor did they consider how the other could have contributed to the welfare of their own organization.

The third command condition is organizational diffusion of responsibility away from the individual and toward the group. Hearing reports from police aviation warning of structural failure, many ranking police officers in the street acted quickly to move their members to safety, yet they never considered telling the fire department. When asked to account for this oversight, they could not explain why they pulled back police officers but

did not also ensure that firefighters were quickly withdrawn. The only rationale they gave was, "I thought the fire department was evacuating, too." Indeed a few of the firefighters and police officers together in the North Tower felt individually responsible to tell each other to evacuate the building, but there is no evidence that detailed messages from the helicopters were ever relayed to the fire personnel. Most disconcerting of all is the fact that police commanders did not feel individually responsible for ensuring that the fire department understood that it was vital to evacuate the North Tower (Figure 15.1).

Similar group dynamics played out in 1964, when 38 people could not explain why they did not phone police as they witnessed the stabbing death of Kitty Genovese in Forest Hills (Gladwell, 2000, p. 27). In these cases, "the presence of others diffused the sense of personal responsibility of any individual" (Zimbardo, 2004, p. 42). When people are in a group, they assume that someone else will make the notification, or, since no one is acting, there is not really an urgent problem.

On 9/11, it was assumed that a police commander had to have told the fire department about the messages from police aviation. Or it was assumed that it was not a problem if the fire department did not receive this exclusive information about the fire on the upper floors because they were evacuating their members anyway. To this day, there has not been a public statement of a sense of personal responsibility by any police commander for not sharing information with the fire department. That absence of acknowledgement supports the theory that people feel less responsible for their behavior when their focus is narrowed by an ingroup mentality. Ironically, if there had been a unified command at the WTC with one fire department incident commander and one police department incident commander, there would have been a sense of responsibility not only for one's own organization but also for the other's. As a result, many more firefighters and other emergency responders would be alive today.

Unified Command

Evaluating the events of 9/11 and the effects of systematic social bias is not intended to assign blame or exonerate any first responder. It is in-

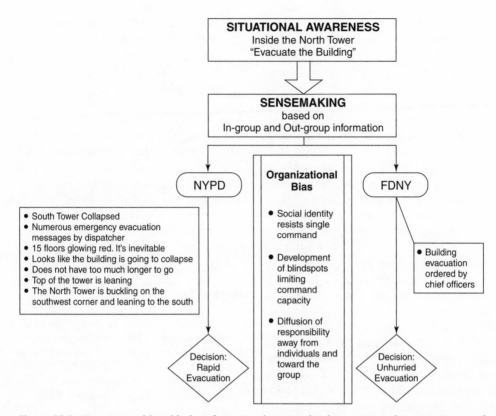

Figure 15.1. Organizational bias blocks information sharing and reduces sense making. Routine use of unified command removes organizational biases.

tended to help develop a command system that is resilient enough to overcome these organizational biases in future crises. The World Trade Center responses demonstrate the shortcomings of advocating a single incident commander or separate parallel commands. After completing its investigation, the 9/11 Commission Report strongly recommended that "when multiple agencies or multiple jurisdictions are involved, they should adopt a unified command" (2004, p. 397).

To overcome organizational bias, agencies with a major role at terrorist events must not seek to control each other but instead work equally in synergistic fashion to command the responses of their members. A unified command allows agencies with different functional responsibilities to work effectively together without affecting their individual authority (National Incident Management System, 2004, pp. 11–12). Incident commanders in a unified command structure will eliminate organizational blind spots by combining their knowledge to build a more robust authority.

Each incident commander will take individual responsibility for jointly sharing information and developing operational objectives. Incident commanders in this unified structure will have prior training and a new sense of control and will be personally responsible to one another for all of the actions taken at an incident.

Today's homeland security efforts of joint exercises under a unified command provide a good first step. However, it may not be enough to overcome these ingrained social biases. It is documented that, as stress increases, people tend to abandon recently learned responses and fall back on overlearned systematic responses (Barthol & Ku, 1959; Weick, 1995). Public service organizations need to repeatedly practice systematically depending on each other at small incidents, as well as at large-scale terrorist events. During these incidents, it is necessary to develop a network of organizations that uses common language and participate in everyday social interaction (Walsh & Ungson, 1991, p. 60). Organizations that seek power over others through their endorsement of a single commander at interagency incidents will revert to an individual group bias during a terrorist event. Only through daily practice of unified command and organizational interdependency can agencies hope to prevail over systematic social biases, thereby enabling organizations to coordinate their strengths in effectively dealing with the next terrorist incident.

Effective commanding during a crisis is dependant upon overcoming organizational biases and strengthening information sharing to maintain a common situational-awareness picture of the crisis venue. When organizations possess critical information, members must feel responsible for sharing it with other emergency responders operating at an incident. Information sharing provides emergency responders with an opportunity to make sense of any emergent ambiguity and to act quickly in response to new messages.

Finally, there is the need for building a synergistic response network for preparedness. This point cannot be overstated. The term *network* implies interconnection into a cohesive fabric. In the context of incident response, this cohesion is possible only through a thorough familiarity with the capabilities and limitations of each member of the network and a willingness to overcome organizational bias to ensure a free flow of information among all of the members.

Conclusion

The actions taken inside and outside the Twin Towers were analyzed for systematic insight on crisis management. It is not my intent to single out the successes and failures of individuals or even particular organizations but rather to use the events of 9/11 to examine emergency response as a whole and determine what is needed to build an integrated response system that will foster future preparedness.

This glimpse of duty at the World Trade Center may give us the greatest opportunity for saving lives in the future. This chapter centers on understanding how organizational biases affect information sharing and decision making when rescue personnel are stretched beyond their capacity by the shock and cumulative stress of a terrorist attack. Failure to carefully examine these issues

may place emergency responders at even greater risk at the next incident.

Commanding complex incidents is directly connected to the systematic development of a unified command at everyday incidents and the construction of a mutual system of respectful interaction. Unless our public service organizations can be integrated into a unified command group, where decisions are made with full awareness of the capabilities and capacities of each of the relevant groups, we are doomed to be governed by our organizational biases and repeat the mistakes of limiting command capacity at the most important times in the lives of the communities we have pledged to serve.

Note

1. The 9/11 Commission Report, the WTC investigation carried out by the National Institute of Standards and Technology (NIST), the NYPD McKinsey Report, and *New York Times* authors Dwyer and Flynn have noted slightly different times for each NYPD helicopter report. However, they agree on content.

References

The 9/11 Commission Report, (2004). *Final Report of the National Commission on Terrorist Attacks Upon the United States.* New York: Norton.

The 9/11 Commission Staff Report #13 (2004, May 18). *Emergency preparedness and response.* Retrieved January 18, 2006, from http://9–11commission. gov/staff_statements/staff_statement_13.pdf.

Barthol, R. P., & Ku, N. D. (1959). Regression under stress to first learned behavior. *Journal of Abnormal and Social Psychology, 59,* 134–136.

Deaux, K. (1996). Social identification. In E. T. Higgins & A. W. Kruglanski (Eds.), *Social psychology: Handbook of basic principles* (pp. 777–798). New York: Guilford.

Dwyer, J., & Flynn, K. (2005). *102 minutes: The untold story of the fight to survive inside the Twin Towers.* New York: Times Books.

Gladwell, M. (2002). *The tipping point: How little things can make a big difference.* New York: Little, Brown.

McKinsey & Company. (2002). *Improving NYPD emergency preparedness and response.* New York: New York City Police Department.

National Incident Management System. (2004). Department of Homeland Security. Washington, D.C.

Retrieved January 18, 2006, from http://www.dhs.gov/interweb/assetlibrary/NIMS-90-web.pdf.

National Institute of Standards and Technology (NIST). (2005). *Federal building and fire safety investigation of the World Trade Center disaster: The emergency response operation.* Retrieved January 18, 2006, from http://wtc.nist.gov/pubs/NISTNCSTAR1-8.pdf.

Starbuck, W. H., & Milliken, F. J. (1988). Executives' perceptual filters: What they notice and how they make sense. In D. C. Hambrick (Ed.), *The executive effect: Concepts and methods for studying top managers* (pp. 35–65). Greenwich, CT: JAI Press.

Walsh, J. P., & Ungson, G. R. (1991). Organizational memory. *Academy of Management Review, 16,* 57–91.

Weick, K. E. (1995). *Sensemaking in organizations.* Thousand Oaks, CA: Sage.

Zimbardo, P. G. (2004). A situationist perspective on the psychology of evil. In A. Miller (Ed.), *The social psychology of good and evil* (pp. 21–50). New York: Guilford.

16

Warfare, Terrorism, and Psychology

L. Morgan Banks
Larry C. James

The history of our species is one of almost continual conflict interspersed with brief periods of peace. Competition, initially between individuals, then tribal units, and finally nation-states and groups of nation-states, is a fundamental theme of our existence. In its most intense and modern form, we refer to this competition as warfare. The purpose of this conflict—of war—is almost never the physical destruction of an opposing group. The real purpose, most often, is for one group to get the other to do something it would not ordinarily do. In military terminology, we say that our purpose is to impose our will on the enemy (Clausewitz, 1993, p. 83). Of course, what we are really talking about is behavior modification. Very rarely has the overall purpose of conflict been to annihilate another group of people (Figure 16.1).

There are certainly exceptions, and the twentieth century had some notable ones, but more often than not, there is a clear political purpose that transcends the military defeat of an enemy. Access to resources is perhaps the most common objective. Be it lebensraum, access to oil, or room for westward expansion, the underlying reason today is usually economic. In one sense this is a circular statement since almost everything that affects a country is essentially economic, but the

point is that the underlying goal is usually *not* one of simple destruction or extermination.

There are some very logical reasons for this. Once a people or a country believe that extermination is the real purpose of a conflict, they will ordinarily fight for survival with fierce determination—not something any enemy usually desires.[1] If simple destruction or killing of the enemy were sufficient, then wars would generally be won or lost based on casualties. As even a brief glimpse of history shows, that is not the case. In fact, it is not uncommon for the victor to accept greater casualties than the side that is defeated (Figure 16.2).

In the U.S. Civil War the North had many more casualties than the South. Now, it is true that since they had larger armies, their disease numbers were higher, even though the rate of disease was actually lower. However, even when looking at battle casualties alone, the number of casualties the North suffered was about 17% greater than what the South endured (Figure 16.3).

The numbers from World War I are equally startling. Although the statistics in Figure 16.4 are not as accurate as we might hope, nevertheless the contrast is stark.

In perhaps the most remarkable case of all—Vietnam—the numbers look like this: The total of

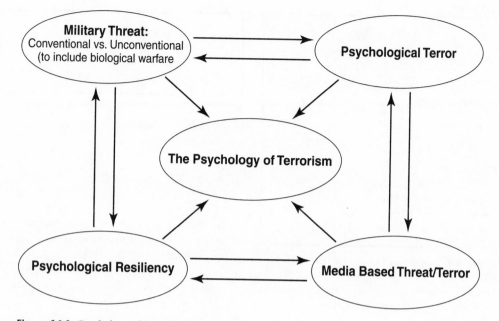

Figure 16.1. Psychology of terrorism model.

all U.S. allied deaths was about one-quarter that experienced by the North Vietnamese/Vietcong (Figure 16.5). And this was a case in which the United States had a tremendous technological advantage.

Of course, there are plenty of examples of the opposite situation, also. With that in mind, we assert that the psychological hardiness—morale, esprit de corps—of a military force is often what will win the day, in spite of fighting a larger foe.

In Singapore in February 1942, Japanese Lieutenant General Yamashita led an attack against the British garrison commanded by Lieutenant General Percival. Yamashita had approximately 40,000 troops, while Percival had more than 107,000. The Japanese troops had very high morale, whereas Percival's troops did not. The British made a number of poor decisions, and after only a few days of fighting, Percival decided to surrender

the garrison. Ironically, when the British surrendered, the Japanese had enough ammunition for only 3 more days of fighting (Perrett, 1993, p. 272).

Contrast that with the Japanese attack on Wake Island in December of 1941. A very small island, isolated and with no chance of reinforcements or relief, had about 400 marine infantry, 12 fighter planes, and about 1,100 civilian construction workers. The first Japanese attack consisted of 1 light cruiser, 2 older cruisers, 6 destroyers, 2 destroyer transports, 2 transports, 2 submarines, and a 450-man naval infantry landing force. The Japanese were repulsed on their first attempt and came back a week later with 2 fleet carriers, 6 heavy cruisers, 6 destroyers, and a 1,000-man naval landing force, with a 500-man reserve. The resulting casualty numbers were 49 marines, 3 seamen, and

---

The best thing of all is to take the enemy's country whole and intact; to shatter and destroy it is not so good.... It is better to capture an entire army than to destroy it.
Sun Tzu, 490 BC

Figure 16.2. *Source:* J. Wintle (Ed.), *The Dictionary of War Quotations* (New York: Free Press, 1989), p. 19.

American Civil War			
North		**South**	
• Battle Deaths	112,000	• Battle Deaths	94,000
• Disease, etc.	227,500	• Disease, etc.	164,000
• Total Deaths	339,500	• Total Deaths	258,000

Figure 16.3. American Civil War casualties.
Source: A. R. Millet & P. Maslowski, *For the Common Defense: A Military History of the United States of America* (New York: Free Press, 1984), 229.

The Great War			
Allies		**Central Powers**	
• Russia	1,700 K	• Germany	1,774 K
• France	1,376 K	• Austria-	1,200 K
		Hungary	
• British Empire	908 K	• Turkey	325 K
• Italy	650 K	• Bulgaria	88 K
• Romania	336 K		
• United States	126 K		
• Serbia	45 K		
• Belgium	14 K		
• Others*	12 K		
• **Total**	**5,167 K**	• **Total**	**3,387 K**
*Portugal, Greece, and Japan			

Figure 16.4. World War I casualties.
Source: S. Everett, *The Two World Wars, Vol. I. World War I* (Greenwich, CT: Bison Books, 1980). Quoted at http://www.worldwar1.com/tlcrates.htm.

70 construction workers killed, versus 4 destroyers, 1 destroyer transport, 1 submarine sunk, and at least 900 Japanese killed (Perrett, 1993, p. 308).

We are not suggesting that morale and psychological hardiness can win every battle. For example, at the battle of the Little Bighorn, Custer lost all 250 members of his attacking element, compared to 50 lost by Chiefs Sitting Bull and Crazy Horse. Having said that, the historical record makes it clear that Custer was not able to maintain appropriate command and control over his forces, nor was he able to effectively use his better disciplined soldiers against the less disciplined, but overwhelming, enemy force.

Vietnam War			
Killed in Action Estimates			
• United States	47,400	• NVA/VC	1,100,000
• ARVN	224,000		
• Other Allies	5,000		
• Total	276,400		1,100,000

Figure 16.5. Vietnam War casualties.
Source: Compiled from U.S. National Archives and Records Administration (2002), Retrieved April 24, 2005, from http://www.archives.gov/research_room/research_topics/vietnam_war_casualty_lists/statistics.html; also at Wikipedia, retrieved February 4, 2006, from http://en.wikipedia.org/wiki/Vietnam_War#casualties.

Supreme excellence consists in breaking the enemy's resistance without fighting.
Sun Tzu, 490 BC

Figure 16.6. *Source:* J. Wintle (Ed.), *The Dictionary of War Quotations* (New York: Free Press, 1989), p. 19.

Rather, the point is that most warfare is essentially psychological in nature. That may sound like an absurd statement since there are usually more than a few nonpsychological injuries that occur on the battlefield. Why then do we cause so much destruction while conducting warfare? We maintain that we ordinarily conduct warfare in the manner we do because of its psychological effects (Figure 16.6).

In other words, we cause destruction because of the psychological effect that it has or that we expect it to have on an opponent. Again, there are some rather well-used (but used for good reason) examples of this.

Japan—Hiroshima, Nagasaki, Tokyo

When the Germans began the bombing of London in World War II, they believed it would cause a great sag in the morale of British citizens. The people of London endured continuous bombing and watched as their modern city was destroyed block by block. There was little of military significance that was destroyed, however.

The same argument applies to the U.S. decision to begin its firebombing campaign in Japan, although it is true that Japan's manufacturing capability was spread throughout its cities. The firebombing of Tokyo on March 9, 1945, killed 83,793 men, women, and children, injured another 40,918, and left more than a million people homeless (Weigley, 1977, p. 364).

In neither case did the bombing have the desired effect. In London, the citizens rallied, and the country appeared to intensify both its opposition to Germany and its determination to win the war. Although today great controversy still surrounds the Tokyo bombing and the subsequent use of atomic weapons on Hiroshima and Nagasaki, the Tokyo firebombing did not immediately end the war with Japan.

On the other hand, the use of atomic weapons did accomplish that objective. In Hiroshima, 70,000–80,000 people died instantly, and an equal number were injured. In Nagasaki, about 35,000 people died at once (Weigley, 1977, p. 365). Why did one cause immediate capitulation and not the other?

Speaking militarily, if the purpose of warfare is to impose our will on the enemy, then we must defeat our adversary. The point, however, is not that we must kill, maim, and destroy the enemy but only that we must defeat our foe. The implied term here is *psychological* defeat.

If any country wishes to impose its will on another, then it must devise a way to psychologically defeat it. One can do this through bloodshed and starvation, as in the U.S. Civil War, or by convincing the enemy that "resistance is futile." In the Gulf war, the United States dropped many bombs on the Iraqi soldiers in the trenches. Although some members of the U.S. Air Force may contest this, the truth is that the bombing killed relatively few Iraqi soldiers. However, the constant bombing and the inability of the Iraqi forces to take any effective action against us produced a response many of us would call learned helplessness. When the ground war began, Iraqi soldiers surrendered by the thousands, and, although there were exceptions, very few put up a stubborn resistance.

In truth, then, defeat—like terrorism—is a psychological concept. Germany was militarily beaten in World War I, but was it defeated? Enemy forces never really set foot in Germany. The people were certainly beginning to feel the effects of the war, but most of them believed they were somehow cheated. The imposed reparations simply added to the buildup of animosity against Britain and France.

At the end of the Vietnam War, the United States was not militarily defeated. We had basically won every battle. Nevertheless, we were psychologically defeated by a strategy that outsmarted us.

George Washington was not a fan of the militia. He believed that it did not have the necessary discipline to fight in a tough battle and would run at the first opportunity (Figure 16.7).

Washington felt that way in part because the militia would not stand up to the British soldiers' bayonet charge. The militia's rifles took a long time to reload and lacked bayonets. Once the militia had fired, the British would charge and be on them with bayonets before they could reload. The very image

> To place any dependence upon militia is assuredly resting upon a broken staff.
> George Washington, letter to Congress, September 1776

Figure 16.7. *Source:* J. Wintle (Ed.), *The Dictionary of War Quotations* (New York: Free Press, 1989), p. 65.

of a line of British soldiers charging with bayonets would make anyone run. In modern warfare, the tank often provokes the same type of response. Military training teaches soldiers that "perception is reality." Our perception of the threat, rather than the threat itself, is the power of terrorism.

Terrorism

How does this concept relate to terrorism? Figure 16.8 presents the army's definition of terrorism, and it is probably as good as most.

As McCauley has pointed out, the distinction between combatants and noncombatants—built up over the centuries—began to erode in the early 1800s with the Grande Armie of Napoleon (McCauley, n.d.). Since then, few wars have been fought only by the military.

The purpose of terrorism is essentially the same as more conventionally oriented warfare, that is, to get governments or societies to do what the terrorist wants. One real difference is that it is conducted by an opponent who does not have the military strength to fight directly. We contend that this type of warfare relies most heavily on the use

> Terrorism
> The calculated use of unlawful violence or threat of unlawful violence to inculcate fear; intended to coerce or to intimidate governments or societies in the pursuit of goals that are generally political, religious, or ideological

Figure 16.8. Definition of terrorism.
Source: Joint Publication 1-02, Department of Defense Dictionary of Military and Associated Terms. Retrieved February 4, 2006, from http://www.dtic.mil/doctrine/jel/doddict/data/t/05394.html.

of psychology. We also believe that Osama bin Laden wanted, as one of his goals, to get the United States out of the Middle East. He calculated that we, as a country, would psychologically run away from the horror he was inflicting on us. (He received bad advice on that.)

In our opinion, there is no better recent example of how one side wished to psychologically defeat another than the overall strategy that bin Laden attempted in his war against us. First, he would demonstrate our vulnerability in what we consider the safest of refuges. He would shock us by killing indiscriminately. In other words, not that he would use this term, he would try to induce learned helplessness in us. Consequently, we would be forced to take some action against him. Then, when we attacked him on his territory, he would maul us—causing many Americans to come home in body bags. His view of the Russian invasion and subsequent departure from Afghanistan was that he and his Mujahedeen had defeated the Russians, and he viewed the Russian military as stronger than the United States. Once we as a country had experienced the horror of war in Afghanistan, he believed that we, too, would leave in defeat—again, just as he had seen in Somalia and just as he believed happened in Vietnam. Because he believed his side was founded on stronger principles—a strong and abiding Islamic faith—there could be no other outcome than the routing of the decadent Western forces. Said another way, bin Laden's goal was not to conquer our military forces (although he actually believed he could do that) but rather to defeat the country psychologically.

Psychology and Psychologists

What does any of this have to do with psychology? As we mentioned earlier, we believe that bin Laden predicted that the United States would recoil from the horror of 9/11. And if we actually sent in ground troops, he would maul us, and we would run away—just as he had seen us do in Somalia and as he had heard we responded in Vietnam.

There is a great deal that would have supported his expectation, especially if one performs a quick review of our psychology literature. For a variety of very good reasons, we focus our energy, research, and treatment on the understanding and remediation of illness. In this context, we have spent a great deal of time studying the effects of traumatic stress. As one might expect, our focus is not usually on the positive aspects of humans under stress but instead is on the negative results of stress and ways to remediate them. (We are certainly not saying that this is a bad thing. One could easily argue that this is the foundation of our science.)

The county in which one of us lives recently went through a severe drought. Mandatory conservation efforts were put into effect, including the use of disposable tableware at restaurants and an appeal to citizens to refrain from watering lawns and washing cars. The most significant request, though, was for voluntary reductions in household water use. As a result of people's response, the rate of water use went from 6.1 million gallons per day to 1.9 million gallons, and most of the decrease was credited to the reductions in household use. This small community pulled together, with neighbor helping neighbor. As Seneca once said, "the good things which belong to prosperity are to be wished, but the good things that belong to adversity are to be admired" (Lucius Annaeus Seneca Quotes, 2005).

Much has been said concerning psychology's focus on pathology. Seligman (1991) has made a strong case that we should review the way in which we address strength and virtue—his work on positive psychology (Seligman, 1991). For 20 years, one of us has been deeply involved in helping soldiers survive the rigors of warfare. As a friend of ours is fond of saying, the goal is to have soldiers moderately aroused while under stresses that would seem to most of us to be unmanageable—such as being in combat. It is not just that we should study strength and virtue. Rather, how do we manage to get men and women to do incredible things under very high levels of stress? How do we resist the forces of terrorism? We maintain that focusing on treating people who have been exposed to this horror as victims is the wrong way to resist.

Unfortunately, over the years we have had to talk to a fair number of people following tragedy. What has always amazed us is the incredible strength that people have. Yes, we know there is a price to be paid. Nothing is free. People who have undergone great tragedy will always carry that with them. However, as Eric Maria Remarque said in his book about a physician living through the Nazi occupation of Paris, "Human beings can stand a great deal" (Remarque, 1945, p. 455). We maintain that it is critical to treat people as though they have resources, not as though they lack them. We must instill competence and confidence to survive another tragedy.

Strength of character, steadfastness in the face of adversity, physical bravery—not just the type that soldiers discuss but that of firefighters and everyday Americans on 9/11—we believe that these are subjects for us to ponder, study, and encourage. We continue to expand our knowledge of the negative effects of stress. At the same time, we need to expand our knowledge of the value of stress and the factors that help develop bravery, courage, and integrity under stress. People are victims only when they decide they have no control over their lives. We are not a nation of victims. We are the most powerful, free, creative, and generous nation on earth because we are doing something right.

A Model for Understanding the Psychology of Terrorism

Understanding the psychology of terrorism can be a daunting task because the act of (as well as the psychology of) terrorism is a complicated process. Those who want to employ psychological terror against us have many ways to enhance our sense of psychological vulnerability and to psychologically attack us. One way to conceptualize this involves a paradigm that examines the dynamics of the military and the psychological threat, perhaps enhanced by a media-influenced perception and our psychological resilience.

Military Threat

Earlier in this chapter we explained how the perception of success or failure, sometimes in direct contradiction to actual success or failure, can be the major determining factor of a battle. The power of this perception has even served to psychologically deter actions of other nations. For example, the United States, during the military buildup of the Cold War era, deterred Eastern bloc countries from attacking with the psychological threat of our overwhelming force and technology—without firing a single missile.

Frequently, the perception of military threat is shaped via a media-based perception of peril. In other words, terrorists will use the media (usually in the form of television or radio news reports) to provide a community, region, or nation with a perceived threat of attack with car bombs, hostage taking, suicide bombers, and so on. Even though the actual military threat to national security may be minimal, the perception is that the threat is real. Modern-day terrorists may not possess as many tanks as the United States during the Cold War, but their threats appear real due to their use of the media in shaping a nation's perception.

Psychological Threat and Terror

In many of the third-world regions, military threat may in fact be less fear provoking than that of the conventional forces of Western society. However, these units from third-world regions employ psychological terror to manipulate and shape the behavior of others. Let us use some recent examples of the application of psychological terror. Shortly after 9/11, anthrax was mailed to a major Washington, D.C., post office building, one of the Senate office buildings, and the post offices at Walter Reed Army Medical Center. A few people died as a result, compared to the thousands of people killed in the World Trade Center bombings. Yet, the psychological terror instilled by the anthrax attack in Washington, D.C., paralleled the horror experienced in New York on September 11. In many cases, the psychological *threat* of biological and chemical weapons can be just as devastating psychologically as an actual attack with major military weapons. Sustained fear rather than death is the goal of psychological threat. When death and physical injuries are objectives as well, terrorists tend to select types of attacks that will kill, as well as provide lingering psychological terror in a particular population.

The Role of Psychological Resilience

Expose two people to the same traumatic event, and they may have very different psychological experiences. Why? One answer appears to have to do with the level of individual resilience. This capability may very well shape not only how people perceive an event but also how they respond at the time and how they physically and psychologically recover from the incident. A resilient person focuses on healthy coping strategies rather than on the event itself and the pathological responses it provokes.

How is resilience related to the psychology of terrorism? As the level of internal flexibility increases, the level of reported ongoing trauma decreases. Thus, it would serve communities well to develop programs that promote and teach resilience training as a response to acts of terrorism. One can argue that such an intervention may very well aid a community in its ability to recover from acts of psychological terror.

Notes

The opinions expressed in this article are those of the authors and do not reflect official policy of either the Department of Defense nor the U.S. Army.

1. For example, some historians have argued that, because the Japanese people believed that the allied forces in World War II wished to completely destroy their culture, the entire country was prepared to fight to the death (Weigley, 1977, p. 310). Certainly, the United States' experience on the islands of Tarawa and Okinawa would support this view. Out of a total of 4,836 Japanese forces, only 146 were captured. The rest died in combat (Perrett, 1993, p. 288).

References

Clausewitz, Carl von. (1993). *On war.* New York: Knopf.

Department of Defense. (2004). Joint Publication 1–02, Department of Defense Dictionary of Military and Associated Terms. Department of Defense, April 12, 2001 (as amended through November 30, 2004).

Lucius Annaeus Seneca Quotes. (2005). Retrieved January 19, 2006, from http://www.brainyquote.com/quotes/quotes/1/luciusanna154988.html.

McCauley, C. R. (n.d.). The psychology of terrorism. Retrieved January 19, 2006, from http://www.ssrc.org/sept11/essays/mccauley_text_only.htm.

Millet, A. R., & Maslowski, P. (1984). *For the common defense: A military history of the United States of America.* New York: Free Press, p. 229.

Perrett, B. (1993). *The battle book: Crucial conflicts in history from 1469 BC to the present.* London: Arms and Armour Press.

Remarque, E. M. (1945). *Arch of triumph* (W. Sorell & D. Lindley, Trans.). New York: Appleton-Century.

Seligman, M. E. P. (1991). *Learned optimism.* New York: Knopf.

U.S. National Archives and Records Administration. (2002). Retrieved April 24, 2005, from http://www.archives.gov/research_room/research_topics/vietnam_war_casualty_lists/statistics.html.

Weigley, R. F. (1977). *The American way of war: A history of United States Military strategy and policy.* Bloomington: Indiana University Press.

Wikipedia. (2005). Retrieved January 19, 2006, from http://en.wikipedia.org/wiki/Vietnam_War#casualties.

Wintle, J. (Ed.). (1989). *The dictionary of war quotations.* New York: Free Press.

IV

Assessment and Treatment

17

Terrorism Stress Risk Assessment and Management

Douglas Paton
John M. Violanti

Acts of terrorism represent a significant risk to mental health. When the World Trade Center and Pentagon were attacked on September 11, 2001, some 100,000 people witnessed the event directly, and millions more through the media. The consequent potential for psychological trauma was immense (Galea et al., 2002; Shuster et al., 2001; Yehuda, 2002). The protective services professionals and disaster mental health workers who respond to the needs of a community as a result of acts of terrorism are not immune from these consequences (Brown, Mulhern, & Joseph, 2002; Creamer & Liddle, 2005; Gorski, 2002; North et al., 2002), and the manner in which the risk to their mental health is conceptualized has acquired a significant new dimension since 9/11.

Protective service professionals (e.g., law enforcement officers, firefighters, military personnel) are in the front line for exposure to acts of terrorism that show no sign of abating. Managing the psychological consequences associated with experiencing these events has implications beyond safeguarding well-being. Stress adversely affects performance in circumstances that demand high levels of attention and creative solutions to emergent problems (Paton & Flin, 1999). Nowhere

are these demands more pronounced than in the context of responding to acts of terrorism (Grant, Hoover, Scarisbrick-Hauser, & Muffet 2003; Jackson, Baker, Ridgely, Bartis, & Linn, 2003; Kendra & Wachtendorf, 2003; Simpson & Stehr, 2003).

Recognition of the risk faced by protective services officers who confront the consequences of terrorist acts is reflected in the development of specific resources to assist them by the American Psychological Association (Carlson, James, Hobfoll, & Leskin, 2004; Leskin, Morland, Whealin, Everly, Litz, & Keane, 2004), and others (Cloak & Edwards, 2004; Gorski, 2002). However, the foundation upon which these resources are based does not represent a comprehensive account of the psychological consequences of response to terrorist events. For example, following the Oklahoma City bombing, North et al. (2002) noted that 77% of the firefighters self-appraised their post–Oklahoma bombing work performance as satisfactory or better. Furthermore, 39% endorsed positive changes from their work compared with 12% who endorsed negative changes (ibid.). The fact that traumatic experiences can be resolved as positive or negative outcomes begs the question of whether it is possible to influence this outcome. The risk management paradigm provides a framework within which we can answer this question.

The Risk Management Paradigm

While usually associated only with loss or deficit outcomes (e.g., PTSD), the risk management paradigm was developed to encapsulate both growth/ adaptation outcomes and deficit/loss outcomes (Dake, 1992; Hood & Jones, 1996). The risk management approach is built on the premise that, if we can identify the factors that predict positive and negative outcomes, we may be able to manipulate them in ways that enable us to make informed choices regarding the psychological consequences of responding to challenging events. According to this conceptualization, we can use our knowledge of these factors and how they interact to estimate stress risk and inform the development of risk management policies and practices. We can then implement these guidelines to increase personal, group, and organizational capacity to adapt to these demands (Creamer & Liddle, 2005; Paton, Violanti, Dunning, & Smith, 2004). That is, by defining event demands and characteristics as risk factors, we can reduce a priori assumptions of an automatic link between adverse events and distress outcomes and provide a more neutral content within which to consider the relationship between people and acts of terrorism. However, to manage this risk, there must exist a capability to make choices regarding outcomes by exercising control over the causes of adverse stress reactions or the factors that influence the way in which people interpret these experiences.

While the process of attempting to comprehend the scale and nature of the consequences of terrorist acts can represent a significant psychological challenge, terrorist stress risk factors can rarely be identified from the event (e.g., detonating a weapon of mass destruction, flying a plane into a building) per se. Stress risk factors can be more readily discerned in the hazardous event characteristics (e.g., threat to health, physical danger, working in protective clothing, confronting biohazardous agents, dealing with human remains, handling infectious materials, making complex and urgent decisions under conditions of uncertainty) that officers encounter when performing their professional role. A combination of these factors arising from sources over which they have little control and the very nature of emergency work precludes preventing exposure to terrorist events as a mitigation strategy. This does not, however, preclude seeking to manage this risk by altering the consequences of exposure to such events. If it is possible to exercise control over the factors that mediate the relationship between this exposure and its psychological consequences, it will be possible to manage stress risk in a proactive manner. There are several ways in which this might be achieved.

One approach would be to use stress inoculation and other training strategies to develop the interpretive mechanisms and competencies (e.g., understand the nature and consequences of critical incident work, decision making) required to accommodate the psychological implications of working in challenging operational environments. These strategies can help protect officers' well-being by providing them with a capacity to render threatening experiences meaningful. They can also facilitate the effective performance of their response role by providing the competencies required to deal with atypical operating demands (Dunning, 2003; Flin, 1996; Paton, 1994). Another approach involves developing organizational practices (e.g., incident management protocols, performance expectations, interagency cooperation) and an organizational culture (e.g., regarding emotional disclosure, reviewing response outcomes as sources of blame versus learning opportunities) that can help mitigate stress risk (Jackson et al., 2003; Paton, 1997; Paton & Jackson, 2002). Once articulated, knowledge of these processes provides a framework within which we can develop and implement stress risk management strategies.

Managing Stress Risk From Threatening Events

Risk can be managed before (primary and secondary prevention) or after (tertiary intervention) exposure. While several personal (e.g., individual competence can be enhanced through selection and training) and organizational (e.g., managing the demands of a multiagency response using interagency team development and decision making) factors are amenable to change prior to exposure, the complexity of terrorist events makes it impossible to mitigate all of the risks, and tertiary strategies are required to manage residual mental health issues (Violanti & Paton, 2006). However, the manner in which tertiary intervention is conceptualized should expand to accommodate the role of social and organizational factors (Paton & Stephens, 1996). Consequently, effective stress risk management will require a comprehensive approach, one that integrates all three perspectives.

While postevent strategies (e.g., debriefing) are routinely provided, the benefits of primary prevention are less well known (Carafano, 2003; Paton, 1994; Paton, Violanti, & Smith, 2003). The fact that protective services officers will be called upon repeatedly to deal with terrorist events and may experience prolonged periods of involvement under hazardous conditions makes a proactive approach particularly important. The importance of primary and secondary prevention is also heightened by the fact that any training and organizational development activities required to mitigate stress risk are not amenable to change through current postevent, tertiary prevention practices (e.g., debriefing). It can be provided only before officers' involvement, making it an essential component of an effective risk management strategy.

In this chapter, the development and implementation of primary prevention strategies is discussed in relation to the choices available at individual and organizational levels. With regard to the former, discussion focuses on the personal competencies and interpretive mechanisms required to render atypical and physically and psychologically threatening aspects of the experience (e.g., the nature of terrorism and its goals, dealing with human remains, exposure to biohazards) meaningful and coherent. The second line of inquiry focuses on identifying the organizational practices (e.g., degree to which authority is devolved, empowerment, interagency collaboration) that reflect sources of risk emanating from the response management paradigm (e.g., command and control, standard operating procedures), which defines how an agency responds to a crisis event. In the next section, the rationale for the inclusion of these perspectives within risk management is discussed.

Personal Factors

The concept of vulnerability has been evoked to explain the range of reactions that accompany exposure to traumatic events (Violanti & Paton, 2006). Blaikie, Cannon, Davis, and Wisner (1994) have defined vulnerability as the combination of characteristics of a person or group in terms of their capacity to anticipate, cope with, resist, and recover from hazardous impacts that threaten their life, well-being, and livelihood. The personal predictors of vulnerability reflect experiential, dispositional, and interpretive factors.

Officers' stress vulnerability is influenced by their history of traumatic experience prior to their employment (Violanti & Paton, 2006), as well as transient factors such as health status, fatigue, and psychological fitness. In their comprehensive account of posttrauma vulnerability, Scotti, Beach, Northrop, Rode, and Forsyth (1995) have identified three categories. The first concerns biological factors and genetically based predispositions (e.g., heightened autonomic and physiological reactivity) and changes in physiological reactivity as a consequence of earlier traumatic exposure. Second, historical antecedents such as learning history, experience of child abuse, preexisting psychopathology, and repetitive exposure to traumatic events also influence vulnerability. Finally, psychological factors such as learned avoidance of threat situations, social skills deficits that limit use of social support, hypervigilance of threat-relevant cues, and inadequate problem-solving behavior are identified for their potential to influence susceptibility to experiencing adverse posttrauma outcomes. However, the diverse nature of dispositional influences on vulnerability renders their organization in ways that can assist risk management problematic. One way in which vulnerability data from these different sources can be quantified and incorporated into the risk assessment process involves using a vulnerability coefficient that is estimated as a constant across a group of individuals (Violanti, 1990; Violanti & Paton, 2006).

While dispositional and personality factors can inform primary prevention through the recruitment and selection processes, the assessment of risk from this quarter has a more prominent role to play in informing the development and deployment of tertiary intervention resources (e.g., peer support). For example, it can be used to assess likely needs and residual risk (that portion of risk that cannot be reduced through primary and secondary intervention) (Violanti & Paton, 2006). It is not discussed further here. There is, however, another individual difference factor capable of influencing stress risk for terrorist events. Risk is influenced by the fact that the mental models or mind-sets that underpin the manner in which people interpret and organize experiences and make predictions about their future (Paton, 1994) have been rendered less applicable by the growing threat of terrorism (Daw, 2001).

Shattered Assumptions of Safety

Despite a long-held belief that their home soil was relatively safe from foreign attack, Americans lost this perception of safety on 9/11. Zimbardo (2001) has stated that the fear generated by terrorism undercuts the sense of trust, stability, and confidence in one's personal world. Moreover, this lost sense of safety and security may be accompanied by feelings of helplessness and anxiety (Figley, 1985). The relationship between exposure to terrorist events and psychological trauma could thus be mediated by individual vulnerabilities as they apply to fear. Fear becomes anxiety when it generalizes to become a more pervasive feeling of personal vulnerability.

The fact that the 9/11 attacks were deliberate human acts made them particularly distressing for Americans and compounded their loss of perceived safety and security. The accuracy of this statement is reflected in the fact that a huge decrease in airline use and travel occurred immediately after the attack. Myers (2001) has stated that the terrorists made progress in their fear war by diverting our anxieties from big risks toward smaller ones. Thus, Americans' illusion of invulnerability was shattered at both the macrolevel and the microlevel of everyday existence. To Americans, the world is now a threatening place—terrorism has come home and is no longer deniable. The fear instilled by terrorism works by breaking down the walls of psychological invulnerability and introducing a new mind-set dominated by preoccupation with the fear of reoccurrence.

Posttraumatic stress reactions can result from a variety of exposures. In the context of these events, *fear* is an important factor in the etiology of PTSD. The *Diagnostic and Statistical Manual of Mental Disorders* (*DSM-IV;* American Psychiatric Association, 1994) lists fear in "criteriion A" for PTSD. Brewin, Andrews, and Rose's (2000) longitudinal analysis of criterion A confirmed its validity. Sixty-one percent of those diagnosed with PTSD reported "intense" trauma-related emotions of fear 6 months after the event. Feelings of vulnerability and fear that result from terrorist acts may be persistent and thus have the potential to pose a much higher risk for PTSD than most other disasters, which are temporary in nature. In addition, unlike natural disasters, the fear and feelings of vulnerability generated by terrorism have the capability to spread to general as well as local populations and persist for considerably longer periods of time.

Managing risk involves first identifying the threatening elements of terrorist events that contribute to this fear. The importance of this activity is emphasized by Cooper's (2001) conclusion that the incidence and destructiveness of acts of terrorism will increase in the future. The ability of the media to instantaneously bring the horrible details of a terrorist event directly into people's homes will no doubt increase not only indirect exposure to terror but also perceived personal vulnerability to its impact, perpetuating this climate of fear. Once one is victimized, it is relatively easy to see oneself in the role again; the experience is now "available," and one sees oneself as "representative" of those who were actually victimized (Maercker & Muller, 2004; Kahneman & Tversky, 1973; Lasker, 2004; North et al., 2005).

Consequently, the United States now sees itself as seriously challenged. The assumptions that had formerly enabled it to function effectively can no longer be relied on as guides for behavior (Janoff-Bulman & Freize, 1983). As a result, Americans must explore a new way of being (Daw, 2001). Samuel Karson (quoted in Murray, 2001), a psychologist for the Federal Aviation Administration, commented that feelings of vulnerability can be assuaged if we deal with our weakness of not knowing our enemies' intention. Massive information is thus needed on the terrorists, their culture, language, and psychology, and this knowledge must be encapsulated in new mind-sets or interpretive mechanisms that can assist us in adjusting to this new reality.

The development of these interpretive mechanisms will be particularly important for protective services officers who may have to repeatedly confront the consequences of terrorism and respond to the challenges it poses to themselves and the communities they serve. Before discussing how this might be accomplished, it is important to consider the fact that protective services officers experience terrorist events and develop their interpretive mechanisms within an organizational context. It is thus pertinent to ask whether this context influences risk. In the next section, this issue is introduced in the context of a brief discussion of the relationship between organizational factors and posttrauma outcomes. In so doing, it also demonstrates the validity of including organizational intervention as the second element in the primary prevention strategy introduced earlier.

Stress Risk From Organizational Sources

Analyses of protective services officers' experience of terrorist events have highlighted the fact that their stress risk does not emanate solely from the nature and scale of these events and their horrific content. It is also influenced by organizational and operational factors (Brake, 2001; Carafano, 2003; Federal Emergency Management Agency [FEMA], 2004; Grant et al., 2003; Jackson et al., 2003; Kendra & Wachtendorf, 2003; McKinsey Report, 2002). What evidence supports a role for organizational factors as predictors of posttraumatic stress risk?

Analysis of the experience of rescue workers following the sinking of an Estonian ferry reveals that perception of organizational culture was the most significant predictor of posttrauma risk for this group (Eränen, Millar, & Paton, 2000; Paton, Smith, Violanti, & Eränen (2000). Compared with dispositional (hardiness), social support, and formal support (debriefing) factors, it was three times more influential as a predictor of traumatic stress outcomes (Figure 17.1). According to this analysis, organizational culture (beta = −0.3) and family dynamics (beta = −0.2) represent the two most significant predictors of stress risk.

Using data from a longitudinal study of police officers, Paton (in press) has demonstrated that not only can this relationship be primarily attributed to the negative elements of organizational culture (e.g., lack of consultation, poor communication, red tape), but these negative elements (beta = 0.23) were also more significant predictors of posttraumatic stress reactions than the traumatic experiences (e.g., shooting incidents, body recovery, dealing with child abuse) (beta = 0.16) per se. Furthermore, he has demonstrated that the negative elements of organizational culture do not predict well-being. In contrast, the positive elements of organizational climate (e.g., empowerment, devolving and delegating responsibility for crisis decision making) do predict positive outcomes (Paton, in press). This means that the organization of risk management strategies requires two components. One manages the negative cultural elements in ways that contribute to mitigating acute stress and posttraumatic stress risk. Another develops those positive cultural elements necessary to promote well-being. Paton et al. (2000) have also identified family dynamics as a significant predictor of posttraumatic outcomes (Figure 17.1)

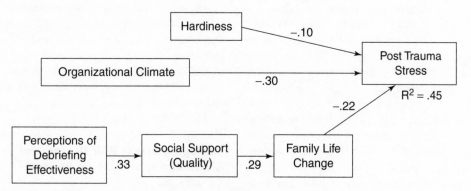

Figure 17.1. The relative contributions of organizational, dispositional, debriefing, social support, and family variables to posttrauma stress outcomes.
Source: Adapted from Eränen et al. (2000) and Paton et al. (2000).

but in ways that are linked to other support resources. In so doing, they also suggest a need for a more comprehensive approach to the provision of tertiary intervention.

Structural equation analysis reveals that, although perceptions of organizational culture had a direct effect on posttraumatic stress scores, the influence of a commonly occurring tertiary intervention (psychological debriefing) did not (Figure 17.1). Rather, the influence of the latter was mediated by social support and changes in family functioning (Figure 17.1). This suggests that, for those who found debriefing to be effective, it was because, first, it enhanced social support quality, which, in turn, enriched the quality of family functioning. The latter had a direct influence on the posttrauma outcome (Figure 17.1). From this we can infer that additional emphasis on developing the quality of social support and family functioning could have beneficial mental health consequences for officers and their family members alike. While this study demonstrates the influence of this change during a 6-month postevent period, organizations have it within their power to develop social support and family functioning resources within the context of a primary prevention program. Indeed, the benefits of the latter can be discerned in other aspects of the work-family relationship.

Shift work, a common component of emergency service work, has a well-documented history as a predictor of the quality of family functioning and provides a good example of an organizational practice capable of influencing family stress risk (Shakespeare-Finch, Paton, & Violanti, 2003). The number and timing of hours worked outside the home significantly influence workers' ability to participate in and enjoy family life. While it is often assumed that the traumatic nature of officers' experiences has a greater influence on this relationship than organizational factors such as shift work (Wraith, 1994), this assumption is incorrect. Shakespeare-Finch and colleagues have discussed how, when shift work was controlled for, there was no difference in family functioning between an emergency services shift work group and a control group composed of nonemergency shift workers. This suggests that shift work, rather than officers' traumatic experience per se, contributes to family problems. While this position is not intended to deny the potential for the psychological consequences of acts of terrorism to contribute to stress risk, the fact that organizations can make choices about their relationship with families (e.g., family friendly policies and support groups, involving family members in recovery planning) provides organizations with the potential to contribute to the proactive management of stress risk.

Overall, the studies discussed in this section demonstrate the value of including organizational and family factors within stress risk assessment and management strategies. The prominence of organizational factors as stressors within the terrorist event response environment (Carafano, 2003; Grant et al., 2003; Kendra & Wachtendorf, 2003) makes it imperative that variables relating to organizational culture and practices be included in the risk assessment and management process. Recognition of the influential nature of these factors and of the fact that they describe variables under the control of the emergency organization also increases the choices available to emergency organizations regarding primary intervention. By making choices about these variables and developing policies and procedures accordingly, organizations can develop strategies that ensure more effective stress risk management (Creamer & Liddle, 2005; Paton et al., 2004). In the sections that follow, discussion centers on the nature of the processes and competencies that can be harnessed in pursuit of this goal. There is, however, one additional variable that must be taken into consideration if a comprehensive overview of terrorism-related stress is to ensue. This additional variable describes changes in officers' involvement over time.

Officers' experience of terrorist events evolves over time as they progress through a series of stages, each with its own unique demands and characteristics and thus implications for stress risk. These stages are the alarm/warning and mobilization phase, the response phase, and the process of reintegration into routine work following the termination of their deployment (Hartsough & Myers, 1985).

Managing Stress Risk During the Alarm and Mobilization Phase

The alarm phase is the period of comprehending and adjusting to the occurrence of a terrorist event.

The demands that typify this phase include, for example, accessing intelligence about what has occurred, differentiating fact from inference, making sense of the confusing and often ambiguous information presented by such events, and negotiating operational arrangements with other agencies and jurisdictions (FEMA, 2004; Grant et al., 2003; Paton & Hannan, 2004). The potential of previous experiences to influence predispositions to interpret accidents (e.g., the New York power outage) as terrorist events can add to the complexity of the response environment for protective services officers.

The final report of the Human Behavior and Weapons of Mass Destruction (HBWMD) Crisis/ Risk Communication Workshop (2001) concluded that, for those in command or coordination roles, terrorist events pose several challenges during this initial phase. The stress of responding under these circumstances can be traced to several factors. In addition to their emanating from the direct effect of experiencing a terrorist attack, acute stress reactions can also be attributed to the demands associated with adapting plans to deal with urgent, emergent, and evolving emergency demands (Brake, 2001; HBWMD, 2001), the need for creative responses to emergent demands (Kendra & Wachtendorf, 2003), and the need for responses to accommodate and integrate the efforts of several agencies across multiple jurisdictions (Brake, 2001; Department of Homeland Security, 2003, 2004; Grant et al., 2003; Paton & Hannan, 2004). A crucial competence in this context is the ability to extract salient cues that assist in adapting plans and response actions to fit unpredictable situational demands. This is situational awareness (Endsley & Garland, 2000), and it is essential to understanding mobilization stress risk (Carafano, 2003; Flin & Arbuthnot, 2002; Paton & Hannan, 2004). Another facet of situation awareness, the capacity to anticipate future demands, has been identified as an important competence for terrorist events (Department of Homeland Security, 2003). High situational awareness facilitates the capability of emergency responders to minimize their exposure to risks, allows more effective use of resources, and enables better command and control by addressing issues such as managing convergence and coordinating operations controlled by multiple agencies (Carafano, 2003; Department of

Homeland Security, 2003; Paton & Hannan, 2004).

Irrespective of the quality of planning for terrorist events, the translation of plans into operational reality remains a contentious issue (Brake, 2001; Department of Homeland Security, 2003; Grant et al., 2003; HBWMD, 2001; McKinsey Report, 2002). The different statutory and regulatory frameworks that prescribe how agencies (e.g., law enforcement, military) define and engage in the response are prominent contributors to this discrepancy (Brake, 2001). Factors such as these complicate the mobilization and coordination of a multiagency response and increase the risk of acute stress reactions for those officers who are involved (Paton, 2003). The TOPOFF 3 exercise (April 2005) examined ways of dealing with this issue. The evaluation of this exercise may provide valuable insights into how these complex issues can be managed. Strategies that can be employed to manage other aspects of a multiagency response are discussed later in the chapter.

Another prominent source of stress risk during the alarm and mobilization phase of terrorist events is their implicit unpredictability (HBWMD, 2001). For example, a terrorist attack that involves the detonation of a conventional bomb will create an event with a clearly defined location, a clear beginning and end, and a finite period of impact. It poses demands that can be accommodated by deployment strategies similar to those used to manage more "routine" emergencies. In contrast, a biohazard attack (e.g., pollution of water supplies, release of a biohazard such as smallpox) may have commenced before its existence has been identified, present more diffuse beginnings and ends, spread in ways dictated by local conditions such as building density, topography, and prevailing weather, and create relatively prolonged periods of impact (Fisher, 2000; HBWMD, 2001; Lasker, 2004). The alarm may be raised some time after the event has actually begun, thus creating greater uncertainty during mobilization. For example, the immediate effects of a disease-causing agent could be dismissed as flu, and its true nature might not become clear until some time after initial contact. This time lag means that protective services professionals will face considerable uncertainty with regard to the nature and magnitude of the problem they face, as well as their own status (particularly if they have come into contact with those affected), and they will, as a result, respond within a more complex societal context (Lasker, 2004; North et al., 2005).

For example, planning for such events assumes that people comply with recommenced actions (e.g., staying where they are until authorities inform them that it is safe to move, going to a vaccination center). The reality may be quite different (Lasker, 2004). Lasker has discussed how the actions that people take are dictated by how they resolve the contradictory demands they experience (e.g., placing a desire to reunite with their children immediately above advice to remain in situ, refusing to go a vaccination center for fear of coming into contact with those already infected). A discrepancy between plan assumptions and actual behavior creates an additional source of uncertainty for protective services officers and further contributes to their stress risk. Response planning should thus be based on more realistic estimates of what people will actually do (Lasker, 2004).

Biohazardous weapons can also generate highly dynamic response scenarios. For example, aerosol dispersion creates a physical hazard whose distribution is a function of both prevailing and changing meteorological conditions. In addition to its direct effects, stress risk is increased by difficulties in knowing where and when to deploy and what protective equipment to take (Department of Homeland Security, 2003). People's uncertainty regarding what they should do to protect themselves can increase their reliance on protective services for information. However, under these circumstances, officers would not have recourse to the normal means of reassuring citizens (Fisher, 2000; Lasker, 2004).

Stress risk is increased if deployment precedes a full appreciation of the nature or implications of a terrorist event. For example, police officers who were immediately deployed to the site of the Lockerbie disaster found it difficult to comprehend the carnage and death they encountered (Mitchell, 1991). While performing similar duties in a similar environment, officers deployed after the cause of the event had been identified (a terrorist bombing) reported significantly lower levels of stress. Being able to define their situation as a criminal investigation allowed them to apply professional schema (e.g., conceptualizing the work of handling human remains as an evidence-gathering procedure) to render the experience more meaningful.

The organizational role is to facilitate this capacity to impose meaning on threatening and challenging demands to limit the likelihood that officers will be overwhelmed by the scale or the horror of the situation they must contend with (Alexander & Wells, 1991; Paton, 1994). To accommodate differing agency definitions of terrorism and their investigative objectives (Brake, 2001), this would have to be done for each organization. In so doing, this strategy could ameliorate stress in each profession, but it could also contribute to coordination stress in multiagency response environments, emphasizing the need to develop a superordinate team structure that accommodates these multiple roles.

For protective services officers, factors such as uncertain dispersal patterns and the possibility of further attacks in unpredictable locations means that the alarm (and subsequent) phase of a terrorist event will be accompanied by significant concerns for their family members (HBWMD, 2001). This marks a significant departure from other emergency events and makes a substantial contribution to the stress risk associated with acts of terrorism. Programs designed to help officers develop a capacity to adapt should also be extended to their family members. These should include ensuring regular and informative communication between agency and families, providing information, offering training that addresses ways to manage their reactions, suggesting ways in which they can assist their partner's recovery, developing support groups, and facilitating their access to, for example, vaccines and mental health resources (HBWMD, 2001; Shakespeare-Finch, Paton, & Violanti, 2003; Violanti & Paton, 2006).

Stress risk during mobilization is greater when officers respond at the end of a shift or when they are affected by transient factors (e.g., illness, occupational stress). The personal and transient nature of these factors renders them difficult to control. Risk management programs that enhance awareness of these limiting factors, their implications for performance, and the need to adopt appropriate response strategies (e.g., increased need for teamwork) can reduce the likelihood of adverse mobilization reactions (Flin, 1996).

It therefore follows that strategies designed to mitigate terrorist stress risk during mobilization must not be based on assumptions derived from routine emergencies or on unrealistic or untested plans (Carafano, 2003; Department of Homeland

Security, 2003; Lasker, 2004; Paton, 1997). Rather, they must be derived from accurate analyses of community (e.g., accommodate the need to reconcile different actions) and professional (e.g., consider concerns for self and family, adapt plans to accommodate emergent issues) response needs and expectations and accommodate the unique demands likely to be encountered. Developing effective stress management plans also requires an understanding of these issues as they arise during the response.

Managing Stress Risk During a Response to Terrorism

Despite having a long and effective history of responding to emergency events, protective services officers face psychological contexts (e.g., vulnerability and assumptions of safety) and demands associated with terrorist events that present them with a unique set of problems (Carafano, 2003; Fisher, 2000; Grant et al., 2003; Jackson et al., 2003; Simpson & Stehr, 2003). For example, greater uncertainty surrounds the timing, duration, and distribution of the consequences of terrorist events, which possess a unique capacity to create a sustained climate of fear. They can also involve hazardous agents (e.g., biohazard and radiological agents) that are difficult to detect, can create significant acute and chronic health problems, and generate consequences that may persist for quite some time. These factors, coupled with the possibility of large-scale destruction and loss of life from the use of weapons of mass destruction (WMD), create a response context whose characteristics differ substantially from those normally encountered. Furthermore, the nature of the threats means that protective services professions are not just protecting the public. They must also protect themselves; thus the need to reconcile the safety of both protective services officers and the public becomes a significant stressor in this context (Department of Homeland Security, 2003).

During the response phase, risk factors emanate from the characteristics of the terrorist incident. However, the psychological consequences of the exposure to these characteristics will be influenced by the personal and organizational competences brought to bear to manage the response (Alper & Kupferman, 2003; Grant et al., 2003;

Kendra & Wachtendorf, 2003; Paton & Hannan, 2004; Simpson & Stehr, 2003).

Event Characteristics

Event causation is a risk factor for terrorist events. Because the causes of terrorist acts can always be attributed to deliberate human action intended to cause harm, they threaten perceived control, a prominent stressor in emergency responders whose training is designed to promote control (MacLeod & Paton, 1999; Myers, 2001).

The magnitude of the death and injury they encounter, which is coupled in many cases with uncertainty regarding the cause of death or whether those they come into contact with are infectious, provides a further source of stress (Jackson et al., 2003). For large-scale events, such as those presented by the aftermath of the World Trade Center collapse, the time frame for body recovery can be prolonged (Simpson & Stehr, 2003). Working in proximity to dead or seriously injured victims, particularly if coupled with a perceived lack of opportunity for effective action, results in officers facing constant reminders of their perceived inability to deal with this loss and suffering. The ensuing reduction in officers' sensitivity to the needs of others as they attempt to shut out these signals can reduce their willingness to utilize support resources (Paton & Stephens, 1996; Raphael, 1986) and increase their risk of experiencing posttraumatic stress reactions. Insufficient, inadequate, or inappropriate resources to perform response tasks can fuel a sense of inadequacy and increase stress vulnerability (Carafano, 2003; Paton, 1994).

Uncertainty regarding the duration of their involvement or additional attacks, for example, heightens officers' stress risk, as does their exposure to personal danger. Officers who respond to the devastation associated with a terrorist bombing would encounter hazards from disrupted sewerage systems, threats associated with working in unstable buildings, exposure to contaminated blood products or infectious diseases, and increased health risks from dust, ash, and asbestos in damaged buildings.

With regard to sources of danger, exposure to events that pose unseen threats (e.g., highly toxic chemical, biological, or radiation hazards) contributes substantially to stress risk by making it more difficult for emergency responders to directly observe what they need to be aware of in order to take protective actions. Separation from family members, if accompanied by continuing concern for their safety, would also constitute a hazard, as would the demands associated with safeguarding the public from threatening circumstances. Terrorist attacks involving weapons of mass destruction can impact over a large and often ill-defined geographical area (e.g., meteorological factors influence the distribution of radioactive plumes) and generate rapidly evolving demands. The scale of destruction increases the risk of death in emergency response personnel. Death or serious injury to a colleague can amplify stress risk associated with an already hazardous environment (Paton & Stephens, 1996).

Environmental factors such as heat, noise, or poor visibility affect stress risk (Vrij, van der Steen, & Koppelaar, 1994), as can the sights, sounds, and especially the smells encountered (Paton, Cox, & Andrew, 1989). The demands associated with environmental factors such as heat may be significant and unexpected as a result of the need to wear protective suits and breathing apparatus as protection from biohazardous agents or toxic dust, for example. Because this need is similar to those that arise in relation to many routine response scenarios, the use of protective clothing and breathing apparatus may be less demanding for fire personnel. It can, however, represent a significant stressor for those (e.g., police, EMT personnel) for whom this would represent a highly novel demand. The need for protective clothing contributes to stress risk both directly (e.g., its use is necessitated by the use of biological or chemical contaminants) and indirectly (e.g., increased heat stress from wearing protective clothing and from additional problems with operating equipment (Carafano, 2003).

This discussion represents a brief summary of event-related stress risk factors. A more comprehensive account can be found in Paton (1997). A key issue here concerns the fact that the demands encountered when responding to terrorist events are qualitatively different from those that characterize routine work. The importance of recognizing this distinction derives from the fact that officers develop mental models from their routine training and experience that prescribe their expectations of how they will respond to events. The degree of fit

between these expectations and what they encounter is a significant indicator of stress risk (Paton, 1994). According to this conceptualization, stress risk will be a function of the degree to which the prevailing mental model or mind-set, derived from socialization, training, and experience in routine contexts, can accommodate these atypical experiences.

Changing the Mind-Set

The events of 9/11 highlighted the fact that, for terrorist events, emergency responders need to make substantive changes to the mind-set or interpretive frameworks they use if they are to develop and implement an effective response to these incidents (Brake, 2001; Kendra & Wachtendorf, 2003). Responders' needs have been underestimated because expectations have been based largely on the experience of responding to routine events or disasters of natural and human origins, which may not be accurate predictors of the conditions that protective services professionals may encounter in a determined, protracted terrorist campaign (Carafano, 2003; HBWMD, 2001; Paton, 1994).

The schema or mental models that guide the response to terrorist events reflect officers' socialization into their profession and organization, their training, the experiences they accumulate over time, and the operating practices that prescribe their response to routine emergencies. These become implicit (or taken for granted) aspects of the mental models officers use to make predictions about future events, organize experiences, and make sense of the consequences of events and their reactions to them. However, their importance as determinants of well-being and performance effectiveness tends to remain unrealized until officers encounter incidents that challenge these implicit assumptions (Paton, 1994). Consequently, training for terrorist events must confront these assumptions and facilitate the development of interpretative competences, or mind-sets, appropriate for the demands likely to be encountered (Flin, 1996; Paton, 1994; Paton & Jackson, 2002). In addition, they must accommodate the legacy (e.g., increased levels of fear in the community, changes in security precautions, perceptions of the world as increasingly threatening) of terrorism into their thinking.

Changes in mind-set are required to accommodate the implications of more complex operating environments (e.g., the response environment could simultaneously be a disaster area, a crime scene, and a mass grave). New ways of conceptualizing the world may be required in order to accommodate the consequences of attacks on elements of strong symbolic value (e.g., the Twin Towers) whose loss can amplify the sense of societal loss associated with acts of terrorism (Simpson & Stehr, 2003).

A combination of the legacy of fear that acts of terrorism leave in their wake and the speed with which information regarding subsequent events is disseminated by media coverage can substantially expand the ripple effect. For example, when many people witness such events both directly and indirectly through the media, as on 9/11 (Shuster et al., 2001; Yehuda, 2002), this additional factor can create contingent demands in areas that may be peripheral to the targeted area or even at some distance from the event (Pfefferbaum et al., 2000), necessitating that officers expand their conceptualization of the social dimensions of a given event relative to that associated with expectations derived from their routine experiences.

New interpretive frameworks are needed to manage events that fall outside the realm of "routine" emergencies. For example, they will be required to accommodate demands associated with agricultural emergencies that threaten the food supply or represent a source of human infectious disease (Carafano, 2003). Officers' mental models must also accommodate the fact that, when responding to terrorist events, the scene could become an intentionally hostile environment for them (Department of Homeland Security, 2003; FEMA, 2004; Maniscalco & Christen, 2002). Several terrorist attacks, such as the Bali bombing, used one bomb to attract responders and evacuees to the location of secondary devices in a manner intended to inflict maximum death and injury on those fulfilling a response role.

Interpretive processes can influence outcome in other ways. For example, the scale or nature of terrorist impact can limit opportunities for effective action. Stress risk increases if these limitations are perceived as a failure attributed to personal inadequacy rather than to environmental constraints beyond an individual's control (e.g., as a result of the sheer scale or complexity of the

event). This process has been labeled *performance guilt* (Raphael, 1986). However, training that develops realistic outcome expectations, an ability to differentiate personal and situational constraints, and interpretive processes that review experiences as learning opportunities that enhance future competence increases adaptive capacity (Dunning, 2003; Paton, 1994; Paton & Jackson, 2002).

Stress risk is particularly pronounced when performing body recovery and identification duties. Following the Oklahoma bombing, firefighters reported being upset by contact with body parts (54%) and body fluids (36%), but encounters with children's remains (72%) were associated with the highest levels of distress (North et al., 2002). The 9/11 attacks on the World Trade Center introduced an additional dimension to risk in this context. Search and rescue personnel had to work in a context defined by considerable diversity with regard to cultural practices associated with the retrieval and treatment of human remains (Simpson & Stehr, 2003).

Positive interpretation (e.g., interpreting body recovery duties in terms of their role in assisting families to begin the grieving process and not as performance failure on their part) can facilitate adaptation to the demands encountered under these circumstances (Paton, 1994; Thompson, 1993). Training and experience in handling body remains lessens stress in those exposed to this activity for prolonged periods but less so for those exposed for relatively short periods (Alexander & Wells, 1991; Deahl, Gillham, Thomas, Searle, & Srinivasan, 1994; Mitchell, 1991; Thompson, 1993). This difference may reflect the time it takes to invoke coping strategies such as imagery. While imagery can be an effective coping strategy during body recovery duties, it can constitute a source of stress following the termination of these duties as personnel review their actions and thoughts (Paton et al., 1989). This highlights the importance of including both positive and negative aspects of experience in postevent reviews.

In general, training that is designed to develop the capability of operational mental models (essential to response planning and organizing action) to impose coherence upon atypical and challenging experiences and to accommodate the demands encountered should be an essential component of stress risk management (Dunning, 2003; Paton, 1994; Paton & Hannan, 2004). A capacity for reframing can be developed using simulations. Simulations provide opportunities to conceptualize and review response activities, construct realistic performance expectations, increase awareness of stress reactions, and rehearse strategies to deal with stressful circumstances and reactions (Crego & Spinks, 1997; Paton, 1994; Paton & Jackson, 2002). They can also identify areas for personal and organizational development.

Developing these more sophisticated psychological structures requires that simulations be constructed using information derived from two sources. One concerns the systematic analysis of the competencies required for effective response to terrorist events. The second involves designing simulations capable of reconciling event characteristics (e.g., exposure to biohazards, personal danger, recovery of human remains, and encounters with cross-cultural aspects of death and loss) with the capabilities required to manage them (e.g., hazard identification and interpretation; adaptation of plans; team and multiagency operations; information and decision management) in ways that promote adaptive capacity (Paton, 1994; Paton et al., 1999; Pollock, Paton, Smith, & Violanti, 2003). The degree to which the choices made within the risk management process are effective in reducing adverse outcomes will influence the quality of officers' adaptation during the postevent, reintegration period.

Discussion in this section has focused on the sources of stress risk. Traditionally, the causes of traumatic stress reactions have been attributed predominantly to the horrific, threatening, or challenging event characteristics (e.g., handling human remains) to which officers are exposed. While this aspect of a terrorist event will remain a prominent predictor of traumatic stress risk, it is not the only one. Organizational factors and the response protocols they prescribe also play a significant role as predictors of stress risk.

Organizational Factors

When responding to terrorist events, protective services officers do so within a context defined by their organizational membership and culture. For example, bureaucratic organizations increase stress risk through the persistent use of established operational and decision procedures (even when responding to different and urgent crisis demands),

internal conflicts regarding responsibility (which can constrain officers' response to emergent demands), and a predisposition to protect the organization from criticism or blame (Gist & Woodall, 2000; Paton, 1997). Organizational culture can also exercise a pervasive influence on stress risk through the procedures it prescribes, such as inadequate consultation, poor communication, and excessive red tape.

However, organizational culture that supports autonomous response systems, a flexible, consultative leadership style, and practices that ensure that role and task assignments reflect incident demands can reduce the risk of adverse stress outcomes (Gist &Woodall, 2000; McKinsey Report, 2002; Paton, 1999). Similarly, managerial practices such as recognizing the value of work in traumatic contexts and delegating responsibility increase adaptive capacity (Dunning, 2003; Paton, in press). Furthermore, because the organization defines the operational paradigm it uses (e.g., command structure, level of autocracy, degree of devolved authority, level of training), stress risk is influenced by the degree to which these polices and practices, which are often extrapolated from those used for routine work, are appropriate for managing the atypical consequences of terrorist events (Carafano, 2003; McKinsey Report, 2002; Kendra & Wachtendorf, 2003; Paton & Hannan, 2004). This supports earlier conclusions regarding the organizational contribution to response effectiveness and stress risk when an organization's members are involved in dealing with the consequences of terrorist acts.

Recognition of the organizational role is important in two respects. First, the role of organizational factors as predictors of traumatic stress outcomes has been underrepresented. Second, they define predictors of stress risk over which emergency organizations have more control. They thus provide the principle means by which emergency organizations can make choices regarding stress risk. These issues are illustrated here by considering communication, decision making, and interagency teamwork.

Information and Decision Management

Communication among agencies responsible for responding to a terrorist attack can be rendered problematic by the loss of infrastructure from their being deliberately targeted or as the result of secondary loss from explosion or contamination (Brake, 2001; Department of Homeland Security, 2003; Carafano, 2003; FEMA, 2004; HBWMD, 2001; McKinsey Report, 2002). Response management is also affected by the quality of information management, that is, the degree to which collaborating agencies can access, interpret, collate, and use information to manage complex events (Alper & Kupferman, 2003; FEMA, 2004; Grant et al., 2003; Jackson et al., 2003; McKinsey Report, 2002; Paton, 2001; Paton et al., 1999). A capacity to make decisions using this nonroutine information is also required.

Terrorist events involve making decisions in a context defined by urgent, emergent (i.e., unique, unexpected, or unpredictable) demands (Brake, 2001; Grant et al., 2003; Kendra & Wachtendorf, 2003; Simpson & Stehr, 2003) and using non-routine data and information from a variety of novel sources to do so. The dynamic and complex nature of terrorist events also generates a need for a level of creative decision making that exceeds that required for response to "routine" emergencies (Jackson et al., 2003; Kendra & Wachtendorf, 2003). Stress risk is also heightened by having to deviate from the standard operational procedures associated with routine work and producing contingent solutions to novel problems. The capacity to do so can be facilitated by the associated stress, particularly if officers are trained in crisis decision making.

For trained personnel, crises enhance alertness and thinking skills (Flin, 1996). However, putting this to good use requires an ability to operate in environments characterized by information overload. Situational awareness—the capability to extract or operate on limited cues within a complex environment and use them to construct mental models of complex events that allows appropriate decisions to be made—is a key adaptive capacity (Carafano, 2003; Endsley & Garland, 2000) and one that contributes to reducing stress risk (Paton & Hannan, 2004). The decision process that is used must also be tailored to this circumstance.

Naturalistic decision making, in which a person recognizes the type of situation at hand and, from previous experience, selects an appropriate course of action, is highly adaptive in events characterized by substantial time pressure and high risk (Flin, Salas, Strub, & Martin, 1997).

Given that responding to events involving WMD and biohazardous weapons can create rapidly changing demands, skill in naturalistic decision making is essential for protecting well-being and facilitating effective responses in those managing the consequences of terrorist acts. Because success in naturalistic decision making is a function of the ability to match current and past situations, decision effectiveness is enhanced by having more options to match. This ability can be developed through experience or simulation. The latter style, however, remains important where time allows. Terrorist events also increase the need for decision making to take place in a multiagency response context.

Team and Interagency Operations

A central characteristic of the response to terrorist acts is the need for a multiagency and multijurisdictional response (Brake, 2001; Department of Homeland Security, 2003; FEMA, 2004; Grant et al., 2003; Jackson et al., 2003; Kendra & Wachtendorf, 2003). Analysis of the interagency activities in Shanksville following the crash of United flight 93 in September 2001 illustrates the benefits of effective coordination of emergency mutual aid assignments (Grant et al., 2003). The possibility that the effectiveness of this activity resulted from the quality of relationships and interagency collaboration that reflect its provincial location cannot be discounted. That is, an equally effective response may not occur so smoothly in large urban settings (McKinsey Report, 2002), and the capacity for interagency communication and decision making operations must be specifically targeted within planning and training processes (Department of Homeland Security, 2003; FEMA, 2004).

The potential scale of terrorist attacks makes this an important issue and one whose implications have been accepted as requiring detailed consideration (Department of Homeland Security, 2003, 2004). Exercises such TOPOFF (1–3) provide good models of the kind of realistic, real-time simulations that are necessary for the development and critical evaluation of a multidisciplinary, multijurisdictional response to complex, large-scale terrorist attacks. The review of the TOPOFF 2 exercise (Department of Homeland Security, 2003) has demonstrated a capacity for the successful integration of agency communications and action relative to the principle federal officials who provided the unified command structure. It also, however, identified a need for improved information management and coordination with regard to making nonroutine decisions such as those associated with the radiological dispersion component of the exercise. A crucial issue here is recognizing that planning for a coordinated response does not guarantee its translation into an effective operational capacity (Department of Homeland Security, 2003). Even in Shanksville, the diverse perspectives applied by different agencies to make sense of the situation generated conflict (Grant et al., 2003). This was often related to the need for protective service agencies to collaborate with nonroutine agencies (e.g., the American Red Cross, Salvation Army).

The complex nature of terrorist events brings together agencies that rarely interact or collaborate with one another under routine circumstances, reducing opportunities to allow shared understanding of their respective roles to develop. For example, the multiagency response to terrorist events could include hazardous materials response teams, urban search and rescue assets, community emergency response teams, antiterrorism units, special weapons and tactics teams, bomb squads, emergency management officials, municipal agencies, and private organizations responsible for transportation, communications, medical services, public health, disaster assistance, public works, and construction workers (Carafano, 2003). To this list could be added experts in radiological plume characteristics and dispersal (Department of Homeland Security, 2003). Given the potential for role conflict and ambiguity under these circumstances, understanding and managing interagency and team issues becomes an important component of the stress risk management process.

For large-scale terrorist events, a cohesive interagency team and a capacity for multijurisdictional management is essential to the effective supervision of events that require coordinated input from several agencies if effective decisions are to be made (Brake, 2001; FEMA, 2004; Grant et al., 2003; Jackson et al., 2003; Kendra & Wachtendorf, 2003). However, simply bringing together representatives of agencies who have little contact with one another under normal circumstances will not guarantee a coordinated response. Rather, such ad hoc arrangements are more likely to increase interagency conflict, result in a blurring of roles and responsibilities, and fuel frustration and feelings of inadequacy and helplessness (McKinsey Report, 2002; Paton, 1994). Thus, irrespective of the quality of the planning that precedes a disaster response, a capacity for cohesive action should not be assumed (Department of Homeland Security, 2003). It can be developed using liaison mechanisms and the integration of respective agency roles through interagency team development (Flin & Arbuthnot, 2002).

This developmental process must take several factors into account. One concerns the way in which each agency defines interagency collaboration. For example, turf protection increases interagency competition and consequently stress risk in situations that require active collaboration (Paton et al., 1999). Organizations must accept the value of collaboration (e.g., the need for diverse perspectives) if they are to understand and manage complex problems. A second factor concerns the patterns of interaction among group members in relation to institutional policies, structures and culture, and the language and terminology they use (Brake, 2001). This would mean conceptualizing terror response as involving a series of superordinate groups whose membership is prescribed by their collective role in managing specific facets of the overall operation, including the development of mechanisms for meaningful (e.g., that supports decision making) communication among them. A third factor involves contextual factors such as the level of understanding of integrated emergency management policies and practices, the status and power accorded to different members, and resource constraints. A fourth issue is the level of trust between partners (Brake, 2001; FEMA, 2004; Grant et al. 2003; Paton et al., 2003).

At one level, these issues reflect the need to match the structural integration between agencies with a corresponding procedural or operational capacity to act in concert during a crisis (Paton et al., 1999). However, it also encompasses participants' understanding of their respective contributions to the same plan and their shared understanding of each member's role in the response (Brake, 2001; FEMA, 2004; Paton & Flin, 1999). This contributes to their ability to share a common understanding of evolving events, to work toward mutual goals over time, and, importantly, to anticipate the needs of those with whom they are collaborating (Department of Homeland Security, 2003; Flin, 1996; Pollock et al., 2003).

Extensive joint planning in conjunction with teamwork activity involving collaborating agencies can reduce the risk of experiencing adverse stress outcomes, particularly when responding in a multiagency context (Brannick, Salas & Prince, 1997; Flin, 1996; Paton et al., 1999; Pollock et al., 2003). The TOPOFF 2 and 3 exercises illustrate this process in practice. A key factor underpinning the benefits that can accrue from these collaborative activities concerns good information sharing (Department of Homeland Security, 2003; Paton, 2003).

In effective teams, members provide more unprompted information, increasing a capability for proactive response management through better decision making and resource allocation when responding to complex acts of terrorism (Department of Homeland Security, 2003; Entin & Serfaty, 1999). For this to occur effectively, team members must share a "team mental model" that facilitates the provision of goal-related information required by decision makers at critical periods (Cooke, Salas, Cannon-Bowers, & Stout, 2000). As the level of teamwork and planning activity increases, officers develop progressively similar mental models of response environments and the roles and tasks performed within them. This, in turn, increases implicit information sharing during high workload periods, enhancing team capacity for adaptive response (Paton & Jackson, 2002; Stout, Canon-Bowers, Salas, & Milanovich, 1999).

The concept of distributed decision making acknowledges the need for contributions from people who differ with respect to their professions, functions, roles, and expertise and who may be in different locations or involved in different levels (e.g., operational vs. tactical) of decision making (FEMA, 2004; Paton & Flin, 1999). The quality of shared understanding and procedural integration thus determines the capability of the multiagency team to utilize its collective expertise, even if dispersed or contributing different perspectives, to manage the response. It also increases the likelihood of their operating with a shared mental model of the situation that facilitates the effective and efficient allocation and use of limited resources. Consequently, high levels of interagency

planning and training are essential components of stress risk management programs. While exercises such as TOPOFF 2 and 3 represent simulations that are capable of testing the effectiveness of interagency and multijurisdictional abilities, an alternative approach is required to develop them in the first place (Paton et al, 1999; Paton, 2001).

Several factors, including pragmatic issues associated with multiagency exercises and the diversity of collaborative relationships (e.g., agencies can be differentiated with regard to those with whom they will collaborate) that will compose the overall response makes developing this capacity a complex task. In an attempt to circumvent these problems, Paton (2001) has proposed a method for accomplishing this by defining decision making and informational needs.

Using realistic decision making scenarios that require input from diverse sources (agencies) to define and resolve problems, it first calls for defining the decisions required to manage anticipated demands. The second stage involves each agency identifying the information it requires to make these decisions. Agency identification of the data and information it needs to acquire (and then to assimilate and translate) to make nonroutine decisions provides a foundation for conceptualizing the need for and benefits of a coordinated multiagency response and understanding how they will relate to other agencies during a crisis if they are to perform effectively.

Building this competence is essential given the complexity of terrorist events. For example, the effective performance of search and rescue operations requires cooperation from biohazard, crime scene security, and quarantine experts. The complexity of the scenario supplies a context within which agencies can develop a model of the relationship between their input and that of other agencies and provides a foundation for developing team mental models whose efficacy can be tested in simulations. A similar approach for managing distributed operations (in which decision makers must coordinate their actions from geographically dispersed locations) when dealing with nonroutine, multiagency response has been proposed by van der Lee and van Vugt (2004). Other models have also been proposed.

Burghardt (2004) has proposed the combined systems model. According to this model, effective response to complex crises can be facilitated by first delegating well-structured tasks to artificial systems, which leaves more time for human decision makers to deal with emergent demands. Second, it argues for employing decentralization mechanisms that delegate control to self-organizing subsystems (e.g., those dealing with radioactive fallout, performing search and rescue role, or managing inoculation centers) who are closer to the scene. Finally, the model advocates the use of decision support systems developed to accommodate the complex psychological, cultural, and political interactions that characterize multiagency response environments. With regard to the latter, Burghardt suggests several mechanisms that can be used to visualize the relationships between evidence and courses of action and the clarification of terminology within these contexts.

To summarize this section, stress risk during response can be managed by developing the interpretative, team, and information and decision-making abilities required to impose a sense of coherence on atypical experiences and to deal with them effectively. It is also important to ensure that these competences are activated within an organizational culture that supports and protects officers' well-being and that establishes response protocols that do likewise. While facilitating the proactive mitigation of stress risk during response, it is, however, important to note that termination of involvement in a specific event does not eliminate risk.

Stress Risk During Reintegration

The unique nature of terrorist events requires new approaches to postevent stress risk management (Carafano, 2003). During reintegration, stress risk management involves managing the emotional correlates of involvement in a terrorist event and providing a framework within which officers can render atypical, threatening experiences meaningful. With regard to the former, support practices that assist positive resolution and growth are discussed elsewhere (Dunning, 2003; Tedeschi & Calhoun, 2003). While the management of stress reactions associated with the event experience itself has dominated postevent practice (e.g., debriefing), stress from this source may, as discussed earlier, represent a less significant source than that emanating from the organizational culture and from family dynamics. Attention to family issues is im-

portant both for their own sake and with regard to their role as a recovery resource. A comprehensive discussion of family intervention can be found in Shakespeare-Finch et al. (2003). Emergency organizations must accept their role in this process and implement resources (e.g., family friendly policies, family support groups, family recovery planning) that contribute to the proactive management of family stress risk.

Managing Stress Risk During Reintegration

The period of transition from responding to an act of terrorism back into routine work and family life poses a unique set of demands. Vulnerability is not restricted to those who had negative event experiences. Positive response experiences can become a risk factor for posttraumatic stress reactions during reintegration if, for example, officers experience a conflict between a period of rewarding personal or professional performance and readjusting to routine duties and catching up with any backlog of work, dealing with reporting pressures, and handling any legal and sociolegal aspects of the response.

During the postevent period, the complex nature of terrorist acts, their causation, and the emergency response may come under intense public and media scrutiny. Sociolegal processes and media coverage can substantially extend the period of event experience and thus stress risk. During this time, officers may have to contend with blame (e.g., media accounts regarding event preventability, response effectiveness) being directed toward them or coming to terms with self-blame as they reflect on their role in the response. There are several ways in which risk can be managed during the reintegration phase, with social support playing a prominent role.

Interpersonal Support and Cohesion

While generally considered to ameliorate stress reactions, the fact that support provision occurs within a social context introduces several factors capable of influencing stress risk (Paton & Stephens, 1996; Solomon & Smith, 1994). Solomon and Smith discuss ways in which the demands on a social network for support occur at a time when all of the members may have support needs, making support provision a highly stressful event in itself, potentially reducing both its availability and quality. This is particularly likely in the aftermath of terrorist events that create substantial ripple effects from the pervasive climate of fear that can affect whole communities and the manner in which events are interpreted or reported. Recovery can be assisted by providing coworker and peer support resources (Paton, 1997; Williams, 1993) capable of managing the diverse issues (e.g., mental health issues, rumination, counterfactual thinking) that characterize the reintegration experience (Gist & Woodall, 2000; MacLeod & Paton, 1999; Paton & Stephens, 1996).

While cohesive teams can constitute a natural protective resource (Park, 1998), team cohesiveness can, ironically, contribute to vulnerability if situational constraints result in a response being perceived as less effective than anticipated. Some level of failure, relative to expectations derived from routine experience, is likely given the unpredictability of terrorist events and their potential to create large-scale destruction. This threat to team integrity may be compounded by the fear and uncertainty that call assumptions of future capability into question. Officers may find it difficult to perceive the positive characteristics in the group necessary to maintain a positive social identity. Under these circumstances, support networks break down (Hartsough & Myers, 1985), a negative social identity develops (Paton & Stephens, 1996; Solomon & Smith, 1994), and the risk of acute stress reactions increases. Countering this possibility requires team processes that facilitate the realistic interpretation of circumstances, including confronting the psychological implications of, for example, the fear that is an explicit goal of terrorist acts and cultural predispositions to martyrdom. It should also involve actively differentiating personal and situational response factors and focus on learning from the experience (Gist & Woodall, 2000; Lyons, Mickelson, Sullivan, & Coyne, 1998; Park, 1998; Paton & Stephens, 1996).

Lyons et al. (1998) describe team resilience as a function of its ability to engage in "communal coping." This is characterized by the members' collective acceptance of responsibility for event-related problems and the existence of mechanisms by which they can cooperate to resolve problems. Acknowledging and building on effective collaboration during the crisis and working together afterward to develop understanding and enhance future preparedness play an important role in mitigating stress and in developing future stress resilience. It should, however, be borne in mind that recovery, reintegration, and support practices occur within an organizational context. The influence of the latter must thus be included in reintegration risk management.

The Organizational Context

Stress risk is increased if reintegration is experienced within an organizational culture that discourages emotional disclosure, focuses on attributing blame to officers, or minimizes the significance of members' reactions or feelings (Paton & Stephens, 1996; MacLeod & Paton, 1999). Positive reintegration experiences are more likely if the organizational culture encourages managers to actively promote reintegration. This is particularly important if it takes place in a context of critical public and media scrutiny regarding event causation (e.g., beliefs that police were less vigilant than they should have been) and response management (e.g., beliefs that response could have been faster or that it involved inadequate resources).

Managers can assist adaptation by helping officers comprehend that they performed to the best of their ability and by reducing performance guilt by realistically reviewing the ways that situational factors constrained performance (Alexander & Wells, 1991; MacLeod & Paton, 1999; Paton, 1997). Managers can also facilitate positive resolution by assisting staff in identifying the strengths that helped them deal with the terrorist emergency and building on this to plan how to deal with future events more effectively. If these actions are not taken, risk management programs should review the climate of relationships between managers and staff (e.g., trust) and seek ways to build this capacity (Gist & Woodall, 2000; Paton et al., 2003). Such analyses can promote future response effectiveness and contribute to the development and maintenance of a resilient organizational climate. Pursuing this objective may require some organizational change.

Organizational Learning and Future Capability

Terrorism will not only increase in the coming years but also become more deadly (Cooper,

2001). Under these circumstances, it is important that emergency organizations learn from experience (both their own and that of others) and commit to developing a capacity to manage the demands associated with acts of terrorism (FEMA, 2004; Jackson et al., 2003; Kendra & Wachtendorf, 2003). What does this mean for organizational learning?

The development of a capacity to effectively manage terrorist events requires that people and organizations confront the assumptions derived from a long history of effective response to routine emergency events and accept the fact of their existence within a changed reality. At the same time, organizations must also accept the influence of organizational culture, procedures, and managerial attitudes, whose nature and influence are directly under their control, on stress risk. Finally, it must use this understanding to make choices regarding these factors in ways that reduce stress risk.

A capability to learn from experience should not be taken for granted (Berkes, Colding, & Folke, 2003; Harrison & Shirom, 1999; Mitroff & Anagnos, 2001; Paton, 1997). For example, bureaucratic inertia, vested political interests, and centralized power and authority conspire to block change. Change is also unlikely if organizations underestimate the consequences for them or assume that their size and existing resources will safeguard them from significant disruption and allow prompt recovery. Change can also be thwarted by managerial expectations regarding operating conditions and outcomes that have become entrenched and insulated from environmental change (Carafano, 2003). Under these circumstances, emergency organizations may underestimate or overlook threats or initiate inadequate actions, thereby reducing their ability to match their capabilities to a changing hazardscape that now includes highly unpredictable acts of terrorism whose occurrence will be a significant predictor of stress risk for their officers. A failure to take appropriate steps to mitigate stress risk not only constrains the exercise of duty of care regarding officers' mental health but also reduces their response effectiveness.

Organizational cultures that embody these characteristics will attempt to render the consequences of terrorist acts understandable by making them fit in with previous experience, which only makes it difficult for managers to consider, far less confront, the demands associated with un-

predictable and dynamic terrorist events. A failure to learn from experience increases the likelihood that response to future events will occur in an ad hoc manner, with effective response occurring more by chance than by sound planning and good judgment.

To enhance the adaptive capacity to deal with complex terrorist events, organizations must learn from past failures and learn to think "outside the square" (Berkes et al., 2003; Kendra & Wachtendorf, 2003; Paton, 1994; Paton & Jackson, 2002). Not only must the organizations learn to live with risk, they must also develop a culture that is appropriate for a contemporary operating environment within which terrorist acts are a fact of life. Recognition of the importance of institutional learning thus becomes an important precursor of cultural change. According to Berkes et al. (2003), this involves first ensuring that the memory of prior terrorist events and the lessons learned, whether positive or negative, are incorporated into institutional memory and accepted as an enduring fact of emergency organizational life. Second, realistic risk estimates should be derived from comprehensive reviews of potential events and accurate audits of competence (Jackson et al., 2003). These risk estimates must form the basis for future officer and organizational development. Finally, recognition of the risk posed by terrorist events and the importance of learning from them must be consolidated into a culture that espouses the policies, procedures, practices, and attitudes required to facilitate a capacity for adaptive response to an uncertain future (Berkes et al., 2003; Brake, 2001; FEMA, 2004; Jackson et al., 2003; Kendra & Wachtendorf, 2003; Paton & Jackson, 2002).

Conclusion

Terrorism adds a new, unique, and challenging dimension to the hazards faced by contemporary protective services organizations and their members and consequently contributes substantially to the risk of acute stress and posttraumatic stress faced by officers. It is possible, however, to develop a proactive approach to managing this risk. The application of the risk management paradigm to managing stress associated with terrorist events affords an opportunity to confront a priori assumptions regarding posttraumatic stress outcomes. That is, the neutral starting point afforded by the risk paradigm can provide a framework within which emergency organizations can identify options that inform their risk management choices. Knowledge of the relationship between the psychologically challenging characteristics of acts of terrorism and the individual and organizational resources mobilized to deal with them can be used to identify those aspects of this relationship about which choices can be made. This constitutes the basis of the risk assessment process. Acting on these choices is risk management.

We have argued here that choices can be made regarding how threatening and challenging experiences and significant operational demands are rendered meaningful. This can be done through training, simulation, and organizational development. Because it is essential that emergency organizations learn from experience and develop a culture that facilitates adaptive capacity, stress risk management should be viewed as an iterative process that encompasses personal and organizational learning in ways that facilitate the capacity to respond effectively to terrorist events and to do so in ways that mitigate stress risk. When these strategies are applied in a holistic manner, estimates of officers' capability to deal with terrorist events will increase substantially, as will confidence in the planning and policies that define organizations' responsibility and their capacity to safeguard the well-being of officers at the front line of protecting the community from the consequences of terrorist acts.

References

Alexander, D. A., & Wells, A. (1991). Reactions of police officers to body handling after a major disaster: A before and after comparison. *British Journal of Psychiatry, 159,* 517–555.

Alper, A., & Kupferman, S. L. (2003). *Enhancing New York City's emergency preparedness.* New York: New York Economic Development Corporation.

American Psychiatric Association. (1994). *Diagnostic and statistical manual of mental disorders* (4th ed.). Washington, DC: Author.

Berkes, F., Colding, J., & Folke, C. (2003). *Navigating social-ecological systems: Building resilience for complexity and change.* Cambridge: Cambridge University Press.

Blaikie, P., Cannon, T., Davis, I., & Wisner, B. (1994). *At risk: Natural hazards, people's vulnerability, and disaster.* London: Routledge.

Brake, J. D. (2001). *Terrorism and the military's role in domestic crisis management: Background and issues for congress.* Washington, DC: Congressional Research Service, Library of Congress.

Brannick, M., Salas, E., & Prince, C. (Eds.). (1997). *Team performance, assessment, and measurement.* Mahwah, NJ: Erlbaum.

Brewin, C. R., Andrews, B., & Rose, S. (2000). Fear, helplessness, and horror in posttraumatic stress disorder: Investigating *DSM-IV* criterion A2 in victims of violent crime. *Journal of Traumatic Stress, 13,* 499–509.

Brown, J., Mulhern, G., & Joseph, S. (2002). Incident-related stressors, locus of control, coping, and psychological distress among firefighters in Northern Ireland. *Journal of Traumatic Stress, 15,* 161–168.

Burghardt, P. (2004). *Combined systems.* Proceedings of ISCRAM 2004. Brussels: Information Systems for Crisis Response and Management (ISCRAM).

Carafano, J. J. (2003). Preparing responders to respond: The challenges to emergency preparedness in the 21st Century. Heritage Lectures no. 812. Washington, DC: Heritage Foundation.

Carlson, L., James, L. C., Hobfoll, S. E., & Leskin, G. A. (2004). *Fostering resilience in response to terrorism: For psychologists working with military families.* APA Task Force on Resilience in Response to Terrorism. Retrieved January 20, 2006, from http://www.apa.org/psychologists/resilience.html

Cloak, N. L., & Edwards, P. (2004). Psychological first aid: Emergency care for terrorism and disaster survivors. *Current Psychiatry Online, 3.* Retrieved February 8, 2006, from http://www.currentpsychiatry.com

Cooke, N. J., Salas, E., Cannon-Bowers, J. A., & Stout, R. J. (2000). Measuring team knowledge. *Human Factors, 42,* 151–173.

Cooper, H. H. A. (2001). Terrorism: The problems of definition revisited. *American Behavioral Scientist, 44,* 881–893.

Creamer, T. L., & Liddle, B. J. (2005). Secondary traumatic stress among disaster mental health workers responding to the September 11 attacks. *Journal of Traumatic Stress, 18,* 89–96.

Crego, J., & Spinks, T. (1997). Critical incident management simulation. In R. Flin, E. Salas, M. Strub, & L. Martin (Eds.), *Decision making under stress.* (pp.85–94). Brookfield, VT: Ashgate.

Dake, K. (1992). Myths of nature and the public. *Journal of Social Issues, 48,* 21–38.

Daw, J. (2001). Responding to the nation's sadness, anger, and fear. *Monitor on Psychology, 32.* Retrieved February 8, 2006, from http://www.apa.monitor/nov01/

Deahl, M. P., Gillham, A. B., Thomas, J., Searle, M. M., & Srinivasan, M. (1994). Psychological sequelae following the Gulf War: Factors associated with subsequent morbidity and the effectiveness of psychological debriefing. *British Journal of Psychiatry, 165,* 60–65.

Department of Homeland Security. (2003). Top Officials (TOPOFF) exercise series: TOPOFF 2. After action summary report. Washington, DC: Author.

———. (2004). *National response plan.* Washington, DC: Author.

Dunning, C. (2003). Sense of coherence in managing trauma workers. In D. Paton, J. M. Violanti, & L. M. Smith (Eds.), *Promoting capabilities to manage posttraumatic stress: Perspectives on resilience* (pp.119–135). Springfield, IL: Charles C. Thomas.

Endsley, M., & Garland, D. (2000). *Situation awareness: Analysis and measurement.* Mahwah, NJ.: Erlbaum.

Entin, E. E., & Serfaty, D. (1999). Adaptive team coordination. *Human Factors, 41,* 312–325.

Eränen, L., Millar, M., and Paton, D. (2000, March 16–19). Organizational recovery from disaster: Traumatic response with voluntary disaster workers. Third World Conference for the International Society for Traumatic Stress Studies, Carlton Crest, Melbourne.

Federal Emergency Management Agency. (2004). *Responding to incidents of national consequence.* Washington, DC: Author.

Figley, C. R. (1985). *Trauma and its wake.* New York: Brunner/Mazel.

Fisher, H. W. (2000). Mitigation and response planning in a bioterrorist attack. *Disaster Prevention and Management, 9,* 360–367.

Flin, R. (1996). *Sitting in the hot seat: Leaders and teams for critical incident management.* New York: Wiley.

———, & Arbuthnot, K. (Eds.). (2002). *Incident command: Tales from the hot seat.* Burlington, VT: Ashgate.

Flin, R., Salas, E., Strub, M., & Martin, L. (Eds.). (1997). *Decision making under stress.* Brookfield, VT: Ashgate.

Galea, S., Ahern, J., Resnick, H., Kilpatrick, D., Bucuvalas, M., Gold, J., et al. (2002). Psychological sequelae of the September 11 terrorist attacks in New York City. *New England Journal of Medicine, 346,* 982–987.

Gist, R., & Woodall, J. (2000). There are no simple solutions to complex problems. In J. M. Violanti, D. Paton, & C. Dunning (Eds.), *Posttraumatic stress*

intervention: Challenges, issues, and perspectives (pp. 81–95). Springfield, IL: Charles C. Thomas.

Gorski, T. T. (2002). Psychological effects of terrorism can affect firefighter performance. GORSKI-CENAPS. Retrieved January 20, 2006, from http://www.tgorski.com

———. (2003). The crash of United Flight 93 in Shanksville, Pennsylvania. In J. L. Monday (Ed.), *Beyond September 11: An account of postdisaster research* (pp. 83–108). Special Publication no. 39. Boulder: Institute of Behavioral Science, Natural Hazards Research and Applications Information Center, University of Colorado.

Harrison, M. I., & Shirom, A. (1999). *Organizational diagnosis and assessment.* Thousand Oaks, CA: Sage.

Hartsough, D. M., & Myers, D. G. (1985). Disaster work and mental health: Prevention and control of stress among workers. DHHS publication no. (ADM) 85–1422. Rockville, MD: U.S. Department of Health and Human Services.

Hood, C., & Jones, D. K. C. (1996). *Accident and design: Contemporary debates in risk management.* London: UCL Press.

Human Behavior and Weapons of Mass Destruction Crisis/Risk Communication Workshop. (2001). Final report. Washington, DC: Defense Threat Reduction Agency, Federal Bureau of Investigation, & U.S. Joint Forces Command.

Jackson, B. A., Baker, J. C., Ridgely, M. S., Bartis, J. T., & Linn, H. I. (2003). *Protecting emergency responders, Vol. 3: Safety management in disasters and terrorism response.* Cincinnati: National Institute for Occupational Safety and Health.

Janoff-Bulman, R., & Freize, I. H. (1983). A theoretical perspective for understanding reactions to victimization. *Journal of Social Issues, 39,* 1–17.

Kahneman, D., & Tversky, A. (1973). On the psychology of prediction. *Psychological Review, 80,* 237–251.

Kendra, J., & Wachtendorf, T. (2003). Creativity in emergency response to the World Trade Center disaster. In J. L. Monday (Ed.), *Beyond September 11: An account of postdisaster research* (pp 121–146). Special publication no. 39. Boulder: Institute of Behavioral Science, Natural Hazards Research and Applications Information Center, University of Colorado.

Lasker, R. D. (2004). *Redefining readiness: Terrorism planning through the eyes of the public.* New York: New York Academy of Medicine.

Leskin, G. A., Morland, L., Whealin, J., Everly, G., Litz, B., & Keane, T. M. (2004). Fostering resilience in response to terrorism: For psychologists working with first responders. APA Task Force on Resilience in Response to Terrorism. Retrieved January

20, 2006, from http://www.apa.org/psychologists/resilience.html

Lyons, R. F., Mickelson, K. D., Sullivan, M. J. L., & Coyne, J. C. (1998). Coping as a communal process. *Journal of Social and Personal Relationships, 15,* 579–605.

MacLeod, M. D., & Paton, D. (1999). Police officers and violent crime: Social psychological perspectives on impact and recovery. In J. M. Violanti & D. Paton (Eds.), *Police trauma: Psychological aftermath of civilian combat* (pp.25–36). Springfield, IL: Charles C. Thomas.

Maercker, A., & Muller, J. (2004). Social acknowledgment as a victim or survivor: A scale to measure a recovery factor of PTSD. *Journal of Traumatic Stress, 17,* 345–351.

Maniscalco, P. M., & Christen, H. T. (2002). *Understanding terrorism and managing the consequences.* Upper Saddle River, NJ: Prentice Hall.

McKinsey Report. (2002, August 19). Improving NYPD emergency preparedness and response. New York: McKinsey and Company. Retrieved February 8, 2006, from http://www.nyc.gov/html/nypd/pdf/nypdemergency.pdf.

Mitchell, M. (1991). The police after Lockerbie: What were the effects? *Police, 23,* 30–31.

Mitroff, I. I., & Anagnos, G. (2001). *Managing crises before they happen.* New York: Amacom.

Murray, B. (2001). It exposed America's vulnerability. *Monitor on Psychology, 32*(10). Retrieved February 8, 2006, from http://www.apa.org/monitor/nov01/exposed.html.

Myers, D. G. (2001). Do we fear the right things? *APS Observer.* Retrieved July 3, 2002, from http://www.psychologicalscience.org/1201/

North, C. S., Pollio, D. E., Pfefferbaum, B., Megivern, D., Vythilingam, M., Westerhaus, E. T., et al. (2005). Capitol Hill staff workers' experiences of bioterrorism: Qualitative findings from focus groups. *Journal of Traumatic Stress, 18,* 79–88.

North, C. S., Tivis, L., McMillen, J. C., Pfefferbaum, B., Cox, J., Spitznagel, E. L., et al. (2002). Coping, functioning, and adjustment of rescue workers after the Oklahoma City bombing. *Journal of Traumatic Stress, 15,* 171–175.

Park, C. L. (1998). Stress-related growth and thriving through coping: The roles of personality and cognitive processes. *Journal of Social Issues, 54,* 267–277.

Paton, D. (1994). Disaster relief work: An assessment of training effectiveness. *Journal of Traumatic Stress, 7,* 275–288.

———. (1997). *Dealing with traumatic incidents in the workplace* (3d ed.) Queensland, Australia: Gull.

———. (1999). Disaster business continuity: Promoting staff capability. *Disaster Prevention and Management, 8,* 127–133.

———. (2001). Information and decision management in an emergency operations centre. Auckland: Auckland City Council.

———. (2003). Stress in disaster response: A risk management approach. *Disaster Prevention and Management, 12,* 203–209.

———. (in press). Posttraumatic growth in emergency professionals. In. L. Calhoun and R. Tedeschi (Eds.), *Handbook of posttraumatic growth: Research and practice.* Mahwah, NJ: Erlbaum.

———, Cox, D., & Andrew, C. (1989). A preliminary investigation into posttraumatic stress in rescue workers. Robert Gordon University Social Science Research Reports no. 1.

Paton, D., & Flin, R. (1999). Disaster stress: An emergency management perspective. *Disaster Prevention and Management, 8,* 261–267.

Paton, D., & Hannan, G. (2004). Risk factors in emergency responders. In D. Paton, J. Violanti, C. Dunning, & L. Smith (Eds.), *Managing traumatic stress risk: A proactive approach* (pp.111–128). Springfield, IL: Charles C. Thomas.

Paton, D., & Jackson, D. (2002). Developing disaster management capability: An assessment center approach. *Disaster Prevention and Management, 11,* 115–122.

Paton, D., Johnston, D., Houghton, B., Flin, R., Ronan, K., & Scott, B. (1999). Managing natural hazard consequences: Information management and decision making. *Journal of the American Society of Professional Emergency Managers, 6,* 37–48.

Paton, D., Smith, L. M., Violanti, J. M., & Eränen, L. (2000). Work-related trauma stress: Risk, vulnerability, and resilience. In J. M. Violanti, D. Paton, & C. Dunning (Eds.), *Posttraumatic stress intervention: Challenges, issues, and perspectives* (pp. 187–202). Springfield, IL: Charles C. Thomas.

Paton, D., & Stephens, C. (1996). Training and support for emergency responders. In D. Paton & J. Violanti (Eds.), *Traumatic stress in critical occupations: Recognition, consequences, and treatment.* Springfield, IL: Charles C. Thomas.

Paton, D., Violanti, J. M., Dunning, C., & Smith, L. M. (2004). *Managing traumatic stress risk: A proactive approach.* Springfield, IL: Charles C. Thomas.

Paton, D., Violanti, J. M., & Smith, L. M. (2003). *Promoting capabilities to manage posttraumatic stress: Perspectives on resilience.* Springfield, IL: Charles C. Thomas.

Pfefferbaum, B., Seale, T. W., McDonald, N. B., Brandt, E. N., Rainwater, S. M., Maynard, B. T., et al. (2000). Posttraumatic stress two years after the

Oklahoma City bombing in youths geographically distant from the explosion. *Psychiatry, 63,* 358–370.

Pollock, C., Paton, D., Smith, L., & Violanti, J. (2003). Team resilience. In D. Paton, J. Violanti, & L. Smith (Eds.), *Promoting capabilities to manage posttraumatic stress: Perspectives on resilience* (pp.74–88). Springfield, IL: Charles C. Thomas.

Raphael, B. (1986) *When disaster strikes.* London: Hutchinson.

Scotti, J. R., Beach, B. K., Northrop, L. M. E., Rode, C. A., & Forsyth, J. P. (1995). The psychological impact of accidental injury. In J. R. Freedy & S. E. Hobfall (Eds.), *Traumatic stress: From theory to practice* (pp.181–212). New York: Plenum.

Shakespeare-Finch, J., Paton, D., & Violanti, J. (2003). The family: Resilience resource and resilience needs. In D. Paton, J. Violanti, & L. Smith (Eds.), *Promoting capabilities to manage posttraumatic stress: Perspectives on resilience* (pp.170–185). Springfield, IL: Charles C. Thomas.

Shuster, M. A., Stein, B. D., Jaycox, L. H., Collins, R. L., Marshall, G. N., Elliott, M. N., et al. (2001). A national survey of stress reaction after the September 11, 2001, terrorist attacks. *New England Journal of Medicine, 345,* 1507–1512.

Simpson, D. M., & Stehr, S. (2003). Victim management and identification after the World Trade Center collapse. In J. L. Monday (Ed.), *Beyond September 11: An account of postdisaster research* (pp.109–120). Special publication no. 39. Boulder: Institute of Behavioral Science, Natural Hazards Research and Applications Information Center, University of Colorado.

Solomon, S. D., & Smith, E. S. (1994). Social support and perceived control as moderators of responses to dioxin and flood exposure. In R. J. Ursano, B. G. McCaughey, & C. S. Fullerton (Eds.), *Individual and community responses to trauma and disaster* (pp. 179–200). Cambridge: Cambridge University Press.

Stout, R. J., Cannon-Bowers, J. A., Salas, E., & Milanovich, D. M. (1999). Planning, shared mental models, and coordinated performance: An empirical link is established. *Human Factors, 41,* 61–71.

Tedeschi, R. G., & Calhoun, L. G. (2003). Routes to posttraumatic growth through cognitive processing. In D. Paton, J. M. Violanti, & L. M. Smith (Eds.), *Promoting capabilities to manage posttraumatic stress: Perspectives on resilience* (pp.12–26). Springfield, IL: Charles C. Thomas.

Thompson, J. (1993). Psychological impact of body recovery duties. *Journal of the Royal Society of Medicine, 86,* 628–629.

van der Lee, M., & van Vugt, M. (2004). *IMI: An information system for effective mutidisciplinary incident management.* Proceedings of ISCRAM 2004. Brussels: ISCRAM.

Violanti, J. M. (1990). Posttrauma vulnerability: A proposed model. In J. W. Reese, J. M. Horn, & C. Dunning (Eds.), *Critical incidents in policing* (pp. 503–510). Washington, DC: U.S. Government Printing Office.

———, & Paton, D. (2006). *Who gets PTSD? Issues of vulnerability to posttraumatic stress.* Springfield, IL: Charles C. Thomas.

Vrij, A., van der Steen, J., & Koppelaar, L. (1994). Aggression of police officers as a function of temperature: An experiment with the fire arms training system. *Journal of Community and Applied Psychology, 4,* 365–370.

Williams, T. (1993). Trauma in the workplace. In J. P. Wilson & B. Raphael (Eds.), *International handbook of traumatic stress syndromes* (pp.925–934). New York: Plenum.

Wraith, R. (1994). The impact of major events on children. In R. Watts & J. D. de la Horne (Eds.), *Coping with trauma* (pp. 101–120). Brisbane: Australian Academic Press.

Yehuda, R. (2002). Posttraumatic stress disorder. *New England Journal of Medicine, 346,* 108–114.

Zimbardo, P. (2001). *The psychology of terrorism: Mind games and healing.* Retrieved January 20, 2006, from http://www.apa.org/science/

18

Evidence-Based Interventions for Survivors of Terrorism

Josef I. Ruzek
Shira Maguen
Brett T. Litz

Although profoundly changed as a result of terrorist acts, most survivors of mass violence or those who have lost loved ones as a result of terrorism do not develop significant mental health problems or disability. As is the case with any trauma, a relatively small but salient percentage of survivors of terror will develop chronic mental health problems, such as posttraumatic stress disorder (PTSD). Any mental health strategy or plan needs to take into account the number of affected individuals, the available treatment resources, and the research literature. If resources were unlimited, we would attempt to hasten recovery and promote adaptive functioning in every survivor of terrorism. However, in most mass violence contexts, too many affected individuals exist, typically coupled with a lack of well-trained professionals. As a result, secondary prevention of chronic mental health problems and functional disability in those most at risk is the priority. In addition, resources should be devoted to providing evidence-based tertiary prevention for those terror survivors who develop chronic psychiatric problems.

A range of interventions may be useful to prevent or address the negative psychological impact of exposure to terrorist incidents. In the following sections we examine findings from the literature on acute stress disorder (ASD) and PTSD in terms of their implications for postterrorism intervention. We also discuss prevention and treatment research related to the management of traumatic bereavement and alcohol problems. Moreover, we review current thinking about disaster mental health care and suggest ways of improving care. Attention is given to individual, group, and community-scale interventions during the emergency, early, and later periods of the terrorist event. Special challenges of service delivery in the postterrorism environment are also explained.

Although mental health practitioners generally agree about the need to use empirically supported intervention methods, to date the outcome research examining services for terrorism and disaster survivors is limited. Few of the components of disaster mental health services have been evaluated, and the methodological base of much of the existing research is not sufficiently strong to support clear recommendations. Therefore, in this chapter we discuss and extrapolate from evidence-based interventions that have been applied to trauma-related psychological problems in contexts other than terrorism and disaster and emphasize intervention methods that, if not evidence based, are at least consistent with current evidence and theory.

Evidence-Based Interventions for Trauma-Related Problems

Evidence-Based Treatment for Posttraumatic Stress Disorder

A considerable body of evidence from randomized controlled trials supports the efficacy of cognitive-behavioral therapy (CBT) for acute and chronic PTSD. CBT entails a package of interventions designed to promote stress and affect management, assimilation and accommodation of the meaning of traumatic experiences, and processing of the emotional residue of trauma. CBT entails prolonged exposure to trauma memories and various forms of cognitive restructuring, which involves challenging maladaptive cognitions related to the trauma and replacing these with healthier alternative thoughts. Prolonged-exposure therapy, which involves a *repeated* therapeutic reliving of traumatic experiences to facilitate emotional processing, is often considered the sine qua non of any effective treatment. However, stress inoculation (applied stress management) and cognitive therapy alone have been shown to be as effective (e.g., Ehlers & Clark, 2003; Foa et al., 1999).

Prolonged-exposure CBT treatments have been found to significantly decrease PTSD symptoms in a range of survivor populations, including Vietnam veterans (Cooper & Clum, 1989; Keane, Fairbank, Caddell, & Zimering, 1989; Boudewyns & Hyer, 1990; Glynn et al., 1999), female sexual assault survivors (Foa, Rothbaum, Riggs, & Murdock, 1991; Foa et al., 1999; Resick, Nishith, Weaver, Astin, & Feuer, 2002), and survivors of varied traumas (Marks, Lovell, Noshirvani, Livanou, & Thrasher, 1998). Cognitive restructuring has been demonstrated to be effective in studies of survivors of mixed traumas (Marks et al., 1998; Tarrier, Pilgrim, et al., 1999), and stress inoculation training (i.e., an anxiety management treatment that makes use of techniques such as breathing, muscle relaxation, and calming self-talk) has performed well with female sexual assault survivors (Foa et al., 1991; Foa et al., 1999). Resick et al. (2002) have demonstrated significant improvements in female rape survivors using cognitive processing therapy, a manualized form of CBT in which elements of exposure and cognitive therapies are combined.

While these studies evaluated individual treatment, there have also been several investigations of group trauma–focused interventions, although only two known studies were randomized controlled trials. Zlotnick et al. (1997) randomly assigned 48 female survivors of childhood sexual abuse with PTSD to either a 15-week affect-management group or a wait-list control condition. Participants received individual therapy and psychotropic medication beginning 1 month before and throughout the study. Those who completed the group reported significantly fewer PTSD symptoms compared to those in the control condition. Schnurr et al. (2003) conducted a multisite randomized and controlled trial of group therapy for PTSD in Vietnam veterans ($n = 360$). Veterans were assigned to either trauma-focused group therapy or to present-centered group treatment, in which participants were explicitly instructed not to discuss their trauma. Weekly groups were held for 30 weeks, followed by a tapered treatment of one session per month for 5 months. Results indicate that PTSD symptoms improved from baseline, with 40% of participants demonstrating significant changes in symptoms; however, there was no significant difference between the trauma-focused and the present-centered groups. When excluding participants who did not attend a sufficient number of treatment sessions, results indicate that avoidance and numbing symptoms were reduced more in trauma-focused group participants, although dropout rates were higher in this group.

Applications to Terrorism

CBT is the prescriptive treatment for PTSD. It is important to note that not everyone is helped by CBT and that positive symptoms (e.g., intrusive thoughts) are more likely to improve than negative symptoms (e.g., avoidance). Furthermore, because PTSD is a chronic problem for many, we should not assume that people necessarily regain their pre-trauma functioning completely. Given these qualifiers, for those who are traumatized as a result of their exposure to a terrorist attack and develop PTSD, some variant of CBT would arguably be useful. Future randomized controlled trials should confirm this expectation.

Studies are needed to demonstrate the efficacy of group treatment following a terrorist attack. The existing studies demonstrate symptom improvement regardless of the modality of therapy. One possibility is that the crucial ingredient in symptom improvement is the support that group therapy offers, given the absence of other forms of treatment. However, in at least one of the group studies, participants were receiving concurrent individual and psychopharmacological interventions. Overall, group therapy seems to be better than no treatment and in and of itself is a cost-effective intervention; however, in the best-case scenario, group therapy should perhaps be utilized in conjunction with individual treatment.

To date, there is only one study of a group intervention for survivors of a terrorist attack. This was conducted in Israel following an attempt to use a Palestinian vehicle filled with explosives to blow up an Israeli bus (Amir et al., 1998). The 15 women participating in group debriefing plus brief group psychotherapy were not injured in the attack and participated in six group sessions in the 2 months following the attack. The group included psychological debriefing (i.e., each woman spoke about her memories of the trauma in a safe environment), normalization of feelings, discussion of coping strategies, cognitive restructuring, and a focus on return to pretrauma functioning.

Symptoms were assessed 2 days, 2 months, and 6 months after the terrorist event. PTSD symptoms improved at 2 and 6 months when compared to 2 days after the event. At the 6-month follow-up, 27% of participants met all of the criteria for a PTSD diagnosis. Due to the lack of a control group and nonrandomized design, it is difficult to ascertain whether improvements in symptoms were due to the natural course of recovery or to the intervention. While this intervention employed a combination of psychological debriefing and group psychotherapy immediately following exposure to a terrorist event, there is emerging consensus that psychological debriefing is contraindicated on empirical and conceptual grounds directly following exposure to trauma (e.g., Litz & Gray, 2004).

Evidence-Based Treatment for Traumatic Grief

Prigerson et al. (1999) have proposed that traumatic grief is a distinct disorder (i.e., separate from PTSD, depression, or other anxiety disorders) and offered a classification system by which clinical problems with traumatic grief or complicated bereavement can be identified. According to this taxonomy, to receive a diagnosis of traumatic grief, a person must experience the death of a loved one

and report three of the following four symptoms: intrusive thoughts about the deceased, yearning for the deceased, searching for the deceased, and/or loneliness as a result of the death. Additionally, the person experiences a host of other possible symptoms (e.g., purposelessness, numbness, difficulty acknowledging the death), with symptoms lasting at least 2 months, and the disturbance needs to cause significant impairment in functioning. Clinically, many of the symptoms and problems of traumatic grief are conflated with PTSD symptoms, but clinicians may mistake traumatic bereavement for PTSD, which is inappropriate because the latter disorder fails to capture the unique problems that result from loss (e.g., Neria & Litz, in press; Raphael, Minkov, & Dobson, 2001). Because of the possible sheer magnitude and the horrific nature of deaths due to terrorism, traumatic grief is important to examine as a separate clinical problem in relation to coping with loss in the context of terrorist events.

There are few systematic and specialized treatments for traumatic grief. Shear et al. (2001) have developed a treatment that is a combination of interpersonal therapy for depression and CBT for PTSD. These researchers conducted an uncontrolled, 16-session pilot study of their treatment with people suffering from traumatic grief. Imaginal and in vivo exposure were the primary strategies for grief reduction (e.g., listening to audiotaped personal accounts of trauma, in vivo hierarchies of painful contexts). Additionally, Shear et al. (2001) used interpersonal therapy techniques to help victims reengage with others. After 4 months of treatment, reduction of grief, depression, and anxiety symptoms was reported; however, the authors have not reported follow-up data, thus the long-term efficacy of this treatment is unknown.

The large dropout rate of those who lost loved ones as a result of a traumatic incident is worrisome; as a result, it is unclear whether this treatment is appropriate for people who may lose a loved one to an act of terror. Additional limitations include the older age of completers, the length of time since the death of the loved one (i.e., the mean was 3 years), and assumptions that participants experience avoidance as a hallmark symptom of traumatic grief, as demonstrated by the decision to employ in vivo hierarchies (i.e., the opposite may be true; people may be constantly thinking about the deceased and/or have intrusive thoughts of the deceased). It is also unclear whether this treatment generalizes to younger people who have unexpectedly lost a loved one as a result of a senseless act of terror rather than losing a spouse or parent to old age.

Two randomized, noncontrolled trials of guided mourning for "morbid grief" (i.e., grief resulting from the loss of a significant other in which symptoms persist for more than a year) resulted in grief symptom improvement for the intervention and control groups, suggesting no differential impact of treatment (Mawson, Marks, Ramm, & Stern, 1981; Sireling, Cohen, & Marks, 1988). Participants received six sessions of either a guided mourning or antiexposure intervention. Those in the guided mourning group were instructed to participate in tasks involving exposure to avoided cognitive, affective, and behavioral cues (e.g., viewing pictures of loved ones, writing letters to the deceased). Conversely, the antiexposure group was encouraged to focus on the future rather than thinking about the past and to avoid all reminders of the deceased. Participants in both groups were assigned between-session tasks and were encouraged to engage in new activities. Results indicate that individuals in both groups demonstrated improvement on a number of variables at several intervals, up to 9 months posttreatment (Sireling et al., 1988). Overall, the exposure group performed significantly better than the antiexposure group only on a bereavement-avoidance task, as well as some measures of distress to bereavement cues (out of a total of 29 outcome measures). One possible conclusion is that support and encouragement to engage in new daily activities are the critical therapeutic ingredients that facilitated improvement. Limitations include failure to report modes of death of loved ones and the assumption that bereaved people avoid thoughts of the deceased (similar to Shear et al., 2001).

There have also been group interventions for those who may experience traumatic grief. For example, Murphy et al. (1998) conducted a 10-week, randomized, controlled trial for parents who lost a child to homicide, suicide, or accident. Parents participated in 2-hour treatment sessions. In the first hour of each group, parents learned skills pertaining to actively confronting problems (e.g., ways to release anger), respecting differences in mourning, closure (e.g., writing down thoughts and

feelings), and self-care. In the second hour, they shared death-related experiences and received emotional support and assistance in reframing the death and its consequences. The intervention resulted in differential effects for mothers and fathers, with mothers improving on 80% of mental distress measures, including depression, anxiety, and fear. Conversely, fathers improved on fewer than 50% of the measures. Additionally, higher self-efficacy, self-esteem, and positive reinterpretation of events at baseline predicted lower mental distress up to 2 years later for both mothers and fathers.

Furthermore, repressive coping predicted greater mental distress for fathers, and Murphy et al. (1998) postulate that repression of feelings in fathers may be difficult to reduce because of gender socialization and may contribute to some of these gender differences. Although mothers seemed to improve, when compared to the control group, there were no significant differences for either parent on any of the outcome measures (i.e., mental distress, trauma, loss accommodation, physical health, and marital satisfaction). When the results were parsed by level of distress, the intervention was beneficial for mothers with higher mental distress and grief at baseline. However, this may be a case of regression to the mean. Conversely, fathers with higher levels of PTSD at baseline did worse than control group fathers, which is of concern and may demonstrate that intervention should vary by gender.

Several potential moderators of treatment outcome were examined in a trial of complicated grief treatment among inpatients ($n = 139$) that were randomized into either interpretive (i.e., exploration of interpersonal and/or intrapersonal conflicts) or supportive (i.e., sharing of coping strategies) short-term group therapy (Ogrodniczuk & Joyce, 2004; Piper, McCallum, Joyce, Rosie, & Ogrodniczuk, 2001). Similar to Murphy et al. (1998), Ogrodniczuk & Joyce (2004) found that women had better outcomes than men following treatment. They report that men were less committed to their therapy groups and perceived by other group members as less compatible than women (Ogrodniczuk et al., 2004), which may suggest that men need different types of treatment or that separate gender groups may be most beneficial.

Several other factors contributed to improvement in symptoms following group including personality factors (Ogrodniczuk, Piper, Joyce, McCallum, & Rosie, 2003), perceived social support from friends (Ogrodniczuk, Piper, Joyce, McCallum, & Rosie, 2002), interpersonal factors (Ogrodniczuk, Piper, McCallum, Joyce, & Rosie, 2002), and level of engagement in the group (Ogrodniczuk & Piper, 2003). More specifically, extraversion, conscientiousness, openness, secure attachment to the deceased, and recent social role functioning were positively associated with symptom improvement, and neuroticism was negatively associated with symptom improvement (Ogrodniczuk, Piper, McCallum, et al., 2002; Ogrodniczuk et al., 2003).

Two group studies were conducted with grieving adolescents. The first included African American adolescents exposed to homicide and consisted of a 10-week group therapy intervention aimed at reducing PTSD symptoms (Salloum, Avery, & McClain, 2001). Participants received psychoeducation about grief and trauma and were encouraged to share their thoughts and feelings about death. They were also taught about normative grief reactions, healthy coping techniques, safety, anger management, and ways to access support, utilize spirituality, and focus on future goals. Following the intervention, group members reported decreased reexperiencing and avoidance symptoms; however, there were no improvements in level of arousal. Interpretation of this study is greatly limited because of the lack of a control group and the absence of randomization. This study was also limited due to a large range of time since death (1–10 years). Rynearson, Favell, Gold, and Prigerson (2002) conducted a similar 10-session adolescent group study with incarcerated youths who had experienced the violent death of a friend or family member. They surveyed a wider range of outcome variables (e.g., depression, grief, and PTSD symptoms), all of which significantly decreased following intervention. Major limitations include lack of a control group and random assignment to condition as well as a small sample size. Additionally, Rynearson et al. (2002) failed to describe the type of treatment provided, although a treatment manual is available upon request.

Applications to Terrorism

Treatment research for traumatic grief is in its infancy, and major methodological problems limit what can be gleaned from this literature. Some promising treatment approaches have been developed (e.g., Shear et al., 2001), but rigorous tests of these approaches are necessary before they can be recommended. Furthermore, given that individual or group treatment studies have not been conducted with people who have lost a loved one due to terrorism, the generalizability to such events is questionable. The one treatment study that included people who suffered *loss from traumatic means* reported the highest dropout rates (Shear et al., 2001). One possibility is that timing is a crucial aspect of these interventions and the most optimal timing of delivery is simply unknown; another is that existing individual treatments for traumatic grief do not generalize to those who have lost a loved one due to traumatic means.

Another possibility is that loss due to traumatic events represents a syndrome that is different from what has been traditionally defined as *complicated bereavement,* which can be associated with any type of loss (many studies of complicated bereavement include large numbers of widows and widowers who lost a loved one due to illness and/or old age). For example, when someone loses a loved one by traumatic means such as terrorism, the person is likely to experience excruciating intrusive thoughts about the deceased and, as a result, is likely to avoid reminders or triggers of these painful memories. In the case of terrorism, the intrusive thoughts will likely involve the means by which the loved one was killed. Thus, arguably, when someone dies as a result of terrorism, the clinical picture of the survivor is an amalgam of traumatic grief and PTSD, with both avoidance of images and reminders and intrusive thoughts of the loved one, especially if the deceased person was horrifically injured in the process.

Murphy et al. (1998) conducted groups with parents who had lost their children, who most closely represent people who have lost a loved one due to traumatic means such as terrorism. Unfortunately, compared to controls, the parents who received the intervention did not improve on any of the outcome measures. One possibility is that the support they received and the skills they were taught through the group were useful, but being exposed to stories of how other children died may have been retraumatizing. Future studies should investigate which treatment modality works best for which group following the loss of a loved one due to terrorism.

Interventions that attempt to create or foster the use of social supports (e.g., support groups of similarly bereaved people) may be especially helpful given that social support is inversely related to symptoms of traumatic grief (Spooren, Henderick, & Jannes, 2000). However, women may benefit from group interventions to a greater extent than men, and these gender differences should be examined.

Arguably, exposure-based interventions may facilitate recovery for those traumatically bereaved individuals who avoid thinking about the deceased, the mode of death, or other reminders of the death (as compared to those who are nonavoidant). However, not everyone who suffers from traumatic grief experiences may exhibit avoidance as a predominant symptom pattern, so this should be carefully assessed, and treatment should be tailored accordingly. In addition, it should not be assumed that avoidance and suppression are necessarily signs of psychopathology. There is emerging consensus in the bereavement literature that evasion of painful affect can lead to positive outcomes from loss (e.g., Bonnano, 2004). It is likely that traditional CBT methods of reducing avoidance, such as imaginal and in vivo exposure, need to be carefully reconsidered. There may be cases that require exposure-based interventions because the functional impairments entail gross restrictions in functioning. Intense forms of emptiness, numbness, and despair may be addressable by behavioral activation strategies that promote active engagement with pleasurable activities.

The optimal timing of delivery of interventions for loss by terrorism is entirely unclear. Indeed, the timing of interventions with a bereaved population has been noted as a confounding variable in several studies (see Schut, Stroebe, van den Bout, & Terheggen, 2001). Some studies highlight the importance of allowing the grieving process to unfold naturally so that the bereaved can heal with time and find sources of support independently of receiving treatment; however, the dearth of controlled studies limits the ability to draw firm conclusions about intervention timing. Although there are clearly significant challenges inherent in conducting randomized clinical trials with this population, more rigorous tests of these approaches with those who have lost loved ones due to terrorism are necessary to evaluate their efficacy (see Litz & Gibson, in press).

Evidence-Based Treatments for Alcohol Abuse

Research has established a link between trauma exposure, chronic PTSD, and alcohol consumption (Ouimette & Brown, 2002). Some evidence also indicates that alcohol consumption may increase following exposure to trauma (e.g., Burnam et al., 1988; Kilpatrick, Acierno, Resnick, Saunders, & Best, 1997) and disaster/terrorism events (North et al., 2002; Vlahov et al., 2002; Grieger, Fullerton, & Ursano, 2003; Vlahov, Galea, Ahern, Resnick, & Kilpatrick, 2004). For example, increases in alcohol consumption were reported by 25% of a sample of Manhattan residents 5–8 eight weeks following the 9/11 attacks (Vlahov et al., 2002), and increased drinking remained in evidence at 6 months (Vlahov et al., 2004). Grieger, Fullerton, and Ursano (2003) also reported increased use of alcohol in survivors of the 9/11 terrorist attack on the Pentagon.

In the context of terrorism and disaster, mental health providers may be confronted by survivors who have increased their consumption of alcohol. For those whose drinking increases to problem levels, it is important for alcohol consumption to be explicitly addressed. In fact, a large literature supports the effectiveness of relatively brief treatments in reducing consumption (e.g., Moyer, Finney, Swearingen, & Vergun, 2002; Dunn, 2003). Not much is yet known about how trauma survivors generally or terrorism survivors in particular will respond to these approaches. One study has demonstrated that a single 30-minute interview with patients admitted to a trauma center for treatment of injury who screen positive for excessive alcohol use can reduce alcohol consumption in those with existing alcohol problems (Gentilello et al., 1999). This intervention consisted of a motivational interview that explored personalized feedback about a patient's drinking habits. Quantity and frequency of consumption were compared to national norms, level of intoxication at admission was related to injury risk, negative consequences of alcohol as indicated on the screening tools were discussed, and negative physical consequences based on abnormal laboratory test results and level of alcohol dependence based on questionnaire assessment were reviewed. The interviewer also stressed individual responsibility for reducing drinking, offered a menu of strategies for change, and provided a list of treatment resources in the local community. While this array of individual assessment information would not be available in crisis counseling situations, the general principles of review of individual drinking habits and consideration of options could be applied.

It is not known how best to provide such education following terrorist attacks. Possibly, brief education to reduce consumption can be supplied by media. A study conducted by Acierno, Resnick, Flood, and Holmes (2003) suggests that a 17-minute educational video delivered shortly following rape may be capable of reducing postrape substance abuse. The low-cost, easily administered educational intervention reduced the likelihood of marijuana abuse at 6 weeks, and there was a trend for the video to be associated with less alcohol abuse among women with a prior history of alcohol or marijuana use. Single-occasion interventions, whether provided via media or face-to-face contact, can be expected to have limited impact for some, and additional follow-up contacts may increase the impact of helping efforts. In another study of an intervention based on motivational enhancement (Miller & Rollnick, 2002), Longabaugh et al. (2001) reported that a 40–60 minute intervention plus a booster session was more effective in reducing alcohol-related negative consequences in patients seeking emergency medical care than standard care or a single-session intervention.

Disaster responders will also see those who may be at elevated risk for relapse into preexisting problems following exposure to a terrorist attack. Those who are in recovery from substance abuse problems, especially those recently abstinent, may benefit from monitoring and intervention to prevent relapse. Those who relapse should be referred for evidence-based treatment.

Conclusions

Given the considerable body of evidence supporting the use of CBT methods in treating PTSD, with some evidence of generalizability of these methods

to terrorism-related PTSD (Gillespie, Duffy, Hackmann, & Clark, 2002), these approaches should perhaps be offered to terrorism survivors who have developed PTSD. Traumatic grief interventions are in the early phase of development and should be regarded as exploratory in the context of terrorism. However, given the need to offer help to those who experience traumatic grief in that context, there may be sufficient anecdotal evidence from the manualized treatment of survivors of 9/11 to warrant consideration. Finally, brief alcohol reduction interventions conducted in a hospital trauma center have been effective, suggesting the possible utility of such interventions among survivors of terrorism and disaster.

Most of the research on the treatment of PTSD is for survivors whose problems have existed for some time. Thus, the current evidence base largely fails to speak to the real world of delivery of terrorism and disaster services, in which services may be provided immediately after an event and in the first weeks and months after a trauma. In the next section, we describe more comprehensively the range of interventions that should be considered and comment on them from the standpoint of current research and theory.

Toward an Integrated Intervention System

Features of a System of Care

Stepped Care

During and after terrorist attacks and in situations of ongoing threat of attack, people's need for assistance will vary widely, depending on aspects of their exposure, history, biology, personal resources, and the recovery environment. While it is expected that most people will continue to function well without intervention or will experience initial acute stress reactions but will recover without formal help, some will not. The challenge is to find better ways of matching people to services based on the nature and degree of their needs.

Many current postterrorism contacts between survivor and helper take place in a relatively informal meeting, on-scene, at an emergency shelter, or in the context of a community outreach visit. In these meetings, the helper offers support, psychological first aid, and brief educational information. In fact, a one- or two-session brief counseling approach characterizes much of current-day disaster crisis counseling.

For those who have developed significant problems, it is likely that multiple-session interventions will be more helpful than a single contact. Some problems may require only two to five sessions. For those who do not improve following this level of help, sustained expert mental health care is indicated. This "stepped-care" approach matches people to a level of care in part based upon response to earlier steps and reduces the likelihood of unnecessary and inappropriate treatment (cf. Haaga, 2000).

Individual and Group Interventions

Interventions to prevent postterrorism problems must be delivered in a variety of interpersonal contexts. Most education and support will likely be provided in the context of individual contacts between disaster mental health workers or other community providers and survivors, and, to date, most of the efforts to develop trauma-related interventions have focused on individual care. However, in many postterrorism environments, individual care may be difficult to deliver (e.g., due to large numbers of affected persons, insufficient availability of mental health providers, or cost constraints), and group interventions provide a potentially cost-effective alternative.

Groups may be used soon after a terrorist attack or disaster to provide education, mobilize social support, and teach skills for coping with stress reactions and other posttrauma challenges. Compared with one-on-one services, they may be able to more effectively harness some important helping processes, including social support and social modeling. When terrorism survivors are part of an existing group that will continue functioning as a unit (e.g., work colleagues), the group will effectively act as part of the ongoing recovery environment, and members can be encouraged to support one another. In such a circumstance, group cohesion may serve a protective function and so may be useful as a target for helping efforts. When group structures permit multisession contact, educational messages can be repeated, supportive relationships among members can be strengthened, and recovery behaviors and skills can be shaped and reinforced. At a later time, group psychotherapies may represent an effective means of treating chronic PTSD (Foy et al., 2000).

To date, terrorism and disaster-specific group interventions require additional development and evaluation. The primary model of early group intervention to reduce the impact of trauma is group stress debriefing (Raphael & Wilson, 2000), but there is no evidence that this approach prevents PTSD (e.g., McNally, Bryant, & Ehlers, 2003), and in our view this approach is inappropriate because it is a single-session intervention that does not screen participants in any way for risk or need and there is no systematic vehicle to stepped care (Litz, Bryant, & Adler, 2002). Other group approaches for early disaster care (e.g., Ruzek, 2002b), disaster-related PTSD (e.g., Young, Ruzek, & Ford, 1999), and disaster-related sleep difficulties (Krakow et al., 2002) have been described.

A special case of group-related social support is the self-help or mutual aid group. When survivors join together to help one another, they can do much to provide mutual emotional support. For example, after the events of 9/11, families who lost loved ones in the World Trade Center attacks linked with families who experienced losses due to the bombing of the Oklahoma City federal building. Mutual aid groups can help members reestablish a sense of control over events and sometimes go beyond support functions to address political or legislative issues affecting themselves and their community.

Generally, in communities affected by terrorism, efforts should be made to restore a sense of control to survivors by helping them to take pragmatic action to improve their situation, strengthen perceived safety, and rebuild their community. Glass and Schoch-Spana (2002, p. 219) have suggested that naturally occurring civic, occupational, or information networks should be seen as "a potential conduit for organizing or facilitating public responses that are beneficial," related to information dissemination, outbreak monitoring, resource distribution, and survivor care. For example, various community networks could be mobilized to distribute antibiotics, convene vaccination gatherings, or organize home visits. A potentially important role for mental health providers is to help facilitate the development of self-help activities by survivor groups. Depending on the situation and the receptivity of the survivors, mental health providers could educate them about reactions to terrorism and ways of coping and provide advice on group structure and function.

Phase-Specific Care

Service delivery needs will evolve over time as on-scene support moves toward acute helping responses, then to the provision of early mental health services, and finally to the detection and delivery of care to those who develop enduring problems as a result of their exposure to terrorism. Services delivered immediately after the act of terrorism or other disaster, those organized in the first weeks and months after the event, and those made available in the longer term will differ greatly. The earliest efforts will focus on psychological first aid appropriate for most survivors. If problems appear severe or disabling or if they persist past the initial postevent period, brief crisis counseling is an option. If brief several-session help is insufficient to resolve problems, referral for mental health treatment may be warranted. Changes in service delivery over time reflect the changing needs of survivor populations and the fact that early posttrauma support may be useful for many survivors, while more intensive help at later times will be required by fewer persons.

Components of Care

Psychological First Aid

There is widespread agreement on the importance of "psychological first aid" (PFA) in the immediate aftermath of terrorist events (National Institute of Mental Health, 2002). PFA is an umbrella term for a variety of helping activities designed to contain distress and reduce acute stress responses. It includes restoration of sleep, reconnection of survivors with loved ones, and direction to helping resources (Litz et al., 2002). Figure 18.1 shows a list of early steps to provide for basic needs and PFA (Veterans Health Administration, 2003). These activities, although difficult to study empirically, are believed to be helpful and are widely judged as unlikely to cause additional harm. Some may lend themselves to more systematic development and delivery. For example, efforts to reduce immediate anxiety may benefit from the application of methods of anxiety management, such as simple training in deep breathing, which may be useful to offer more systematically to disaster survivors experiencing hyperarousal.

For a variety of reasons, there is a growing reluctance to go beyond this kind of pragmatic help to provide more formal mental health interventions in the first days following exposure. Exceptions include providing treatment to those who are in danger (e.g., psychotic, suicidal) and those whose initial responses are extreme (e.g., intense panic) and who may benefit from short-term medications. However, with regard to most survivors, no single-session interventions that can be administered very soon after trauma have yet been shown to be effective in preventing later problems (Bisson, 2003).

Screening, Triage, and Referral

In the immediate aftermath of terrorist events, helping resources are likely to be very limited; thus more intensive psychological care must be reserved for those most in need. Initial triage efforts depend on the ability to differentiate between those whose problems require immediate help and those who may not require urgent care. When terrorist events involve biological or chemical attacks, the identification of those in need of more intensive care will be especially difficult. Emergency medical facilities may be overwhelmed by large numbers of help seekers. For example, following the Aum Shinrikyō cult sarin attacks in 15 Tokyo subway stations, approximately 5,000 people sought emergency care; almost 75% of those who were seen had not been exposed to sarin (Bowler, Murai, & True, 2001). Also, reactions to various biological or chemical agents may mimic stress reactions or psychiatric problems (Ursano, Norwood, Fullerton, Holloway, & Hall, 2003), making differential diagnosis difficult.

In addition to initial triage efforts, some approaches to early posttrauma intervention include an effort to identify those who are expected to be at risk for development of chronic problems so that preventive interventions can be delivered (Ruzek, in press). There is, however, a limited current ability to accurately differentiate in the first weeks between those whose distress and traumatic stress reactions will improve without help and those whose symptoms are unlikely to remit. After several months have passed, accuracy improves.

Nonetheless, identification of those who may be in need of mental health intervention occurs at all stages of response. Gross indicators of risk may be sufficient in some circumstances. These include severe direct exposure to the aftermath of violence, destruction, and traumatic loss. For example, in the aftermath of 9/11, such groups included bereaved families, those evacuated from workplaces, and those involved in the recovery of remains. In the context of face-to-face interactions, outreach workers and mental health counselors routinely make judgments about whom to refer for counseling. In current disaster mental health practice, people who are using FEMA-funded crisis counseling services typically receive brief counseling (e.g., 1–3 sessions), and if they determine the need, crisis counselors refer these help seekers to more intensive mental health counseling. However, most disaster mental health training materials devote relatively little attention to evidence-based criteria for referral (Young, Ruzek, & Pivar, 2001), and little is known about how these determinations of need for referral are actually made.

While triage decisions are necessitated in many postdisaster environments, there is ongoing debate about the application of systematic screening to identify those who may need more intensive

---

- Provide for basic survival needs and comfort
- Help survivors achieve restful, restorative sleep
- Preserve an interpersonal safety zone protecting basic personal space (privacy, quiet, personal effects)
- Provide nonintrusive ordinary social contact
- Address immediate physical health problems or exacerbations of prior illnesses
- Assist in locating separated loved ones and friends and verifying their safety
- Reconnect survivors with loved ones, friends, trusted others
- Help survivors take practical steps to resume day-to-day life
- Help them take practical steps to resolve pressing problems caused by the trauma (e.g., housing, finances)
- Facilitate resumption of normal family, community, school, and work roles
- Provide opportunities for grieving
- Help them reduce problematic tension or anxiety to manageable levels
- Support helpers with training in common reactions and stress management techniques
  Source: Veterans Health Administration (2003).

Figure 18.1. Some elements of management of acute stress reaction

mental health services. Wessely (2003) maintains that screening that is intended to facilitate the prevention of posttrauma psychological disorders should meet a variety of conditions, including that spontaneous recovery is unlikely, that those who are screened would not have presented for care in the absence of screening efforts, that there is a proven intervention for those detected, that the anticipated benefits of screening outweigh the negative consequences, that screening and treatment are acceptable to those screened, that a validated screening tool is available, and that evidence indicates that early treatment will lead to better outcomes than late treatment.

At present, these questions cannot be answered in the affirmative for early screening. Our ability to accurately identify those who are at risk for chronic problems is limited. Early symptom levels are not necessarily indicative of risk, and predictors of PTSD may vary significantly across trauma populations (Brewin, Andrews, & Valentine, 2000); moreover, the challenge is to predict other problems in addition to PTSD, including other anxiety, substance use, and mood disorders (Yehuda, McFarlane, & Shalev, 1998). Bryant (2003) has suggested that it may be premature to identify people for intervention before 2 weeks posttrauma, that active cognitive-behavioral intervention should not be offered earlier than 2 weeks, and that delay in intervention may be recommended in part because it may allow time for survivors to marshal resources and deal with practical problems.

With regard to posttraumatic stress symptoms, screening is possibly most effective several months posttrauma. In this context, validated screening tools and evidence-based treatment for PTSD have been developed. Following the World Trade Center attacks in New York, Project Liberty created a range of services intended to help the community; in its second year of operation, a paper-and-pencil screening tool was used to identify those who might benefit from a referral for more advanced services. Also in New York, Difede, Roberts, Jaysinghe, & Leck (n.d.) have developed a screening program for emergency relief workers who responded to the attacks. They used a battery of well-validated measures to screen for PTSD and other mental health disorders. There is a need for systematic evaluation of both early and later screening initiatives, related to their predictive validity, impact, and cost-effectiveness.

Selected Follow-Up With Survivors

One approach worth considering is the delivery of routine telephone follow-up monitoring of survivors who appear to be at risk for continuing posttrauma problems on the basis of known risk factors. This "screen and treat" (Brewin, 2003) approach has several potential benefits. It would identify those who should be monitored, not those who require early intervention. A simple request for permission to recontact a survivor at a later date may be less stigmatizing or less likely to engender negative responses from oneself and others. It is probable that such a follow-up opportunity will be welcomed and seen as a sign of significant interest and commitment on the part of the practitioner and parent organization. Those who do not wish to be followed up can simply deny permission. People will differ in their receptivity to offers of counseling at different points in time, and this approach may provide the survivor with multiple opportunities to seek services. If a survivor continues to report mental health problems 3 months after the terrorist event, counselors may have more confidence in the person's need for more formal help.

Survivor Education

One practice that remains widely supported at all stages of terrorism and disaster response is education for survivors and the community at large. However, it is important to note that this practice has not been empirically validated. Nonetheless, brief educational efforts are relatively nonstigmatizing and generally appreciated by survivors; they are low-cost forms of care that may be delivered through informal conversations or in structured formal presentations. After terrorist events that affect large numbers of people, such educational information will need to be delivered via cost-effective public media presentations, written materials, and group educational activities. Generally, educational content is selected for the following reasons:

- to help survivors better understand a range of posttrauma responses
- to normalize responses so that survivors come to view their posttrauma reactions as typical (e.g., not as reactions to be feared, signs of personal weakness, or signs of mental illness)
- to increase survivors' use of social support

- to increase adaptive ways of coping with the trauma and its effects and decrease problematic forms of coping (e.g., alcohol consumption, social isolation)
- to increase survivors' ability to help family members cope (e.g., information about how to talk to children about what happened) and, in some cases, include entire families in educational efforts
- to help survivors recognize the circumstances under which they should consider seeking counseling and to reduce obstacles to seeking therapeutic help (e.g., misperceptions of helping services, perceived stigma)
- to inform survivors where they can obtain additional help, including mental health counseling

An important early goal of educational intervention is the normalization of stress reactions, and research is needed to examine the normalization process and our ability to influence it; indeed, the emphasis on reducing fear and misinterpretation of acute stress responses is consistent with some current theories of PTSD (e.g., Ehlers & Clark, 2003). It is important that mental health responders ask about survivors' perceptions of their own reactions and help them better understand and manage them. Efforts should be made to reduce shame or embarrassment at seeking help, and mental health services should be described as commonsense and practical opportunities for support.

A challenge will be to combine education about stress and coping with information about the aftermath of the event. In bioterrorist incidents, mental health providers will need to work with medical educators to provide accurate and timely information about issues such as the biological agents, infection control, the care of seriously ill persons, and the unfolding situation itself in ways that are consistent with media-delivered public health messages. Another challenge will be to provide care for families, who in some cases may need the information conveyed at several different developmental levels.

Enhancement of Social Support

Postterrorism care should include significant efforts to increase social support for survivors. Although the ways in which support can help or hinder recovery are not well understood, research does indicate that perceived social support is related to posttrauma and postdisaster outcomes. Lack of social support after a trauma is a risk factor for PTSD (Brewin, Andrews, & Valentine, 2000), and greater received and perceived social support has been associated with less distress among disaster survivors (Norris, Friedman, Watson, Byrne, Díaz, et al., 2002). Declines in social support account for a large share of disaster victims' subsequent declines in mental health (Norris et al., 2002).

Rather than seeking out mental health professionals, those affected by terrorist events primarily turn for help to nonprofessional sources such as family, friends, and colleagues (Luce & Firth-Cozens, 2002). As a result, mental health professionals must work with natural helping networks to increase support over time. In the immediate aftermath of a terrorist event, it is standard practice to make efforts to reestablish contact between disaster and terrorism survivors and their loved ones. Disaster workers also advise survivors to spend time with family and friends and to seek and offer support. Support groups are often established by helping professionals, and self-help groups sometimes provide significant opportunities for mutual helping.

In addition to the routine enhancement of social support with affected people, families, and communities, mental health providers should undertake to identify those who are socially isolated or lacking in social support and, if judged appropriate, take steps to increase their access to support. They should also routinely assess the interpersonal functioning of survivors and make efforts to maintain interpersonal functioning in those whose relationships are suffering as a result of exposure to the terrorism or disaster stressors. Exposure to terrorism and the development of PTSD and other problems may impair the survivors' relationships with significant others, including spouses or partners (North et al., 1999). This impairment may be common, for example, among emergency workers and their spouses.

Coping Skills Training

Disaster mental health responders routinely provide written materials about coping and review ways of coping with survivors. This instruction is primarily conveyed through brief advice and is a simple low-intensity element of stepped care that reaches large numbers of survivors. When disaster mental health counseling settings provide opportunity for multiple contacts with survivors who are experiencing significant postevent problems, it is possible to go beyond the simple sharing of information to provide coping skills training. Such guidance can help survivors learn how to do the things that will support their recovery by delivering a cycle of instruction that includes education, modeling, coaching, repeated practice, and feedback. It can also include between-session task assignments with diary self-monitoring and real-world practice of these coping mechanisms. Skills taught in this way can include anxiety management (breathing retraining and relaxation), challenging maladaptive thoughts, emotional "grounding" (Najavits, 2002), anger management, and problem-solving skills. As noted previously, stress inoculation training (anxiety management) has been effective as a treatment for chronic PTSD (e.g., Foa et al., 1999).

To date, attempts to train survivors in these skills have not been systematically undertaken or evaluated in the context of disaster and terrorism. However, a single session of telephone-delivered anxiety management training has been shown to decrease anxiety among Israeli citizens who were worried about the possibility of a Scud attack (Somer, Tamir, Maguen, & Litz, 2005). When citizens called a hotline as a result of Scud-related distress, they were randomized to either cognitive-behavioral intervention or a standard hotline counseling (unconditional positive regard, empathic listening, validation, social support) control group. The intervention lasted around 15 minutes and included normalization of stress responses, instruction in diaphragmatic breathing and cognitive restructuring, phone practice of the latter techniques, and assignments to practice at home. Compared with standard hotline practice, the experimental intervention was associated with significantly less distress, anxiety, and worry about missile attack 3 days after the counseling. In addition to its innovative telephone delivery system, this project is significant for its demonstration of the utility of anxiety management skills training for those affected by disasters and terrorism. Also important is the fact that paraprofessional hotline counselors were trained in the anxiety reduction intervention via a single 5-hour training workshop.

Interventions for Survivors Experiencing Significant Problems

As noted in the context of coping skills, some people whose problems do not respond to simple advice or education may benefit from multiple-session or intermediate-intensity interventions. For example, ASD has been established as a relatively strong predictor of development of chronic PTSD, and a cognitive-behavioral approach that includes education, anxiety management training, imaginal exposure therapy, in vivo exposure, and cognitive restructuring (cognitive therapy) has been shown to be significantly more effective in preventing PTSD and in decreasing depressive symptoms than simple education and support. To date, this approach has been tested with individual survivors of motor vehicle accidents, industrial accidents, and nonsexual assault that meet criteria for a diagnosis of ASD (Bryant, Harvey, Dang, Sackville, & Basten, 1998; Bryant, Sackville, Dang, Moulds, & Guthrie, 1999). It has been delivered over the course of four to five individual therapy sessions and initiated about 2 weeks after the trauma. In a long-term follow-up of those receiving their intervention, Bryant, Moulds, and Nixon (2003) reported that, 4 years after being helped, participants who had received the CBT intervention showed a lower intensity of PTSD symptoms than those receiving education and support.

Intermediate intensity services may hold promise for incorporating effective behavior-change methods (e.g., cognitive restructuring, anxiety management, therapeutic exposure, skills training, self-monitoring, social reinforcement) while requiring fewer resources than full mental health treatment, but they have not been tested with mass violence or disaster survivors as an early phase postdisaster intervention. However, Gillespie et al. (2002) conducted an open trial of a cognitive-behavioral therapy delivered between 1 and 34 months (median 10 months) postattack with survivors of the 1998 Omagh terrorist bombing in Northern Ireland who had developed PTSD. Ninety-one patients who met the criteria for PTSD resulting from the bombing received 2–78 sessions (with a mean of 8) of a treatment that combined imaginal exposure with cognitive therapy; 37% of

the survivors were treated in 5 or fewer sessions. Seventy-eight patients demonstrated significant pre-post improvement on standardized measures of symptoms from the treatment, with an effect size for improvement in PTSD symptoms of 2.47 (a magnitude of change comparable to or larger than controlled trials of CBT for PTSD). In this demonstration study, intensity of care (i.e., number of sessions) was determined by response to intervention and varied from a few sessions to many.

A cognitive-behavioral intervention was also delivered to some of the survivors of the New York City World Trade Center attacks, beginning approximately 18 months after 9/11, as part of an "enhanced" service offered under the auspices of Project Liberty crisis counseling programs. Composed of psychoeducation, coping skills training, and cognitive restructuring delivered in 9–12 sessions, it was provided to users of crisis counseling services who screened positive on a paper-and-pencil selection tool and was well received by providers and survivors (Norris et al., in press). Clinicians reported that this intervention was well received by clients, but no formal outcome assessment has been conducted to date.

In the years following an event affecting large numbers of survivors, many can be expected to develop chronic problems, including PTSD, despite the availability of crisis counseling services. Affected communities should continue to detect and treat PTSD in survivors who have not sought or benefited from access to these services. Postterrorism mental health response must therefore be extended in time and incorporate the implementation of screening programs in key community settings where survivors may present for help (e.g., primary care) and training of mental health providers in the evidence-based treatments discussed earlier. Such screening and treatment practices do not currently represent standard care in medicine and mental health.

Toward Terrorism-Related, Situation-Specific Interventions

Those who provide mental health services in the wake of terrorist attacks may be challenged to extend conventional disaster mental health approaches to meet the challenges associated with specific postterrorism situations. For example, specific interventions for people who have experienced actual and perceived toxic exposure are not part of conventional disaster mental health training and require more development. In fact, the physical interventions that may be needed in terrorism environments—barrier environments, quarantine, restricted travel, mass immunization, use of gas masks, decontamination, and destruction of personal clothing and property—may increase stress levels among survivors (Holloway, Norwood, Fullerton, Engel, & Ursano, 1997; Norwood, 2001), and mental health activities may need to focus on assisting survivors in coping with these interventions. For example, in situations involving the delivery of vaccinations (or other medical prophylaxis), survivors may benefit from interventions that include assistance with decision making or address adherence to a physician's instructions. The wearing of gas masks has been associated with anxiety and panic in some people (e.g., Carmeli, Liberman, & Mevorach, 1991; Rivkind et al., 1999), and mental health providers may be called upon to assist people in adapting to this equipment. Those who are evacuated due to environmental risk may represent a high-risk group and may benefit from support and training before, during, and after their move.

Terrorist events can also involve ongoing exposure to legal proceedings, and mental health providers may need to help survivors manage trial-related stressors and exacerbation of distress. For example, following the bombing of Pan Am Flight 103 over Lockerbie, Scotland, those affected were provided with a Lockerbie trial handbook, opportunity to observe the trial proceedings via remote closed-circuit viewing, and funds to enable victims' family members to receive mental health counseling throughout the trial process (Smith, Kilpatrick, Falsetti, & Best, 2002). In some postterrorism environments, the risk of community violence can be expected to increase. This may be due to a breakdown in societal order or may affect particular segments of the community. For example, after the attacks of 9/11, violence and threats of violence against Arab Americans increased, meaning that mental health response was charged both with attempting to prevent or reduce anger and perpetration of violence and with helping Islamic families cope with situations of increased risk of harm.

Coping With the Continuing Threat of Terrorism

Although some interventions exist to help individuals cope with the *aftermath* of trauma and terrorism, there is scarce information about how to help people deal with the ongoing and *potential* threat of terrorism, especially in communities at risk. In order to better understand how to intervene in these communities, it is important to understand which types of coping styles produce the best mental health outcomes, especially in those who demonstrate resilience amid the threat of terror.

Following the tragedies of 9/11, the possibility of another terrorist attack in the United States was a looming threat, and U.S. citizens were warned to be on constant alert for suspicious activity. In this context, Silver, Holman, McIntosh, Poulin, and Gil-Rivas (2002) examined coping styles in a national sample and reported that, 6 months after the attacks, active coping (e.g., taking action to improve the situation) was inversely associated with distress and general anxiety. Conversely, denial, self-blame, and behavioral disengagement (i.e., giving up) predicted higher levels of distress. Furthermore, PTSD symptom severity 6 months after 9/11 was predicted by acceptance (e.g., learning to live with the situation), behavioral disengagement, denial, seeking social support, self-blame, and self-distraction (e.g., turning to work to take one's mind off of the situation). Overall, active coping seemed to lead to the best adaptation to the ongoing terrorist threat.

Given that most people will indeed cope well with the threat of ongoing terror and prove to be resilient, understanding the conditions that promote adaptation is a key ingredient in intervening appropriately with those who are not able to cope effectively. In the context of the attacks on 9/11, a prospective study was conducted in which people were surveyed prior to the terrorist attacks and again after they had occurred. Fredrickson, Tugade, Waugh, and Larkin (2003) determined that resilient individuals were able to find positive meaning in daily hassles and stressors and also reported more positive emotions and fewer negative ones following the attacks. Furthermore, there was an inverse relationship between resilience and depression symptoms, and this relationship, as well as that between resilience and growth in psychological resources, was mediated by positive emotions.

Positive emotions seem to be an important component in coping with the ongoing threat of terrorism and serve as a protective factor against negative psychological symptoms and distress.

There have also been a number of studies conducted internationally that help shed light on effective coping amid the threat of terror. Israel is a country in which the threat of terrorism is a chronic concern; it is an environment that is quite different from the United States, where overt terrorist acts are still a rarity. Consequently, Israelis have been living with the threat much longer than citizens in many other countries, which provides a unique perspective on how people cope with ongoing threat. In two studies, both adults and children who employed problem-focused coping, as compared to emotion-focused coping, did worse in the long run. Weisenberg, Schwarzwald, Waysman, Solomon, and Klingman (1993) surveyed children who were at risk for Scud attacks, and Gidron, Gal, and Zahavi (1999) surveyed adults who were at risk of transportation explosions. Measurement limitations (i.e., unstandardized measures of coping), administration timing (i.e., measuring coping directly following a terrorist event that obfuscates whether the types of coping measured are beneficial in acute versus chronically threatening situations), and specificity of coping reaction (i.e., whether ways of coping were evaluated generally versus encompassing methods specific to the terrorist events that preceded the surveys) were among some of the limitations of these studies.

Researchers have also measured coping in Ireland and France. In Northern Ireland, Cairns and Wilson (1989) found that those who were living in higher-violence areas used more distancing. Regardless of the actual violence in their neighborhood, people who appraised the violence as more severe used more social support seeking and less distancing (i.e., these were the two types of coping examined in this study). Therefore, those living in areas with greater potential for violence tended to distance themselves from the situation in order to cope. Limitations of the study included failure to test for association with mental health outcomes and failure to include a wider variety of ways of coping. In France, following a terrorist attack in a Parisian subway, Jehel, Duchet, Paterniti, Consoli, and Guelfi (2001) surveyed

victims of the bombing attack 6 and 18 months later and found that emotion-focused coping was positively associated and problem-focused coping was negatively associated with PTSD symptoms. Both of these studies surveyed individuals about 6 months after the attacks and occurred in countries that do not have to confront chronic terrorist attacks (i.e., these horrific situations were novel). These results are similar to those of Silver et al. (2002).

The need to focus on promoting positive emotionality in the context of coping with the threat of terrorism is an important intervention method that emerges from existing research. Indeed, positive emotionality has been demonstrated to be a resilience factor in several recent studies involving people who have been exposed to stressful events (e.g., Tugade & Fredrickson, 2004), and positive emotionality is consistently associated with growth following trauma (Liney & Joseph, 2004). Therefore, promoting positive emotionality in the context of coping with the threat of terror will perhaps allow people to be more resilient in the context of ongoing threat. With regard to optimal types of coping, study results are challenging to disentangle, given the diversity of environments and situations in which the studies were conducted. Many more studies should also be conducted before firmly drawing any conclusions about coping with an ongoing threat of terrorism. Nonetheless, one possibility is that emotion-focused coping may promote better health in chronically terror-ridden environments immediately following a terrorist event. Conversely, problem-focused coping may be more helpful in environments where terrorism is rarer in order to cope with the threat many months after a terrorist event.

Given the scarcity of studies that examine coping with the threat of potential terror, conclusive recommendations are difficult to make; however, at least one study has demonstrated that, although most people will have adequate resources and support to cope with the threat of terrorism on their own, cognitive-behavioral techniques such as relaxation training and modifying irrational beliefs about the threat may be helpful to people who require further assistance (Somer et al., 2005). Even for the average person who is not unduly burdened with the threat of potential terror, challenging occasional maladaptive thoughts and relaxation techniques may be helpful.

Actual and Perceived Toxic Exposure

Biological terrorism is a serious threat that may be especially frightening for affected populations. Noy (2002) maintains that a primary prevention program is the most important component in the protection of citizens against biological warfare and that failure to implement such a program will result in maladaptive coping and an unnecessary increase in somatic and psychological casualties. Previous studies have suggested the importance of not only educating the masses about how to recognize the signs of a biological attack, which is an important goal in and of itself, but also preparing psychologically for such an attack (i.e., how to regulate anxiety about the threat of an attack). For example, during the Scud attacks in 1992, Israelis were taught how to use gas masks in preparation for biological warfare, given instructions on preparing sealed rooms, and provided with guidance about when to self-administer antidote injections. When Scud missiles were eventually launched, they did not contain biological warheads as feared. Nonetheless, the missiles caused widespread destruction, in some cases resulting in death. A study reviewing the medical records of patients who were hospitalized as a result of the attacks determined that 43% of these cases resulted from the victims' psychological response to the assault (Bleich, Dycian, Koslowsky, Solomon, & Wiener, 1992). Furthermore, 27% of those who were hospitalized had mistakenly injected themselves with an antidote, and there was a great deal of overlap between mistaken antidote injections and individuals classified as psychological casualties.

Given these high rates of psychological hospitalization, one specific intervention recommendation would be to systematically educate citizens about psychological reactions to the threat of terrorism. This could be done in conjunction with education about different biological agents, how to recognize signs of a biological attack, and specific behavioral steps that should be taken in the event of such an attack. Educating the public about psychological responses and how to counteract them (e.g., challenging irrational thoughts, relaxation training) is arguably an important step toward minimizing psychological casualties in the event that such an attack should occur and may

reduce the burden of preventable admissions. Benedek, Holloway, and Becker (2002) contend that lucid, consistent, easily available, dependable, and redundant information that is distributed from reliable sources will curtail uncertainty and fear about the cause of a symptom and that the absence of such information is likely to be associated with unnecessary treatment and use of resources. Particular attention should be given to special populations, such as patients with preexisting anxiety disorders who may have difficulty following instructions that would ensure their survival. As was the case in Israel, individuals with preexisting anxiety disorders may develop anxiety attacks when faced with taking steps to ensure their safety, such as utilizing a gas mask during a possible attack (e.g., Rivkind et al., 1999).

Education also should be provided concerning which types of samples to submit for further testing, given that public health laboratories may otherwise be overburdened with samples, thus taxing existing resources. For example, following the deaths due to anthrax, one state public health laboratory received 1,496 environmental submissions of anthrax, all of which tested negative for bioterrorism agents (Dworkin, Ma, & Golash, 2003). Education is important not only to prevent putting an unnecessary burden on the public health system but also to ensure that suspected outbreaks are reported in a timely and efficient manner. For example, Ashford et al. (2003) have reported that, for six outbreaks in which bioterrorism or intentional contamination was possible, reporting was delayed for up to 26 days, arguing that education and frontline work by healthcare professionals and local health departments are crucial to the dissemination of critical information.

Health

Many of those affected by terrorist events will complain of health or somatic symptoms, especially in connection with events involving possible exposure to chemical, biological, or radiological toxins. Both medical professionals and mental health professionals will face the challenge of distinguishing symptoms of actual exposure from stress-related somatic symptoms, and the relationships between stress and health difficulties will be difficult to interpret in many cases. Having the best possible information is important if mental and medical health providers are to help reduce anxiety-eliciting misinformation and rumor (Hyams, Murphy, & Wessely, 2002).

For those with inexplicable health problems, Fischoff and Wessely (2003) have outlined some simple principles of patient management that may be useful in the context of terrorist attacks: Focus communication around patients' concerns; organize information coherently; give risks as numbers; acknowledge scientific uncertainty; use universally understood language; and focus on relieving symptoms. Although relatively little is known about treating these problems, a recent clinical trial comparing treatments for Gulf War illness may have some relevance to similar complaints associated with terrorist incidents. Donata et al. (2003) have reported that both cognitive-behavioral group therapy (CBGT) and exercise were effective; CBGT improved physical function, whereas exercise led to improvement in many of the symptoms of Gulf War veterans' illnesses. Both treatments improved cognitive symptoms and mental health functioning, but neither improved pain. In this study, CBGT was specifically targeted at physical functioning and included time-contingent activity pacing, pleasant activity scheduling, sleep hygiene, assertiveness skills, confrontation of negative thinking and affect, and structured problem-solving skills. The low-intensity aerobic exercise intervention was designed to increase activity level by having veterans exercise once per week for 1 hour in the presence of an exercise therapist and independently two to three times per week.

It is likely that most of those who seek help for stress-related complaints will focus on physical symptoms and present in emergency medicine (Ruzek, Young, Cordova, & Flynn, 2004) and primary care medical settings rather than to crisis counseling services. This can be expected both immediately following possible exposure, when large numbers of people have begun to worry even before the extent of actual community and individual exposure is known, and in the months and years postdisaster, when people visit their physicians with stress-related health concerns (e.g., headaches, sleep difficulties). For the primary care provider, this means that patients will require screening for exposure to traumatic events and posttraumatic symptomatology. In the months and years following an event, systematic screening can lead to better identification of stress-related pro-

blems and increased rates of referral for mental health care (cf. Leskin, Ruzek, Friedman, & Gusman, 1999).

Service Delivery Challenges in the Postterrorism Environment

The Context of Ongoing Threat

As mentioned earlier, many terrorism situations present a continuing possibility of additional attacks. Circumstances of ongoing threat may create anticipatory fears (Piotrowski & Brannon, 2002; Silver et al., 2002), sustain anxiety, and potentially interfere with recovery in those who have survived a previous attack. Some evidence suggests that the disrupted daily routines created by these circumstances may be associated with PTSD symptomatology (Shalev, Tuval-Mashiach, Frenkiel, & Hadar, 2004). Because interventions that are designed for the treatment of PTSD have been applied primarily under conditions of relative safety (i.e., threat of continued harm is minimal), questions can be raised about their generalizability to some terrorist-threat environments. If realistic ongoing exposure to continued attacks is part of the environment in which traumatic stress reactions must be managed, this may have implications for mental health services. Shalev et al. (2003) have described modifications in the delivery of cognitive-behavioral treatment for PTSD related to terrorist attacks in Israel, designed to reflect a terror-ridden environment. During in vivo exposure assignments, survivors were encouraged to expose themselves to situations that were clearly safe but not to those widely considered dangerous and avoided by most of the populace (e.g., city centers where repeated bombings had occurred).

They also noted that differences in cognitions underlying avoidance by the general population compared with avoidance by those with PTSD. Members of the latter group were thinking, "if I go, there will definitely be another attack, and this time I will definitely die," whereas those without PTSD were thinking, "the risk is very small, but I really don't need to go and buy a book—it is not worth the risk" (Shalev et al., 2004, p. 182). Cognitive therapy was applied to help the members of the PTSD group modify their beliefs. Finally, terror survivors in treatment were frequently exposed to additional traumatic events during therapy. They were advised to limit indirect media exposure by not watching detailed news reports, their appropriate avoidance was characterized as "positive safety behaviors," and their goal was achieving "normal fear." It can be anticipated that such pragmatic flexibility in the modification of interventions will be needed to provide care in the midst of continuing danger and other challenging aspects of the postterrorism environment.

Availability of Evidence-Based Services

A second contextual constraint in the postdisaster environment is the likelihood of limited availability of evidence-based care for PTSD. Most mental health providers have not been trained in evidence-based treatments, and in most affected communities, the demand is likely to outstrip the supply. However, recent evidence suggests that mental health professionals can rapidly be trained in the delivery of these treatments.

In an important first demonstration of the feasibility of training indigenous mental health providers in evidence-based treatments, Gillespie et al. (2002) conducted an open trial of cognitive therapy with survivors of the 1998 Omagh terrorist bombing in Northern Ireland. Therapists were National Health Service mental health providers with no previous experience in treating trauma. The study suggests that this intervention can easily be disseminated and effectively implemented and is promising for the potential delivery of CBT interventions by a range of mental health professionals and paraprofessionals following disasters.

Following the attacks of 9/11, several efforts to train mental health providers in evidence-based treatments were undertaken. Neria, Suh, and Marshall (2003) described their efforts to provide systematic training and supervision in PTSD prolonged-exposure treatment for New York City therapists (Foa & Rothbaum, 1998). Training was initiated approximately 2 months after the attacks, and over a 12-month period, more than 500 local clinicians were trained. This project is notable for its use of a theory of behavior change to guide the design of dissemination efforts and its evaluation of the impact of training activities on changes in provider attitudes, behaviors, and self-efficacy.

Together, these efforts demonstrate the feasibility of the dissemination of evidence-based

methods of care after an event has taken place, as well as their potential for reducing PTSD symptoms. They also suggest that such efforts will require workshop-style training, ongoing supervision and consultation, and the development of strategies to maintain delivery of services (cf. Young, Ruzek, Wong, Salzer, Naturale, et al., in press). In the New York City training program mentioned earlier, clinicians perceived clinical case demonstration as the most valuable training mode; they also considered role plays as very useful, and lectures were rated as the least valuable (although they were seen as useful in giving theoretical information). Generally, the selection, training, and support of providers are critical parts of postterrorism response. Preplanned, systematic procedures can be expected not only to improve the quality of care but also to help in answering common service-delivery questions: how to ensure that the large numbers of volunteers who show up after disaster events are competent to offer help; how to incorporate important local systems resources (e.g., local clergy) who do not possess standard disaster training or credentials; and how to decide which volunteers to turn away.

Obstacles to Mental Health Providers' Access to Survivors

Reluctance of Survivors to Seek Available Mental Health Care

In most disasters, many of those who are affected do not use the available crisis counseling programs or the more conventional mental health services. For example, 3–6 months after the World Trade Center attacks in New York City, only 27% of those reporting severe psychiatric symptoms had obtained mental health treatment (Delisi et al., 2003). Following the terrorist bombing of Pan Am 103 over Lockerbie, Scotland, relatively few family members of those who perished sought counseling despite significant levels of distress (Smith et al., 2002). This reluctance to use mental health services appears to extend to emergency workers (e.g., North et al., 2002) and medical staff (e.g., Luce & Firth-Cozens, 2002).

Some of this reluctance to use services may represent an acceptance of posttraumatic distress that reflects an awareness that some stress symptoms are to be expected and that life can go on nonetheless. Some people who endorse high levels of PTSD symptoms may not label themselves as significantly distressed or disabled, as has been found with Israeli citizens exposed to continuous terror (Shalev et al., 2004). As Shalev and colleagues have noted, PTSD symptoms are to be expected in communities that are subjected to ongoing terrorist attacks and may not represent maladaptive reactions. However, stigma and other obstacles likely play an important role as well. For those who lost family members in the Lockerbie bombing, the most frequent reasons given for not using counseling included thinking that they could handle it with help from family, friends, and their religious faith; that mental health counseling is a sign of weakness and felt stigmatizing; that they could not afford it financially; or that they could not admit to having a problem (Smith et al., 2002).

It is important to recognize that not everyone needs mental health treatment and that, for some, seeking help from one's family, friends, and/or religious faith is adequate and offers sufficient support. However, those who attempt to offer evidence-based terrorism and disaster interventions must acknowledge this underutilization of services and take steps to reduce any obstacles to appropriate utilization by those in need. Disaster mental health practice has evolved to address this reality by including significant outreach components. Much help is provided at places where survivors congregate as mental health responders offer "therapy while walking around." Outreach workers seek out survivors in shopping malls, on doorsteps, in workplaces, and at religious gatherings. At large events, the mass media are harnessed to market crisis counseling programs; in New York, the services of Project Liberty were advertised via major public education campaigns that involved television spots in which well-known celebrities appeared.

Relatively little is know about how to encourage the use of services and how survivors make decisions about self-referral. In much postterrorism/disaster education, information is presented to help survivors differentiate between normal reactions to the event and those that may warrant counseling. These efforts are appropriate, but it is not known whether they are effective in encouraging appropriate self-referral. More efforts should be made to understand the perspectives of survivors themselves. For example, Difede et al. (n.d.) have reported that, among emergency services workers who responded to the World Trade Center collapse, distress at trauma reminders was seen as a normal reaction to the events and not a reason to seek treatment. Rather, anger, irritability, and sleep problems were seen as reasons to seek help.

A better understanding of what motivates people who need help to actually seek it might be useful in marketing these services, increasing engagement in counseling, and widening acceptance of mental health referral. Since many disaster and terrorism survivors will talk to their primary care practitioners, ways of addressing mental health in these settings will be important. Others will seek assistance in emergency rooms. More generally, efforts to destigmatize help seeking are in need of creative development. One possibility involves having a mental health worker available at the emergency room or within a medical practice to help patients struggling with issues that are more psychological in nature (i.e., a "one-stop shopping" model of care). The idea is that, once the patient meets with the mental health professional and rapport is established, transition to short-term problem-focused therapy will occur with greater ease.

Restrictions on Physical Access to Survivors

In some events, it may be difficult for mental health providers to establish face-to-face contact with survivors. This may be due to restrictions on travel by authorities, perceptions of ongoing environmental danger (e.g., continuing risk for terrorist attack or toxic exposure), or, possibly, quarantine. In situations of ongoing risk of exposure to biological toxins, providers themselves may be reluctant to work with possibly infected survivors. Telephone- or Internet-delivered services may be useful in these circumstances. Both cognitive-behavioral telephone (Greist et al., 2000; Mohr et al., 2000; Somer et al., 2005) and Internet interventions (Gega, Marks, & Mataix-Cols, 2004) have proven helpful with a variety of mental health problems. Future research should focus on testing these modalities of help following a terror event, especially given their ability to provide a convenient and stigma-reducing vehicle to promote self-management (Gega, Marks, & Mataix-Cols, 2004).

Providers as Survivors

Especially in large-scale terrorist attacks, many of those who are called upon to provide mental health services will themselves be affected by the event. For example, following the 9/11 terrorist attack, many employees of the Pentagon's Family Assistance Center were in the building when it was hit or lost friends and colleagues (Huleatt, LaDue, Leskin, Ruzek, & Gusman, 2002). In some events, mental health workers may be concerned about the well-being of their loved ones. The fact that, in some scenarios, workers will have been exposed to the terrorist event and will themselves be experiencing stress reactions may affect their ability to respond and provide care. For example, in a simulation of a biological outbreak, some responders and their spouses disagreed about reporting for duty (DiGiovanni Jr., Reynolds, Harwell, Stonecipher, & Burkle Jr., 2003). In the 1994 outbreak of plague in Surat, India (Ramalingaswami, 2001), doctors were among the estimated 600,000 people who fled the city, believing that nothing could be done to effectively treat the outbreak. In designing mental health response postterrorism, it will be important to anticipate that staff will experience conflict between their work and personal/family roles. Systematic staff care procedures should be developed, and steps should be taken to minimize the extent to which staff members may be distracted by concerns about their family and/or community (e.g., by establishing systems to enable staff contact with loved ones).

Future of Mental Health Response in Terrorism

Changing Models of Disaster Mental Health Service Delivery

Psychological research on prevention of PTSD and other posttrauma problems has implications for delivery of postterrorism care. Potentially valuable is an effort to synthesize lessons learned from different groups of trauma survivors, for whom early intervention services have often evolved independently with resulting differential strengths (Ruzek, in press). However, ways of integrating psychological treatment and disaster mental health "resilience" perspectives requires development and experimentation. In the context of terrorism and other community disasters, emphasis on the identification of vulnerable or high-risk individuals and

groups conflicts with an evident need to view affected people and communities as survivors and to emphasize capacity and commitment to resist efforts at intimidation and to overcome adversity (Hyams et al., 2002).

On the other hand, in the aftermath of the events of 9/11, there was considerable questioning of the fit between the disaster mental health crisis counseling program model (with its emphasis on normalization and low-level interventions for many people) and the significant mental health impact of such a high-magnitude terrorist event (Norris et al., in press). Much concern was expressed about the adequacy of such brief interventions for survivors who were the most severely affected. The inclusion of enhanced, moderate-intensity services is part of an ongoing evolution of disaster mental health practice to meet the needs of such groups (Gibson et al., in press).

Many of the procedures that have been developed as mental health interventions are based on an educational, skills-training model. Cognitive-behavioral interventions for posttraumatic stress in particular are based on a model that stresses that posttrauma problems are the outcomes of normal adaptive learning processes (Follette & Ruzek, in press) and interventions derived from the model are often relatively brief, pragmatic, and goal directed, features that lend themselves to application following disasters and terrorism.

Technology and Terrorism Response

Communication technologies will be increasingly harnessed to provide interventions for individuals and groups in future terrorist attacks and disasters. The Project Liberty 800-number hotline operating in New York was widely hailed as a major source of support and referral information for survivors and a key useful feature of 9/11 response (Norris et al., in press), and it can be assumed that similar efforts will be widely implemented in the future. The demonstration that anxiety management may be effectively undertaken via telephone will only accelerate exploration of phone services. Similarly, the Internet saw significant use during 9/11 that prefigures wider application. The Project Liberty website (http://www.projectliberty.state.ny.us/) provided information and other services to crisis counselors and terrorism survivors alike, and the

National Center for PTSD site (http://www .ncptsd.org) attracted a heavy volume of traffic. Because of their capacity to reach large numbers of affected individuals and their relative ease of use and circumvention of concerns about stigma and confidentiality, these technologies have significant potential to become a key element of stepped care, supplement face-to-face care, and improve post-disaster response (Ruzek, 2002a).

Summary

No individual victims, groups of victims, or communities victimized by terrorism escape unscathed. However, most people will not develop formal long-term mental health disturbances. The key practical, ethical, logistic, clinical, and administrative challenge in the aftermath of mass violence is to identify those who are most at risk for chronic posttraumatic mental health problems and functional impairments. Secondary prevention of these problems is critical because the life-course impact of trauma for those most at risk is pernicious and disabling. Unfortunately, risk and resilience research is in its infancy. However, there are rules of thumb to guide efforts at devoting resources to those most at risk following a terrorist attack; the most important risk factors are, in order of importance, degree of life threat and loss of life, traumatic loss, direct exposure to the aftermath of violence (e.g., seeing the dead and dying), and loss of personal and social resources as a result of the terrorist event. In this chapter we have described the evidence to support various clinical interventions and strategies to address those most in need. When there was no evidence to address a given problem, we offered a set of practical and least restrictive options for treating survivors of terror.

References

Acierno, R., Resnick, H. S., Flood, A., & Holmes, M. (2003). An acute post-rape intervention to prevent substance use and abuse. *Addictive Behaviors, 28,* 1701–1715.

Amir, M., Weil, G., Kaplan, Z., Tocker, T., & Witztum, E. (1998). Debriefing with brief group psychotherapy in a homogenous group of non-injured victims of a terrorist attack: A prospective study. *Acta Psychiatrica Scandinavica, 98,* 237–242.

Ashford, D. A., Kaiser, R. M., Bales, M. E., Shutt, K., Patrawalla, A., McShan, A., et al. (2003). Planning against biological terrorism: Lessons from outbreak investigations. *Emerging Infectious Diseases, 9,* 515–519.

Benedek, D. M., Holloway, H. C., & Becker, S.M. (2002). Emergency mental health management in bioterrorism events. *Emergency Medicine Clinics of North America, 20,* 393–407.

Bisson, J. I. (2003). Single-session early psychological interventions following traumatic events. *Clinical Psychology Review, 23,* 481–499.

Bleich, A., Dycian, A., Koslowsky, M., Solomon, Z., & Wiener, M. (1992). Psychiatric implications of missile attacks on a civilian population: Israeli lessons from the Persian Gulf War. *Journal of the American Medical Association, 268,* 613–615.

Bonanno, G. A. (2004). Loss, trauma, and human resilience: Have we underestimated the human capacity to thrive after extremely aversive events? *American Psychologist, 59,* 20–28.

Boudewyns, P. A., & Hyer, L. (1990). Physiological response to combat memories and preliminary treatment outcome in Vietnam veteran PTSD patients with direct therapeutic exposure. *Behavior Therapy, 21,* 63–87.

Bowler, R. M., Murai, K., & True, R. H. (2001, January/ February). Update and long-term sequelae of the sarin attack in the Tokyo, Japan subway. *Chemical Health and Safety,* 1–3.

Brewin, C. R. (2003). *Post-traumatic stress disorder: Malady or myth?* London: Yale University Press.

————, Andrews, B., & Valentine, J. D. (2000). Meta-analysis of risk factors for posttraumatic stress disorder in trauma-exposed adults. *Journal of Consulting and Clinical Psychology, 68,* 748–766.

Bryant, R. A. (2003). Cognitive behaviour therapy of acute stress disorder. In R. Orner & U. Schnyder (Eds.), *Reconstructing early intervention after trauma: Innovations in the care of survivors* (pp. 159–168). Oxford: Oxford University Press.

Bryant, R. A., Harvey, A. G., Dang, S. T., Sackville, T., & Basten, C. (1998). Treatment of acute stress disorder: A comparison of cognitive-behavioral therapy and supportive counseling. *Journal of Consulting and Clinical Psychology, 66,* 862–866.

Bryant, R. A., Moulds, M. L., & Nixon, R. D. V. (2003). Cognitive behaviour therapy of acute stress disorder: A four-year follow-up. *Behaviour Research and Therapy, 41,* 489–494.

Bryant, R. A., Sackville, T., Dang, S. T., Moulds, M., and Guthrie, R. (1999). Treating acute stress disorder: An evaluation of cognitive behavior therapy and supportive counseling techniques. *American Journal of Psychiatry, 156,* 1780–1786.

Burnam, M. A., Stein, J. A., Golding, J. M., Siegel, J. M., Sorenson, S. B., Forsythe, A. B., et al. (1988). Sexual assault and mental disorders in a community population. *Journal of Consulting and Community Psychology, 56,* 843–850.

Cairns, E., & Wilson, R. (1989). Coping with political violence in Northern Ireland. *Social Science and Medicine, 28,* 621–624.

Carmeli, A., Liberman, N., & Mevorach, L. (1991). Anxiety-related somatic reactions during missile attacks. *Israel Journal of Medical Sciences, 27,* 677–680.

Cooper, N. A., & Clum, G. A. (1989). Imaginal flooding as a supplementary treatment for PTSD in combat veterans: A controlled study. *Behavior Therapy, 20,* 381–391.

Delisi, L. E., Maurizio, A., Yost, M., Papparozzi, C. F., Fulchino, C., Katz, C. L., et al. (2003). A survey of New Yorkers after the Sept. 11, 2001, terrorist attacks. *American Journal of Psychiatry, 160,* 780–783.

Difede, J., Roberts, J., Jaysinghe, N., & Leck, P. (manuscript submitted for publication). Evaluation and treatment of firefighters and utility workers following the World Trade Center attack.

DiGiovanni, C., Jr., Reynolds, B., Harwell, R., Stone-cipher, E. B., & Burkle, F. M., Jr. (2003). Community reaction to bioterrorism: Prospective study of simulated outbreak. Emerging Infectious Diseases (serial online). Retrieved January 22, 2006, from http://www.cdc.gov/ncidod/EID/v019n06/02–0769.htm

Donata, S. T., Clauw, D. J., Engle, C. C., Guarino, P., Peduzzi, P., Williams, D. A., et al. (2003). Cognitive behavioral therapy and aerobic exercise for Gulf War veterans' illnesses: A randomized controlled trial. *Journal of the American Medical Association, 289,* 1396–1404.

Dunn, C. (2003). Brief motivational interviewing interventions targeting substance abuse in the acute care medical setting. *Seminars in Clinical Neuropsychiatry, 8,* 188–196.

Dworkin, M. S., Ma, X., & Golash, R. G. (2003). Fear of bioterrorism and implications for public health preparedness. *Emerging Infectious Diseases, 9,* 503–505.

Ehlers, A., & Clark, D. M. (2003). Early psychological interventions for adult survivors of trauma: A review. *Biological Psychiatry, 53,* 817–826.

Fischoff, B., & Wessely, S. (2003). Managing patients with inexplicable health problems. *British Medical Journal, 326,* 595–597.

Foa, E. B., Dancu, C. V., Hembree, E. A., Jaycox, L. H., Meadows, E. A., & Street, G. P. (1999). A comparison of exposure, therapy, stress inoculation training, and their combination for reducing posttraumatic stress disorder in female assault victims. *Journal of Consulting and Clinical Psychology, 67,* 194–200.

Foa, E. B., & Rothbaum, B. O. (1998). *Treating the trauma of rape: Cognitive-behavioral therapy for PTSD.* New York: Guilford.

————, Riggs, D. S., & Murdock, T. B. (1991). Treatment of posttraumatic stress disorder in rape victims: A comparison between cognitive-behavioral procedures and counseling. *Journal of Consulting and Clinical Psychology, 59,* 715–723.

Follette, V. M., & Ruzek, J. I. (in press). *Cognitive-behavior therapies for trauma* (2d ed.). New York: Guilford.

Foy, D. W., Glynn, S. M., Schnurr, P. P., Jankowski, M. K., Wattenberg, M. S., Weiss, D. S., et al. (2000). Group therapy. In E. B. Foa, T. M. Keane, & M. J. Friedman (Eds.), *Effective treatments for PTSD: Practice guidelines from the International Society for Traumatic Stress Studies* (pp. 155–175). New York: Guilford.

Fredrickson, B. L., Tugade, M. M., Waugh, C. E., & Larkin, G. R. (2003). What good are positive emotions in crisis? A prospective study of resilience and emotions following the terrorist attacks on the United States on September 11th, 2001. *Journal of Personality and Social Psychology, 84,* 365–376.

Gega, L., Marks, I., & Mataix-Cols, D. (2004). Computer-aided CBT self-help for anxiety and depressive disorders: Experience of a London clinic and future directions. *Journal of Clinical Psychology, 60,* 147–157.

Gentilello, L. M., Rivara, F. P., Donovan, D. M., Jurkovich, G. J., Daranciang, E., Dunn, C. W., et al. (1999). Alcohol interventions in a trauma center as a means of reducing the risk of injury recurrence. *Annals of Surgery, 230,* 473–483.

Gibson, L., Ruzek, J. I., Naturale, A., Bryant, R. A., Hamblen, J., Jones, R., et al. (in press). Early intervention. Paper presented at SAMHSA/NIMH Screening and Assessment, Outreach, and Intervention for Mental Health and Substance Abuse Needs Following Disasters and Mass Violence meeting, August 26–28, 2003, Bethesda, MD.

Gidron, Y., Gal, R., & Zahavi, S. (1999). Bus commuters' coping strategies and anxiety from terrorism: An example of the Israeli experience. *Journal of Traumatic Stress, 12,* 185–192.

Gillespie, K., Duffy, M., Hackmann, A., & Clark, D. M. (2002). Community-based cognitive therapy in the treatment of post-traumatic stress disorder following the Omagh bomb. *Behaviour Research and Therapy, 40,* 345–357.

Glass, T. A., & Schoch-Spana, M. (2002). Bioterrorism and the people: How to vaccinate a city against panic. *Clinical Infectious Diseases, 34,* 217–223.

Glynn, S. M., Eth, S., Randolph, E. T., Foy, D. W., Urbaitis, M., Boxer, L., et al. (1999). A test of behavioral family therapy to augment exposure for combat-related posttraumatic stress disorder. *Journal of Consulting and Clinical Psychology, 67,* 243–251.

Greist, J. H., Marks, I. M., Baer, L., Kobak, K. A., Wenzel, K. W., Hirsch M. J., et al. (2002). Behavior therapy for obsessive-compulsive disorder guided by a computer or by a clinician compared with relaxation as a control. *Journal of Clinical Psychiatry, 63,* 138–145.

Grieger, T. A., Fullerton, C. S., & Ursano, R. J. (2003). Posttraumatic stress disorder, alcohol use, and perceived safety after the terrorist attack on the Pentagon. *Psychiatric Services, 54,* 1380–1382.

Haaga, D. A. (2000). Introduction to the special section on stepped-care models in psychotherapy. *Journal of Consulting and Clinical Psychology, 68,* 547–548.

Holloway, H. C., Norwood, A. E., Fullerton, C. S., Engel, C. C., & Ursano, R. J. (1997). The threat of biological weapons: Prophylaxis and mitigation of psychological and social consequences. *Journal of the American Medical Association, 278,* 425–427.

Huleatt, W. J., LaDue, L., Leskin, G., Ruzek, J., & Gusman, F. (2002). Pentagon Family Assistance Center interagency mental health collaboration and response. *Military Medicine, 167*(Suppl.), 68–70.

Hyams, K. C., Murphy, F. M., & Wessely, S. (2002). Responding to chemical, biological, or nuclear terrorism: The indirect and long-term health effects may present the greatest challenge. *Journal of Health Politics, Policy, and Law, 27,* 273–291.

Jehel, L., Duchet, C., Paterniti, S., Consoli, S. M., & Guelfi, J. D. (2001). Prospective study of post-traumatic stress in victims of terrorist attacks. *Encephale, 5,* 393–400.

Keane, T. M., Fairbank, J. A., Caddell, J. M., & Zimering, R. T. (1989). Implosive (flooding) therapy reduces symptoms of PTSD in Vietnam combat veterans. *Behavior Therapy, 20,* 245–260.

Kilpatrick, D. G., Acierno, R., Resnick, H. S., Saunders, B., & Best, C. L. (1997). A two-year longitudinal analysis of the relationships between violent assault and substance use in women. *Journal of Consulting and Clinical Psychology, 65,* 834–847.

Krakow, B., Melendrez, D. C., Johnston, L. G., Clark, J. O., Santana, E. M., Warner, T. D., et al. (2002). Sleep dynamic therapy for Cerro Grande fire evacuees with posttraumatic stress symptoms: A preliminary report. *Journal of Clinical Psychiatry, 63,* 673–684.

Leskin, G. A., Ruzek, J. I., Friedman, M. J., & Gusman, F. D. (1999). Effective clinical management of PTSD in primary care settings: Screening and treatment options. *Primary Care Psychiatry, 5,* 3–12.

Linley, P. A., & Joseph, S. (2004). Positive change following trauma and adversity: A review. *Journal of Traumatic Stress, 17,* 11–21.

Litz, B. T., & Gibson, L. (in press). Conducting research on early interventions. In E. C. Ritchie, P. J. Watson, & M. J. Friedman (Eds.), *Mental health intervention following disasters or mass violence.* New York: Guilford.

Litz, B. T., & Gray, M. J. (2004). Early intervention for trauma in adults. In B. Litz (Ed.), *Early intervention for trauma and traumatic loss* (pp. 87–111). New York: Guilford.

———, Bryant, R., and Adler, A. B. (2002). Early intervention for trauma: Current status and future directions. *Clinical Psychology: Science and Practice, 9,* 112–134.

Longabaugh, R., Woolard, R. E., Nirenberg, T. D., Minugh, A. P., Becker, B., Clifford, P. R., et al. (2001). Evaluating the effects of a brief motivational intervention for injured drinkers in the emergency department. *Journal of Studies on Alcohol, 62,* 806–816.

Luce, A., & Firth-Cozens, J. (2002). Effects of the Omagh bombing on medical staff working in the local NHS trust: A longitudinal survey. *Hospital Medicine, 63,* 44–47.

Marks, I., Lovell, K., Noshirvani, H., Livanou, M., & Thrasher, S. (1998). Treatment of posttraumatic stress disorder by exposure and/or cognitive restructuring: A controlled study. *Archives of General Psychiatry, 55,* 317–325.

Mawson, D., Marks, I., Ramm, E., & Stern, R. (1981). Guided mourning for morbid grief: A controlled study. *British Journal of Psychiatry, 138,* 185–193.

McNally, R., Bryant, R. A., & Ehlers, A. (2003). Does early psychological intervention promote recovery from posttraumatic stress? *Psychological Science in the Public Interest, 4,* 45–79.

Miller, W. R., & Rollnick, S. (2002). *Motivational interviewing: Preparing people for change* (2d ed.). New York: Guilford.

Mohr, D. C., Likosky, W., Bertagnolli, A., Goodkin, D. E., van der Wende, J., Dwyer, P., et al. (2000).

Telephone-administered cognitive-behavioral therapy for the treatment of depressive symptoms in multiple sclerosis. *Journal of Consulting and Clinical Psychology, 68,* 356–361.

Moyer, A., Finney, J. W., Swearingen, C. E., & Vergun, P. (2002). Brief interventions for alcohol problems: A meta-analytic review of controlled investigations in treatment-seeking and non-treatment-seeking populations. *Addiction, 97,* 279–292.

Murphy, S. A., Johnson, C., Cain, K., Dimond, M., Das Gupta, A., Lohan, J., et al. (1998). Broad-spectrum group treatment for parents bereaved by the violent deaths of their 12-to-28-year-old children: A randomized controlled trial. *Death Studies, 22,* 1–27.

Najavits, L. M. (2002). *Seeking safety: A treatment manual for PTSD and substance abuse.* New York: Guilford Press.

National Institute of Mental Health. (2002). Mental health and mass violence: Evidenced-based early psychological intervention for victims/survivors of mass violence. A workshop to reach consensus on best practices. NIM publication no. 02–5138. Washington, DC: U.S. Government Printing Office.

Neria, Y., & Litz, B. (in press). Bereavement by traumatic means: The complex synergy of trauma and grief. *Journal of Loss and Trauma.*

Neria, Y., Suh, E. J., & Marshall, R. D. (2003). The professional response to the aftermath of September 11, 2001, in New York City: Lessons learned from treating victims of the World Trade Center attacks. In B. Litz (Ed.), *Early intervention for trauma and traumatic loss* (pp. 201–215). New York: Guilford.

Norris, F. H., Friedman, M. J., Watson, P. J., Byrne, C. M., Díaz, E., & Kaniasty, K. (2002). 60,000 disaster victims speak: Part 1: An empirical review of the empirical literature, 1981–2001. *Psychiatry, 65,* 207–239.

Norris, F. H., Hamblen, J. L., Watson, P. J., Ruzek, J. I., Gibson, L. E., Price, J. L., et al. (in press). Toward understanding and creating systems of postdisaster care: Findings and recommendations from a case study of New York's response to the World Trade Center disaster. In E. C. Ritchie, P. J. Watson, & M. J. Friedman (Eds.), *Mental health intervention following disasters or mass violence.* New York: Guilford.

North, C. S., Nixon, S. J., Shariat, S., Mallonee, S., McMillen, J. C., Spitznagel, E. L., et al. (1999). Psychiatric disorders among survivors of the Oklahoma City bombing. *Journal of the American Medical Association, 282,* 755–762.

North, C. S., Tivis, L., McMillen, J. C., Pfefferbaum, B., Spitznagel, E. L., Cox, J., et al. (2002). Coping, functioning, and adjustment of rescue workers after the Oklahoma City bombing. *Journal of Traumatic Stress, 15,* 171–175.

Norwood, A. E. (2001). Psychological effects of biological warfare. *Military Medicine, 166*(Suppl. 2), 27–28.

Noy, S. (2002). Early dissemination of information: An essential ingredient in the prevention of biological warfare. *Harefuah, 141,* 119.

Ogrodniczuk, J. S., & Piper, W. E. (2003). The effect of group climate on outcome in two forms of short-term group therapy. *Group Dynamics: Theory, Research, and Practice, 7,* 64–76.

———, & Joyce, A. S. (2004). Differences in men's and women's responses to short-term group psychotherapy. *Psychotherapy Research, 14,* 231–243.

Ogrodniczuk, J. S., Piper, W. E., Joyce, A. S., McCallum, M., & Rosie, J. S. (2002). Social support as a predictor of response to group therapy for complicated grief. *Psychiatry, 65,* 346–357.

———. (2003). NEO-five factor personality traits as predictors of response to two forms of group psychotherapy. *International Journal of Group Psychotherapy, 53,* 417–442.

Ogrodniczuk, J. S., Piper, W. E., McCallum, M., Joyce, A. S., & Rosie, J. S. (2002). Interpersonal predictors of group therapy outcome for complicated grief. *International Journal of Group Psychotherapy, 52,* 511–535.

Ouimette, P., & Brown, P. J. (2002). *Trauma and substance abuse: Causes, consequences, and treatment of comorbid disorders.* Washington, DC: American Psychological Association.

Piotrowski, C. S., & Brannon, S. J. (2002). Exposure, threat appraisal, and lost confidence as predictors of PTSD symptoms following September 11, 2001. *American Journal of Orthopsychiatry, 72,* 476–485.

Piper, W. E., McCallum, M., Joyce, A. S., Rosie, J. S., & Ogrodniczuk, J. S. (2001). Patient personality and time-limited group psychotherapy for complicated grief. *International Journal of Group Psychotherapy, 51,* 525–552.

Prigerson, H. G., Shear, M. K., Jacobs, S. C., Reynolds, C. F., III, Maciejewski, P. K., Davidson, J. R. T., et al. (1999). Consensus criteria for traumatic grief: A preliminary empirical test. *British Journal of Psychiatry, 174,* 67–73.

Ramalingaswami, V. (2001). Psychological effects of the 1994 plague outbreak in Surat, India. *Military Medicine, 166,* 29–30.

Raphael, B., Minkov, C., & Dobson, M. (2001). Psychotherapeutic and pharmacological intervention for bereaved persons. In M. S. Stroebe, W. Stroebe, R. O. Hansson, & H. Schut (Eds.), *New handbook of bereavement: Consequences, coping, and care* (pp. 587–612). Washington, DC: American Psychological Association.

Raphael, B., & Wilson, J. P. (2000). *Psychological debriefing: Theory, practice and evidence.* New York: Cambridge University Press.

Resick, P. A., Nishith, P., Weaver, T. L., Astin, M. C., & Feuer, C. A. (2002). A comparison of cognitive-processing therapy with prolonged exposure and a waiting condition for the treatment of chronic posttraumatic stress disorder in female rape victims. *Journal of Consulting and Clinical Psychology, 70,* 867–879.

Rivkind, A. I., Eid, A., Weingart, E., Izhar, U., Barach, P., Richter, E. D., et al. (1999). Complications from supervised mask use in post-operative surgical patients during the Gulf War. *Prehospital and Disaster Medicine, 14,* 107–108.

Ruzek, J. I. (2002a). Dissemination of information and early intervention practices in the context of mass violence or large-scale disaster. *Behavior Therapist, 25,* 32–36.

———. (2002b). Providing "brief education and support" for emergency response workers: An alternative to debriefing. *Military Medicine, 167*(Suppl.), 73–75.

———. (in press). Models of early intervention following mass violence and other trauma. In E. C. Ritchie, P. J. Watson, & M. J. Friedman (Eds.), *Mental health intervention following disasters or mass violence.* New York: Guilford.

———, Young, B. H., Cordova, M. J., & Flynn, B. W. (2004). Integration of disaster mental health services with emergency medicine. *Prehospital and Disaster Medicine, 19,* 46–53.

Rynearson, E. K., Favell, J. L., Gold, R., & Prigerson, H. (2002). Bereavement intervention with incarcerated youth. *Journal of the American Academy of Child and Adolescent Psychiatry, 41,* 893–894.

Salloum, A., Avery, L., & McClain, R. P. (2001). Group psychotherapy for adolescent survivors of homicide victims: A pilot study. *Journal of the American Academy of Child and Adolescent Psychiatry, 40,* 1261–1267.

Schnurr, P. P., Friedman, M. J., Foy, D. W., Shea, M. T., Hsieh, F. Y., Lavori, P. W., et al. (2003). Randomized trial of trauma-focused group therapy for posttraumatic stress disorder: Results from a Department of Veterans Affairs cooperative study. *Archives of General Psychiatry, 60,* 481–489.

Schut, H., Stroebe, M. S., van den Bout, J., & Terheggen, M. (2001). The efficacy of bereavement interventions: Determining who benefits. In M. S. Stroebe, W. Stroebe, R. O. Hansson, & H. Schut

(Eds.), *New handbook of bereavement: Consequences, coping, and care* (pp. 705–737). Washington, DC: American Psychological Association.

Shalev, A. Y., Adessky, R., Boker, R., Bargai, N., Cooper, R., Freedman, S., et al. (2003). Clinical intervention for survivors of prolonged adversities. In R. J. Ursano, C. S. Fullerton, & A. E. Norwood (Eds.), *Terrorism and disaster: Individual and community mental health interventions* (pp. 162–188). New York: Cambridge University Press.

Shalev, A. Y., Tuval-Mashiach, R., Frenkiel, S., & Hadar, H. (2004). Psychological reactions to continuous terror. Paper under review.

Shear, M. K., Frank, E., Foa, E., Cherry, C., Reynolds, C., Bilt, J., et al. (2001). Traumatic grief treatment: A pilot study. *American Journal of Psychiatry, 158,* 1506–1508.

Silver, R. C., Holman, E. A., McIntosh, D. N., Poulin, M., & Gil-Rivas, V. (2002). Nationwide longitudinal study of psychological responses to September 11. *Journal of the American Medical Association, 288,* 1235–1244.

Sireling, L., Cohen, D., & Marks, I. (1988). Guided mourning for morbid grief: A controlled replication. *Behavior Therapy, 19,* 121–132.

Smith, D. W., Kilpatrick, D. G., Falsetti, S. A., & Best, C. L. (2002). Postterrorism services for victims and surviving family members: Lessons from Pan Am 103. *Cognitive and Behavioral Practice, 9,* 280–286.

Somer, E., Tamir, E., Maguen, S., & Litz, B. T. (2005). Brief cognitive-behavioral phone-based intervention targeting anxiety about the threat of attack: A pilot study. *Behaviour Research and Therapy, 43,* 669–679.

Spooren, D. J., Henderick, H., & Jannes, C. (2000). Survey description of stress of parents bereaved from a child killed in a traffic accident. A retrospective study of a victim support group. *Omega, 42,* 171–185.

Tarrier, N., Pilgrim, H., Sommerfield, C., Faragher, B., Reynolds, M., Graham, E., et al. (1999). A randomized trial of cognitive therapy and imaginal exposure in the treatment of chronic posttraumatic stress disorder. *Journal of Consulting and Clinical Psychology, 67,* 13–18.

Tarrier, N., Sommerfield, C., Pilgrim, H., & Humphreys, L. (1999). Cognitive therapy or imaginal exposure in the treatment of post-traumatic stress disorder. *British Journal of Psychiatry, 175,* 571–575.

Tugade, M. M., & Fredrickson, B. L. (2004). Resilient individuals use positive emotions to bounce back from negative emotional experiences. *Journal of Personality and Social Psychology, 86,* 320–333.

Ursano, R. J., Norwood, A. E., Fullerton, C. S., Holloway, H. C., & Hall, M. (2003). Terrorism with weapons of mass destruction: Chemical, biological, nuclear, radiological, and explosive agents. In R. J. Ursano & A. E. Norwood (Eds.), *Annual Review of Psychiatry, Vol. 22* (pp. 125–154). Washington, DC: American Psychiatric Association.

Veterans Health Administration. (2003). Management of post-traumatic stress. Publication 10Q-CPG/PTSD-04. Washington, DC: Clinical Practice Guideline Working Group, Office of Quality and Performance, Department of Veterans Affairs and Health Affairs, Department of Defense. Retrieved January 22, 2006, from http://www.oqp.med.va.gov/cpg/PTSD/PTSD_Base.htm

Vlahov, D., Galea, S., Ahern, J., Resnick H., & Kilpatrick, D. (2004). Sustained increased consumption of cigarettes, alcohol, and marijuana among Manhattan residents after September 11, 2001. *American Journal of Public Health, 94,* 253–254.

Vlahov, D., Galea, S., Resnick H., Ahern, J., Boscarino, J. A., Bucavalas, M., et al. (2002). Increased use of cigarettes, alcohol, and marijuana among Manhattan, New York, residents after the September 11th terrorist attacks. *American Journal of Epidemiology, 155,* 988–996.

Weisenberg, M., Schwarzwald, J., Waysman, M., Solomon, Z., & Klingman, A. (1993). Coping of school-age children in the sealed room during Scud missile bombardment and postwar stress reactions. *Journal of Consulting and Clinical Psychology, 61,* 462–467.

Wessely, S. (2003). The role of screening in the prevention of psychological disorders arising after major trauma: Pros and cons. In R. J. Ursano, C. S. Fullerton, & A. E. Norwood (Eds.), *Terrorism and disaster: Individual and community mental health interventions* (pp. 121–145). New York: Cambridge University Press.

Yehuda, R., McFarlane, A., & Shalev, A. (1998). Predicting the development of posttraumatic stress disorder from the acute response to a traumatic event. *Biological Psychiatry, 44,* 1305–1313.

Young, B. H., Ruzek, J. I., & Ford, J. D. (1999). Cognitive-behavioral group treatment for disaster-related PTSD. In B. H. Young & D. D. Blake (Eds.), *Group treatments for post-traumatic stress disorder* (pp. 149–200). Philadelphia: Brunner/Mazel.

Young, B. H., Ruzek, J. I., & Pivar, I. (2001). Mental health aspects of disaster and community violence: A review of training materials. Menlo Park, CA: National Center for PTSD; Washington, DC: Center for Mental Health Services.

Young, B. H., Ruzek, J. I., Wong, M., Salzer, M., Naturale, A., & Wisher, R. (in press). Disaster mental health training: Guidelines, considerations, and recommendations. In E. C. Ritchie, P. J. Watson, & M. J. Friedman (Eds.), *Mental health intervention following disasters or mass violence.* New York: Guilford.

Zlotnick, C., Shea, T. M., Rosen, K., Simpson, E., Mulrenin, K., Begin, A., et al. (1997). An affect-management group for women with posttraumatic stress disorder and histories of childhood sexual abuse. *Journal of Traumatic Stress, 10,* 425–436.

19

Neurobiological and Behavioral Consequences of Terrorism

Distinguishing Normal From Pathological Responses, Risk Profiling, and Optimizing Resilience

Rachel Yehuda
Richard Bryant
Joseph Zohar
Charles R. Marmar

Some people are vulnerable to the development of psychopathology following exposure to events that elicit terror and helplessness, but the majority experience transient symptoms that for the most part resolve within weeks or months. One of the major gaps in our knowledge is the difficulty in predicting long-term responses to trauma on the basis of the nature and time course of the acute response to any traumatic event—particularly for any given person. This chapter summarizes current knowledge about differentiating normal from pathological responses and predicting psychopathologic responses following exposure to terrorism and highlights promising areas for future research.

It is important to determine the generalizability of findings on the effects of trauma exposure arising from other contexts to terrorism and mass violence. In one sense terrorism is a prototypic traumatic event, particularly for those who directly experience a threat to their lives or physical integrity or experience traumatic loss. Those directly exposed to terrorism are candidates for the development of acute stress disorder (ASD) or posttraumatic stress disorder (PTSD), and knowledge about the impact of other traumatic events may be helpful in defining their psychological outcomes.

On the other hand, terrorism is not only about life threat to individuals or even a small group of people but is also designed to instill fear in society at large. Those who are not in immediate proximity to the attack or who were not directly affected by the loss of someone important to them can also be affected, in part because terrorist attacks receive repeated coverage in the media. Terrorism can threaten the sense of safety and security of everyone in the society attacked because they are aware that terrorists may strike again in unpredictable locations. The mental health consequences in those who are indirectly exposed but show symptoms may be qualitatively or quantitatively different from those of people who have suffered direct exposure and also different from those of people who experienced near misses. The cumulative effect of anticipatory anxiety of future incidents in those who have been directly exposed is also not known. The real threat of imminent attack may be related to how quickly they can recover from its effects.

A critical issue in differentiating normal from pathological responses is the passage of time. This is particularly true in considering outcomes such as PTSD, a diagnosis that requires symptoms and functional disturbances to have persisted for at least a month following trauma exposure. However, terrorist acts usually initiate anxiety about future attacks. If a terrorist event represents the beginning or continuation of a situation or threat—as it often does—the timetable for recovery may be shifted. Thus, in considering whether the effects of terrorism are pathological, it may be appropriate to conceptualize normal responses to be present for more than 30 days after the initial trauma. In the context of ongoing terrorist threat, identifying persistent disorder may be more accurately defined only after the immediate threat is substantially reduced. This caveat does not suggest that people do not have mental health needs that should be met within this timeframe. Instead, it acknowledges that a normative response may involve strong and persistent symptomatic reactions if actual threat persists.

In trying to delineate the mental health consequences of terrorism, researchers have generally conducted surveys or interviews in which they inquire about expectable emotional reactions. These include difficulties in sleeping and concentrating, irritability, nightmares, distressing thoughts about the event, or distress at reminders of the event (Schuster et al., 2001), that is, symptoms suggestive of PTSD. In the immediate aftermath of terrorism most people will exhibit these symptoms. The question becomes whether having time-limited high levels of symptoms at a time when most of those directly exposed also have them constitutes, let alone predicts, pathology.

Although hypervigilance to future attacks or persistent worry about exposure to anthrax may have been widely present following the attacks of 9/11, is it best to consider these symptoms as indicative of a pathological or normative response in a terrorist environment? Most mental health models regard acute stress reactions as a mental disorder, but it may be erroneous to attribute symptoms of anxiety to a mental disorder when the context suggests that such reactions are warranted. The question of how to think about such symptoms is important from a public health perspective since it raises the even greater issue of whether the presence of early symptoms requires intervention. The question resonates with commentators who have noted that a definition of disorder should recognize the extent to which a condition is dysfunctional in the context of the situation in which the individual is functioning (Wakefield, 1996).

A longitudinal perspective provides insight into the pathological nature of acute responses to terrorism. It is now clear that most people recover from early posttraumatic symptoms. This phenomenon can be illustrated by results of surveys conducted by the New York Academy of Medicine following the attacks of September 11 in New York City. Five to eight weeks after the attacks, 7.5% of randomly sampled subjects living south of 110th Street had reportedly developed PTSD (Galea et al., 2002), with those who experienced the most severe exposure or personal loss at higher risk than others. When another randomly sampled group was studied 6 months after the attacks, only 0.6% of those living south of 110th Street met all of the diagnostic criteria for PTSD, and an additional 4.7% met the criteria for subsyndromal PTSD (Galea, Boscarino, Resnik, & Vlahov, 2003). As a whole, the Manhattan community recovered substantially from the initial effects of the September 11 attacks. However, an important question raised by these findings is whether the initial estimates of PTSD based on early symptoms constituted a real clinical syndrome requiring treatment or rather was simply a reflection of temporary distress. Obviously, in those who did not recover or had persistent features of PTSD even if they partially recovered, these symptoms may have been the earliest manifestations of psychopathology, raising a second important question of the extent to which early symptoms of postterrorism are predictive of later ones.

Predictors of Pathological Responses

Those with minimal symptoms in the immediate aftermath of a traumatic event are at low risk for the development of subsequent PTSD or other forms of psychopathology (Shalev, 1992). Greater symptom severity from 1–2 weeks posttrauma and beyond is positively associated with subsequent symptom severity (Harvey and Bryant, 1998, Murray, Ehlers, & Mayou, 2002; Shalev et al., 1997). Those who do show high-magnitude PTSD symptoms in the days immediately posttrauma represent two distinct subgroups: those in whom symptoms will abate within days to weeks and those in whom symptoms will persist (McFarlane, 1989; Shalev, 1992). These findings support the idea that the "pathologic process" involved in PTSD and possibly other posttraumatic mental health reactions are in part a reflection of a failure to recover from early symptoms. Yet because high levels of PTSD symptoms in the first days after a trauma predict failure to recover in some but not other trauma victims, the findings point to the importance of identifying additional early markers of longer-term pathology.

One possible predictor of long-term psychopathology may be peritraumatic dissociation. Numerous studies have found an association between peritraumatic dissociation and the subsequent development of PTSD (e.g., Marmar et al., 1994; Ehlers, Mayou, & Bryant, 1998; Koopman, Classen, & Spiegel, 1994; Marmar, Weiss, Metzler, Delucchi, & Best, 1999; Murray et al., 2002; Shalev et al., 1998; Marmar, Metzler, & Otte, 2004; Marmar et al., 2005). Peritraumatic dissociation refers to a dissociative experience that occurs at the actual time of the traumatic event and includes features of depersonalization, derealization, and altered time sense. A meta-analysis by Ozer, Best, Lipsey, and Weiss (2003) indicates that peritraumatic dissociation was the single best predictor ($r = .35$) of PTSD among trauma-exposed individuals, but this view has not been unanimously supported in prospective studies (e.g., Dancu, Riggs, Hearst-Ikeda, Shoyer, & Foa, 1996; Marshall & Schell, 2002).

In 2003, McNally asserted that findings of the predictive power of peritraumatic dissociation are difficult to interpret because many studies do not adequately distinguish between true peritraumatic dissociation and subsequent depersonalization and derealization in the first weeks after exposure, which are required for a diagnosis of ASD, and which do not appear to be predictive of PTSD over and above the acute reexperiencing, and presence of avoidance and arousal symptoms. Studies of peritraumatic dissociation usually do not covary for cognitive ability, which in itself is a risk factor for PTSD that is linked with dissociation (McNally, 2003). Thus, it may be that peritraumatic dissociation predicts PTSD because it is highly linked with other risk factors for this disorder, in particular peritraumatic panic (Brunet et al., 2001; Marmar et al., 2005).

Another potentially important predictor of pathological outcomes following trauma exposure is the presence of a panic attack during and/or immediately after trauma exposure. There is evidence that such panic attacks occur in 53%–90% of trauma survivors who experience severely traumatic events (Bryant & Panasetis, 2001). More than half of those who meet the criteria for ASD report peritraumatic as well as subsequent panic attacks (Nixon & Bryant, 2003). Galea et al. found peritraumatic panic to be the best predictor of PTSD in the post-9/11 survey of 1,008 residents living south of 110th Street in Manhattan. This observation is consistent with recent observations from a study of 747 police officers, in which panic reactions and related emotional distress during exposure were highly predictive of pre-9/11 PTSD symptoms (Brunet et al., 2001) and in a prospective study of 311 NYPD officers also predictive of post-9/11 symptoms (Marmar et al., 2005).

McNally has suggested that both peritraumatic dissociation and peritraumatic panic can result in a catastrophic interpretation of the event and or the erroneous conclusion that the symptoms are harbingers of more serious problems (McNally, 2003). Indeed, some investigators have demonstrated the power of negatively appraising any aspect of the event in the peritraumatic period to predict long-term pathology. For example, having a negative perception of other people's responses (e.g., "I feel that other people are ashamed of me now") predicts PTSD beyond what can be predicted from initial symptom levels (Dunmore, Clark, & Ehlers, 2001). People with ASD show enhanced anxiety sensitivity. For example, they are prone to catastrophize about somatic cues (Smith & Bryant, 2000) and also respond to a hyperventilation challenge test by engaging in more dysfunctional thoughts about somatic responses (Nixon & Bryant, in press). Similarly, attributions of exaggerated responsibility for a trauma in the acute posttrauma phase predicts PTSD (Andrews, Brewin, Rose, & Kirk, 2000; Delahanty et al., 1997). In the context of terrorism, the presence of these attributions provides a way of distinguishing between being external events that attempt to terrorize and internal reactions of actually being terrified. Those who are exposed to a traumatic event are not traumatized unless they are deeply distraught at the time of the event and then make ongoing catastrophic interpretations.

Peritraumatic panic may favor the development of PTSD for neurobiological reasons as well as cognitive misattributions. Basic science research on memory consolidation and fear conditioning have demonstrated that heightened adrenergic activation can promote the consolidation and retrieval of fear-provoking memories (Bohus & Lissak, 1968). Building on this preclinical work, conditioning models of trauma response propose that PTSD is the result of strong associative learning whereby people who will go on to develop PTSD initially react to a traumatic event (unconditioned stimulus) with high levels of sustained arousal and fear, as occurs in peritraumatic panic reactions (unconditioned response). People with PTSD then continue to show arousal (conditioned response) when confronted with trauma-related cues (conditioned stimuli).

It has been hypothesized that extreme sympathetic arousal at the time of a traumatic event may result in the release of stress-related neurochemicals (including norepinephrine and epinephrine) in the cortex, mediating an overconsolidation of trauma memories (Pitman, Shalev, & Orr, 2000). The majority of trauma survivors will engage in extinction learning in the weeks after trauma exposure, in which they associate the conditioned stimuli with safe consequences and thereby actively inhibit the fear response through new learning. In contrast, the minority of people who will develop PTSD have impaired extinction learning and overconsolidated memories of the trauma. Both dissociation (Simeon, Guralnik, Knutelska, Yehuda, & Schmeidler, 2003) and panic reactions (Charney, Deutch, Krystal, Southwick, & Davis, 1993; Southwick et al., 1997) have been associated with increased catecholamine states. It is plausible that people who experience panic, dissociation, or other forms of intense emotional distress during and immediately after a traumatic event have higher levels of catecholamines than those who do not respond in this manner. An enhanced elevation of catecholamines in the immediate aftermath of a traumatic event may increase the probability of intrusive recollections in the first few days and weeks posttrauma (Pitman, 1989; Charney et al., 1993).

One of the major gaps in our knowledge concerns the interplay of biologic responses at the time of a traumatic event and cognitive factors. Indeed, it is easy to see how an increased catecholaminergic response to trauma could be the proximal cause of intense panic. Furthermore, it seems plausible that those who find themselves in a more intense biologic state of fear might be likely to appraise a situation as more immediately dangerous. On the other hand, it may be that preexisting cognitive factors or exaggerated threat appraisals at the time of exposure drive the catecholaminergic response to the trauma that leads to the panic. These preexisting cognitive factors, in turn, may or may not be the cause, result, or correlate of a preexisting biological alteration that sets the stage for an extreme response.

In summary, those who are exposed to terrorism or other catastrophic events, do not panic or dissociate during the event and in the first hours afterward, and have low levels of PTSD-like symptoms in the first days and weeks after exposure are most likely to have a normal stress reaction and not to develop PTSD. Among those who experience high levels of symptoms in the first days or weeks, some will recover and some will not. Prolonged and sustained peritraumatic panic (Brunet et al., 2001; Galea et al., 2002; Marmar et al., 2005), as well as peritraumatic dissociation (Ozer et al., 2003; Marmar, Metzler, and Otte, 2004), are strong predictors of those who will not recover.

Clarifying the causes of high levels of immediate and long-term symptoms will no doubt lead to ideas about potential preventative treatments. For example, to the extent that panic reactions are associated with increased catecholamine responses at the time of trauma, aggressive intervention with adrenergic blocking agents such as propranolol (Pitman et al., 2002; Vaiva et al., 2003) or cognitive behavioral stress management techniques emphasizing anxiety management rather than emotional catharsis or retelling (i.e., reexposure, as in some forms of debriefing) may be the most appropriate immediate interventions for those who panic at the time of exposure and in the hours immediately following a traumatic experience. For those who are not in a position to receive intervention within several hours or days posttrauma, it will be necessary to determine the impact of posttraumatic risk factors such as lack of social support and subsequent adverse life events on the longitudinal course of pathologic responses to trauma.

It is important to note that there is not a perfect one-to-one correspondence between the level of acute stress reactions and longer-term adjustment. A small proportion of people can apparently develop PTSD or other disorders after a delayed period of time following the traumatic event. The *Diagnostic and Statistical Manual of Mental Disorders* (*DSM-IV*) identified delayed-onset PTSD when the disorder becomes apparent at least 6 months after the precipitating event (American Psychiatric Association, 1994). Large-scale studies of civilian trauma have reported delayed-onset PTSD in a small minority of cases (around 5%; Bryant & Harvey, 2002; Buckley, Blanchard, & Hickling, 1996; Ehlers et al., 1998; Mayou, Bryant, & Duthrie, 1993). Evidence indicates that people who develop delayed-onset PTSD experience more persistent stressors after the initial trauma, which may contribute to PTSD development (Ehlers et al., 1998; Solomon, Kotler, Shalev, & Lin, 1989; Green et al., 1990).

It is possible that ongoing stressors in the aftermath of an initial terrorist attack (for example, the ongoing threat of terrorist attacks and later terrorist acts of violence elsewhere in the world) may contribute to the development of delayed-onset PTSD. Alternately, fear-conditioning models posit that initial conditioning may persist in a latent form, restrained by new fear extinction learning, until sufficient cues or increased stressors perhaps elicit a conditioned response in the form of PTSD (Charney et al., 1993). Fear-conditioning models suggest that some form of fear reaction should occur in the acute phase and that this should be exacerbated under certain circumstances that reinstate the initial fear-related cues. This proposal is supported by evidence that most people who develop delayed-onset PTSD do display elevated stress reactions and higher resting heart rates in the acute phase after trauma exposure (Bryant & Harvey, 2002).

Differentiating Normal From Pathological Responses in the First Weeks Following Exposure

One of the formal attempts to recognize initial pathological responses to trauma was the introduction of the ASD diagnosis in *DSM-IV* (American Psychiatric Association, 1994). This diagnosis was intended to fill what was considered to be a diagnostic gap because the PTSD diagnosis requires that symptoms be present for at least a month. A second purpose of the diagnosis was to identify acutely traumatized people who were likely to de-

velop chronic PTSD (Koopman, Classen, Cardena, & Spiegel, 1995). The ASD diagnosis attempts to differentiate between the majority of trauma survivors who display a transient stress reaction and recover within a few weeks to months and those who are in the initial phase of a chronic disorder.

The ASD diagnosis was strongly influenced by the perspective that dissociative reactions are a crucial mechanism in posttraumatic adjustment (Spiegel, Classen, & Cardena, 2000). The argument that ASD reflects a "disorder" is based in part on the belief that dissociative responses after trauma lead to psychopathological responses because they impede access to and processing of traumatic memories. Dissociative reactions in the acute aftermath of trauma exposure are predicted to limit or disorganize emotional processing of the traumatic memories, leading to psychically unmetabolized traumatic memories and chronic symptoms.

There are now 12 longitudinal cohort studies of adults that have addressed the extent to which ASD within the initial month after trauma exposure predicts subsequent PTSD (Brewin, Andrews, Rose, & Kirk, 1999; Bryant & Harvey, 1998; Creamer et al., 2004; Difede et al., 2002; Harvey & Bryant, 1998, 1999, 2000b; Holeva, Tarrier, & Wells, 2001; Kangas, Henry, & Bryant, in press; Murray et al., 2002; Schnyder, Moergeli, Klaghofer, & Buddeberg, 2001; Staab, Grieger, Fullerton, & Ursano, 1996). Most of these studies demonstrate that the majority of trauma survivors who display ASD— approximately 75% across studies—subsequently develop PTSD. However, only a minority of people who eventually developed PTSD initially met the criteria for ASD. It appears that a major reason the ASD diagnosis does not adequately identify the majority of people who develop PTSD is the requirement that three dissociative symptoms be displayed (Bryant, 2003). Evidence suggests that there are multiple pathways to developing PTSD that may or may not involve dissociation (Harvey & Bryant, 2002).

Identifying Those at Greater Risk

Although being able to predict long-term pathology from the acute response, such as peritraumatic panic, is of paramount importance, understanding the development of pathologic responses will also necessitate understanding the risk factors for those early responses. The finding that only a percentage of those exposed to trauma develop short-term symptoms and that only a minority of those with high levels of acute symptoms will develop a chronic severe form of PTSD justifies a search for individual differences in resilience and vulnerability. A wide variety of risk factors, including developmental, familial, situational, and even genetic risk factors for PTSD, have now been identified (McFarlane, 1989; Yehuda, 1997; Brewin, Andrews, & Valentine, 2000; Ozer et al., 2003).

Retrospective studies suggest that those who are at greatest risk for developing PTSD following a traumatic event are people with a personal or family history of psychopathology (Breslau, Davis, Andreski, & Peterson, 1991), prior exposure to trauma, especially during childhood (Nishith, Mechanic, & Resick, 2000; Breslau, Chilcoat, Kessler, & Davis, 1999), cognitive factors, such as lower IQ (Silva et al., 2000), female gender (Breslau et al., 1999), stressful life events in the year preceding the traumatic event, and certain preexisting personality traits, such as proneness to experiencing negative emotions and having poor social supports (Brewin et al., 2000). To a large extent, prospective studies have supported these findings, in that individuals with greater initial distress and less recovery over time had more of these risk factors than those with less distress. However, when such risk factors have been used in discriminant function analyses to predict subsequent PTSD in prospective studies, no single variable emerged as a strong predictor. This may reflect the fact that retrospective studies use a narrower range of subjects that are classified based on the dichotomy of presence or absence of PTSD, whereas prospective studies usually include a broader range of people with generally lower levels of PTSD symptoms, reducing the power of such predictions.

Recent work has begun to identify risk factors by assessing populations that are likely to be exposed to trauma before and after such exposure actually occurs. A prospective study by Marmar et al. (2005) of New York police officers has found that elevated symptoms of PTSD assessed several years before 9/11 predicted greater 9/11-related PTSD symptoms several years after the WTC attacks. A study by Guthrie & Bryant (2005) of startle responses has found that skin conductance and eyeblink (electromyographic [EMG]) startle responses before trauma exposure in a cohort of firefighter trainees predicted acute stress reactions after subsequent trauma exposure. Further, slower extinction learning after aversive conditioning before trauma exposure strongly predicted chronic posttraumatic stress after trauma exposure (Guthrie & Bryant, manuscript submitted for publication). Collectively, these findings point to the importance of psychophysiological reactivity prior to trauma exposure as a risk factor for subsequent fear conditioning and development of posttraumatic stress.

Family and genetic studies are pointing toward the role of genetic contributions to posttraumatic stress reactions. Compared to adult children of Holocaust survivors without PTSD, adult children of Holocaust survivors with PTSD show a greater prevalence of PTSD to their own traumatic events (Yehuda, Schmeidler, Wainberg, Binder-Brynes, & Duvdevani, 1998). It is difficult to know to what extent that increased vulnerability to PTSD in family members of trauma survivors with PTSD can be attributed to being raised by a parent with this disorder (Yehuda, Halligan, & Bierer, 2001), to exposure of the fetus to the mother's stress hormones during pregnancy, or to genetic factors.

Several studies on twins support the role of genetic contribution, given the increased prevalence of PTSD in monozygotic compared with dizygotic twins (True et al., 1993). Further, a study by Orr et al. (2003) compared startle responses in pairs of Vietnam combat veterans and their monozygotic twins who were not exposed to battle. They found evidence of more slowly habituating skin conductance startle responses in veterans with PTSD and their non-combat-exposed twins, compared to veterans without PTSD and their non-combat-exposed twins. This finding suggests that more slowly habituating skin conductance responses to acoustic startle stimuli may represent a pretrauma vulnerability factor for PTSD (Orr et al., 2003). This model is supported by the prospective findings of greater skin conductance and eyeblink EMG startle responses before trauma exposure in firefighter trainees with greater acute stress reactions after duty-related traumatic exposure (Guthrie & Bryant, 2005).

The issue these risk factors raise is whether they need to be part of an initial assessment in the immediate aftermath of a trauma, and this is currently an open question. Studies have clearly demonstrated that people with both high PTSD symptoms in the first week and additional risk factors—childhood trauma, low educational attainment, personal or family history of anxiety or mood disorders, history of heavy alcohol use in the months prior to an incident, poor social supports in the posttraumatic period, and greater levels of exposure during the incident—are less likely to recover than those who do not. However, if the panic and related emotional distress at the time of the traumatic event—or if a high level of PTSD symptoms that substantially interfere with occupational and relationship functioning within the first few weeks after an event—are sufficiently predictive of longer-term symptoms, it may not be necessary to assess pretraumatic risk factors for the purpose of triage and timely intervention. Rather, those risk factors might prove important in understanding and possibly differentiating among various types of acute reactions and in providing stress inoculation training as a prophylaxis.

Biological Markers Differentiating Normal From Pathological Responses to Trauma

There appears to be a distinct set of biological markers of PTSD. These markers have been found to differentiate those with PTSD from trauma-exposed individuals without PTSD and from psychiatric controls. These findings suggest that the biology of PTSD is not simply a reflection of a normative stress response but rather a distinct pathologic condition (Yehuda and McFarlane, 1995).

In concert with observations of the phenomenology and psychology of PTSD, neurobiological examinations of trauma survivors also support the possibility that the development of PTSD is facilitated by a runaway stress response at the time of the trauma, resulting in a cascade of biological alterations that lead to intrusive, avoidance, and hyperarousal symptoms. In contrast to the normal fear response, which is characterized by a series of biological reactions that help the body cope with, and gradually recover from, stress (e.g., high cortisol levels), some recent prospective biologic studies have demonstrated that people who develop PTSD or greater PTSD symptoms appear to have attenuated cortisol increases in the acute aftermath

of a trauma (Resnick, Yehuda, Foy, & Pitman, 1995; Delahanty, Riamonde, & Spoonster, 2000). Moreover, those who develop PTSD show higher heart rates in the emergency room and at 1 week posttrauma compared to those who ultimately recover (Bryant, Guthrie, & Moulds, 2000; Shalev et al., 1998, Zatzick et al., 2005), suggesting a greater degree of sympathetic nervous system activation. These findings imply that biologic response to acute trauma are distinct in those who do and do not go on to develop PTSD.

Further supporting the distinction between normal and pathological responses to trauma are sensitization models of PTSD. Post, Weiss, and Smith (1995) have proposed that, with chronic repeated stimulation by trauma reminder cues, the reexperiencing of symptoms begins to occur spontaneously, rather than requiring triggering, in a kindling-like process. Consistent with this model, Shalev and colleagues (2000) have reported that elevated heart rate and more slowly habituating skin conductance and EMG responses to startle stimuli were observed at 1 and 4 months following trauma but not at 1 week after trauma in those who subsequently developed PTSD. These results suggest a progressive neuronal sensitization associated with heightened physiological reactivity underlying PTSD development.

The precise origin and onset of any of the biologic alterations associated with PTSD have not been elucidated. Recent findings suggest that at least some of the biologic alterations observed (e.g., low cortisol levels, smaller hippocampal volumes) may represent a genetic or early developmental risk factor for the disorder rather than either a consequence of trauma exposure or development of PTSD (Yehuda et al., 2000; Gilbertson et al., 2002). It is important to first develop models and then testable hypotheses for how such preexisting risk factors might explain the development of PTSD. Low cortisol may favor the development of PTSD for several reasons. Cortisol inhibits its own release through negative feedback at the level of the pituitary and the hypothalamus. Lower levels of cortisol at the time of a traumatic event would disrupt the process of stress recovery by failing to inhibit the activation of the pituitary, resulting in increased hypothalamic corticotropin-releasing factor (CRF) stimulation in synergy with other neuropeptides, such as arginine vasopressin, resulting in a higher magnitude ACTH response, which might further stimulate the sympathetic nervous system (Holsboer, 2001). Further, glucocorticoid release inhibits norepinephrine secretion from the sympathetic nerve terminals; as a result, lower cortisol levels may have the consequence of prolonging norepinephrine availability to synapses both in the periphery and in the brain (Pacak, Palkovitz, Kopin, & Goldstein, 1995). Ultimately, low cortisol levels might result in an upregulation or increased sensitivity of glucocorticoid receptors in response to the detection of a greater internal demand by the pituitary, which would further strengthen negative feedback inhibition. Alternatively, an enhanced negative feedback inhibition may be present at the time of the trauma and may contribute to the premature suppression of ACTH and cortisol, leading to undermodulated catecholamines responses (Yehuda, 2002).

There may be consequences of increased catecholamine levels in the acute aftermath of the trauma for promoting the consolidation of the traumatic memory. Indeed, adrenergic activation in the face of a low cortisol level has been shown to facilitate learning in animals (Cahill, Prins, Weber, & McGaugh, 1994). If this were also occurring in trauma survivors, the memory of the event would not only be strongly encoded but also associated with extreme subjective distress. The distress, in turn, could facilitate the development of altered perceptions and thoughts in the aftermath of the event, particularly those associated with one's own perception of danger or ability to cope with threat. These altered beliefs could serve to further delay recovery by leading to a failure to modulate fearful responses, which would further serve to strengthen, rather than reduce, both maladaptive cognitions in response to trauma and fear responses, thus perpetuating the intrusive, avoidance, and hyperarousal symptoms described earlier. In this context, there is evidence that, in the initial month after trauma, survivors with ASD display greater theta EEG activity than non-ASD trauma survivors (Felmingham, Bryant, & Gordon, in press). Theta EEG activity has been associated with overconsolidation of memories (Klimesch, Doppelmayr, Russegger, & Pachinger, 1996).

PTSD has been associated with numerous other biologic alterations, including immune (Maes and colleagues, 1999), catecholaminergic (Southwick et al., 1997), and psychophysiologic (Orr, 1997) alterations, as well as changes in sleep architecture (Neylan et al., 2003). Structural and functional neuroimaging studies of PTSD have demonstrated changes in brain volume, neuronal metabolism, and/or activation in regions such as the hippocampus and the amygdala (Rausch, Shin, & Pitman, 1997; Schuff et al., 2001). One model proposes that PTSD is influenced by excessive amygdale activation resulting from diminished inhibitory regulation of the central nucleus of the amygdala by the rostral anterior cingulate (Bush, Luu, & Posner, 2000; Shin et al., 2001). Hippocampal abnormalities may also preexist trauma exposure and serve as risk factors (Gilbertson et al., 2002). It is also possible that there are important individual differences in biologic systems in PTSD. In support of individual differences in biological responses, Southwick and colleagues demonstrated that in certain PTSD patients, panic attacks and flashbacks were elicited by the manipulation of the noradrenergic system with yohimbine, whereas in others they were elicited by the manipulation of serotonergic neurotransmission with m-chlorophenylpiperazine (mCPP) (Southwick et al., 1997).

Low GABA plasma levels immediately after trauma are also predictive of subsequent PTSD (Vaiva et al., 2003). GABA agonists reduce fear reactions (Zangrossi, Viana, & Graeff, 1999). Lower GABA levels shortly after trauma may suppress glutamatergic functioning, and thereby lead to PTSD. This interpretation is consistent with the finding that intoxication at the time of trauma can reduce the risk for PTSD (Maes, Delmeire, Mylle, & Altamura, 2001).

It remains to be determined which of these are risk factors and which evolve with exposure to traumatic stressors or with the development acute and chronic PTSD. It is conceivable that any one of a number of biologic risk factors would have the effect of facilitating a biological sensitization to subsequent traumatic events by allowing for greater physiologic arousal, greater terror during exposure, and, as a result, greater fear conditioning and memory consolidation. Biological characteristics of those at risk for developing PTSD appear to potentially involve preexisting alterations that might compromise adaptive cognitive processing at the time of the event (e.g., lower IQ, prior trauma) and/ or preexisting alterations that might impede containment of the biologic response to fear (e.g., lower cortisol or additional neuropeptides that might fail to contain sympathetic nervous system arousal). It is not known whether these biologic risk factors are related to biologic factors, such as increased catecholamines, that may be present in tandem with and influence levels of peritraumatic panic or distress. It is now critical to determine in prospective studies the relationships between biologic alterations in PTSD and symptoms and particularly between biologic alterations that may have been present before or during trauma exposure and the subsequent development of pathologic responses.

Limitations in the Use of Behavioral and Biological Markers for Risk Profiling, Diagnosis, and Prognosis of PTSD Following Terrorist Acts

If the results of the World Trade Center attack studies are generalizable, most people who are distressed in the first few months will substantially recover from the effects of terrorism, with estimates of PTSD rates dropping from 7% at 2 months to 0.5% at 6 months (Galea, Ahern, & Resnick, 2002; Galea, Boscarino, Resnik, & Vlahov, 2003; Galea, Nandi, & Vlahov, 2005). At the same time among those who no longer met the criteria for PTSD, more than half manifested subsyndromal PTSD, suggesting caution about a long-term course. Those with partial PTSD may be particularly susceptible in the event of future attacks in New York or elsewhere in the United States. Those at risk for long-term symptoms appear to have a more intense reaction at the time of the trauma, for example, peritraumatic dissociation or peritraumatic panic, associated with a more negative appraisal of danger. It is not clear whether and to what extent pretraumatic risk factors (e.g., preexisting psychopathology, prior adversity, family history of psychopathology including PTSD and panic disorder, low IQ and other cognitive risk factors, preexisting personality traits such as avoidance and/or neuroticism) influence the intensity of peritraumatic responses to trauma, but presumably these risk factors are more relevant in situations where exposure is less severe.

Posttraumatic risk factors, such as lack of social support and newly occurring stressful life events, also seem to be important predictors of psychopathology, but the extent to which these may be influenced by pre- or even peritraumatic

risk factors and levels of posttraumatic symptoms is currently unknown. Those with greater PTSD symptoms following a terrorist attack may be more likely to withdraw from social support, disrupt close relationships, and struggle to meet occupational demands leading to a domino progression of losses. They may also become nihilistic (e.g., "Why drive with a seat belt when you can be wiped out any time?") or counterphobic (e.g., "I survived the collapse of the towers, so I am immune to normal dangers") and as a consequence engage in increased risk-taking behavior leading to subsequent retraumatization.

The conclusion that PTSD is specifically associated with neuroendocrine, neurotransmitter-related, and neuroanatomic alterations is warranted, as there has been a good degree of replication across different groups of trauma survivors at different phases of the chronic PTSD condition. However, no single biologic marker or even pattern of biologic markers have been demonstrated to be sufficiently sensitive and specific to constitute a reliable and valid diagnostic test of PTSD. Furthermore, it is not yet clear whether these biologic alterations constitute preexisting risk factors for the disorder rather than consequences of trauma exposure or failure to recover from the biologic responses to stress. Studies examining biologic alterations prospectively beginning soon after trauma exposure have produced reproducible, but not universal, results and primarily only in studies evaluating more homogenous groups of trauma survivors (e.g., following the trauma of rape or motor vehicle accidents).

Indeed, biologic alterations in the peri- and posttraumatic periods are likely to be highly influenced by many individual differences in both stress exposure and personal characteristics. Difficulties in recruiting subjects for detailed biologic studies in both the immediate aftermath of trauma and more chronic PTSD studies can result in a selection bias with respect to subjects both willing and eligible to participate. Whether biologic alterations observed in other groups of subjects with PTSD would be similar to those observed in victims of terrorism with mental health symptoms is not currently known and represents a critical frontier. Certainly, to the extent that biologic alterations represent either specific risk factors for trauma exposure or PTSD, it is imperative to determine whether pathologic responses to terrorism are similar, from a biologic perspective, to those observed in other groups with PTSD related to combat, rape, accidents, or other forms of interpersonal violence. It is also important to determine whether there are biologic alterations associated with the more nonspecific effects of terrorism, such as anticipatory anxiety, that might contribute to adverse psychological and medical outcomes.

There is also agreement about the predictive power of peritraumatic dissociation and peritraumatic panic attacks. What remains somewhat disputed is whether peritraumatic dissociation and panic are proxies for other PTSD risk factors such as negative appraisal or cognitive performance or, alternatively, whether the experiences of dissociation and panic during exposure characterize the state of being traumatized and drive subsequent negative appraisals regarding self-efficacy, and safety. Because these studies generally call for retrospective analysis (usually within days or weeks of the traumatic event, however), it is possible that some bias is introduced. That is, very few studies report on actually observing peritraumatic dissociation or panic occurring in real time since investigators are not generally at the scene of a traumatic event to witness this firsthand. Also, the majority of studies documenting peritraumatic dissociation and panic attacks have not been direct examinations of survivors of terrorism.

Research Priorities in Mental Health Consequences of Terrorism

The following are pressing research priorities: (1) Determine whether individual differences in genetic, familial, cognitive, behavioral, and personality risk factors for the development of psychopathology following exposure to trauma require different interventions or surveillance in the immediate aftermath of terrorism; (2) determine the role of adverse outcomes other than PTSD including major depression, panic disorder, generalized anxiety disorder, substance abuse, somatic symptoms, and physical illnesses, particularly hypertension, asthma, chronic pain syndromes, and other psychosomatic illnesses (Boscarino, 1996); (3) determine the interplay of biological and behavioral variables in risk for PTSD, using prospective, longitudinal designs following terrorism; (4) determine whether the contribution of peritraumatic dissociation or

panic in the development of chronic disorder may be moderated by the relationship of these factors to pretrauma vulnerability factors, such as childhood abuse (Keane, Kaufman, & Kimble, 2001; Otte et al., 2005); (5) determine whether resilience is associated with biologic and behavioral mechanisms that are different from those involved in vulnerability to PTSD; (6) conduct research on novel strategies for building resilience, including stress inoculation training; (7) differentiate between pathologic responses in those directly exposed and among those who become anxious and impaired because they are frightened by eyewitness news coverage or secondhand reports of what happened as told by survivors or because they are afraid of subsequent attacks; (8) conduct studies addressing the risks and benefits of the mass media, the Internet, and other public education tools; (9) determine the characteristics of those most likely to seek treatment; and (10) determine whether chronic intrusion and avoidance in the absence of hyperarousal and disability are pathological.

Without a coordinated intellectual framework for the effects of psychological trauma, public policy makers cannot design effective public health responses to terrorism, and public education will result in the presentation of contradictory or incomplete information. The mental health response to the two main terrorist attacks in this country (the Oklahoma City bombing and the 9/11 attacks) was not guided by evidence-based medicine and psychology but largely by clinical lore and prior practices. Because almost no systematic research was done on the nature of those who needed or received services, it is not even clear to what extent the responses were successful or what should be done differently next time. As many opinion leaders raised the possibility that some interventions, including "hot debriefings" of those in acute distress, may have been contraindicated (McNally, 2003), it is clear that it is critical to obtain and to disseminate the proper information to mental health response teams on a large scale.

What we currently know justifies that, at a minimum, public health agencies should ensure that the natural recovery process is not impaired through any interventions provided in the initial stage. Although evidence is limited, it appears appropriate to provide educational information that supports activities that enhance safety, security, and social support and promotes the reduction of hyperarousal in the immediate phase. Often referred to as "psychological first aid," this approach does not presume that trauma survivors have a mental disorder or in fact that a mental disorder needs to be prevented; instead, it assumes that the majority of people are resilient and that meeting their immediate needs is the most appropriate step. Surveillance may be the key in the acute phase, so that people can be tracked and that, when resources are needed, they can be provided. This, coupled with a general education approach about adaptive coping strategies, can be delivered as a public health rather than a clinical intervention. Proper training might help to reduce the risk of pathological responses. The role of proper instructions in mass media tools needs to be studied.

References

American Psychiatric Association. (1994). *Diagnostic and statistical manual of mental disorders* (4th ed.). Washington, DC: Author.

Andrews, B., Brewin, C. R., Rose, S., & Kirk, M. (2000). Predicting PTSD in victims of violent crime: The role of shame, anger, and blame. *Journal of Abnormal Psychology, 109,* 69–73.

Bohus, B., & Lissak, K. (1968, July). Adrenocortical hormones and avoidance behaviour of rats. *International·Journal of Neuropharmacology, 7*(4), 301–306.

Boscarino, J. A. (1996). Posttraumatic stress disorder, exposure to combat, and lower plasma cortisol among Vietnam veterans: Findings and clinical implications. *Journal of Consulting and Clinical Psychology, 64,* 191–201.

Breslau, N., Chilcoat, H. D., Kessler, R. C., & Davis, G. (1999). Previous exposure to trauma and PTSD effects of subsequent trauma: Results from the Detroit area survey of trauma. *American Journal of Psychiatry, 156,* 902–907.

Breslau, N., Davis, G. C., Andreski, P., & Peterson, E. (1991). Traumatic events and posttraumatic stress disorder in an urban population of young adults. *Archives of General Psychiatry, 48,* 216–222.

Brewin, C. R., Andrews, B., Rose, S., & Kirk, M. (1999). Acute stress disorder and posttraumatic stress disorder in victims of violent crime. *American Journal of Psychiatry, 156,* 360–366.

Brewin, C. R., Andrews, B., & Valentine, J. D. (2000). Meta-analysis of risk factors for posttraumatic stress disorder in trauma-exposed adults. *Journal of Consulting and Clinical Psychology, 68,* 748–766.

Brunet, A., Weiss, D. S., Metzler, T. S., Best, S. R., Neylan, T. C., Rogers, C., et al. (2001). The Peritraumatic Distress Inventory: A proposed Measure of PTSD Criterion A2. *American Journal of Psychiatry, 158,* 1480–1485.

Bryant, R. A. (2003). Early predictors of posttraumatic stress disorder. *Biological Psychiatry, 53,* 789–795.

———, Guthrie, R., & Moulds, M. (2000). A prospective study of acute psychophysiological arousal, acute stress disorder, and posttraumatic stress disorder. *Journal of Abnormal Psychology, 109,* 341–344.

Bryant, R. A., & Harvey, A. G. (1998). Relationship of acute stress disorder and posttraumatic stress disorder following mild traumatic brain injury. *American Journal of Psychiatry, 155,* 625–629.

———. (2002). Delayed-onset posttraumatic stress disorder: a prospective study. *Australian and New Zealand Journal of Psychiatry, 36,* 205–209.

Bryant, R. A., & Panasetis, P. (2001). Panic symptoms during trauma and acute stress disorder. *Behaviour Research Therapy, 39,* 961–966.

Buckley, T. C., Blanchard, E. B., & Hickling, E. J. (1996). A prospective examination of delayed onset PTSD secondary to motor vehicle accidents. *Journal of Abnormal Psychology, 105,* 617–625.

Bush, G., Luu, P., & Posner, M. I. (2000). Cognitive and emotional influences in anterior cingulate cortex. *Trends in Cognitive Sciences, 4,* 215–222.

Cahill, L., Prins, B., Weber, M., & McGaugh, J. L. (1994). Adrenergic activation and memory for emotional events. *Nature, 371,* 702–704.

Charney, D. S., Deutch, A. Y., Krystal, J. H., Southwick, S. M., & Davis, M. (1993, April). Psychobiologic mechanisms of posttraumatic stress disorder. *Archives of General Psychiatry, 50*(4), 295–305.

Creamer, M., O'Donnell, M. L., & Pattison, P. (2004). The relationship between acute stress disorder and posttraumatic stress disorder in severely injured trauma survivors. *Behaviour Research and Therapy, 42,* 315–328.

Dancu, C. V., Riggs, D. S., Hearst-Ikeda, D., Shoyer, B. G., & Foa, E. B. (1996). Dissociative experiences and posttraumatic stress disorder among female victims of criminal assault and rape. *Journal of Traumatic Stress, 9,* 253–267.

Delahanty, D. L., Herberman, H. B., Craig, K. J., Hayward, M. C., Fullerton, C. S., Ursano, R. J., et al. (1997). Acute and chronic distress and posttraumatic stress disorder as a function of responsibility for serious motor vehicle accidents. *Journal of Consulting and Clinical Psychology, 65,* 560–567.

Delahanty, D. L., Riamonde, A. J., & Spoonster, E. (2000). Initial posttraumatic urinary cortisol levels predict subsequent PTSD symptoms in motor vehicle accident victims. *Biological Psychiatry, 48,* 940–947.

Difede, J., Ptacek, J. T., Roberts, J. G, Barocas, D., Rivers, W., Apfeldorf, W. J., et al. (2002). Acute stress disorder after burn injury: A predictor of posttraumatic stress disorder. *Psychosomatic Medicine, 64,* 826–834.

Dunmore, E., Clark, D. M., & Ehlers, A. (2001). A prospective investigation of the role of cognitive factors in persistent PTSD after physical and sexual assault. *Behavior Research Therapy 39,* 1063–1084.

Ehlers, A., Mayou, R. A., & Bryant, B. (1998). Psychological predictors of chronic PTSD after motor vehicle accidents. *Journal of Abnormal Psychology, 107,* 508–519.

Felmingham, K., Bryant, R. A., & Gordon, E. (in press). Tonic arousal in acute stress disorder. *Psychiatry Research.*

Galea, S., Ahern, J., Resnick, H., Kilpatrick, D., Bucuvalas, M., Gold, J., et al. (2002). Psychological sequelae of the September 11 terrorist attacks. *New England Journal of Medicine, 346,* 982–987.

Galea, S., Boscarino, J., Resnik, H., & Vlahov, D. (2003). Trends of probable post-traumatic stress disorder in New York City after the September 11 terrorist attacks. *American Journal of Epidemiology, 158,* 514–524.

Galea, S., Nandi, A., & Vlahov, D. (2005). The epidemiology of post-traumatic stress disorder after disasters. *Epidemiolic Reviews, 27*(1), 78–91.

Gilbertson, M. W., Shenton, M. E., Ciszewski, A., Kasai, K., Lasko, N. B., Orr, S. P., et al. (2002). Smaller hippocampal volume predicts pathologic vulnerability to psychological trauma. *Nature Neuroscience, 5,* 1242–1247.

Green, B. L., Lindy, J. D., Grace, M. C., Gleser, G. C., Leonard, A. C., Korol, M., et al. (1990). Buffalo Creek survivors in the second decade: Stability of stress symptoms. *American Journal of Orthopsychiatry, 60,* 43–54.

Guthrie, R. M., & Bryant, R. A. (in press). A study of auditory startle response in firefighters before and after trauma exposure. *American Journal of Psychiatry.*

————. Impaired extinction learning before trauma exposure predicts posttraumatic stress. Manuscript submitted for publication.

Harvey, A. G., & Bryant, R. A. (1998). Relationship of acute stress disorder and posttraumatic stress disorder following motor vehicle accidents. *Journal of Consulting and Clinical Psychology, 66,* 507–512.

————. (1999). A two-year prospective evaluation of the relationship between acute stress disorder and posttraumatic stress disorder. *Journal of Consulting and Clinical Psychology, 67,* 985–988.

————. (2000). A two-year prospective evaluation of the relationship between acute stress disorder and posttraumatic stress disorder following mild traumatic brain injury. *American Journal of Psychiatry, 157,* 626–628.

————. (2002). Acute stress disorder: a synthesis and critique. *Psychological Bulletin, 128,* 892–906.

Holeva, V., Tarrier, N., & Wells, A. (2001). Prevalence and predictors of acute stress disorder and PTSD following road traffic accidents: thought control strategies and social support. *Behavior Therapy, 32,* 65–83.

Holsboer, F. (2001). The corticosteroid receptor hypothesis of depression. *Neuropsychopharmacology, 23,* 477–501.

Kangas, M., Henry, J. L., & Bryant, R. A. (in press). The relationship between acute stress disorder and posttraumatic stress disorder following cancer. *Journal of Consulting and Clinical Psychology.*

Keane, T. M., Kaufman, M. L., & Kimble, M. O. (2001). Peritraumatic dissociative symptoms, acute stress disorder, and the development of posttraumatic stress disorder: Causation, correlation or epiphenomena. In L. Sánchez-Planell & C. Diez-Quevedo (Eds.), *Dissociative states* (pp. 21–43). Barcelona: Springer.

Klimesch, W., Doppelmayr, M., Russegger, H., & Pachinger, T. (1996). Theta band power in the human scalp EEG and the encoding of new information. *Neuroreport, 7,* 1235–1240.

Koopman, C., Classen, C., Cardena, E., & Spiegel, D. (1995). When disaster strikes, acute stress disorder may follow. *Journal of Traumatic Stress, 8,* 29–46.

Koopman, C., Classen, C., & Spiegel, D. (1994). Predictors of posttraumatic stress symptoms among survivors of the Oakland/Berkeley, Calif., firestorm. *American Journal of Psychiatry, 151,* 888–894.

Maes, M., Delmeire, L., Mylle, J., & Altamura, C. (2001). Risk and preventive factors of post-traumatic stress disorder (PTSD): Alcohol consumption and intoxication prior to a traumatic event diminishes the relative risk to develop PTSD in response to that trauma. *Journal of Affective Disorders, 63,* 113–121.

Maes, M., Lin, A. H., Delmeire, L., Van Gastel, A., Kenis, G., De Jongh, R., et al. (1999). Elevated serum interleukin-6 (IL-6) and IL-6 receptor concentrations in posttraumatic stress disorder following accidental man-made traumatic events. *Biological Psychiatry, 45,* 833–839.

Marmar, C., Metzler, T., Chemtob, C., Delucchi, K., Liberman, A., Fagan, J., et al. (2005, July 18–20). Impact of the World Trade Center attacks on New York City police officers: A prospective study. Annual Conference on Criminal Justice Research and Evaluation, Washington, DC.

Marmar, C., Metzler, T., & Otte, C. (2004). The peritraumatic dissociative experiences questionnaire. In J. P. Wilson & T. M. Keane (Eds.), Assessing psychological trauma and PTSD. 2d ed. New York: Guilford.

Marmar, C., Weiss, D., Metzler, T., Delucchi, K., & Best, S. (1999). Longitudinal Course and Predictors of Continuing Distress in Emergency Services Personnel. Journal of Nervous and Mental Disease, 187, 15–22.

Marmar, C., Weiss, D., Schlenger, W., Fairbank, J., Jordan, B., Kulka, R., et al. (1994). Peritraumatic dissociation and post-traumatic stress in male Vietnam theater veterans. American Journal of Psychiatry, 151, 902–907.

Marshall, G. N., & Schell, T. L. (2002). Reappraising the link between peritraumatic dissociation and PTSD symptom severity: Evidence from a longitudinal study of community violence survivors. Journal of Abnormal Psychology, 111, 626–636.

Mayou, R., Bryant, B., & Duthrie, R. (1993). Psychiatric consequences of road traffic accidents. British Medical Journal, 307, 647–651.

McFarlane, A. C. (1989). The aetiology of post-traumatic morbidity: Predisposing, precipitating, and perpetuating factors. British Journal of Psychiatry, 154, 221–228.

McNally, R. J. (2003, May 1). Psychological mechanisms in acute response to trauma. Biological Psychiatry, 53(9), 779–788. Review.

Murray, J., Ehlers, A., & Mayou, R. A. (2002). Dissociation and post-traumatic stress disorder: Two prospective studies of road traffic accident survivors. British Journal of Psychiatry, 180, 363–368.

Neylan, T. C., Lenoci, M., Maglione, M. L., Rosenlicht, N. Z., Metzler, T. J., Otte, C., et al. (2003). Delta sleep response to metyrapone in post-traumatic stress disorder. Neuropsychopharmacology, 28, 1666–1676.

Nishith, P., Mechanic, M. B., & Resick, P. A. (2000). Prior interpersonal trauma: The contribution to current PTSD symptoms in female rape victims. Journal of Abnormal Psychology, 109, 20–25.

Nixon, R., & Bryant, R. A. (2003). Peritraumatic and persistent panic attacks in acute stress disorder. Behaviour Research and Therapy, 41, 1237–1242.

———. (in press). Induced arousal and reexperiencing in acute stress disorder. Journal of Anxiety Disorders.

Orr, S. P. (1997). Psychophysiologic reactivity to trauma-related imagery in PTSD: Diagnostic and theoretical implications of recent findings. In R. Yehuda & A. C. McFarlane (Eds.), Psychobiology of posttraumatic stress disorder (pp. 114–124). New York: New York Academy of Sciences.

———, Metzger, L. J., Lasko, N. B., Macklin, M. L., Hu, F. B., Shalev, A. Y., et al. (2003). Physiologic responses to sudden, loud tones in monozygotic twins discordant for combat exposure: Association with posttraumatic stress disorder. Archives of General Psychiatry, 60, 283–288.

Otte, C., Neylan, T. C., Pole, N., Metzler, T., Best, S., Henn-Haase, C., et al. (2005). Association between childhood trauma and catecholamine response to psychological stress in police academy recruits. Biological Psychiatry, 57, 27–32.

Ozer, E. J., Best, S. R., Lipsey, T. L., & Weiss, D. S. (2003). Predictors of posttraumatic stress disorder and symptoms in adults: A meta-analysis. Psychological Bulletin, 129, 52–73.

Pacak, K., Palkovitz, M., Kopin, I. J., & Goldstein, D. S. (1995). Stress-induced norepinephrine release in the hypothalamic paraventricular nucleus and pituitary-adrenocortical and sympathoadrenal activity: In vivo microdialysis studies. Frontiers in Neuroendocrinology, 16, 89–150.

Pitman, R. K., Post-traumatic stress disorder, hormones, and memory. (1989). Biological Psychiatry, 26, 221–223.

———, Sanders, K. M., Zusman, R. M., Healy, A. R., Cheema, F., Lasko, N. B., et al. (2002). Pilot study of secondary prevention of posttraumatic stress disorder with propranolol. Biological Psychiatry, 15(51), 189–192.

Pitman, R. K., Shalev, A. Y., & Orr, S. P. (2000). Posttraumatic stress disorder: Emotion, conditioning, and memory. In M. D. Corbetta & M. S. Gazzaniga (Eds.), The new cognitive neurosciences (pp. 687–700). New York: Plenum.

Post, R. M., Weiss, S. R., & Smith, M. A. (1995). Sensitization and kindling: Implications for the evolving neural substrates of post-traumatic stress disorder. In M. J. Friedman, D. S. Charney, & A. Y. Deutch (Eds.), Neurobiological and clinical consequences of stress: From normal adaptation to posttraumatic stress disorder (pp. 203–224). Philadelphia, Lippincott-Raven.

Rausch, L. S., Shin, L. M., & Pitman, R. K. (1997). Evaluating the effects of psychological trauma using neuroimaging techniques. In R. Yehuda (Ed.), Psychological trauma: Annual review of psychiatry, Vol. 17 (pp. 67–96). Washington, DC: American Psychiatric Press.

Resnick, H. S., Yehuda, R., Foy, D. W., & Pitman, R. (1995). Effect of prior trauma on acute hormonal response to rape. *American Journal of Psychiatry, 15,* 1675–1677.

Schnyder, U., Moergeli, H., Klaghofer, R., & Buddeberg, C. (2001). Incidence and prediction of posttraumatic stress disorder symptoms in severely injured accident victims. *American Journal of Psychiatry, 158,* 594–599.

Schuff, N., Neylan, T. C., Lenoci, M. A., Du, A. T., Weiss, D. S., Marmar, C. R., et al. (2001, December 15). Decreased hippocampal N-acetylaspartate in the absence of atrophy in posttraumatic stress disorder. *Biological Psychiatry, 50*(12), 952–959.

Schuster, M. A., Stein, B. D., Jaycox, L., Collins, R. L., Marshall, G. N., Elliott, M. N., et al. (2001, November 15). A national survey of stress reactions after the September 11, 2001, terrorist attacks. *New England Journal of Medicine, 345*(20), 1507–1512.

Shalev, A. Y. (1992). Posttraumatic stress disorder among injured survivors of a terrorist attack: Predictive value of early intrusions and avoidance symptoms. *Journal of Nervous and Mental Disease, 180,* 505–509.

———, Freedman, S., Peri, T., Brandes, D., Sahar, T., Orr, S. P., et al. (1997). Predicting PTSD in trauma survivors: Prospective evaluation of self-report and clinician-administered instruments. *British Journal of Psychiatry, 170,* 558–564.

———. (1998). Prospective study of posttraumatic stress disorder and depression following trauma. *American Journal of Psychiatry, 155,* 630–637.

Shalev, A. Y., Peri, T., Brandes, D., Freedman, S., Orr, S. P., & Pitman, R. K. (2000). Auditory startle response in trauma survivors with posttraumatic stress disorder: A prospective study. *American Journal of Psychiatry, 157,* 255–261.

Shalev, A. Y., Sahar, T., Freedman, S., Peri, T., Glick, N., Brandes, D., et al. (1998). A prospective study of heart rate response following trauma and the subsequent development of posttraumatic stress disorder. *Archives of General Psychiatry, 55,* 553–559.

Shin, L. M., Whalen, P. J., Pitman, R. K., Bush, G., Macklin, M. L., Lasko, N. B., et al. (2001). An fMRI study of anterior cingulate function in posttraumatic stress disorder. *Biological Psychiatry, 50,* 932–942.

Silva, R. R., Alpert, M., Muñoz, D. M., Singh, S., Matzner, F., & Dummitt, S. (2000). Stress and vulnerability to posttraumatic stress disorder in children and adolescents. *American Journal of Psychiatry, 157,* 1229–1235.

Simeon, D., Guralnik, O., Knutelska, M., Yehuda, R., & Schmeidler, J. (2003). Basal norepinephrine in depersonalization disorder. *Psychiatry Research, 121,* 93–97.

Smith, K., & Bryant, R. A. (2000). The generality of cognitive bias in acute stress disorder. *Behaviour Research and Therapy, 38,* 709–715.

Solomon, Z., Kotler, M., Shalev, A., & Lin, R. (1989). Delayed onset PTSD among Israeli veterans of the 1982 Lebanon war. *Psychiatry, 52,* 428–436.

Southwick, S. M., Krystal, J. H., Bremner, J. D., Morgan, C. A., III, Nicolaou, A. L., Nagy, L. M., et al. (1997). Noradrenergic and serotonergic function in posttraumatic stress disorder. *Archives of General Psychiatry, 54,* 749–58.

Spiegel, D., Classen, C., & Cardena, E. (2000). New *DSM-IV* diagnosis of acute stress disorder. *American Journal of Psychiatry, 157,* 1890–1891.

Staab, J. P., Grieger, T. A., Fullerton, C. S., & Ursano, R. J. (1996). Acute stress disorder, subsequent posttraumatic stress disorder, and depression after a series of typhoons. *Anxiety, 2,* 219–225.

True, W. R., Rice, J., Eisen, S. A., Heath, A. C., Goldberg, J., Lyons, M. J., et al. (1993). A twin study of genetic and environmental contributions to liability for posttraumatic stress disorder. *Archives of General Psychiatry, 50,* 257–264.

Vaiva, G., Thomas, P., Ducrocq, F., Fontaine, M., Boss, V., Devos, P., et al. (2003). Low posttrauma GABA plasma levels as a predictive factor in the development of acute posttraumatic stress disorder. *Biological Psychiatry, 55,* 250–254.

Wakefield, J. C. (1996). *DSM-IV:* Are we making diagnostic progress? *Contemporary Psychology, 41,* 646–652.

Yehuda, R. (Ed.). (1997). *Psychological trauma: Annual review of psychiatry, Vol. 17.* Washington, DC: American Psychiatric Press.

———. (2002). Posttraumatic stress disorder. *New England Journal of Medicine, 346,* 108–114.

———, Bierer, L. M., Schmeidler, J., Aferiat, D. H, Breslau, I., & Dolan, S. (2000). Low cortisol and risk for PTSD in adult offspring of holocaust survivors. *American Journal of Psychiatry, 157,* 1252–1259.

Yehuda, R., Halligan, S. L., & Bierer, L. M. (2001). Relationship of parental trauma exposure and PTSD to PTSD, depressive and anxiety disorders in offspring. *Journal of Psychiatric Research, 35,* 261–269.

Yehuda, R., & McFarlane, A. C. (1995). Conflict between current knowledge about posttraumatic stress disorder and its original conceptual basis. *American Journal of Psychiatry, 152,* 1705–1713.

Yehuda, R., Schmeidler, J., Wainberg, M., Binder-Brynes, K., & Duvdevani, T. (1998, September). Vulnerability to posttraumatic stress disorder in adult offspring of Holocaust survivors. *American Journal of Psychiatry, 155*(9), 1163–1171.

Zangrossi, H., Jr., Viana, M. B., & Graeff, F. G. (1999). Anxiolytic effect of intra-amygdala injection of midazolam an 8-hydroxy-2-(di-n-propylamino) tetralin in the elevated T-maze. *European Journal of Pharmacology, 369,* 267–270.

Zatzick, D. F., Russo, J., Pitman, R. K., Rivara, F., Jurkovich, G., & Roy-Byrne, P. (2005). Reevaluating the association between emergency department heart rate and the development of posttraumatic stress disorder: A public health approach. *Biological Psychiatry, 57,* 91–95.

20

Older Adults and Terrorism

Lisa M. Brown
Donna Cohen
Joy R. Kohlmaier

Within 24 hours following the 9/11 terrorist attacks, animal advocates were on the scene rescuing pets, yet abandoned older and disabled people waited for up to 7 days for an ad hoc medical team to rescue them.

Nora O'Brian, Director of Partnerships,
International Longevity Center

The importance of preparing our country to counter and respond to terrorism has been paramount since the 9/11 attack on the World Trade Center, the Pentagon, and United Flight 93 in Pennsylvania. In contrast to the large body of empirical studies describing the emotional and behavioral consequences of natural and human-caused disasters, the existing literature on the psychological consequences of terrorism is small. Likewise, our knowledge about the differential impact of specific forms of terrorism (e.g., explosives; chemical, biological, radiological, or nuclear weapons), which determine how long the effects of the attack last, the number and distribution of victims, the types of first responders, quarantine and decontamination requirements, and clinical interventions, is almost nonexistent (Stein et al., 2004). Therefore, it is not surprising that studies specific to the effects of terrorist attacks on the psychological health of older adults are even more limited in scope and detail. The methods used include large-scale epidemiological studies examining age effects between older and younger adults (Boscarino, Adams, & Figley, 2004; Chen, Chung, Chen, Fang, & Chen, 2003; Schlenger et al., 2002; Silver, Holman, McIntosh, Poulin, & Gil-Rivas, 2002) and small, exploratory, qualitative investigations de-

scribing psychological reactions to the terrorist events of 2001 (Chung, 2004; Strug, Mason, & Heller, 2003). Only one study had pre-9/11 measures of depression to compare with postevent levels in older adults living in Manhattan who were participating in a research project examining the relationship between depression and vision loss (Brennan, Horowitz, & Reinhardt, 2004).

Two important reports sponsored by the Institute of Medicine (Butler, Panzer, & Goldfrank, 2003; Hooke & Rogers, 2005) give scant attention to the special vulnerabilities and needs of older populations. The 2003 report extensively reviews issues related to the prevention and treatment of emotional and behavioral consequences in children and adolescents, but it mentions older persons only three times throughout the volume, acknowledging that they have special needs. The 2005 report again mentions older adults only four times, recognizing their vulnerability due to social isolation and the special requirements for emergency responses to terrorism.

The available literature on the aftermath of terrorist attacks indicates that the ratio of people who develop serious adverse psychological effects relative to those who sustain illness or physical injuries ranges from 4–5:1. Therefore, it is imperative that effective mental health interventions be developed that can readily be implemented by health care professionals and trained volunteers from relief organizations to help restore psychological functioning. Mental health intervention may be particularly important for vulnerable populations of older adults, including, but not limited to, those who are more socially isolated, frail, physical disabled, and cognitively impaired and have a history of exposure to an extreme and prolonged traumatic stressor.

This chapter reviews empirical research and theoretical perspectives regarding psychological consequences of terrorist events on different populations of older adults. It also examines the effects of natural disasters on long-term health care systems serving vulnerable older populations. Additionally, we identify the challenges of responding to the needs of older people and their families in the community, describe strategies to assess the vulnerabilities and mental health risks of various older populations, and provide an overview of interventions that can be used at the personal, family, community, and health care system level.

The Effects of Natural and Human-Made Disasters on Older Adults

Natural and human-made disasters share characteristics with terrorist attacks. Occurring with unexpected swiftness and overwhelming force, they adversely affect ordinary people who happen to be in the wrong place at the wrong time. In contrast to the experience of individual trauma (e.g., accidents or criminal acts), which affect one person and intimate family members, the occurrence and aftermath of a terrorist attack adversely affect social structures and dynamics, which in turn threaten the existence and functioning of communities, cities, and larger geographic areas (Butler, et al., 2003; Fullerton, Ursano, Norwood, & Holloway, 2003). When a large-scale traumatic event occurs, every aspect of community life is disrupted, causing a breach in an individual's emotional, social, physical, and environmental support system. Moreover, homes, worksites, health care facilities across the continuum of care, schools and other educational institutions, as well as law enforcement, fire fighting, and other emergency operations may have been destroyed. Large numbers of people

may be injured, ill, or dead. Lives are irrevocably altered. Mass catastrophes shatter core personal assumptions of individual control, safety, and the predictability of life (Parkes, 2002).

The immediate deadly consequences of terrorism cause a series of powerful emotional reactions in adults of all ages: feelings of shock, horror, and disbelief; concerns that other attacks will occur; intense personal emotions (e.g., anxiety, apprehension, fear, anger); and the need to find and help family, pets, neighbors, and friends. Whereas most healthy older persons will be able to react and cope with the immediate emergencies, there are vulnerable older adult populations who are at high risk for immediate, short-term, and long-term negative consequences. These include but are not limited to those who are socially isolated, frail, chronically ill, and cognitively impaired and have a history of exposure to an extreme and prolonged traumatic stressor (e.g., refugees from terrorist regimes, holocaust survivors).

Although distinctions can be drawn between intentional acts of terrorism, human-caused disasters, and natural disasters, there are some commonalities in psychological consequences, social disruption, and destruction of personal and community property (Fullerton et al., 2003; Butler, et al., 2003). However, ample research indicates that psychological symptom profiles in the population following human-made disasters are different from those after natural disasters (Baum, Fleming, & Singer, 1982; Frederick, 1987; Green, 1990; Norris, Byrne, Diaz, & Kaniasty, 2002; Phifer & Norris, 1989). Norris, Byrne, Díaz, and Kaniasty (2001) have reported that the presence of at least two of the following four conditions increased the negative mental health consequences of an event: the occurrence of a human-made disaster, widespread damage to property and community, economic hardship, and high prevalence of threat to life, injury, and loss of life. In general, disasters caused by malicious human intent are more disturbing than other human-made and natural disasters (Beaton & Murphy, 2002; North et al., 1999; Norris et al., 2001). In these circumstances there may be a greater need for delivery of mental health services to avoid lasting, severe, and pervasive psychological disturbances. Table 20.1 presents the similarities and differences among natural and human-made disasters at each stage (i.e., pre-, during, and postevent) in more detail.

Table 20.1. Differences and similarities between human-made intentional, human-made unintentional, and natural disasters

Timing and Event Characteristics	Human-Made Intentional Act	Human-Made Unintentional	Natural Disaster	Pandemic Flu
Pre-Event				
Advance Warning	No	Rarely	Yes—hurricanes Oftentimes—tornadoes No—earthquakes No—mudslides/avalanche Sometimes—fire Sometimes—tsunami	Likely—Ongoing monitoring by public health officials and the World Health Organization to detect human infection
Predictability	No	No	Seasonal activity: hurricanes, tornadoes, fire, mudslides/avalanche No—earthquakes No—tsunami	Some—Ongoing monitoring by public health officials and the World Health Organization to detect infection
Psychological preparedness of population	No	No	Sometimes; prior exposure to event resilence/inoculation training	No
High perceived threat to life prior to event	Yes	No	Sometimes—variable	Yes
Uncertainty if exposure to toxin occurred	Yes	Sometimes	No	Uncertainty if infected
Preventability of event	Sometimes—with sufficient monitoring and intervention	Sometimes—with sufficient monitoring and training	Loss of life and psychological distress can be reduced with advanced warning	Limited—existing treatments may not work as influenza viruses have the ability to change
Information stress from media coverage	Sometimes—elevated warning	No	Yes—only in affected area	Yes

Event

Local fear	Yes	Yes	Yes	Yes
National Fear	Yes	Yes	No	Yes
Information stress from media coverage	Yes—only in affected area	Yes—only in affected area	Yes—only in affected area	Yes
Controllability	No	No	No	Limited—existing treatments may not work as influenza viruses have the ability to change
Loss of life	Yes	Sometimes	Likely	Yes
Physical injury or harm	Yes	Sometimes	Likely	Yes
Exposure to dead	Yes	Sometimes	Sometimes	Likely
Post-Event				
Information stress from media coverage	Yes	Yes—more so in affected area	Yes—only in affected area	Yes
Behavioral disturbance	Yes	Yes—more so in affected area	Yes—only in affected area	Yes
Psychological distress/illness	Yes	Yes—more so in affected area	Yes—only in affected area	Yes
Disruption of social networks	Yes—more so in affected area	Yes—only in affected area	Yes—only in affected area	Yes
Disruption of community	Yes—more so in affected area	Yes—only in affected area	Yes—only in affected area	Yes
Altered sense of safety	Yes	Yes	Yes	Yes
Healthcare systems overwhelmed	Yes—more so in affected area	Yes	Sometimes	Yes
Loss of faith in institutions	Likely	Likely	Sometimes	Likely
National bereavement	Yes	Yes	Sometimes	Yes
Loss of property	Sometimes	Sometimes	Likely	No

Green (1990) described several factors that mediate negative psychological outcomes of disasters. People who report significantly more concerns about being at risk for death or injury and those who have a closer temporal or physical proximity to the event are at higher risk for adverse psychological functioning. Personal injury and physical harm, exposure to dead and mutilated bodies, and the violent, sudden death of family, friends, and coworkers are potent mediators of acute and long-term sequelae of traumatic stress. Norris (2001), in a comprehensive review of the literature, has also found a number of studies that reported a proximity dose-relationship with mental health status. However, two additional studies that have examined mental health functioning following the events of 9/11 and the Florida hurricanes found that the nature of the recovery phase, more so than actual proximity to the event, was associated with adverse mental health consequences (Brown, Schinka, Borenstein, & Mortimer, 2005; Silver, Poulin, et al., 2004). While the type and severity of catastrophic disasters influence psychological outcomes, the premorbid existence of psychiatric symptoms or emotional distress is the best overall predictor of long-term maladaptive psychological functioning (Kessler et al., 1999; Knight, Gatz, Heller, & Bengston, 2000; Phifer & Norris, 1989).

Although an extensive body of research suggests that older adults typically fare better in terms of emotional and psychological functioning when compared to younger adults, they still experience decrements in mental health in the aftermath of a disaster (Bolin & Klenow, 1983). However, for the majority of older adults, most untreated psychological distress that occurs shortly after a disaster will abate in time (Blanchard et al., 1995; Krause, 1987; Raphael, 2003). For those who require more than psychological first aid following a terrorist event, special efforts may be required to overcome personal and system barriers to treatment. For example, some older adults in the community may be reluctant to admit they feel overwhelmed, confused, or distressed in the aftermath of a disaster because they fear that such an admission may lead to loss of freedom or institutionalization in a long-term care facility. Others may refuse to ask for help because of the stigma associated with mental health treatment. Some may believe that only seriously mentally ill people receive treatment from mental health clinicians, fear that their reaction to the event is a sign that they are becoming demented, or perceive acceptance of psychological treatment as a sign of personal weakness. Finally, some may resist asking for help because they suppose that others have fared far worse than they and therefore are less willing to actively pursue or accept available mental health intervention. A step in overcoming a number of these barriers includes educating those at risk for adverse psychological outcomes about typical reactions to disaster and providing information about the nature of mental health intervention.

Along with directing survivors to available services such as water, food, shelter, and medical care, triage for mental health problems should be included in the hierarchy of basic disaster response. Older adults may be more willing to be assessed for potential mental health problems if the screening is conducted with a medial evaluation or provided with other basic necessities. Early mental health assessments should effectively screen those at greater risk for developing acute stress disorder, PTSD, depression, and complicated bereavement. Depending on timing, situation, and circumstances, it may be appropriate for some individuals to receive group treatment. A more comprehensive discussion of treatment issues specific to older adults is presented later in this chapter. Nevertheless, even without the onset of serious psychological impairment, many older adults will require assistance in preparing, responding, and recovering from such events.

Theoretical Frameworks: Psychological Responses to Disasters and Mass Violence in Older Populations

Early work suggested that disasters would have a disproportionate effect on older adults, who would be more vulnerable to psychological distress than younger adults. Friedsam (1960, 1961) concluded from his review of the disaster literature that older adults were least likely to receive warning about impending disasters, more reluctant to evacuate, more disturbed by disruption in daily life, and more likely to become physical casualties, thus experiencing a greater sense of deprivation in response to losses. In another review of the literature, Kilijanek & Drabek (1979) reported that older disaster victims were at greater risk for incurring debt, economic losses, physical injury, and disrupted employment relative to younger adults. However, this and a later review of the literature did not find sufficient support for the relative deprivation hypothesis (Fields, 1996; Kilijanek & Drabek, 1979). Since then, several theories have attempted to explain the response of older adults to traumatic events. We briefly describe a number of theories that have appeared in the literature.

Age is one of many predisaster, within-disaster, and postdisaster risk factors that mediate the severity of adverse consequences (Norris et al., 2002). Analyses of the relationship of age and mass violence have revealed that school-aged children are the most vulnerable to severe mental health problems throughout the world (Norris et al., 2002). In all of the published U.S. studies, middle-aged people (40–60 years) sustained the most adverse effects, whereas individuals older than age 60 were more resilient. Cross-cultural research has suggested that age effects are mediated by sociopolitical, economic, historical, and cohort effects (Norris et al., 2002). In the aftermath of the 1995 bombing of the Oklahoma City federal building, posttraumatic stress disorder increased with age in Asian and Middle Eastern immigrants (Trautman et al., 2002). At least one study of Bosnian refugees has shown that increased mortality rates in older persons were associated with mass violence (Mollica et al., 1990).

Many theoretical frameworks, presented as theories, models, or hypotheses, are useful in organizing the results of empirical studies that investigate the relationship of advanced age to adaptive versus maladaptive emotional and behavioral outcomes: resilience and coping theories, inoculation theory, burden theory, the maturational hypothesis, residual stress vulnerability, conservation of resources, and social deterioration models.

Resilience and Coping

A significant body of research indicates that age is a protective factor and that older adults tend to be more resilient than younger adults in responding to stressful events, including disasters and mass violence (Huerta & Horton, 1978; Norris, Byrne, Díaz, & Kaniasty, 2002). Resilience is defined as the ability to adapt quickly or recover from illness, difficult life experiences, misfortune, and traumatic events (Rutter, 1987). Older adults have an extensive and varied accumulation of life experiences that affect short- and long-term vulnerability or resilience following exposure to traumas. They may adapt to certain life stressors with relative ease yet experience difficulty responding to and recovering from other types of traumatic events. Although older adults may endure a more severe exposure to disaster, have poorer health, and have fewer social and economic resources, they have a lifetime of learning how to cope with stressful events as well as fewer currently unresolved stressful experiences, both of which promote adaptation to disasters (Phifer, 1990).

For older Americans, a lifetime of experience also provides many opportunities to make comparisons between current and previous stressors and evaluate the effectiveness of different coping strategies. Cognitive strategies facilitate the ability to maintain a perspective on goals and outcomes and manage negative emotions to prevent overreaction to stressful situations. Active coping strategies are frequently used to avoid negative situations and maladaptive interactions under times of extreme stress (Folkman, Lazarus, Dunkel-Schetter, DeLongis, & Gruen, 1986; Janoff-Bulman, 1992). Problem-focused coping focuses on altering the person-environment transaction or managing the source of stress, in contrast to emotion-focused coping centering on the regulation of emotional responses elicited by the situation (Folkman & Lazarus, 1980).

In a study of the frequency and impact of potentially traumatic events, Norris (1992) reported not only that older adults were more resilient but also that younger adults had the highest rates of PTSD in response to 9 of 10 potentially traumatic events. Many older adults have learned that they can overcome difficult or challenging life events, adapt to adversity, and return to prior levels of psychological functioning. In describing the resilience of the old-old (i.e., those who are 75–84), Phifer (1990) noted several factors that could account for this age group's ability to overcome adversity in the aftermath of a natural disaster. The nature and severity of the traumatic event, personal history and experiences, and psychological characteristics affect individuals' psychological outcomes (King, King, Fairbank, Keane, & Adams, 1998).

Maturation Hypothesis

The maturation hypothesis is based on the premise that psychological maturation is protective (i.e., more mature coping styles associated with advancing age protect older adults against the harmful effects of stressors). Older adults are thought to be less emotionally reactive to stressful events than younger adults, and the maturation hypothesis helps to explain the lower levels of depressed mood in older adults following a traumatic event. The maturation theory was not supported by a study that examined the presence of depressed mood in adults before and after the 1994 Northridge earthquake (Knight et al., 2000). Although Knight and colleagues found support for the inoculation theory, age did not moderate the relationship between rumination and damage exposure.

Inoculation Theory

The main premise of the inoculation hypothesis is that prior experience with stressful circumstances, including disasters, inoculates people against intense emotional reactions to future disaster-related stressors. Therefore, the greater the exposure to disasters, the higher the level of protection to future disasters (Knight et al., 2000). Since older persons have had a lifetime of opportunities for stressful experiences, coping capacities should increase with advancing age.

Support for the age relationship to an inoculation effect is mixed. Knight et al. (2000) found partial support for this hypothesis when they reported that prior earthquake experience was associated with lower levels of postearthquake depression in both young and old adults. Although the results of a study of older adults following the 1997 Red River flood showed no changes in psychological functioning (Ferraro, 2003), the authors interpreted the findings to reflect the constant exposure of residents to many earlier floods in that location. Phifer and Norris (1989) reported that older adults' reactions to the 1984 Kentucky flood were influenced by previous experience with a flood in 1981 and that those with past exposure showed better psychological adaptation than their inexperienced counterparts.

Although the inoculation hypothesis has received substantial support, Thompson, Norris, and Hanacek (1993) noted that it failed to explain differences between middle-aged and older adults. The authors proposed that disaster impact and age were not characterized by an inverse linear relationship (that is, young adults are affected the most, and older adults the least). Instead, a curvilinear relationship applies, with middle-aged adults being affected the most by disasters, due to their responsibilities to children, parents, and employers.

Burden Theory

The Burden theory posits that middle-aged adults have multiple roles and responsibilities as parents, caregivers, and employees and therefore feel more burden relative to younger and older persons with fewer responsibilities. The results of several studies have found that middle-aged adults showed more distress in response to disasters than younger or older adults (Phifer, 1990; Verger et al., 2004). Verger and associates (2004) have reported that the risk of PTSD following the 1995–1996 bombings in France was significantly higher among people aged 35–54 compared to younger and older adults. Phifer (1990) reported that, following the 1984 Kentucky flood, those aged 55–64 were at greatest risk of experiencing psychological symptoms compared to those age 65–74 and 75 years and older.

Residual Stress Vulnerability

Although older adults tend to be resilient in the face of life challenges, including disasters, some older adults may be particularly vulnerable (e.g., Holocaust survivors, prisoners of war, persons exposed to interpersonal violence, persons abused as a child or adult) (Bremner et al., 1992; Breslau et al., 1998; Eaton, Sigal, & Weinfeld, 1982; Green et al., 2000; Nishith, Mechanic, & Resnick, 2000; Yehuda et al., 1995). Exposure to extreme, prolonged stress may result in permanent developmental effects that increase vulnerability to future traumatic events throughout the lifespan. Dougall and colleagues (2000) hypothesized that trauma history sensitizes people to new stressors, thus potentiating its effect.

Several studies of survivors of the Nazi Holocaust have helped elucidate the vulnerabilities of older persons. Yehuda and colleagues (1995) reported that the presence and severity of PTSD symptoms were related to many factors, including the immediate trauma, as well as current and lifetime stressors. In a similar study, Holocaust survivors were more likely to have mild psychiatric symptoms than controls, and the levels of psychiatric symptoms were greatly amplified in those survivors who had recently perceived an increase in anti-Semitism in the community (Eaton, Sigal & Weinfeld, 1982). Port, Engdahl, Frazier, and Eberly (2002) have reported an increase in PTSD symptoms among older men who had been prisoners of war. These authors emphasized the importance of assessing for additional late-life stressors, including decreased social support, negative health changes, and lower death acceptance, which may impact trauma-related symptomatology.

Conservation of Resources

According to the conservation of resources (COR) theory, psychological stress results when there is a threat to or an actual loss of existing resources (Hobfoll, 1989; Hobfoll, Dunahoo, & Monnier, 1995). Resources include physical possessions, social roles, personal resources, and financial resources. The attendant losses from disasters tend to be most closely related to survival, and they are usually profound and numerous. This theory suggests that the use of psychological interventions immediately after a traumatic event is not especially helpful. The focus should be on more pressing needs, such as the rapid replacement of necessary resources (e.g., food, water, shelter) (Hobfoll et al., 1995). When basic needs are met, older adult disaster survivors have the potential for developing a new sense of self-efficacy and mastery or learning new coping skills as they recover from a disaster.

Social Deterioration Model

Acts of terrorism and disasters result in social deterioration and pose a threat to the existing social order. Following a disaster, personal loss may result in an intense but short-term effect on older adults' depressive symptomatology, but destruction of communities and loss of social support networks produces long-term psychological distress (Kaniasty & Norris, 1993). This is most likely because older adults are in need of continued support from family, personal social networks, and the community at large after a cataclysmic event and because interruption and breakdown in these systems create distress. In particular, the perception of support from nonrelatives was found to mediate the impact of disaster stress on depression. For older adults, deeper and broader social support networks play a significant role in ameliorating the negative impact of traumatic life events (Tyler & Hoyt, 2000; Watanabe, Okumura, Chiu, & Wakai, 2004).

The Role of Social Support Networks

Most social networks are composed of family, close friends, neighbors, and community associates (Cantor, 1979). As it is not uncommon for families to provide 70%–80% of in-home care for older adults with chronic health conditions, informal caregivers, such as family, neighbors, and friends, are often first on the scene following a disaster and can be instrumental in securing shelter, medical care, food, and water and providing support. For older adults, these social connections typically play a role in buffering or mitigating the negative effects of normal life stressors. During times of crisis, social support systems are critical to the psychological well-being of older adults. Several studies have found that anticipated or perceived support, the belief that significant others care and will provide assistance, if required, is predictive of better psychological outcomes following a disaster than the receipt of actual assistance (Cook & Bickman, 1990; Krause, 2001). Additionally, the degree of social embeddedness, that is the size, closeness, and activeness of the older adult's social network, is also directly related to mental health functioning. These socially protective resources are particularly vulnerable to disruption and decline following a disaster. Significant deterioration of the social support system is likely to result in adverse short- and long-term psychological consequences (Kaniasty & Norris, 1993).

To offset potential mental health problems, provisions for preparing for, responding to, and recovering from a disaster need to be adequate. Social support can come from various sources, but not every type of support may be available or appropriate (Watanabe et al., 2004). It is not unusual for dysfunctional family interactions to worsen during stressful circumstances. Although family members are more likely than friends to provide instrumental support to older adults, in some instances family relational behaviors may have a negative impact on perceived social support (Wright and Query, 2004). Sometimes members of an older adult's family may feel obliged to assume a supportive role because of relational ties as opposed to a true desire to provide care. Friendships, because they tend to be formed voluntarily, are not as affected by a sense of familial obligation (Wright and Query, 2004). Friends and close neighbors are often a source of assistance to older adults who need help in accomplishing disaster-related tasks (Crohan & Antonucci, 1989).

Although social support is often mobilized when an older person's life or health is threatened after a natural disaster, assistance is less available when property is damaged or destroyed, electricity or phone communication is lost, or daily routines are disrupted (Kaniasty and Norris, 1993). It is probable that many members of an older adult's social support network will also be victims of the same disaster. Social network members may be dead, have relocated, or be unable to assist because their immediate needs exceed their current resources. Compounding the situation, disruption and destruction of community services diminishes the availability of other formal resources that provide social support, such as senior center activities and Meals on Wheels. As a result, the need for support and services for all of the disaster survivors may surpass the availability of existing resources, leaving traditional networks unable to provide much-needed support to older adults.

Even though social networks may be depleted, crisis intervention workers can provide temporary support and assistance in rebuilding these systems. Steps to reestablish and strengthen the support networks include educating family members about the range of normal psychological reactions to disaster, such as irritability, stress, and fatigue. Because survivors accurately recognize the grave danger they were exposed to during the disaster, mild to moderate stress reactions during the postevent phase are not uncommon. If appropriate, family members should be encouraged to talk about their feelings and experiences. Contact with others who have undergone the same trauma can buffer the negative psychological effects of disaster

(Boscarino, 1995). Setting realistic expectations about the quantity or quality of family support provided in the aftermath of a disaster may decrease the potential for interpersonal conflict and minimize negative interactions. To the extent possible, resuming normal daily activities and maintaining social connectedness help preserve social embeddedness and foster recovery.

The Impact of Disasters and Terrorism on Older Adults

In the late summer and early fall of 2004, four major hurricanes devastated Florida in a period of 44 days, resulting in the deaths of 117 people and more than $60 billion in damages. Florida experienced more adverse effects from this series of hurricanes than any other state had sustained from natural disasters in the same period of time. The consequences of the hurricanes exceeded the state's capabilities and resources because of insufficient time for recovery between storms and because all 67 counties were severely impacted. Many areas faced extensive and continued loss of electrical power, lack of food, and potable water. Homes, hospitals, nursing homes, hotels, businesses, and airports were severely damaged from wind, flooding, and heavy rains. Indeed, entire communities throughout the state were devastated. Voluntary and mandatory evacuation forced thousands of people to evacuate several times, leaving their homes and communities for extended periods to live with family and friends and in hotels.

Systems that provide care and services to older adults were significantly strained during this 6-week period. Among the many challenges were difficulties in securing transportation to evacuate older adults from areas that lay in the path of the hurricanes and learning that buildings designated to serve as shelters were severely damaged and unusable. The residents of many nursing homes and assisted-living residents had to be evacuated many times during the 6 weeks, and patients in damaged hospitals had to be triaged and relocated to other counties. Locating and assisting older residents who were living at home (many in trailer parks) was complicated. In the immediate aftermath, these services included finding people, locating sufficient temporary housing for them, recovering pets, identifying and treating medical problems, getting medications, providing food and water, protecting against the natural elements (e.g., heat, high humidity, and hornets that were released from overturned trees), and assisting people with cleaning up and getting insurance payments, aid from the Federal Emergency Management Agency (FEMA), and other assistance.

In the months to come, it became apparent that recovery from these four hurricanes was to be measured in months and years, not days and weeks. It also became painfully clear that state as well as city and county disaster assistance plans were not adequately developed to deal with the multiple direct hits throughout Florida or to deal with the special needs of vulnerable older populations. Numerous meetings and conferences were held by state authorities, local government and nonprofit agencies, and long-term care providers to attempt to handle this challenge. Existing disaster preparation guidelines were reviewed, and the preparation and response capabilities of older adults and care providers to deal with prolonged disruption were evaluated.

Similar meetings were also held by various agencies in New York City shortly after the events of 9/11, resulting in a report that described shortcomings in the existing emergency response system and presented a disaster response plan to meet the needs of older New York City residents more effectively (O'Brien, 2003). Reviews of the proceedings from the meetings held in Florida and New York reveal two conclusions: (1) Older adults in the community, frail and homebound persons, and older adults living in long-term care facilities often had distinctively different needs, and (2) current emergency response plans did not adequately address those differences. The special disaster considerations identified in long-term care or home health environments included but were not limited to the level of care and assistance needed by patients or residents, the resources and equipment required to provide care, and the ability of patients and residents to assist themselves or others during a disaster. Because these environments provide specialized care, they, in turn, require unique emergency preparedness plans.

Older Adults in the Community

Problems encountered in providing emergency assistance to older New York City residents subsequent to 9/11 included a lack of appropriate emergency management services, inadequate city-wide coordinated community services, the absence of a system to identify and locate older adults, and the lack of mechanisms to convey pertinent information before and after emergencies. Emergency organizations such as FEMA and the American Red Cross were not prepared to assist older and disabled people living near Ground Zero. For 7 days or more after the attacks, older and disabled people were still unidentified and neglected in the surrounding residential buildings (O'Brien, 2003, p. 2).

In contrast to younger adults, older adults are less likely to complain, ask for support, and receive services or resources following a disaster (Fields, 1996). Not surprisingly, after the events of 9/11 and the hurricanes, older adults who were not affiliated with a community service agency or registered with the county for special needs shelters were at risk for not receiving services from emergency providers. Many resisted preenrolling in programs designed to identify vulnerable adults, fearing they might be forced to move from their home to a long-term care facility. However, with each passing hurricane, more people signed registries identifying themselves as requiring the services of a special needs shelter because they increasingly recognized the benefit (Ott, 2005).

Ideally, older adults in the community should have at least one person in their social support network who will be willing and able to assist them during or after a terrorist event. For predictable events such as hurricane or tornado season, many older adults will appreciate assistance with purchasing emergency supplies (food, water, medication), preparing their home for the event (tarps, window protection, weather radio), registering with the county for housing at a special needs shelter, identifying evacuation routes and securing transportation, if needed, and cleaning up, if the event occurs. The list of recommended items for an adequately stocked disaster supply kit is extensive. (Items recommended for a standard emergency supply kit can be found at http://www.ready.gov/america/get_a_kit.html.)

To facilitate contact with members of the social support network and to secure medical treatment if needed, older adults should develop a list that provides contact and background information before a disaster occurs. At a minimum this list should include personal contacts (relatives, friends, and neighbors), health care providers (physician, pharmacist, and mental health clinician), medical conditions, disabilities, medications, treatments (e.g., dialysis, oxygen), allergies, and insurance information (health, home, car). Depending on the situation, duplicate copies of this list might be kept by trusted family members or friends. A free form to create emergency reference cards is available at http://www.ready.gov. Some individuals with cognitive impairment, such as Alzheimer's disease, may have registered with the Safe Return program, wear an identification bracelet (similar to a medic alert bracelet), or carry an identification card that notes their memory loss. In times of disaster, detailed contact and medical information should be attached to those who may not be able to communicate because of memory impairment or other condition, such as speech or hearing loss.

Many older adults, especially those age 85 and older, have chronic physical illnesses and disabilities that affect their ability to prepare for a disaster (Davis, 2004; Gignac, Cott, & Badley, 2003). Approximately one-fifth of the U.S. population has one or more disability (Davis, 2004). Chronically ill or disabled people of all ages may require help with emergency preparedness and assistance during and after a disaster (Orr & Pitman, 1999). Davis (2004) has reported that 61% of those with disabilities did not have a plan to evacuate from their home quickly and safely, and 58% admitted they did not know who to contact in an emergency. People with service dogs may find that their animal is hurt or too frightened to work immediately following a disaster. Furthermore, it may be difficult to reach a veterinarian or purchase pet food. A disaster-planning kit for service animals should be prepared and include collar, harness, identification tags, vaccination records, medications, and animal food.

Older adults who require assistance may be confused about whom to call for aid and unsure about which organizations are available to provide help. Material providing information and telephone numbers, describing how to prepare for a disaster, and detailing steps to take in the event of a disaster should be developed and widely disseminated by government and nonprofit agencies, the media, and other community-based organizations such as churches and synagogues. Emergency directives should be available as print material since more than 29% of the older population

(approximately 11 million) are hard of hearing or deaf (Holt & Hotto, 1994). Backup communication systems need to be developed to disseminate emergency information to the entire population following a disaster. Communication systems were severely impacted by the destruction of the World Trade Towers. Cell phones, telephones, email, television, and radio service was disrupted throughout the city (O'Brien, 2003). Similarly, cell phone and telephone service was interrupted in many communities that were hit by the hurricanes.

Before a disaster occurs, emergency contact numbers such as 911, the police department, fire station, hospital, as well as family and close friends, should be programmed into all phones. A communications plan that utilizes family and friends should be in place so that contact can be made with a person outside the area, as well as with local family, friends, and neighbors. Following a disaster, a caller is more likely to connect with a long-distance number outside the affected area than with a local phone number. Additionally, older adults should learn how to forward their home number to their cell phone in the event of an evacuation.

In the aftermath of a human-made or natural disaster, survivors may experience a sense of unreality and dissociation, although the event is over and the area is calm. However, older adults are not in a position to benefit from psychological interventions in the period immediately succeeding a disaster since most will have legitimate worries about meeting basic needs. The ability of older adults to adjust and cope after a disaster is mitigated by their capacity to access tangible support. Obtaining water, food, and a safe place to stay are the initial concerns following a traumatic event: "Physical care is psychological care, and this is the prime and essential function of relief organizations" (Kinston & Rosser, 1974, p. 450).

However, some older adults may be reluctant to accept assistance from government agencies, or they may find the task of completing the necessary paperwork daunting. Some may be more willing to receive assistance from the Salvation Army, Red Cross, or church groups than from government agencies. Penner (2003) has recommended that mental health crisis workers be knowledgeable about existing service providers and provide older adults with assistance in identifying organizations that can help with disaster response and recovery. A useful reference for mental health providers is a comprehensive list of websites that provide information and resources for older adults who have been exposed to terrorism (Cohen & Brown, 2004).

After the Florida hurricanes, stores that supplied medication, disposables to manage diabetes, and incontinence supplies were damaged or destroyed. The results of a study conducted shortly after the first of the four destructive hurricanes, Hurricane Charley, indicated that medical care was disrupted because of damaged or destroyed medical facilities, which resulted in the worsening of medical conditions in about one-third of the survey respondents (Little et al., 2004). Since older adults may be forced to seek medical treatment, supplies, and medication outside the community, programs need to be in place to coordinate services among agencies that provide care, identify community residents who might be in need of such services, and assist with transportation needs.

Homebound Older Adults

In an ideal world, home health aides would continue to provide daily care during disaster evacuations and accompany frail older adults to temporary or long-term shelters. However, the probability of service interruptions to the homebound is high, and during the 2004 Florida hurricane season, there was a gap between what should have happened and what actually took place. A total of 29 home health agencies were damaged or destroyed during the hurricanes (Gregory, 2004), and many homebound older adults found themselves alone at special needs shelters because their home health aide was dealing with personal or family needs (Ott, 2005). A survey of New York City public health nurses who were attending an emergency preparedness program revealed that 90% of the attendees reported at least one barrier (e.g., family responsibilities, transportation problems, personal health issues) to their ability to report to duty in the event of an emergency (Qureshi, Merrill, Gershon, & Calero-Breckheimer, 2002).

Other obstacles in providing continued care to this population were evident after 9/11:

> Service personnel lacked access to older and frail residents living in the "frozen areas." Essential services, such as meals for the homebound and home health care, were not delivered because staff had no official authorization to carry out

responsibilities. Emergency workers believed the buildings had all been evacuated, but disabled people who were unable to leave their apartments were left behind with no electricity (and therefore no television, radio, lights, elevators, refrigerators, etc.), no running water, and no information about what was happening and what they should do. Home health aides were unable to check on whether or not their patients had been rescued. (O'Brien, 2003, p. 2)

In reviewing the events that followed the 2004 hurricanes, people raised concerns about how some communities had triaged frail, older persons and moved them from shelter to shelter, creating relocation anxiety in those who were already highly stressed from the disaster (Ott, 2005). The literature on the relocation of older adults includes a number of reports that describe the negative effects on mental and physical health and social networks (Raid & Norris, 1996; Sanders, Bowie, & Bowie, 2003). Relocated people were found to be more distressed than other survivors of the disaster (Bland et al., 1997; Gleser, Green, & Winget, 1981). For vulnerable older adults who were sheltered without home health aids, lack of physical mobility, confinement to a wheelchair, and vision impairment further compounded disaster-related stresses.

Other problems may arise during the recovery phase of a disaster or terrorist event. Without assistance, vulnerable homebound adults may not have the ability to access public or private transportation. Lack of transportation and physical impairments that restrict mobility may limit their opportunities to seek help from disaster assistance centers and replenish food and water. Furthermore, people who are poorly educated, have limited financial resources, and have weak social networks are unlikely to use community services (Rosenzweig, 1975). Outreach programs will need to locate older adults who may not have the knowledge needed to access services or the physical ability to leave their homes and stand in line for assistance.

Institutionalized Older Adults

The ability of Florida's long-term care providers to prepare for, respond to, and recover from disasters or acts of terrorism is critical since 18% of the population is 65 years of age and older and nursing homes and assisted-living facilities care for

70,000–77,000 residents, respectively. Facilities that were damaged or destroyed during the 2004 hurricanes included 114 of the 276 hospitals, 60 of the 699 nursing homes, and 85 of the 2,287 assisted-living facilities (Gregory, 2004). Many of these institutions were closed for an extended period of time, forcing residents to receive shelter outside their community.

During the hurricanes, the difference in the level of assistance provided to those in nursing homes compared to those in assisted-living facilities was pronounced. State regulations for nursing homes specify staff duties and responsibilities, evacuation procedures, and required resource reserves, whereas assisted-living facilities are not under the same obligation to assist residents with evacuation and care during the storms. Several special needs shelters were overwhelmed when assisted-living facilities dropped off residents with dementia or communication impairments, without accompanying staff to provide care or identification to relocate residents after the storms (Ott, 2005). A number of older adults with cognitive impairment were briefly lost in the system because they were unable to describe where they had been living before they arrived at the shelter.

Emergency relocation of people with significant cognitive impairment presents a unique set of challenges. Older adults with cognitive impairment are more likely to require institutional care and are especially vulnerable in disaster situations. Approximately 4 million Americans are afflicted with Alzheimer's disease, and this number is expected to exceed 16 million by the year 2050. Most people survive an average of 8–10 years after being diagnosed with Alzheimer's disease, and many will spend 5 of those years living in a skilled nursing facility (Hendrie, 1998). After the 2004 hurricanes, it was suggested that shelters be designated to provide the level of care required for this at-risk population. Although nursing homes with transfer agreements were able to move patients with Alzheimer's disease to other facilities, the wander guard system used by the home facility was not always compatible with the system used by the host facility. This presented a problem for staff, already short in numbers, who had to monitor residents closely to prevent elopement during and after the storm.

Since many long-term care staff were unable to report to work because of family or personal needs, staff shortages and extended work hours further strained the system. Cross-training the staff to provide services outside their daily routines before the hurricanes was helpful. For example, nurses and physical therapists who had obtained a license to drive buses were able to transport residents and staff from the facility to the shelter.

Several facilities that were forced to evacuate at night because of heat, heavy traffic, and changing weather conditions required more time to move their residents. One long-term care facility reported that rousing sleeping residents, who had taken hypnotics or psychotropic medications with sedative effects, greatly slowed their evacuation during the first hurricane. However, staff were better prepared during the second hurricane strike and moved residents who received sleep medication to locations that were close to emergency exits.

Not all counties were equally prepared to respond to the hurricane. A survey of 670 nursing homes and 500 assisted-living providers was conducted shortly after the 2004 Florida hurricane season to understand their experiences in preparing for, responding to, and recovering from this series of disasters (Hyer, Brown, Polivka-West, & Bond, 2005). Difficulties with evacuation and transportation, as well as extended power loss, were among the major problems the long-term care facilities encountered. The buildings that housed the emergency operating centers in Charlotte and Polk counties were badly damaged, and this greatly impeded their ability to assist in coordinating services. Moreover, emergency transport companies were overwhelmed and unable to meet their agreements with nursing homes as hospitals had top priority for services.

The loss of electrical power was also a significant problem for many long-term facilities that remained in operation. Not all of the facilities had working generators, sufficient fuel to operate them for extended periods of time, or adequate power to operate multiple areas within the facility. Those that lost electrical power were entitled to receive priority restoration of services, but not all parts of the state recognized priority reconnection for nursing homes, and a handful of facilities that were providing skilled care to frail, vulnerable persons went days without power.

Despite many difficulties with the disaster response system, many dedicated people worked diligently with a number of agencies to provide continued care to this vulnerable population. It is to their credit that, despite the severity of these storms, there was no immediate loss of resident or staff life directly related to the hurricanes. Before the 2004 hurricane strike, the Florida Health Care Association had established a disaster preparedness committee and had widely disseminated published guidelines delineating steps to be taken in response to a variety of natural and human-made disasters. During the hurricanes, this organization sent out daily email alerts that contained information about past and pending storms, queried facilities about their needs for supplies and assistance, located needed resources, and coordinated relief efforts.

The experience of dealing with several hurricanes proved emotionally and physically stressful for residents and staff alike, and the disruptions contributed to the need for disaster mental health services. Long-term care facilities varied in their ability to provide mental health services to residents. Some had a social worker on staff, whereas others had to refer residents elsewhere for mental health services. Immediately after a serious disaster or terrorist event, a multidisciplinary team that includes psychologists, physicians, social workers, nurses, and other mental health paraprofessionals is an ideal way to quickly identify high-risk groups to promote recovery from acute stress and decrease the likelihood of long-term adverse effects. Mental health clinicians that arrive from outside the facility benefit from working collaboratively with staff who can provide information about residents' premorbid functioning and assist in screening. Those who provide relief and mental health services should possess basic knowledge about how mental health problems manifest in older adults (O'Brien, 2003).

Priority Issues in the Assessment of Older Persons

As noted earlier, the experiences that accumulate over a lifetime provide most older people with the knowledge and skills they need to cope with and adapt to the many changes, losses, and painful emotions associated with mass violence and disasters. Different cohorts of older persons have various characteristics and life experiences that shape their vulnerability and resilience in the future. The population age 65 and older have absorbed the impact of the terrorist attacks with a perspective that comes only from surviving a lifetime of experiences, including living though World War II and the Korean War. Many displayed resilience as well as a historical and personal perspective on good and evil, love and hate, living and dying, and war and peace.

Although older people as a population adapt better than younger adults, there are certain vulnerable subgroups, including but not limited to the following: those who are very old and frail; those who have multiple, disabling health problems; those who have grown old with developmental disabilities and mental retardation; those with Alzheimer's disease and related dementias; those who already have psychiatric problems; and those who have endured a serious traumatic circumstance (e.g., Holocaust survivors).

A sudden, threatening, traumatic event induces fear, helplessness, and a vulnerability in everyone affected, but when an older person already feels increasingly susceptible because of impaired health, mobility, and declining sensory and cognitive abilities, the feelings of powerlessness and helplessness may be overwhelming (Young, Ford, Ruzek, Friedman, & Gusman, 1998). Unexpected evacuations from nursing homes, assisted-living facilities, retirement communities, senior apartments, or trailer parks, as well as moves from one facility to another, can be frightening experiences that cause disorientation, confusion, and anxiety. Cognitive and sensory impairments usually make it harder for older people to understand evacuation instructions or emergency assistance information, cope with a chaotic environment, and respond to emergency workers and friends who want to assist them (Massey, 1997).

The untimely deaths of children or grandchildren are among the most difficult situations for older persons, not only because of the unexpected, violent death of a loved one but also because of a sense of broken continuity within the family, including its traditions, ceremonials, and legacies. Family support and contact for older relatives may decrease in the immediate aftermath of a tragedy while everyone in the family and community is consumed with the struggle of dealing with immediate losses, injuries, and deaths. When family support is less available, it is common for older people, especially those with health problems, to fear being moved into an institution, which prompts them to withhold their personal concerns, difficulties, and emotional reactions.

Grandparents may find themselves taking on parenting roles and responsibilities for their grandchildren when adult children have been killed. This increases emotional stress not only as older adults grieve for an adult child and help grandchildren cope with the loss of a parent but also as they significantly alter their lifestyles and routines to integrate the needs of young grandchildren. Frailty, chronic illness, housing, and financial insecurity are other factors that affect the ability of grandparents to deal with the aftermath of a disaster.

Mass violence and terrorism in their many forms have profound effects on the immediate victims and communities, as well as on others removed from the event. There are many common emotional, cognitive, behavioral, and physical reactions following mass disaster and violence. Table 20.2 provides an overview of symptoms that may be expressed in each of these domains.

These are normal reactions in the face of sudden mass violence caused by explosives and chemical, biological, radiological, or nuclear weapons. Individuals may experience all or only a few of these responses, but as time passes, these symptoms and difficulties should diminish as the normal routines of daily life are restored. Because there are significant differences in people's histories and in the way they express grief, fear, and anger, the recovery time will vary across the population. However, some vulnerable persons are at a greater risk for manifesting symptoms of PTSD, other anxiety disorders, depressive disorders, and substance abuse disorders.

The psychological effects of severe violence and mass trauma have not been well studied in the older population (Cook, Arean, Schnurr, & Sheikh, 2001). Older people who are geographically distant from the attack appear to recover faster than younger adults, but the recovery rate for those in affected areas will vary depending on the many circumstances discussed in the previous section. Although older persons may not meet all of the diagnostic criteria for PTSD or other anxiety disorders, they may manifest clinical symptoms that interfere with biopsychosocial functioning (e.g.,

partial or subthreshold PTSD). The existing literature suggests that a small group of older people will develop full-blown PTSD, but the prevalence of subsyndromal PTSD could be a serious consequence of mass disasters.

The few studies that have examined the prevalence of PTSD in older adults suggest that it either is often not identified or is incorrectly diagnosed (Davidson, 2001; Port, Engdahl, & Frazier, 2001). Some researchers have hypothesized that older adults go undiagnosed because they do not associate their posttrauma difficulties (e.g., sleep disturbance, intrusive thoughts) as abnormal (e.g., friends and family are experiencing the same thing). Furthermore, because PTSD is often comorbid and a variety of mental illnesses can and do occur with PTSD, it may also be that healthcare clinicians attribute the symptoms that older adults experience and report as related solely to alcoholism, depression, or anxiety disorders (Goenjian et al., 1994). Within the spectrum of criteria defined in *DSM-IV* there are a number of posttraumatic responses that fall short of meeting full PTSD diagnostic criteria. Even though a full PTSD syndrome may not be present, older adults can and do experience significant functional impairment following traumatic exposure (Bramsen & van der Ploeg, 1999; Spiro et al., 1994).

Assessment of Risk

Everyone should be screened for risk factors for developing PTSD. Certain factors (e.g., history of significant traumatic stressors, psychiatric history, and gender) place a person at greater risk for PTSD but are not mutable, whereas other factors (e.g., loss of resources and social support) can be modified by intervention. Knowledge of these modifiable factors can be useful when developing future interventions. Given the high prevalence of psychiatric comorbidity, assessment for depression is also warranted. It is the responsibility of the mental health clinician to differentiate between normal and abnormal reactions to terrorism. Interviewing older persons to assess this complex set of issues requires a careful process of therapeutic enjoining to develop the trust and rapport necessary to accurately assess mental health needs. Table 20.3 summarizes the information that should be included in a screening assessment.

Table 20.2. Normal emotional, cognitive, behavioral, physiological, and interpersonal reactions to stress

Emotional	Physiological
Anger	Aches, pains, muscle soreness
Anxiety	Choking, smothering sensation, "lump" in throat
Apathy	Cold or hot spells/chills or sweating
Blame	Dizziness
Denial or constriction of feelings	Fatigue and weakness
Depression	Fine motor tremors
Dissociation	GI upset
Fear about present and future	Headaches
Feeling overwhelmed	Heart palpitations and chest pain
Guilt	Hyperventilation
Helplessness and powerlessness	Lightheadedness
Irritability	Nausea
Rage	Paresthesias (numbness, tingling sensation)
Sadness or grief	Reduced immune response/vulnerable to illness
Shock and disbelief	Tachycardia
Terror	Tics
Cognitive	**Behavioral**
Calculation difficulties	Crying easily or for no apparent reason
Confusion	Decreased libido
Concentration problems	Excessive alcohol or drug use
Decision-making difficulties/slowness of thought	Hyperactivity
Difficulty with verbal expression	Hyperarousal
Disbelief	Hypervigilance
Disorientation	Inappropriate humor
Emotional numbing	Inertia
Intrusive thoughts/memories	Insomnia
Loss of pleasure	Over- or undereating
Memory problems/forgetfulness	Nightmares
Perseveration	Pacing
Reduced attention span	Ritualistic behavior
Self-blame	Startle response
Worry	
Interpersonal	
Alienation	
Distrust	
Externalization of blame	
Externalization of vulnerability	
Family problems	
Feelings of being abandoned	
Increased relational conflict/reduced intimacy	
Overprotectedness	
Social withdrawal	

Table 20.3. Issues to Consider During the Screening Assessment

Connection with individual

Medical needs/health status/exposure to toxic contamination

Signs of traumatic stress/individual responsiveness

Current or previous psychiatric illness

Weather exposure/extreme fatigue

Frailty/disability/cognitive impairment

Mobility

Cultural background/demographics

Living situation

Proximity of family members

Availability of other social supports

Determination of appropriate level of care

Injury or death of family members as victims

Assessment of danger/safety of self and others

Previous exposure to serious trauma

Availability of transportation and communication

Extent of terrorism or disaster preparedness (e.g., food, water, medications)

Normalization of responses/psychoeducation

Perception of trauma

Coping methods

Religious beliefs

Drug/alcohol use

Suicide/homicide risk

Note: Issues are not ranked in order of importance.

Older adults may refuse mental health screening and rarely make use of mental health services following a disaster (Lindy, Grace, & Green, 1981). After 9/11, there was a surge in visits among patients who were in therapy before the terrorist attacks, but there was no significant increase in mental health service use by younger and older adults who were not previously receiving mental health care, despite the availability of free services (Boscarino, Adams, & Figley, 2004). Older adults may turn to religious leaders, family members, informal social networks, or their personal physician for relief from their distress. Somatic symptoms associated with PTSD, depression, and anxiety may motivate some older adults to ask for medication from their physician. For those that seek care from a medical provider, this is encouraging in that it indicates a willingness to receive treatment. Primary care physicians have increased their efforts to screen for trauma among older adults who seek medical care for somatic complaints after disasters (Green, Epstein, Krupick, & Rowland, 1997).

Interventions After Terrorism or Mass Violence

Crisis intervention services are now widely recognized as an effective treatment modality for emergency mental health care to individuals and groups. Guidelines published by the Centers for Disease Control (CDC, n.d.) recommend that, following a traumatic event, clinicians allow people to talk when they are ready, validate their emotional reactions, avoid diagnostic and pathological language, and communicate person to person rather than expert to victim. The American Psychological Association (APA) has suggested several levels of intervention for older people after a terrorist attack. These include building resilience with psychosocial and behavioral support, performing therapeutic interventions for persons with psychopathology, and also using older people as community resources to cope with community needs and restore normalcy (APA, n.d.). The timely delivery of appropriate treatment is imperative following the acute crisis phase to mitigate the potential for psychopathology (e.g., acute stress disorder, PTSD, and other forms of anxiety and depression). Although older people are at low risk for mental health problems, those who do develop serious psychiatric distress may go unrecognized or untreated or be inadequately treated following a terrorist attack.

Several practical strategies and tactics that older persons can use to build their resilience include the following: educating themselves about normal reactions to terrorism; maintaining routines as much as possible; maximizing self-care (e.g., sleeping, eating appropriately, exercising, following good hygiene practices, engaging in pleasurable activities, staying connected to family and friends, talking with others about feelings, writing a journal or diary, reaching out for help if needed, prioritizing problems, developing a concrete plan of what needs to be done and taking action one step at a time, volunteering, examining personal strengths, and finding personal meaning in the experience). All of these simple but critical approaches are essential to work though during the immediate and short-term aftermath of mass disasters.

Secondary Exposure

News broadcasts of the horrific events on 9/11 engendered considerable distress in most television viewers, and research that was conducted to examine the impact of the media in creating collective traumatic stress in people who were not present at the actual event revealed a dose-response effect; that is, those who watched the most television coverage reported the highest levels of distress (Ahern et al., 2002; Schuster et al., 2001). People who lost friends or family were found to be particularly vulnerable to vicarious traumatization from frequent viewing of disturbing images (Ahern et al., 2002). Older adults in institutional settings, as well as those who were living in the community, were more likely to watch television coverage of traumatic events for prolonged periods of time. Because intentional death and harm are considered especially heinous, they elicit strong reactions that appear to enhance the retention of information, even in those with Alzheimer's disease (Budson et al., 2004).

A study investigating memory and emotions among older adults for the September 11, 2001, terrorist attacks showed that those with Alzheimer's dementia were more likely to remember personal (e.g., how they heard the news) rather than factual information (e.g., details of the attack), compared to those with mild cognitive impairment or cognitively intact older adults. Notably, people with Alzheimer's disease did not differ from cognitively intact adults in their level of emotional intensity for six emotions (sadness, anger, fear, frustration, confusion, and shock) that were measured in response to the terrorist attacks (Budson et al., 2004).

Conclusion

Older adults appear to be more willing to accept help on many levels from families or in familiar settings, including senior centers and religious institutions. The challenge to mental health professionals and trained volunteers is to find a balance in responding to the special needs of vulnerable populations, as well as supporting the resilience of others in the greater affected communities. Responding professionals need to be trained to understand that older adults with mental health problems are responsive to psychotherapies, group therapies, counseling, and psychotropic medications, when necessary (APA, 1998). However, older people may be especially reluctant, ashamed, or embarrassed to admit and discuss mental health problems, given the mass devastation, injury, and deaths in the aftermath of disaster. Education to decrease the misattribution of somatic symptoms and increase the acceptance of mental health treatment should be provided. Effective screening measures need to be validated with older adult populations so that those at risk for postdisaster psychopathology can be quickly and accurately identified. Programs to reduce stigma and enhance the attractiveness of mental health interventions need to be developed. Following acts of terrorism, intervention should be focused on building a recovery environment that returns people to their usual sources of social support and restores normalcy.

Although exposure to traumatic stressors can be potentially hazardous to one's psychological well-being, times of crisis may lead to personal growth (Tedeschi, Park, & Calhoun, 1998, p. 2). Gerald Caplan, the founder of modern crisis intervention, argued that crisis is a necessary precursor to growth (1961, p. 19). The coping process, a time when an individual strives for equilibrium or stability in response to a stressor, provides a venue for achieving either a higher or lower level of functioning than the precrisis state and creates a foundation for future development (Brown, Shiang, & Bongar, 2003). This appears to support the data on older persons exposed to mass violence and disasters who largely show greater resilience and adaptation than middle-aged and younger adults.

The older population is an underutilized community resource to assist with everything that must be done to assist victims and families, restore normal routines, deliver basic necessities of life, cook, provide child care, and canvas neighborhoods. Thompson and colleagues have proffered that "intervention efforts should be directed at shifting some of the burden towards older people" (1993, p. 615). Older adults have significant generative roles and responsibilities with which to assist children and other adults in coping with short- and long-term effects. Indeed, older people, by their very existence, are a symbol that life goes on and that there are many ways to survive.

References

Ahern, J., Galea, S., Resnick, H., Kilpatrick, D., Bucuvalas, M., & Gold, J., et al. (2002). Television images and psychological symptoms after the September 11 terrorist attacks. *Psychiatry, 65*(4), 289–300.

American Psychological Association. (1998). APA working group on the older adult: What practitioners should know about working with older adults. *Professional Psychology: Research and Practice, 29,* 413–427.

————. (n.d.). Fostering resilience in response to terrorism: For psychologists working with older adults. Fact sheets. Washington, DC: Author.

Baum, A., Fleming, R., & Singer, J. E. (1982). Stress at Three Mile Island: Applying social psychology to psychological impact analysis. In L. Bickman (Ed.), *Applied social psychology annual: Vol. 3.* Beverly Hills, CA: Sage.

Beaton, R., & Murphy, S. (2002). Psychosocial responses to biological and chemical terrorist threats and events: Implications for the workplace. *Journal of the American Association of Occupational Health Nurses, 50,* 182–189.

Blanchard, E. B., Hickling, E. J., Vollmer, A. J., Loos, W. R., Buckley, T. C., & Jaccard, J. (1995). Short-term follow-up of post-traumatic stress symptoms in motor vehicle accident victims. *Behaviour Research and Therapy, 33*(4), 369–377.

Bland, S. H., O'Leary, E. S., Farinaro, E., Jossa, F., Krough, V., & Violanti, J. M., et al. (1997). Social network disturbances and psychological distress following earthquake evacuation. *Journal of Nervous and Mental Disease, 185,* 188–194.

Bolin, R., & Klenow, D. J. (1983). Response of the elderly to disaster: An age-stratified analysis. *International Journal of Aging and Human Development, 16,* 283–296.

Boscarino, J. A. (1995). Post-traumatic stress and associated disorders among Vietnam veterans: The significance of combat exposure and social support. *Journal of Traumatic Stress, 8*(2), 317–336.

————, Adams, R. E., & Figley, C. R. (2004). Mental health service use 1 year after the World Trade Center disaster: Implications for mental health care. *General Hospital Psychiatry, 26*(5), 346–358.

Bramsen, I., & van der Ploeg, H. M. (1999) Fifty years later: The long-term psychological adjustment of ageing World War II survivors. *Acta Psychiatrica Scandinavica, 100,* 350–358.

Bremner, J. D., Southwick, S., Brett, E., Fontana, A., Resenheck, R., & Charney, D. S. (1992). Dissociation and posttraumatic stress disorder in Vietnam combat veterans. *American Journal of Psychiatry, 149,* 328–332.

Brennan, M., Horowitz, A., & Reinhardt, J. P. (2004). The September 11th attacks and depressive symptomatology among older adults with vision loss in New York City. *Journal of Gerontological Social Work, 40*(4), 55–71.

Breslau, N., Kessler, R. C., Chilcoat, H. D., Schultz, L. R., Davis, G. C., & Andreski, P. (1998). Trauma and posttraumatic stress disorder in the community: The 1996 Detroit area survey of trauma. *Archives of General Psychiatry, 55*(7), 626–632.

Brown, L. M., Schinka, J. A., Borenstein, A. A., & Mortimer, J. A. (n.d.). Predictors of psychological status following the 2004 Florida hurricanes in a cohort of older adults. Manuscript submitted for publication.

Brown, L. M., Shiang, J., & Bongar, B. (2003). Crisis intervention: Theory and practice. In G. Stricker & T. A. Widiger (Eds.), *Comprehensive handbook of psychology, Vol. 8. Clinical psychology* (pp. 431–451). New York: Wiley.

Budson, A. E., Sullivan, A. L., Solomon, P. R., Simons, J. S., Beier, J. S., Scinto, L. F., et al. (2004). Memory and emotions for the September 11, 2001: Terrorist attacks in patients with Alzheimer's disease, patients with mild cognitive impairment, and healthy older adults. *Neuropsychology, 8*(2), 315–327.

Butler, A. S., Panzer, A. M., & Goldfrank, L. R. (Eds.). 2003. *Preparing for the psychological consequences of terrorism: A public health strategy.* Sponsored by the Committee on Responding to the Psychological Consequences of Terrorism, Board on Neuroscience and Behavioral Health, Institute of Medicine. Washington, DC: National Academies Press.

Cantor, M. H. (1979). Neighbors and friends: An overlooked resource in the informal support system. *Research on Aging, 1*(4), 434–463.

Caplan, G. (1961). *An approach to community mental health.* New York: Grune and Stratton.

Centers for Disease Control and Prevention (CDC). Coping with a traumatic event: Information for health professionals. Atlanta, Georgia. Retrieved February 20, 2006, from http://www.bt.cdc.gov/masstrauma/copingpro.asp.

Chen, H., Chung, H., Chen, T., Fang, L., & Chen, J. P. (2003).The emotional distress in a community after the terrorist attack on the World Trade Center. *Community Mental Health Journal, 39*(2), 157–165.

Chung, I. (2004). The impact of the 9/11 attacks on the elderly in NYC Chinatown: Implications for culturally relevant services. *Journal of Gerontological Social Work, 40*(4), 37–53.

Cohen, D., & Brown, L. M. (2004). Terrorism and older persons: Websites for geriatric mental health professionals. *Journal of Mental Health and Aging, 9,* 139–143.

Cook, J. D., & Bickman L. (1990). Social support and psychological symptomatology following a natural disaster. *Journal of Traumatic Stress, 3*(4), 541–556.

Cook, J. M., Arean, P. A., Schnurr, P. P., & Sheikh, J. (2001). Symptom differences of older depressed primary care patients with and without history of trauma. *International Journal of Psychiatry in Medicine, 31,* 415–428.

Crohan, S. E., & Antonucci, T. C. (1989). Friends as a source of social support in old age. In R. G. Adams & R. Blieszner (Eds.), *Older adult friendship: Structure and process* (pp. 129–146). Newbury Park, CA: Sage.

Davidson, J. R. (2001). Recognition and treatment of posttraumatic stress disorder. *Journal of the American Medical Association, 286*(5), 584–588.

Davis, E. (2004). The emergency preparedness initiative: Guide on the special needs of people with disabilities for emergency managers, planners, and responders. Washington, DC: National Organization on Disability's Emergency Initiative Guide. Retrieved February 18, 2005, from http://www.nod.org.

Dougall, A. L., Herberman, H. B., Delahanty, D. L., Inslicht, S. S., & Baum, A. (2000). Similarity of prior trauma exposure as a determinant of chronic stress responding to an airline disaster. *Journal of Consulting and Clinical Psychology, 68,* 290–295.

Eaton, W. W., Sigal, J. J., & Weinfeld, M. (1982). Impairment in Holocaust survivors after 33 years: Data from an unbiased community sample. *American Journal of Psychiatry, 139*(6), 773–777.

Ferraro, R. F. (2003). Psychological resilience in older adults following the 1997 flood. *Clinical Gerontologist, 26*(3/4), 139–143.

Fields, R. B. (1996). Severe stress in the elderly: Are older adults at increased risk for posttraumatic stress disorder? In P. E. Ruskin & J. A. Talbott (Eds.), *Aging and posttraumatic stress disorder* (pp. 79–100). Washington, DC: American Psychiatric Press.

Folkman, S., & Lazarus, R. S. (1980). An analysis of coping in a middle-aged community sample. *Journal of Health and Social Behavior, 21,* 219–239.

———, Dunkel-Schetter, C., DeLongis, A., & Gruen, R. (1986). The dynamics of a stressful encounter. *Journal of Personality and Social Psychology, 50,* 992–1003.

Frederick, C. J. (1987). Psychic trauma in victims of crime and terrorism. In G. R. VandenBos & B. Bryant (Eds.), *Cataclysms, crises, and catastrophes: Psychology in action* (pp. 59–108). Washington, DC: American Psychological Association.

Friedsam, H. J. (1960). Older persons as disaster casualties. *Journal of Health and Human Behavior, 1*(4), 269–273.

———. (1961). Reactions of older persons to disaster-caused losses: A hypothesis of relative deprivation. *Gerontologist, 1,* 34–37.

Fullerton, C. S., Ursano, R. J., Norwood, A. E., & Holloway, H. H. (2003). Trauma, terrorism, and disaster. In R. J. Ursano, C. S. Fullerton, & A. E. Norwood (Eds.), *Terrorism and disaster: Individual and community mental health interventions* (pp. 1–20). New York: Cambridge University Press.

Gignac, M. A., Cott, C. A., & Badley, E. M. (2003). Living with a chronic disabling illness and then some: Data from the 1998 ice storm. *Canadian Journal of Aging, 22*(3), 249–259.

Gleser, G., Green, B., & Winget, C. (1981). *Prolonged psychosocial effects of disaster: A study of Buffalo Creek.* New York: Academic Press.

Goenjian, A. K., Najarian, L. M., Pynoos, R. S., Steinberg, A. M., Manoukian, G., & Tavosian, A., et al. (1994). Posttraumatic stress disorder in elderly and younger adults after the 1988 earthquake in Armenia. *American Journal of Psychiatry, 151,* 895–901.

Green, B. L. (1990). Defining trauma: Terminology and generic dimension. *Journal of Applied Social Psychology, 20,* 1632–1642.

———, Epstein, S. A., Krupnick, J. L., & Rowland, J. H. (1997).Trauma and medical illness: Assessing trauma-related disorders in medical settings. In J. P. Wilson & T. M. Keane (Eds.), *Assessing psychological trauma and PTSD* (pp. 160–191). New York: Guilford.

Green, B. L., Goodman, L. A., Krupnick, J. L., Corcoran, C. B., Petty, R. M., Stockton, P., et al. (2000). Outcomes of single versus multiple trauma exposure in a screening sample. *Journal of Traumatic Stress, 13*(2), 271–286.

Gregory, S. (2004, November). Preparing your health care facility for the next hurricane(s). Paper presented at the Florida Health Care Association, In the eye of the storm: Lessons learned from Charley, Frances, Ivan, and Jeanne. Tampa, FL.

Hendrie, H. C. (1998). Epidemiology of Alzheimer's disease. *American Journal of Geriatric Psychiatry, 6,* S3–S18.

Hobfoll, S. E. (1989). Conservation of resources: A new attempt at conceptualizing stress. *American Psychologist, 44,* 513–524.

———, Dunahoo, C. A., & Monnier, J. (1995). Conservation of resources and traumatic stress. In J. R. Freedy & S. E. Hobfoll (Eds.), *Traumatic stress: From theory to practice* (pp. 29–47). New York: Plenum.

Holt, J., & Hotto, S. (1994). *Demographic aspects of hearing impairment: Questions and answers* (3d ed.). Washington, DC: Gallaudet University Press.

Hooke, W., & Rogers, P. G. (Eds.). 2005. *Public health risks of disasters: Communication, infrastructure, and preparedness.* Sponsored by the Roundtable on Environmental Health Sciences, Research, and Medicine, Board on Health Sciences Policy, Institute of Medicine and Disasters Roundtable, National Research Council. Washington, DC: National Academies Press.

Huerta, F., & Horton, R. (1978). Coping behavior of elderly flood victims. *Gerontologist, 18,* 541–546.

Hyer, K., Brown, L. M., Polivka-West, L., & Bond, J. Preparation, response, and recovery of long-term care facilities staff and residents: The 2004 Florida hurricane season. Manuscript submitted for publication.

Janoff-Bulman, R. (1992). *Shattered assumptions: Toward a new psychology of trauma.* New York: Free Press.

Kaniasty, K., & Norris, F. H. (1993). A test of the support deterioration model in the context of natural disaster. *Journal of Personality and Social Psychology, 64,* 395–408.

Kessler, R., Sonnega, A., Bromet, E., Hughes, M., Nelson, C., & Breslau, N. (1999). Epidemiological risk factors for trauma and PTSD. In R. Yehuda (Ed.), *Risk factors for posttraumatic stress disorders* (pp. 23–60). Washington, DC: American Psychiatric Press.

Kilijanek, T. S., & Drabek, T. E. (1979). Assessing long-term impacts of a natural disaster: A focus on the elderly. *Gerontologist, 19,* 555–566.

King, L. A., King, D. W., Fairbank, J. A., Keane, T. M., & Adams, G. A. (1998). Resilience-recovery factors in post-traumatic stress disorder among female and male Vietnam veterans: Hardiness, postwar social support, and additional stressful life events. *Journal of Personality and Social Psychology, 74,* 420–434.

Kinston, W., & Rosser R. (1974). Disaster: Effects on mental and physical state. *Journal of Psychosomatic Research, 18,* 437–456.

Knight, B. G., Gatz, M., Heller, K., & Bengston, V. L. (2000). Age and emotional response to the Northridge earthquake: A longitudinal analysis. *Psychology and Aging, 15,* 627–624.

Krause, N. (1987). Exploring the impact of a natural disaster on the health and psychological well-being of older adults. *Journal of Human Stress, 13,* 61–69.

———. (2001). Social support. In R. H. Binstock & L. K. George (Eds.), *Handbook of aging and the social sciences* (5th ed.) (pp. 273–294). San Diego: Academic Press.

Lindy, J. D., Grace, M. C., & Green, B. L. (1981). Survivors: Outreach to a reluctant population. *American Journal of Orthopsychiatry, 51,* 468–478.

Little, B., Gill, J., Schulte, J., Young, S., Horton, J., Harris, L., et al. (2004) Rapid assessment of the needs and health status of older adults after Hurricane Charley: Charlotte, DeSoto, and Hardee counties, Florida, August 27–31, 2004. *Journal of the American Medical Association, 292,* 1813–1814.

Massey, B. A. (1997). Victims or survivors? A three-part approach to working with older adults in disaster. *Journal of Geriatric Psychiatry, 30,* 193–202.

Mollica, R. F., Wyshak, G., Lavelle, J., Truong, T., Tor, S., & Yang, T. (1990). Assessing symptom change in Southeast Asian refugee survivors of mass violence and torture. *American Journal of Psychiatry, 147,* 83–88.

Nishith, P., Mechanic, M. B., 25.

Norris, F. H. (1992). Epidemiology of trauma: Frequency and impact of different potentially traumatic events on different demographic groups. *Journal of Consulting and Clinical Psychology, 60,* 409–418.

———, Byrne, C. M., Díaz, E., & Kaniasty, K. (2001). The range, magnitude, and duration of effects of natural and human-caused disasters: A review of the empirical literature. A National Center for PTSD Fact Sheet. Retrieved January 23, 2006, from http://www.ncptsd.org/facts/disasters/fs_range.html

Norris, F. H., Friedman, M. J., & Watson, P. J. (2002). 60,000 disaster victims speak: Part 2. Summary and implications of the disaster mental health research. *Psychiatry, 65,* 240–260.

———, Byrne, C. M., Díaz, E., & Kaniasty, K. (2002). 60,000 disaster victims speak: Part 1. An empirical review of the empirical literature, 1981–2001. *Psychiatry, 65,* 207–239.

Norris, F. H., Kaniasty, K., Conrad, L. M., Inman, G. L., Murphy, A.D. (2002). Placing age differences in cultural context: A comparison of the effects of age on PTSD after disasters in the United States, Mexico, and Poland. *Journal of Clinical Geropsychology 8*(3), 153–173.

North, C. S., Nixon, S. J., Shariat, S., Mallonee, S., McMillen, J. C., Spitznagel, E. L., et al. (1999). Psychiatric disorders among survivors of the Oklahoma City bombing. *Journal of the American Medical Association, 282,* 755–762.

O'Brien, N. (2003, January/February). *Emergency preparedness for older people.* (Issue Brief). New York: International Longevity Center USA.

Orr, S., & Pitman, R. (1999). Neurocognitive risk factors for PTSD. In R. Yehuda (Ed.), *Risk factors for post traumatic stress disorders* (pp. 125–142). Washington, DC: American Psychiatric Press.

Ott, D. C. (2005, March 10–13). The changing face of elder disaster response: Hurricane season 2004.

Paper presented at the annual joint conference of the American Society on Aging and the National Council on the Aging, Philadelphia.

Parkes, C. M. (2002). Postscript. In J. Kauffman (Ed.), *Loss of the assumptive world: A theory of traumatic loss* (pp. 237–242). New York: Brunner-Routledge.

Penner, N. R. (2003). Collaborating with relief agencies: A guide or hospice. In M. Lattanzi-Licht & K. J. Doka (Eds.), *Living with grief: Coping with public tragedy* (pp. 277–288). New York: Brunner-Routledge.

Phifer, J. F. (1990). Psychological distress and somatic symptoms after natural disaster: Differential vulnerability among older adults. *Psychology and Aging, 5*(3), 412–420.

————, & Norris, F. H. (1989). Psychological symptoms in older adults following natural disaster: Nature, timing, duration, and course. *Journals of Gerontology, 44*(6), S207–S217.

Port, C. L, Engdahl, B., & Frazier, P. (2001) A longitudinal and retrospective study of PTSD among older prisoners of war. *American Journal of Psychiatry, 158*(9), 1474–1479.

————, & Eberly, R. (2002). Factors related to the long-term course of PTSD in older ex-prisoners of war. *Journal of Clinical Geropsychology, 8,* 203–214.

Qureshi, K. A., Merrill, J. A., Gershon, R. M., & Calero-Breckheimer, A. (2002). Emergency preparedness training for public health nurses: A pilot study. *Journal of Urban Health: Bulletin of the New York Academy of Medicine, 79*(3), 413–416.

Raid J., & Norris, F. (1996). The influence of relocation on the environmental, social, and psychological stress experienced by disaster victims. *Environment and Behavior, 28,* 163–182.

Raphael, B. (2003). Early intervention and the debriefing debate. In R. J. Ursano, C. S. Fullerton, & A. E. Norwood (Eds.), *Terrorism and disaster: Individual and community mental health interventions.* New York: Cambridge University Press.

Rosenzweig, N. (1975). Some differences between elderly people who use community resources and those who do not. *Journal of the American Geriatrics Society, 23,* 224–233.

Rutter, M. (1987). Psychosocial resilience and protective mechanisms. *American Journal of Orthopsychiatry, 57,* 316–331.

Sanders, S., Bowie, S. L., & Bowie, Y. D. (2003). Lessons learned on forced relocation of older adults: The impact of Hurricane Andrew on health, mental health, and social support of public housing residents. *Journal of Gerontological Social Work, 40*(4), 23–35.

Schlenger, W. E., Caddell, J. M., Ebert, L., Jordan, B. K., Rourke, K. M., Wilson, D., et al. (2002).

Psychological reactions to terrorist attacks: Findings from the National Study of Americans' Reactions to September 11. *Journal of the American Medical Association, 288*(5), 581–588.

Schuster, M. A., Stein, B. D., Jaycox, L. H., Collins, R. L., Marshall, G. N., Elliott, M. N., et al. (2001). A national survey of stress reactions after the September 11, 2001, terrorist attacks. *New England Journal of Medicine, 345,* 1507–1512.

Silver, R. C., Holman, E. A., McIntosh, D. N., Poulin, M., & Gil-Rivas, V. (2002). National longitudinal study of psychological responses to September 11. *Journal of the American Medical Association, 288*(10), 1235–1244.

Silver, R. C., Poulin, M., Holman, A. E., McIntosh, D. N., Gil-Rivas, V., Pizarro, J. (2004). Exploring the myths of coping with a national trauma: A longitudinal study of responses to the September 11th terrorist attacks. *Journal of Aggression, Maltreatment & Trauma, 9*(1–2), 129–141.

Spiro, A., Schnurr, P. P., & Aldwin, C. M. (1994). Combat-related posttraumatic stress disorder symptoms in older men. *Psychology and Aging, 9*(1), 17–26.

Stein, B. D., Tanielian, T. L., Eisenman, D. P., Keyser, D. J., Burnam, M. A., & Pincus, H. A. (2004). Emotional and behavioral consequences of bioterrorism: Planning a public health response. *Milbank Quarterly, 82*(3), 413–455.

Strug, D. L., Mason, S. E., & Heller, F. E. (2003). An exploratory study of the impact of the year of 9/11 on older Hispanic immigrants in New York City. *Journal of Gerontological Social Work, 42*(2), 77–99.

Tedeschi, R. G., Park, C. L., & Calhoun, L. G. (1998). Posttraumatic growth: Conceptual issues. In R. G. Tedeschi, C. L. Park, & L. G. Calhoun (Eds.), *Posttraumatic growth: Positive changes in the aftermath of crisis* (pp. 1–22). Mahwah, NJ: Erlbaum.

Thompson, M. P., Norris, F. H., & Hanacek, B. (1993). Age differences in the psychological consequences of hurricane Hugo. *Psychology and Aging, 8*(4), 606–616.

Trautman, R., Tucker, P., Pfefferbaum, B., Lensgraf, S. J., Doughty, D. E., Buksh, A., et al. (2002). Effects of prior trauma and age on posttraumatic stress symptoms in Asian and Middle Eastern immigrants after terrorism in the community. *Community Mental Health Journal, 38*(6), 459–474.

Tyler, K., & Hoyt, D. R. (2000). The effects of an acute stressor on depressive symptoms among older adults: The moderating effects of social support and age. *Research on Aging, 22,* 143–164.

Verger, P., Dab, W., Lamping, D. L., Loze, J. Y., Deschaseaux-Voinet, C., Abenhaim, L., et al.

(2004). The psychological impact of terrorism: An epidemiologic study of posttraumatic stress disorder and associated factors in victims of the 1995–1996 bombings in France. *American Journal of Psychiatry, 161,* 1384–1389.

Watanabe, C., Okumura, J., Chiu, T., & Wakai, S. (2004). Social support and depressive symptoms among displaced older adults following the 1999 Taiwan earthquake. *Journal of Traumatic Stress, 17*(1), 63–67.

Wright, K. B., & Query J. L. (2004). Handbook of communication and aging research. In J. F. Nussbaum & J. Coupland (Eds.), *Handbook of communication and aging research* (2d ed.) (pp. 499–519). Mahwah, NJ: Erlbaum.

Yehuda, R., Kahana, B., Schmeidler, J., Southwick, S. M., Wilson, S., & Giller, E. L. (1995). Impact of cumulative lifetime trauma and recent stress on current posttraumatic stress disorder symptoms in Holocaust survivors. *American Journal of Psychiatry, 152*(12), 1815–1818.

Young, B. H., Ford, J. D., Ruzek, J. I., Friedman, M. J., & Gusman, F. D. (1998). *Disaster mental health services: A guidebook for clinicians and administrators.* Menlo Park, CA: Department of Veteran Affairs, National Center for PTSD.

21

Children and Terrorism

A Family Psychoeducational Approach

Maureen Underwood
John Kalafat
Nicci Spinazzola

Since the terrorist bombing of the Alfred P. Murrah Federal Building in Oklahoma City in 1995, there has been a growing body of mental health literature emphasizing the critical importance of addressing the needs of families and children who were directly impacted by this type of traumatic event (Webb, 2004; Gist & Lubin, 1999). Borrowing from interventions in countries such as Israel that deal with chronic terrorism (e.g., Itzhaky & York, 2005), the approaches utilized in the United States have included both indicated interventions for those exhibiting significant stress responses (Saltzman, Layne, Steinberg, Arslanagic, & Pynoos, 2003) and selective interventions for those who are exhibiting subclinical reactions to exposure and loss, which characterize the majority of responses to traumatic events (Kelly, Berman-Rossi, & Palombo, 2001).

The unprecedented events of 9/11 necessitated the adaptation of these as well as a variety of other approaches in response to a myriad of complicated mental health issues related to the massive numbers of deaths, the ongoing trauma exposure of the first responders, and the continuing threat of future terrorist events. The impact on families in the New York metropolitan area has been documented as substantially greater than in other parts of the

country as measured by exposure to the event, continuing media coverage, and loss of a family member (e.g., Galea, Ahern, & Resnick, 2002; Schlenger, Caddell, et al., 2002). Several northern New Jersey communities that stretch along the commuter rail line into New York City were particularly impacted. In one town, for example, 18 residents, most of whom were the fathers of large, young families, lost their lives. Moreover, the impact of the attacks was felt in many ways unknown to the rest of the country, such as commuter lots filled with unclaimed cars and smoke rising from the ruins that lingered for weeks, creating a constant reminder.

As in most communities, there was a dearth of trained mental health practitioners to address the challenging trauma recovery tasks presented by these families (Gurwitch, Sitterle, Young, & Pfefferbaum, 2002). Well-intentioned practitioners attempted to fill the breach in services, sometimes with uninformed interventions that made families question the wisdom of mental health services (Padgett, 2002). Examples from our experience include one mother who reported that a therapist had created towers of blocks for her 6- and 8-year-old children, then crashed a toy plane into them and asked the children where they thought their father was located. Another told the story of a counselor who asked her 3- and 5-year-olds which child missed their father more.

Immediately after 9/11, Underwood, Milani, & Spinazzola (2004), who are practitioners in one of the most affected communities, provided debriefings and consultations to local schools with students who had experienced deaths of family members to assist in both student management and the processing of staff responses. With a recognized expertise in crisis intervention and the impact of traumatic death on children, they responded to requests for in-service training programs at schools and mental health agencies statewide and developed written guidelines for crisis response that were published on the University of Medicine and Dentistry of New Jersey website. Inundated with these service requests, they joined with a third associate and approached colleagues to explore the possibility of designing and implementing a community-based group intervention for these local families.

In this chapter Underwood, Kalafat, & Spinazzola describe a psychoeducational approach for helping children and families cope with the 9/11 terrorist attacks in New York City that is based on ongoing work with children and families who lost a family member on that day. First, is a review of the conceptual framework that informed the intervention, followed by a description of the program derived from these applied intervention principles.

Conceptual Framework

In selecting the intervention approach, Underwood & Kalafat drew on their experience in developing community-based psychoeducational programs for families living with cancer (Joannides, Underwood, & Kalafat, 1986), adults and children dealing with the impacts of divorce (Kalafat, Underwood, Fiedler, & Neigher, 1990), those who had experienced traumatic events in schools (Kalafat & Underwood, 1989; Underwood & Dunne-Maxim, 1997), and children exposed to natural disasters (Shepherd-Levine, Underwood, & Cernak, 2000). The basic strategy for developing such programs consists of initially engaging and observing members of the affected population in order to inductively capture their experiences, issues, and needs. Following this grounded, qualitative approach, each of these in-terventions was informed by a consistent set of relevant conceptual and empirical sources:

- crisis intervention, which emphasizes the provision of structure, mobilization of supports, and the avoidance of pathologizing, which were originally found to be effective during wartime (Butcher & Maudal, 1976, p. 678)
- community education, which applies adult learning principles such as collaborative, active learning relevant to current issues in participants' lives (Knowles, Swanson, & Holton, 2005)
- ecological emphasis, which focuses on interactions between people and their environments, as opposed to strictly person-centered approaches (Kelly, 2000)
- empowerment (Rappaport, 1981), which emphasizes the enabling of community (Iscoe, 1974), family (Dunst, Trivette, & Deal, 1988), and individual (Bonanno, 2004) competence and resilience. In this context, Gitterman (2001) has noted that resilience is an ecological concept reflecting complex person-environment transactions and not simply a personal attribute.
- group approaches, which, in addition to mutual support (Lieberman & Borman, 1979), provide classic healing factors such as universality, altruism, imitation learning, socializing techniques, information, feedback, and cohesiveness (Yalom, 1995). Additional group mediators have been posited for trauma groups, including reducing isolation and promoting reconnections to family and other supports, validation of the trauma experience, rebuilding trust, reality testing, and correcting distortions in one's assumptive world created by disasters, practice of nurturing (including self-nurturing behaviors), and grieving (Dembert & Simmer, 2000; Buchele & Spitz, 2004).

Even in the face of the challenges presented by the unprecedented events of 9/11, we saw no reason to abandon these established approaches, which had effectively informed our work to date.

Our review of the literature on the current status of responses to trauma and disasters affirmed these approaches and further informed our family group interventions. There have been several reviews of the psychosocial impacts of 9/11

(Galea et al.,2002; Groves, 2002; Schlenger et al., 2002), as well as the impacts of disaster and trauma on children and families (Berkowitz, 2003; Catherall, 2004; Joshi & Lewin, 2004; Pynoos, Steinberg, & Wraith, 1995; Pynoos & Nader, 1988; Vernberg & Vogel, 1993; Weingarten, 2004). These reviews report sequelae such as risk factors for and the incidence of PTSD; the responses of children at different ages; the fact that families can, in addition to giving support, transmit anxiety and transgenerational effects of exposure to violence; the fact that early coping responses predict later adjustment; and the plasticity and, hence, vulnerability of children's physical and psychological development. These findings have led to recommendations for early, family-focused interventions and the ongoing monitoring of children and families' responses.

At the same time, these reviews note that, even in the face of events such as 9/11, while children and families may experience transitional perturbation in normal functioning, their resilience is so common as to constitute the norm rather than the exception (Bonanno, 2004; Padgett, 2002). The implication of this is an emerging consensus for interventions that acknowledge and address families' crises, stress, and grief in a nonpathologizing way and focus on enabling family strength and resilience. Joshi et al. (2004) have warned against "overmedicalizing normal reactions" (p. 715) and noted that not all children exposed to traumatic events develop PTSD and can actually be resilient. They contend that programs that effectively build resilience focus either on protective factors or on what works in children's lives instead of risk factors or what does not work.

In their own review of evidence-based interventions for trauma, Litz, Gray, Bryant, and Adler (2002) have concluded that the most appropriate early intervention should be "conceptualized as supportive and non-interventionist, but definitely not as therapy or treatment" (p. 128). They further conclude that this approach includes group support that responds to the need that arises for people to share their experience while respecting those who do not wish to focus on what happened. Berkowitz (2003) notes that parental support is quite amenable to early intervention and salient in preventing poor functioning in children, while O'Donnell, Schwab-Stone, and Muyeed (2002) have stated that factors related to family environment and children's social milieu are among the most stable predictors of resilience in youth exposed to violence. Kumpfer and Alvarado (2003), in their contribution to *American Psychologist*'s special section on prevention, which deals with children and youth, report that family-focused prevention efforts have a greater impact than strategies that focus only on parents or children.

Finally, in a review of evidence-based early interventions for victims of mass violence, the National Institute of Mental Health (2002) identified key intervention components: nurturing resilience and recovery by fostering—but not forcing—social interactions, providing coping skills training, promoting natural supports, and offering group and family interventions. Several resources are now available for implementing these recommendations for enabling resilience through family and group interventions (Underwood, 2004; Buchele & Spitz, 2004; Kelly et al., 2001; Klein & Schermer, 2000; Stoiber, Ribar, & Wass, 2004).

The Family GOALs Project

Sustained, visual media coverage of the events of 9/11 created a myopic preoccupation with the circumstances of the trauma, and many families felt that life had stopped for them in those tragic moments. The choice of a community-based intervention reflected the goal of reconnecting members of a traumatized community through shared healing activities, rather than through continued emphasis on the disaster. The use of community resources was also a way to concretely engage the community in healing and provide an antidote to the pervasive sense of helplessness initially reported by the community at large (Van den Eynde & Veno, 1999).

Underwood, Milani, & Spinazzola (2004) also recognized that, because the postdisaster recovery environment exerts such a powerful effect on children's reactions to disasters, an essential component in long-term adjustment would be the augmentation of the systemic connections with possible protective and resilience effects. It was decided that the focus of the interventions would be on the engagement of community resources in support of family life. The name of the project, Families Going On After Loss (GOALs), was chosen to reflect this intention.

Another objective of community healing was to situate the program in an accessible community location. The initial site selected was the local YMCA, although it was clear at the first meeting that there was a palpable contrast between the families attending the "Y" for fun events and those gathering there in grief, which disturbed the leaders. A multinational corporation, located in the same community, was approached and agreed to host the project at its corporate headquarters. The local mental health center was intentionally avoided because leaders were concerned that there might be an unspoken stigma attached to services provided in a clinical location. They felt it would be easier to address mental health concerns and to make potential referrals for clinical services in a neutral setting. Neighborhood schools were also not considered because leaders did not want children, especially those who had become somewhat school phobic, to associate their grief with the school environment.

The community focus was evident not just in the intervention's location but also in the businesses, organizations, and community groups that donated supplies and services. Community outreach became the responsibility of one of the staff members, and there was a generous outpouring of support and assistance from sources as diverse as the United Way and the local pizzeria for the myriad of things that needed to be done to make the project really work.

Phase 1

Basic Considerations

Consistent with the strength-based or resilience paradigm, the initial goal was to acknowledge the families' and children's pain, fear, and loss and then to identify and emphasize strengths and effective coping methods. The latter consist of a positive and hopeful outlook and active rather than passive or avoidant coping strategies (Bonanno, 2004; Nation et al., 2003). In addition, a central issue for the program was how to frame these approaches so that children could understand and apply them to their concerns.

Given that most of the existing program models targeted children and adults either separately or in individual family units, project leaders felt that one aspect of a more effective model of service delivery should focus on bringing together all of the members of the nuclear family affected by the loss. Research indicates that the existing family structure is at least temporarily altered by a traumatic loss event such as 9/11 (Berkowitz, 2003; Kissane & Bloch, 1994). Parents face multiple communication challenges as they struggle to find words to explain what happened to themselves and to their children. The children must also find ways to communicate at a time when their life experiences do not provide them with a frame of reference either for what has occurred or what they are feeling. Vital executive functions in the family can also be disturbed as surviving parents strive to remain available for emotional nurturing, education, and protection when they themselves are in great need of similar support and guidance (Cook & Dworkin, 1992; Curry, 2002; Vernberg & Vogel, 1993).

With this increase in the emotional and physical demands on the surviving parent, supervision in the household often decreases or is delegated to surrogate caregivers. Because the family's sense of invulnerability has been shattered, the family may become fatalistic and expect the worst from life (Janoff-Bulman, 1985). As a result of these worries, parents often become overprotective of their children and impede the development of autonomy, which can create anxiety in their children. Because each member of the family understandably deals with the trauma and grief differently, the many good things the family shares can get lost in the sense of isolation and confusion created by the traumatic event The initial outpouring of support immediately following a traumatic incident is discontinued long before the family's recovery is complete. People get back to the business of living their own lives, leaving families who have experienced the trauma feeling that there is a lack of understanding of the deeper meaning of the loss.

Project leaders felt strongly that creating an intervention model that included all of the members of the nuclear family, even the youngest children, might moderate some of the more deleterious effects of the trauma on family life. Since families are often divided by each member's unique style of grieving, Underwood, Milani, & Spinazzola (2004) also felt that the intervention plan should contain similar learning objectives for the entire family, although the activities designed to accomplish these objectives needed to be developmentally relevant for each member. This similarity would provide the family with opportunities for joining together in some aspects of their grief.

The resulting psychoeducational support group model included entire families that were combined into multifamily groups, which addressed many of the aforementioned concerns and enhanced several other therapeutic factors of groups (Stoiber, Ribar, & Waas, 2004):

1. Families that felt isolated and stigmatized by the traumatic event could be reassured by the presence of other families who had undergone similar experiences (Curry, 2002).
2. Groups would provide an opportunity for validation and normalization of feelings through comparison with others (Gordon, Farberow, & Maida, 1999).
3. In addition to active participation, groups would provide an opportunity for vicarious learning (Bloch & Crouch, 1985).
4. Groups would expose children to age-mates who might be at different stages in trauma resolution.
5. Youths might accept both support and shared learning from peers that they would not accept from adults (Terr, 1989).
6. Family members would have an opportunity to help others in the group, which might counteract some of the feelings of helplessness generated by the trauma (Bloch & Crouch, 1985).
7. Families in need of additional services could be assessed and referred (Terr, 1989).
8. The use of a psychoeducational format could help organize the tasks of recovery (Harkness & Zador, 2001).

The project leaders were also sensitive to the limitations of groups in situations of mass trauma (Nader, 2004). They recognized that some aspects of the trauma experience, like specific discussions about what type of remains had been recovered, might be very personal and private and thus inappropriate topics for group discussion. They were also alert to the tendency of youth to be influenced by their perceptions of others' expectations, which predisposed the leaders to exclude certain aspects of trauma resolution such as the construction of personal narratives from the curriculum.

The timing of the intervention was also critical. Because Underwood, Milani, & Spinazzola (2004) knew that the 6-month anniversary of 9/11 would present a barrage of trauma and loss reminders, they wanted to have an intervention in place that would help the families both anticipate the challenges of that day and plan a family response that would contain their grief and honor the memory of the deceased. The leaders also saw this as an opportunity to model for the families ways in which the 1-year anniversary could be commemorated. The series was therefore scheduled to begin in late February 2002. Up to that time, most of the families were still struggling to accept the reality of what had happened, adjust to the changes in family life precipitated by the loss, plan and carry out private memorial services, and deal with the Thanksgiving and December holidays. In addition, the families were invited to a plethora of public activities related to 9/11. Special concerts, sporting events, meetings with local and national elected officials, and plans for various public memorials occupied their time and energies. Because midwinter schedules seemed more open, the leaders felt that group intervention held at this time of the year would help families make their way into the busy spring.

Recognizing the competing demands of school, extracurricular events, and grief-related activities, the project leaders decided to employ a closed-group format and limit the group series to six sessions of 90 minutes each. Because the groups included a psychoeducational component with an assumption of accumulated learning, the closed format seemed to be better designed to achieve this objective. It also facilitated the development of cohesiveness and supportive connection among the families who reported feeling isolated and stigmatized in the community at large.

Participants

The participants for this intervention were drawn from a population that shared risk factors for posttraumatic stress identified by Gurwitch et al. (2002) in their review of the aftermath of terrorism. These include degree of exposure, television reexposure, relationship to the victim (with children most affected by the loss of a parent), and bereavement (i.e., trauma and grief interact with posttraumatic stress to complicate the grieving process and interfere with children's efforts to both address the loss and adapt to subsequent life changes). Gurwitch et al. also found that the parents' responses to the events affected the children's reactions and, specifically, that family support mitigated the development of PTSD symptoms.

Considering these factors, recruitment focused on the population of families with school-aged children within three geographically contiguous New Jersey communities that had been particularly impacted by 9/11 casualties. Initial screening revealed that all of these families were Caucasian; the primary loss for these families had been the death of the husband and father, which became the primary admission criteria. Thus, the need for services seemed particularly acute in families where the father had been lost, as has been documented in other disasters (Gurwitch et al., 2002).

Twenty families who met the criteria were identified by individual therapists, schools, and the agencies providing support services to 9/11 families. They were contacted by telephone in late January 2002 by one of the group's leaders. She explained the purpose of the groups as providing information and support to assist the family in managing its loss and inquired about the family's level of interest. All of the contacted families were receptive to the program, but three of them felt too overwhelmed with the single parenting of very young children to take on another activity at the time the groups were being offered. With the remaining families, the leader ascertained the number and ages of the children, whether the family was involved in any type of counseling or receiving formal support services, and how the children were performing in school. Although minimal information was obtained in these phone conversations, most of these discussions lasted for more than an hour as each woman told the leader her personal 9/11 story. An unintended positive consequence of this telephone outreach was that the leader was able to personally engage these women. Thus, when they arrived at the first group, they were already feeling some sense of connection. Seventeen adults with 27 children, ages 5 to 15, signed up for the first group series.

Group membership was closed after the first session, although preregistered families who were unable to attend that session were included in subsequent ones as long as they were able to attend session two. The leaders stressed the importance of attendance at each session. Because of the sudden nature of the losses on 9/11, the leaders were sensitive to the impact of unexplained absences, especially on the younger children. If

a family could not attend a session, the leaders would contact the family member who was in their group to explain what had happened during the missed session. This outreach served to reinforce group cohesion, and the younger children in particular were usually surprised and pleased to get such a call from the "grown-up" leaders.

An aspect of group structure that is perhaps related to group composition (i.e., families struggling to regain homeostasis after a devastating event) was a need for continuing outreach. Many of the participating families had contact with the group leaders between sessions, especially during the first series. They brought questions related to their children's' adjustment, school-related dilemmas, and the need for validation in the face of the continuing demands of the trauma. Although it was not an intentional aspect of the initial group design, this outreach component seemed to be very helpful in maintaining the group's continuity and in expanding the families' support networks.

Staff

Because there was no funding base for the initial program, staffing was provided by volunteer mental health practitioners who were recruited from a variety of settings, including schools, mental health centers, hospitals, and private practice. The recruits were, in general, well qualified and had some level of prior experience with trauma and crisis intervention with youth, as well as skill in leading groups. September 11, however, was a daunting and unprecedented event that required an as yet unknown set of intervention skills. Thus the high degree of experience and expertise in the recruitment criteria perhaps reflected the need to generate confidence in the project through the combined experience base of the staff. Table 21.1 outlines the specific characteristics of staff members involved in the first group series.

Staff recruitment also considered the ideal leadership paradigm for each group. A developmental perspective was utilized in selecting female leaders for the prekindergarten group to provide some of the maternal nurturing that may have been compromised by the mothers' grief. The leaders used a systemic perspective in selecting both a male and a female leader for the elementary, middle, and high school groups. Because all of the participants had experienced the death of a father, the leaders felt a male presence was essential to counterbalance the

Table 21.1. Characteristics of staff: First group series

Group Role	Training	Age	Sex	Years of Professional Experience
Project coordinator	MSW	50+	F	35
Leader: adults	Professional counselor, hospice volunteer	50+	F	10
Leader: adolescents	Professional counselor, marriage & family therapist	40+	F	25
Coleader: adolescents	Doctor of psychology	50+	M	35
Leader: latency	School psychologist, professional counselor	40+	M	20
Coleader: latency	Professional counselor	40+	F	5
Leader: early kids	Professional counselor	40+	M	20
Coleader: early kids	Professional counselor	40+	F	3
Leader: pre-K	MSW	30+	F	12
Coleader: pre-K	MSW	30+	F	10
Interns	Social work, professional counseling	20+	F	3, 5
Volunteers	Education, business, homemakers, high school students	16–50	M (4); F (3)	

father loss in the family system. In the adult group, which was composed of young widows, female leaders were the choice to model the female paradigm shift from nurturer to nurturer/provider in support of the reconstituted matriarchal, single-parent family.

The project leaders also attempted to balance older staff with younger assistants, whom the children would not view as parent figures. Volunteers who ranged in age from senior citizens to high school students rounded out the staffing picture, which modeled an extended family system. In the groups with the youngest children, each group member would be paired with an assistant who was available to help that child with activities, especially those that required writing or drawing. This assistant also helped with bathroom breaks or, if the child experienced any separation anxiety at all, took the child on short trips to see the youngster's mother. Because many of these families had children below the age of three, staff members also had to be available for babysitting. The most successful babysitters were high school boys, who seemed to energetically manage the tired children at the end of the day, and these youngest children would often be the first members of their families to arrive in the group room each week, eagerly looking for their "sitters."

Although the leaders preferred that the volunteers maintain the same assignments each week, reassignment was considered under some circumstances. The leaders anticipated that the content of the adult group's discussion would challenge the ability of the leaders and volunteers to remain open and empathic to the intensity of feelings expressed by group members without becoming personally overwhelmed. In pregroup interviews, potential members were quite clear about their frustration when people to whom they told their stories began to cry or respond emotionally. This response made them feel as if they had to take care of the other person's feelings and that they could no longer talk about themselves. "This is worse than unhelpful," one woman stated. Unfortunately, during the first session, one of the volunteers in the adult group had trouble containing her feelings, getting tears in her eyes as the group members told their stories. Unsurprisingly, the group process became restrained and stilted. In a private debriefing the leaders spoke with the volunteer and decided the group's needs would be best served if she were moved to one of the children's groups. The change was announced at the next session. The explanation given was that, although the tragedy had created lots of helping roles, it sometimes took time to determine where a person could make the best contribution. The careful consideration of the timing of the group, the staff members' qualifications, and the participants' developmental needs also reflect evidence-based principles of effective prevention programs (Nation et al., 2003) and recommendations for support groups after a community disaster (Dembert & Simmer, 2000).

Program Design

The initial planning meetings, held in a local school, began in January 2002. They focused on the staff's personal reactions to 9/11 and its sequelae before exploring perceived needs for services. The project leaders felt that it was critical for staff members to recognize their reactions and feelings at every step of the process to mitigate against the "compassion fatigue" so commonly associated with trauma work (Figley, 1999). To emphasize this point, strategies for self-care were discussed over a meal before the discussion about the needs of the targeted community even began. Moreover, in this situation, in which the leaders themselves were members of the affected community, personal reflection and processing were vital. There was a continued focus on the feelings and reactions of the project staff at every step of the project development to ensure as much objectivity as possible in responding to the participants' articulated needs.

When a myriad of opportunities arose for qualified mental health professionals to assist in support activities at Ground Zero, the leaders made a conscious choice to limit the scope of the project to assisting survivor families in their natural community settings. The leaders felt that providing services at Ground Zero would compromise the delicate degree of emotional distance that would be needed in order to maintain the strategic posture between empathy and disengagement that is necessary for clinically sound trauma-related interventions. Finally, in recognition of the dangers of compassion fatigue, the leaders felt that any successful intervention would need to incorporate staff support and debriefing into every aspect of the project design.

From the beginning session, the leaders knew that the groups' needs would exact an extraordinary emotional demand on all of the staff members and volunteers, regardless of their previous training or experience. At the conclusion of each group session, it was essential for leaders and volunteers to review what had happened. The project leaders saw one of

their roles as modeling self-disclosure by sharing their personal reactions in the debriefings, which they hoped would encourage staff and volunteers to do the same. Staff members were also required to complete written reports of each session that included not just information about members' participation but also recorded their personal reflections on that group's content and dynamics. The project leaders would review these notes and provide feedback and consultation when necessary. Other simple touches, such as serving food at every project meeting and giving each leader and volunteer a journal for personal reflection, were additional techniques the project leaders employed to nurture the staff and acknowledge the emotional challenges inherent in this work.

Group Design

The project leaders provided the framework for the proposed psychoeducational support group interventions, which included disaster mental health, grief theory, family systems work, group work process and dynamics, and resilience, and then reviewed these theoretical bases to ensure that all of the staff members held the same frame of reference for intervention design. Using these theoretical foundations, the leadership team and staff arrived jointly at specific objectives for the project which were then divided into topic-focused group sessions that, addressed the following content areas: development of group cohesiveness; education about grief and trauma responses; identification of and attention to individual and family needs related to the traumatic circumstances of the death; encouragement of personal and family problem solving; enhanced recognition of personal and family resilience; and the development of coping skills. Activities to address each objective were then designed in consideration of the developmental skills of the specific age groups: prekindergarten (4–5), early childhood (6–8), latency (9–11), adolescents (12 and older), and adults.

The groups used activities and discussions that were grounded in cognitive-behavioral theory. By utilizing these techniques, group leaders could identify and foster relevant coping skills (Bryant, Harvey, Dang, Sackville, & Basten, 1998). These techniques included writing, drawing, storytelling, and arts and crafts. Their aim was to provide the participants with a concrete way to organize the "disorganized" experience of the trauma and death, as well as allow them to maintain as much emotional distance from the topic as they needed to feel safe (Appleton, 2000). The language of metaphors, which speaks to the unconscious and stretches abstract reasoning skills, was the choice for most of the activities in order to provide a safe approach to potentially threatening topics and to invite each participant to decide on a personal meaning for content areas (Underwood & Clark, 2004; Barker, 1985). Especially after a traumatic event such as 9/11, which shattered people's assumptions about personal and family safety, the provision of group content that reinforced survivors' emotional safety was of paramount concern (Burrough & Mize, 2004).

For several reasons, the project leaders decided to omit from curriculum activities a content area that was particularly relevant to trauma interventions. That activity was the construction of a trauma narrative (Neimeyer & Levitt, 2000). The creation of such narratives would ultimately be essential to helping participants integrate the experience and receive social validation for their account of their losses. Nevertheless, the story of what had transpired on September 11 was still evolving, and families were still learning new facts about what had happened to their loved one that day. In addition, most of the families had yet to receive personal remains, which the leaders felt was an essential element of their narratives. They also did not want a member's personal narrative to be influenced by what other group members might construct. Moreover, as members themselves of the affected communities, the project leaders—albeit unconsciously at the time—had yet to complete their own narratives, which made it difficult for them to help others in this essential task. They did feel, though, that there were enough other aspects of the trauma recovery process that the project could address to make it both helpful and meaningful for the participating families. Others have concurred with this decision. Berkowitz (2003) contends that reexposing participants to the details of the event by asking them to review what occurred is not appropriate for crisis models. Mayou, Ehlers, and Hobbs (2000) have noted that exposure to internal and external stimuli without clear and obvious symptomatology may interfere with the natural recovery process.

Each session was carefully structured to have a beginning, a middle, and an end, which symboli-

cally modeled the progression of the grief process and provided sharp contrast to the unstructured trauma experience. Sessions would begin with ritualized, emotionally nonthreatening, introductory activities that provided members with an opportunity to reengage in the group after the week's break between sessions. The youngest children recited a short reading called "Our Circle," which reminded them of the group's goals. "We have come together," it began, "to listen to each other, to support each other, to care about each other, to understand each other because special people in our lives have died and we need each other" (Underwood, Milani, & Spinazzola, 2004). Latency-aged children and adolescents began their groups by randomly tossing a skein of yarn among the members to create a "web of connection." Each week's toss was accompanied by a "question of the week," which was designed to increase group cohesiveness through self-disclosure.

Even the adult group had a ritualized beginning. Small, plastic garbage pails were placed in the center of each group circle, and the participants were given scraps of paper on which they were instructed to write down all of the "junk" that had happened to them during the past week. Each participant would stuff her weekly "junk" into the garbage pail, and it was shredded ceremoniously at the last group session. This activity was also used with success in the prekindergarten group, where the personally decorated garbage can often occupied a place of honor in the child's room. Several months after the group's conclusion, one mother reported she had observed her 4-year-old son explaining to a playmate that he used his garbage can to "throw away all the sad and mad stuff that happens." These opening rituals were similar to those in a closed-membership trauma and grief group developed at the National Center for Child Traumatic Stress at UCLA (Saltzman, Layne, Steinberg, & Pynoos, in press).

The middle portion of the session contained the material directly related to the trauma as it was addressed in that week's objectives. Personally reflective activities such as writing to the deceased or illustrating difficult feelings were balanced by the inclusion of a less emotionally demanding activity such as cookie decorating or a scavenger hunt (Burrough & Mize, 2004). The content was infused with creative activities, which the leaders felt were essential to approaching the emotionally difficult content in a nonthreatening manner (Barker, 1985). Providing an opportunity for the participants to establish emotional distance from the challenging material would facilitate the containment of painful affect. Creative techniques also helped break down complex issues and emotional responses into manageable pieces; they were selected to emphasize strength and resilience, another of the project's themes.

The thread of metaphor tied most of the group activities together. The leaders chose this frame of reference because it facilitated individual interpretation of the same material in ways that reflected the emotional tolerance and understanding of individual participants. Because specific stories that addressed the challenges of trauma recovery through metaphor were not readily accessible for a proposed family storytelling activity, one of the leaders collaborated with a personal friend to create "Adventures on Maple Street," a collection of short stories with specific curriculum-related themes. These included the use of cognitive restructuring as a coping technique, the responsibility to always do one's best despite the intrinsic unfairness of life, the importance of learning to trust oneself, the function of caring adults in the support systems of children, and the power of holding memories of the deceased in one's heart (Underwood, Milani, & Spinazzola, 2004). The stories, which were read aloud in an engaging fashion by guest speakers, served as the beginning activity at several of the group sessions in both the first and the second series to provide continuity between the curricula of the two group series. Copies of these stories were given to all of the families at the series' conclusion to encourage review of group learning, and many families reported that they had read the stories again on more than one occasion.

Having all of the families meet together for certain activities such as the storytelling or cookie decorating was included in the curriculum design so that the participants could see how they could use simple activities at home to address the continuing challenges of grief or honor the memory of the deceased. Again, even though serious topics were addressed in an activity such as how to identify and hold on to memories of the deceased (exemplified through the decoration of cigar boxes to serve as containers for tokens of memories) or in a discussion of the importance of acknowledging support system members who had provided help (demonstrated in the decoration of sugar cookies that the participants gave to people who had been helpful), they were carried out with a mixture of fun and seriousness that the leaders hoped would facilitate their replication by the family at home.

The ending of each group session was also ritualized to demonstrate how to contain the content discussed in that session and to practice the use of coping techniques and resiliency skills. All of the groups, regardless of age, made use of personal affirmations to conclude the sessions with a positive focus. For the youngest children, affirmations such as "All of my feelings are okay" or "I am special" were often combined with scavenger hunts or written on pieces of colorful paper and wrapped around lollipop sticks. The adults were provided with a list that included statements such as "What I need to heal will be given to me" or "I am stronger than I think I am" and asked to choose the most relevant affirmation to read aloud in the closing circle. By the conclusion of the sessions, the adults were asked to create affirmations for both themselves and other group members.

Several sessions incorporated closing rituals that gathered all of the families together. The leaders knew that most of the families had participated in large, impersonal ceremonies on local, state, national, and even international levels, so, in the absence of common cultural rituals, they wanted to create a more personal model of a memorial that the families could replicate at home. They were strongly committed to the importance of the use of ritual in healing and recovery (Rando, 1988). The leaders knew that, because of the lack of personal remains, many of the families would be deprived of the comfort sometimes provided by a burial site, so the knowledge of how to create personal memorial rituals in other places might facilitate their grieving. Each ritual always began with each family member speaking the name of the special person who had died and then addressing a question that was related to that session's particular theme. For example, there might be questions related to a lesson the deceased had taught the family about courage or something that remained special about the family despite the death of this important person. Music, candles, light sticks, bubble blowing, and balloon launching were some of techniques that were used to symbolize the continuing light of the family's strength and the transcendent presence of the deceased. Despite the different religious and cultural beliefs about death that some of the group members presented, these rituals were all well received, perhaps because they were cloaked in metaphor and symbolism.

Since all of the participants had experienced sudden, traumatic deaths of family members without the opportunity for good-byes, the final session in each group series was given careful consideration. The theme of closure was reinforced in the activities for each small group, which included both acknowledgements of everyone's contributions, as well as symbolic parting wishes for one another. All of the children were given small, wrapped boxes with fist-sized holes cut in the top to hold what the leaders called "palancas." The Spanish word for "lever," "palanca" was the name given to describe the short notes that participants were asked to write to each other about something they admired about that other person. Just as a lever enables a person to move something that is beyond one's normal strength, the palancas, which were placed in the boxes, could be removed and read whenever the group member needed extra encouragement.

Members of the adult groups were given "success kits," small hand-decorated boxes that included the following items: a stick of gum to help the family stick together, a roll of Life Savers candy for the days when life seems overwhelming, confetti as a reminder to celebrate personal success, a rubber band to reinforce the importance of flexibility, and a chocolate kiss for love. A concluding celebration brought all of the family members together for a dinner during which a slide show of pictures taken during the sessions was shown. The project leaders acknowledged the contribution of each staff member and volunteer, and the family members used this opportunity to express their gratitude and presented the leaders with an album of letters of special thanks written by each family.

Special Curriculum Issues

Because the objectives for all of the groups were the same, the staff was faced with the creative challenge of designing a developmentally relevant curriculum for the youngest children that addressed some of the more abstract curriculum concepts such as the importance of trust or coping with the unfairness of life. Holding a pretend birthday party during which some of the children were given bigger pieces of cake than others helped even the 4-year-olds to understand the abstraction of the latter topic. The

children, in fact, elaborated on the subject and provided a range of examples of unfairness like "when someone else plays with your presents first" or "two people give you the same present, and you really don't like it in the first place."

The activities that were chosen to help the children understand these topics were described to parents in letters that the leaders distributed at the end of each group. These letters provided suggestions for continuing that group's lessons through specific conversation between the parent and the child about the activities. For example, a letter might suggest that the parent ask the child about a particular memory the youngster had shared at the group meeting and then encourage the parent to share a similar memory. The leaders felt it was essential to reinforce the importance of open channels of family communication and thought that reviewing the activities that had taken place in the children's' groups would facilitate this. Letters were not given to the parents of the adolescents, however, as the leaders believed the teens would appreciate respect for their individuation.

Despite the curriculum's structure, a seminal point upon which it rested was the recognition of the ongoing nature of the trauma and the potential need to modify session content based on temporal events. During the course of the group series, for example, a change in the excavation location at Ground Zero resulted in the uncovering of a significant amount of human remains. The leaders recognized that the groups needed to address the ways in which the families had been impacted by these discoveries.

A staff meeting was scheduled before that week's session to process the staff's reactions to the events and to prepare guidelines for discussion, especially with the children. The next week, the mother of a 9-year-old boy reported that, when she and her son returned home from that particular session, he had climbed into bed with her, and they lay in the darkened bedroom, sharing what they had talked about in their groups. Their ability to approach the difficult subject of the way in which the child's father's remains would be handled, the mother felt, was a result of their conversations that night in their respective groups. Subsequent group series were modified to address heightened terrorist threats in the New York area, extensive media coverage of plans for the Ground Zero memorial, and the declaration of war against

Iraq. Each time it seemed prudent to adjust a session's content to reflect current events or specific trauma-related issues in participants' lives, a pregroup meeting was held so that the group leaders could process their own reactions before they processed those of the group.

Phase 2

At the conclusion of the series, the participants clearly articulated the need for additional sessions, so two special "pulsed" interventions, designed for potentially challenging times of the year such as Father's Day and the winter holidays, were developed. An additional 6-week series that used the same format as the first was also created in response to participants' requests and delivered the following fall. The age range for this second series was lowered to 3 years, both in response to parental requests for a program for their younger children and the availability of a social worker with a clinical specialty in infant and prekindergarten mental health. Tables 21.2–21.4 outline the objectives for each series and for the pulsed interventions. Since these objectives were reviewed for staff and volunteers in the training sessions that took place before each series began, the rationale for the selection of each objective was discussed in order to reinforce the grounding of the project objectives in specific theory bases.

When the second group series concluded after the pulsed intervention in December 2002, many of the participants expressed a need for additional meetings. Because their children had aged, they wanted them to be exposed to the older children's curriculum. So, with support from Project Phoenix, the New Jersey FEMA project, and the New Jersey Division of Mental Health Services, a third group series began in February 2003. The curriculum for this series expanded upon themes that had been addressed in earlier sessions and included topics such as the differences in family expressions of grief, personal and family resilience, self-care, and social support. At the conclusion of that series, the parents of the young girls aged 6–8 stated that they believed that continued groups would be beneficial for these children. The leaders had themselves observed the unusual cohesiveness among the girls and were impressed that many of them maintained contact with each other outside the groups. Consequently, the project leaders initiated a monthly group meeting for girls aged 5–11 that began in the fall of 2003.

The leaders considered the monthly 90-minute session as a pilot program to evaluate the effectiveness of this less-concentrated form of intervention. Ratings of satisfaction from the 14 participants were extremely positive, and each girl indicated she had learned at least one new coping strategy during the 9-month series. Several of the girls also reported they felt they had been helpful to other members of the group and that they especially liked meeting without boys.

Another pilot intervention that began when the GOALs series ended in spring 2003 was a biweekly adult support group. With an unstructured, open format, this group provided members with an opportunity to address contemporaneous concerns that related to either themselves or their children. The parenting of young children and the challenge of recognizing their grief developmentally were common discussion topics. These concerns, however, were frequently interspersed with conversations about the continuing retrieval of personal possessions from Ground Zero or the difficulties in dealing with the government's financial settlement, which was designed to provide the families with monetary compensation for their losses. Compensation was to be based on a complicated formula that included the deceased's salary, lifetime earning potential, life insurance, supplemental benefits, and family membership. In addition, the families were asked to provide personal information about the deceased that reflected the degree of loss the family experienced. The vagueness of the criteria troubled the women, as did the emotional challenge of gathering data to support the impact of the death on the family. They clearly welcomed the opportunity the group provided to discuss these issues with each other because they understandably felt that no one else could really empathize.

In spring 2003, Project Phoenix funded the dissemination of the project to other counties in New Jersey that had been severely affected by 9/11. They also funded the publication of the curriculum for greater distribution (Underwood, Milani, & Spinazzola, 2004). This expansion of the project required a clearer delineation of the less codified elements of the project, such as the leaders' qualifications and training, membership screening, and guidelines for curriculum adaptation.

Table 21.2. Session objectives and selection rationale for series 1

Session Number	Objectives	Selection Rationale
1. "Getting to Know One Another"	1. Develop group cohesiveness.	1. In order for the group process to be effective, the members must form a cohesive identity. In closed, short-term groups, this process can be accelerated by specific activities that are designed to help members focus on shared goals.
	2. Identify the tasks of grief prompted by traumatic loss.	2. The tasks of grief are the foundation upon which all mourning occurs. These tasks are complicated when the loss is sudden and traumatic and are prolonged for children who must experience them at each new developmental passage. Explaining these tasks to participants is helpful in providing structure and order to a process that can seem confusing and even chaotic.
	3. Identify personal resilience and competencies.	3. At a time when the bereaved can feel that life is out of control, it is imperative to help them identify the skills and competencies that characterized their lives before the loss. These resiliencies are available to help them through the present challenges.
	4. Teach the use of affirmations as a coping strategy.	4. Personal coping techniques are critical life skills that are even more important in stressful circumstances and are reinforced in each group session.
2. "Living With Our Feelings"	1. Identify personal feelings of grief.	1. The second task of grieving is to experience the feelings of loss. Because there is wide range of "normal" feelings, it's important to review and validate them. Although every member of the family has experienced the death of the same person, their feelings about and reactions to the loss will be individual and unique. Understanding these differences can be an important factor in uniting families.
	2. Review strategies for expression of feelings.	2. Problem-solving skills are often compromised by grief, so it's important to review a variety of alternative techniques for dealing with the complicated feelings generated by loss.
	3. Introduce the technique of cognitive restructuring.	3. Research shows that being able to look at life situations from different, more positive perspectives can assist in the development of coping strategies.
3. "Patching Together Our Memories"	1. Identify personal memories of the deceased.	1. Identifying and sharing memories is one way of keeping the deceased alive. Children, in particular, have memories of them that are personal and unique and may be lost if they are not highlighted and recorded.
	2. Identify family memories of the deceased.	2. Holding on to memories of the deceased is a critical step in the grieving process.
	3. Review ways to capture memories.	3. Because they are such critical components in grief resolution, techniques for preserving memories are reviewed and practiced.
	4. Learn a third coping strategy.	4. One of the important elements in a resilient personality is the ability to create a personal repertoire of coping techniques. Additional age-appropriate strategies are reviewed in this session.

(continued)

Table 21.2. (Continued)

Session Number	Objectives	Selection Rationale
4. "The Way We Were and the Way We Are"	1. Review ways in which family life may now be different. 2. Identify reactions to those changes. 3. Anticipate future changes. 4. Learn a fourth coping strategy.	1. The third task is to adjust to an environment without the deceased. Because family life may be chaotic after a traumatic loss, family members may not have taken the time to identify the specific changes they face. 2. It's important to give permission to the bereaved to identify and express their feelings about the changes in their lives, especially those that may be positive. Sharing these feelings can normalize and validate them. 3. One of the challenges that families face after a distressing loss is traumatic reminders. The anticipatory stress model helps prepare them for these reminders, especially the anniversary of the event. 4. Coping techniques to deal with changes and challenges are highlighted.
5. "Getting by with a Little Help From…"	1. Review the importance of developing a strong support system. 2. Enhance family resilience. 3. Practice coping strategies.	1. Mental health literature is clear that support systems are crucial elements for both mental and physical health. Even young children are encouraged to develop and use these systems. 2. The next task of grieving is to adjust to the environment without the deceased. Since so many changes take place in a family when a special person dies, it is important to identify these changes and how each family member might address them. Also important is the recognition of the socioemotional roles the deceased filled since these are often overlooked by the immediacy of dealing with concrete tasks. 3. To enhance skill acquisition, coping techniques are reviewed and practiced.
6. "What We Hold in Our Hearts"	1. Review the grief process and validate its individuality. 2. Explore the concept of "moving on." 3. Review coping strategies. 4. Effectuate group closure.	1. Remind each family member that the grief process will be different for each of them and that the children will continue the process at each developmental stage; community resources are available if the family needs help or support in the future. 2. Often used in an attempt to provide the bereaved with some type of consolation, the phrase "moving on" often generates anger in the bereaved. It's important for the family to articulate what the process of going on with life means to them and how they will choose to express that sentiment. 3. While each member of the family will have individual coping techniques, the family members will be given a chance to share those personal approaches and also develop some family coping strategies. 4. Because group members are coping with traumatic losses for which there was no closure, this process takes on added importance at the conclusion.

Table 21.3. Session objectives and selection rationale for series 2

Session Number	Objectives	Selection Rationale
1. "Looking Back, Going Forward"	1. Review group rules and agenda.	1. Understanding the structure of the program will provide participants with an understanding of the relevance of its content and the way in which one session builds upon another.
	2. Catch up on current status of former participants and introduce new members.	2. Structured introductions can facilitate the development of group cohesiveness.
	3. Recognize seasonal changes as reflections of beginnings and endings and focus attention on personal intentions for the coming season.	3. Recognize that changes in feelings often accompany seasonal changes; provide a context for understanding these feelings if they occur. Intentional thinking reinforces a sense of control over the reactions to seasonal and life changes.
2. "Learning To Trust Ourselves"	1. Acknowledge the violation of trust presented by a sudden or traumatic loss.	1. One of the consequences of a sudden or traumatic death is the perception that the world is no longer a safe place and that people cannot be trusted. It is important to directly confront this perception since it will impede the resolution of grief if it is not resolved.
	2. Use metaphor to enhance resiliency skills.	2. Resiliency skills are founded on the ability to trust one's intuition and to make decisions about trusting others.
	3. Identify trustworthy people in the environment.	3. Support systems are an essential element in nurturing and maintaining effective coping in the face of life challenges, especially for children.
3. "Finding Our Wings and Learning to Fly"	1. Identify the aspects of grief that seem the most challenging.	1. Identifying and confronting the challenges one faces in the grieving process can make these challenges feel more manageable. We always have more control over the problems we can identify.
	2. Develop a plan to address at least one of these challenges.	2. Problem solving, even if the solution will be implemented at a future time, increases a sense of resiliency and coping.
	3. Identify the challenges other family members have faced and negotiated successfully.	3. Validating family strengths and growth in the face of traumatic loss shifts the family's focus from the event per se to the positive ways in which all members of the family, even the youngest children, have responded.

(continued)

325

Table 21.3. (*Continued*)

Session Number	Objectives	Selection Rationale
4. "Remembering Our Joys and Celebrating Our Strengths"	1. Help families recall and name significant family times and events.	1. Recognizing that the family had a history before the traumatic death can help the family focus on its previous accomplishments and strengths.
	2. Create an opportunity for the sharing of family stories.	2. In many families, each member will have personal memories of the deceased that are not necessarily known by the other members. Sharing these stories increases the memory bank of everyone in the family and may give added dimension to the life of the deceased.
	3. Remind families that they remain intact despite the loss of an important member.	3. Families can be so preoccupied with the deceased member that they lose their definition of an extended family. Concentrating on the larger family system enhances the families' recognition of a larger base of support.
5. "When Life Isn't Fair"	1. Address the need to continue to do one's best despite the unfair things that happen in life.	1. Another consequence of traumatic loss is the recognition that terrible and unfair things happen in life. It is important to realize that unfairness is ever present to some degree. Recognition of this is a critical element of growth and maturation.
	2. Understand that life's unfairness is not personal.	2. Perceiving life's unfairness as personally directed can lead to feelings of victimization and helplessness. Recognizing their arbitrary nature is essential to healing and recovery. It is important to understand that, while we may be powerless to stop the unfairness, we always have control over how we choose to respond when it happens.
6. "Holding On and Letting Go"	1. Review the resiliency concepts covered in the groups.	1. It is important to give structure and organization to the resiliency concepts reviewed in the groups to facilitate their use by participants.
	2. Reinforce self-care skills and suggest strategies for expanding upon them in the future.	2. Self-soothing is a critical element in resilience.
	3. Bring closure to the group experience.	3. It is important that participants have the opportunity to say good-bye to each other and identify what they will carry with them from the group experience.

Table 21.4. Special sessions: "Pulsed" interventions

Spring Session: "We Are Family"	1. Create a container for family memories of the decreased.	1–3. Scheduled near Mother's or Father's Day, this special session reflects an awareness that the feelings of grief may resurface with intensity around the holidays that celebrate family. The memory of the deceased is acknowledged in the creation of "spirit boxes" and the continued, albeit changed, strengths of the current family unit.
	2. Review family strengths.	
	3. Celebrate continuing family resilience.	
Fall Session: "Seasons of Strength"	1. Provide the family with an opportunity to identify their unique strengths.	1. The change of the seasons is often a time when the death of a family member is felt more keenly. Families can benefit from an opportunity to get special support from others and from the chance to focus on their continuing strengths.
	2. Take time to acknowledge support systems.	2. Acknowledging sources of support helps the family to recognize and name all of the kindnesses the family has received in the aftermath of the death. It is also a way to help families restore a feeling of balance by giving back to others in addition to receiving from them.
	3. Celebrate their continued connection with other members of the GOALs group.	3. Acknowledging the bonding that has taken place between families during the course of the groups affirms their connections and encourages continuing relationships.

To standardize the instruction of group leaders, the project leaders used their expertise in the development and implementation of training to develop a written didactic and experiential training protocol (ibid.). This 8-hour training reviewed the theoretical basis of the GOALs Project, with specific emphasis on the process of grief, the impact of traumatic loss on children and family systems, the significance of resiliency skills as part of recovery, and the ways in which a psychoeducational support group can assist in the grief process. It also focused on leadership tasks and skills and the importance of self-assessment in preventing compassion fatigue. The training sessions always included participation in several of the curriculum activities to help potential leaders anticipate ways in which group members might respond to a particular task. The instruction was modeled after the GOALs group paradigm, with a discrete opening and ending activity to bookend the didactic content. The participants received written copies of all of the training materials for review and reference. Table 21.5 provides an outline of a typical training session.

With regard to specific qualifications, the project leaders recommended that all of the potential group facilitators meet the criteria for 'certified group psychotherapist' as set forth by the American Group Psychotherapy Association. These criteria include an advanced clinical degree, extensive experience in running groups, a specified number of hours of supervision, and certain academic courses in group theory and dynamics. Although the groups are based on a psychoeducational support model, the leaders felt that a facilitator with group therapy expertise and clinical credentials would best be able to deal with the complications of traumatic loss and its potential effects on group dynamics. The project leaders were especially sensitive to the mental health complications of grief after trauma and felt that staff with clinical training would be in the best position to make assessments and referrals for additional mental health services if needed. These rigorous standards were not, however, as necessary for group assistants, although previous experience in working with children was considered essential for anyone involved in the project at any level.

The project leaders suggested more detailed screening for future group members and felt that the best candidates for this intervention would be families who had acknowledged the reality of their loss even if their level of acceptance was

Table 21.5. Staff training outline

Activity	Rationale
1. Opening Exercise: "Web of Connection"	1. Using this activity, which is part of the adolescent curriculum, models how it is conducted. It also visually reinforces the connections that already exist between leaders by asking participants to introduce themselves by providing their names as well as one personal characteristic they bring to their involvement in the GOALs project.
2. Review of the GOALs Project: Video Presentation	2. To capture the essence of the groups as well as describe the theoretical foundations upon which they are based, participants are shown a 30-minute videotape (Shepherd-Levine, Underwood, Spinazzola, & Milani, 2003).
3. Experiential Exercise: Personal Awareness of Death	3. Understanding one's personal relationship to death and the process of grief is essential to assisting group members in accomplishing the tasks death presents to them. Participants are asked to complete a short personal loss inventory to help them assess their experience with death and traumatic events. Discussion of this questionnaire can also assist project staff in their assessment of participants in relation to their possible roles in the groups.
4. Didactic Presentation and Discussion: The Tasks of Grief and How They Are Complicated by Trauma	4. Since grief theory is one of the cornerstones of all group content, it is reviewed in a lecturette. This group model uses the "tasks of grief" outlined by Worden (1992). The work of Eth and Pynoos (1985) is used to describe some of the complications of traumatic loss.
5. Experiential Exercise: How Children Grieve	5. As a way to acknowledge and recognize the skills participants bring to the groups, a small-group exercise asks them to identify grief reactions at different ages.
6. Didactic Presentation: Looking at Death in a Family Context and Using Resilience to Heal.	6. Because this model focuses on the recovery of the entire family, the impact of traumatic death on the family system is discussed, with emphasis on a wellness model that emphasizes family strength and resilience.
7. Group Discussion: Leader's Role	7. Even though most of the participants will have had prior experience running groups, it's important to review the leader's role in this psychoeducational support group model (Underwood, in press).
8. Curriculum Review	8. Goals and objectives for each session are reviewed.
9. Experiential Exercise: Team Totem Poles	9. An exercise from the curriculum is adapted for the training to help build cohesiveness among the participants, model a group activity that reinforces family resilience, and demonstrate ways in which leaders can facilitate group process and content.
10. Closing Activity: Personal Affirmations	10. The training borrows from the groups in its use of a closing affirmation ritual.

intermittent. They felt that families who were still struggling to accept what had happened to them might be too challenged by the group's objectives, which included specific acknowledgement of the reality of the death. Because families needed at least 4–6 months after the death to assimilate the reality of the changed family structure, group membership

before this time would probably not be beneficial. Families also needed to have enough internal organization to be able to commit to regular attendance. Since parents and caretakers with extreme mental health needs, such as severe depression or posttraumatic stress disorder, would not necessarily have the reserves of emotional strength required for group interaction, the group leaders needed to possess the appropriate clinical skills to be able to make these eligibility determinations.

The project leaders also decided to expand the pool of members from exclusively 9/11 families to include families that had experienced deaths under other circumstances. While the similarities shared by the 9/11 families had initially been more profound than their differences, this had begun to fade after the second anniversary of the event. Before that time, the similarities in the experiences of the 9/11 families were so intense and pervasive that including families that had experienced losses under other circumstances was contraindicated. For example, all of the 9/11 families were invited to almost weekly supportive and/or political events; they shared the same deadlines for the filing of legal papers and other documents related to the disaster; and many of them were consistently retraumatized by the continuing media coverage of the event. After the second anniversary, most of the families had settled into a new routine with fewer disaster-related interruptions. Their issues and challenges began to share commonalities with families that had experienced death under other circumstances, and the leaders felt that all of the families could benefit from the perspective of varied losses.

The project leaders also believed that, by inviting families into the groups that had recently experienced traumatic loss events, the 9/11 families would be integrated into this larger, existing community of grieving families, which was seen as beneficial for several reasons. First, the stigma associated with the events of 9/11 could be diminished, and the family changes that accompany any death could be normalized. Second, the opportunity for sharing various methods of dealing with the ubiquitous challenges of single parenting would be increased. Finally, the 9/11 families would have the opportunity to serve as role models for other families who were not as far along in the grieving process. Self-help literature makes it clear that this type of opportunity can assist the more experienced group members in recognizing and sharing the skills they have accumulated throughout the mourning process (Reissman & Carroll, 1995).

This inclusion of families with different loss events required minor adjustments to the curriculum. Specific references to 9/11 were replaced with more generic language that recognized a variety of loss circumstances over a wider span of time. Ob-

viously, the groups needed to spend more time on the development of cohesiveness because of the differences presented by the circumstances of members' losses, although the project leaders felt that all of the participants would share the tasks of grief recovery, regardless of when or how the death had taken place. When members who had experienced other types of loss events were finally invited into the third GOALs group series in the autumn of 2003, the perspective that other losses could provide was evident in the unanimous agreement among the 9/11 families that the new members whose spouses had completed suicide faced even more challenges than they themselves had.

Clarification of the project's community health orientation was as important to successful program replication as increased specificity in both program content and delivery. Because the GOALs model is grounded in belief in the resilience of an impacted community, replications of the project needed to validate and involve both formal and informal community resources and be congruent with belief in that community's inherent strengths. The project leaders were aware that a degree of territoriality often existed in community agencies that had received funding for trauma-related services and believed it was important to make this up-front acknowledgement to other communities interested in replication. Making sure that input from these divergent sources was included in project planning might mitigate some of the negative impact of community competition.

Project Replication

With support from the Emergency Management Office of the New Jersey Division of Mental Health and Hospitals, leader training sessions were carried out in the spring of 2003 in the seven New Jersey counties most affected by 9/11: Essex, Bergen, Morris, Somerset, Monmouth, Union, and Passaic. More than 65 mental health practitioners from a variety of professional disciplines were trained in the GOALs model. Four of the participating counties subsequently went on to conduct their own groups, with GOALs staff providing supervision and technical assistance throughout each series. These groups exhibited some cultural diversity, but the affected population in the service areas remained mostly Caucasian. In the counties that tried unsuccessfully to launch programs, most of the reported challenges and difficulties were the result of political turf issues that had developed among agencies providing 9/11 relief. Thus, while expansion of service delivery was not universal, having a cadre of trained professionals met a critical component of New Jersey's strategic commitment to increasing the knowledge and skills of mental health practitioners as they relate to the impact of traumatic loss events on children and families.

In addition, project staff provided training on the GOALs model to a variety of agencies and organizations within the New York metropolitan area, including the counseling department of the Fire Department of the City of New York, the trauma team of St. Vincent's Hospital, the New Jersey chapter of the National Association of Social Workers, and the interfaith council of the Jersey City mayor's office. The instruction reviewed the theoretical basis of the project, outlined the objectives and curriculum, and provided suggestions for the adaptation of the material to local needs. Training also covered the ways in which the program could address issues of cultural diversity. Project leaders held the perspective that, despite cultural and ethnic differences in the expression of grief, the feelings generated in the grief process were as universal as was its impact on the daily functioning of the family. Because these universal issues were at the project's core, minor adjustments in activities would facilitate respect for differing ethnic approaches to death.

Phase 3

Continuing and Unmet Needs

The final phase of the GOALs project acknowledges the importance of ending direct services such as the groups in a way that integrates the traumatic experiences and the lessons learned from them into the life of the larger community (Van den Eynde & Veno, 1999). To this end, the project leaders reviewed what they considered to be unmet community needs, as well as the development of specific interventions that would reflect the empowerment and resilience of the affected families and communities.

The families themselves stated what they considered to be their continuing needs for service. With several types of formal support having been withdrawn in what disaster mental health experts refer to as the "disillusionment stage" of trauma

recovery, many of the families reported feelings of abandonment and voiced concerns about having to continue the process of recovery on their own. They still faced decisions about the disposal of remains, legal and financial questions, and the evolving impact of single-family life.

In particular, the members in the biweekly women's group stated that the government's financial settlement was an aspect of their recovery that has carried significant and unexpected negative consequences. To a one, the group members reported feeling "stigmatized" and "judged" by what outsiders seemed to feel was their instant status as millionaires. "The minute a stranger hears I'm a 9/11 widow," one woman reported, "the typical comment I hear is 'you may not have your husband, but at least you're financially well off for life.'" Public misinformation about the settlements, which had been discussed for months in the media, had also contributed to what several widows described as a "backlash against us." "People think we all got six million dollars," another woman complained, a figure that was frequently cited in the press as the amount of the largest settlement.

Unfortunately, these settlements also created a chasm that these widows felt separated them from people who experienced losses under other circumstances. They described feeling guilty in other support groups because they knew that people with other types of losses often found their standard of living changed by the death of the family's breadwinner. They expressed strong sentiments about having continued access to the peer support of their group and began to explore ways to continue meeting when the GOALs program concluded.

When a spouse began dating, other families found themselves coping with the impact on the family. The developmental manifestations of grief in the growing children was another topic of increasing concern. In addition, a population that had not been addressed in the existing GOALs model or in any other formally provided support services included members of the extended family, who often reported to their 9/11 FEMA advocates that they felt excluded and unrecognized for their losses. Even the group process within the GOALs series had reflected this same sense of disenfranchisement by the relatives, which often had a negative impact on the nuclear family. Surviving spouses reported tensions with in-laws, and children often mentioned the paternal grandparents and other relatives with whom they were no longer in contact. An important project direction, it seemed, would be the provision of a supportive and healing forum that brought all of the family members together. The project leaders considered arranging half-day programs called "Days of Helping and Healing," which would present guest speakers to address the challenges to family reconciliation occasioned by traumatic loss.

The final area of direct service need that had been previously unmet was continuing support services for boys between the ages of 5 and 11. Because the monthly pilot groups had been limited to girls, parents requested that this program be expanded to include the boys as well.

In the larger community, the project leaders felt that educators in the primary and secondary schools in the service area were ill equipped to recognize or manage the manifestations of long-term grief in children. It seemed critical to provide training to help these teachers distinguish the symptoms of grief from normal developmental changes in order to increase their capacity to become active partners in longer-term recovery. There also seemed to be a need to alert teachers to curriculum material that might create trauma or loss reminders and thereby compromise the learning of affected students. Table 21.6 shows an outline of the specific interventions the leaders designed to address these needs.

Evaluation

While the planners sought to derive the intervention from their experience with conceptually and empirically grounded approaches, a substantial evaluation component was not associated with the intervention. In fact, attempts to evaluate the intervention may be considered a case study of issues in the evaluation of a grass-roots response to an unprecedented event. The initial GOALs groups started in the spring of 2002, and the planners focused on the timely development of an appropriate response. Hence, as with many community-based interventions, evaluation was not built in from the start. Also, the initial intervention was considered a pilot and thus not at an evaluable level (Wholey, 1979). Moreover, aside from participant feedback, the imposition of evaluation was considered culturally insensitive in that context.

Before the fall of 2003, GOALs staff members consulted with a national expert on the evaluation of prevention programs who attempted to locate funding for program evaluation. Her contacts declined due to concerns about the lack of control groups and the fact that the program had started before the development of a research protocol. A local evaluator was subsequently retained who attempted to employ psychometrically sound measures to assess the impact of the groups. Initially, the Behavior Assessment System for Children (BASC) (Reynolds & Kamphaus, 1992) was administered during the fall of 2003 in response to the mothers' expressed concerns about their children's current levels of adjustment. Results from the BASC did not reveal any significant clinical symptomatology among the respondents. This result is in line with previously reviewed findings on the lack of pathology in children and families' reactions to trauma (Bonanno, 2004; Joshi & Lewin, 2004; Padgett, 2002).

Subsequently, the State Hope Scales for Children (Snyder et al., in press) and Adults (Snyder et al., 1996) were selected as having sound psychometric properties and measuring a proposed impact of the GOALs program: an increase in hope expressed as a sense of ability to initiate and sustain action toward a desired goal. These measures were administered to a group of participants before and after the spring of 2004 in a six-session program for 20 children and 17 adults. There were significant increases in hope for both children ($t = 3.04$, $p < .007$) and adults ($t = 4.00$, $p < .001$). Because of a lack of control groups, this provided limited support for the proposed program logic.

For the program staff, the ongoing observations of and feedback from group members, while not empirical data, reinforced the importance of the program. From the parent who reported that his 4-year-old daughter would read from her box of palancas before bedtime every night to the teenaged girl who wore her "web of connection" bracelet until it fell off her wrist, stories of how the lessons have been incorporated into the participants' everyday lives continued to surface months after the formal groups had ended. One anecdote in particular seems to capture the intention that was central to the project's creation. A 9-year-old girl had been introduced to the monthly groups in November 2003. Quiet and shy and still recovering from her mother's death, the group leaders were unsure of what she took away from the sessions. Several days after the girl's attendance at her third session, the

Table 21.6. Phase 3 activities

Identified Need	Intervention	Rationale
Adults		
1. Support for widows and widowers 2. Information about the complicated grief process for adults 3. Information about the impact of grief on children 4. Recognition of the permanent impact of 9/11 on the family system 4. Enhancement of coping skills	Continuation of biweekly community-based support and psychoeducation groups that began meeting in January 2004. The first group meets during the day, while the second group meets in the evening to accommodate working parents. The groups will use following techniques: • creative activities (e.g., writing, art) • bibliotherapy and handouts; consultation with group leaders • discussion and handouts • review of cognitive behavioral techniques	Using an empowerment theory of community intervention, these support groups recognize the importance of providing continuing support to those families who suffered losses on 9/11. Techniques in the group recognize the resilience of the participants and use cognitive techniques to address some of the challenges created by complicated bereavement.
Boys aged 6–11		
1. Support to normalize the grief process 2. Information about grief 3. Strategies to facilitate the mourning process 4. Enhancement of coping skills	Biweekly community-based support group, with male and female coleaders who use the following techniques: • creative activities (e.g., writing, art, exercise, storytelling, music) • cognitive techniques such as cognitive restructuring	This biweekly group series is the companion to a similar series for young girls. It prepares children for some of the continuing challenges in the grief process through education and problem solving, reinforces the use of cognitive behavioral techniques to enhance coping, and strengthens support systems.
Family units		
1. Family support at challenging times of the year 2. Opportunity for reconnection with other group members	"Family Days" Continuation of special programs held at selected intervals that bring families together to engage in creative activities, reinforce family strengths, and recognize the deceased as a continuing part of family life. Activities include creative art projects, writing exercises, meals, and special rituals to honor the deceased.	Strategically timed interventions allow families to practice skills learned during group series and provide an opportunity for families to share an activity that incorporates the memory of the deceased.

Entire family

1. Opportunity to increase feelings of connection between extended family and nuclear family members

2. Opportunity for extended family members to join in healing activities

"Days of Helping and Healing"

Four workshops with guest speakers address issues related to grief and transcendence, spirituality, the importance of respecting differences in grieving styles, personal strategies for accessing healing energy, and adjusting to the changes in family structure and functioning. Participants also form small groups based on their role in the family (sibling, parent, widow, etc.) to receive individualized support and an opportunity to discuss the impact of their loss within their perspective in the family system. Participants complete needs assessments to determine additional topics for future discussion.

Traumatic deaths can fracture family systems, creating challenges in role functioning and communication patterns. In particular, the inequities of formal support provided to different types of family members after 9/11 added to family tension and dysfunction. These workshops will bring all of the family members together to explore neutral topics that can assist in family recovery.

Educators

1. Accurate information about the grieving process in children, especially as it relates to developmental differences

2. Practical strategies to facilitate grief work within their limited range of responsibility

3. Knowledge about ways in which to access additional school and community resources

4. Recognition of the ways in which regular curriculum can create trauma and/or loss reminders and strategies to address these reminders in the classroom

"Train the Teachers"

Half-day workshops are offered to educators to address these identified needs. Workshops use didactic information, video material, and interactive exercises to accomplish learning objectives.

Teacher focus groups generate examples of curriculum reminders. A short pamphlet is written and distributed to all local schools that summarizes the groups' findings and addresses educator remediation strategies.

Since children spend most of their structured time within the school setting, educators are on the front line to provide appropriate support and identify potential problems. Educator empowerment is always facilitated through the provision of information.

leader received a phone call from the child's aunt, who related the following story: "We were out running errands, when, out of the blue, my niece began talking about the kind of car she wanted to drive when she grew up. She even said she knew what she wanted to have on a personalized license plate. When I asked her what she wanted, my niece responded, 'GOALs. That means "going on after loss," and that's what I'm doing: going on after loss.'"

Summary and Conclusions

This chapter has described the development, implementation, modification, and dissemination of community-based psychoeducational programs for families that lost their fathers in the 9/11 terrorist attacks on New York City. The urgent need to respond to the community-wide impacts of this event precluded the application of an orderly, deductive, laboratory-based methodology. As a result, the GOALs program, a grass-roots intervention, drew upon its creators' extensive experience in the development and provision of community-based interventions that apply existing clinical principles and related empirical findings. As such, this program incorporated nearly all of the essential components of the current knowledge as identified by reviews of family and group interventions in response to terrorism and community violence (Gurwitch et al., 2002; Saltzman et al., in press) and trauma (Catherall, 2004; Klein & Schermer, 2000); evidence-based prevention programs for youth (Nation et al., 2003); family strengthening and resilience (Kumpfer & Alvarado, 2003); and research on mediators of effective group approaches (Buchele & Spitz, 2004) (exceptions were mainly the exclusion of some of the clinical, indicated interventions). For example, research on group processes (Bloch & Crouch, 1985; Worchel, 1994), has concluded that factors such as universality, altruism, and vicarious learning affect group outcomes. Saltzman et al. (in press) have cited studies involving traumatized adolescents in high-crime communities in Southern California (Saltzman et al., 2001a, 2001b), in postwar Bosnia (Layne et al., 2001), and in the domestic school-based application of the program (Saltzman et al., 2001a, 2001b), as providing evidence of the effectiveness of the UCLA Trauma/Grief Group Psychotherapy Program. Although these programs are intended for youths who are evidencing significant stress reactions, they share many elements with the Family GOALs project.

References

Appleton, V. (2000). Avenues of hope: Art therapy and the resolution of trauma. *Art Therapy: Journal of the American Art Therapy Association, 19*(1), 6–13.

Barker, P. (1985). *Using metaphors in psychotherapy.* New York: Brunner-Mazel.

Berkowitz, S. J. (2003). Children exposed to community violence: The rationale for early intervention. *Clinical Child and Family Psychology Review, 6,* 293–302.

Bloch, S., & Crouch, E. (1985). *Therapeutic factors in group psychotherapy.* New York: Oxford University Press.

Bonanno, G. A. (2004). Loss, trauma, and human resilience: Have we underestimated the human capacity to thrive after extremely aversive events? *American Psychologist, 59,* 20–28.

Bryant, R. A, Harvey, A. G., Dang, S. T., Sackville, T., & Basten, C. (1998) Treatment of acute stress disorder: A comparison of cognitive-behavioral therapy and supportive counseling. *Journal of Consulting and Clinical Psychology, 66,* 862–866.

Buchele, B. J., & Spitz, H. I. (Eds.). (2004). *Group interventions for treatment of psychological trauma.* New York: American Group Psychotherapy Association.

Burrough, C., & Mize, D. (2004). Ongoing, long-term grief support groups for traumatized families. In N. B. Webb (Ed.), *Mass trauma and violence: Helping families and children cope* (pp. 142–166). New York: Guilford.

Butcher, J. A., & Maudal, G. R. (1976). Crisis intervention. In I. B. Weiner (Ed.), *Clinical methods in psychology* (pp.591–648). New York: John Wiley.

Catherall, D. R. (Ed.). (2004). *Handbook of stress, trauma, and the family.* New York: Brunner-Routledge.

Cook, A. S., & Dworkin, D. S. (1992). *Helping the bereaved.* New York: Basic Books.

Curry, C. (2002). *Keeping your kids afloat when it feels like you're sinking.* Ann Arbor: Servant.

Dembert, M. L., & Simmer, E. D. (2000). When trauma affects a community: Group interventions and support after a disaster. In R. H. Klein & V. L. Schermer (Eds.), *Group psychotherapy for psychological trauma* (pp. 239–264). New York: Guilford.

Dunst, C. J., Trivette, C. M., & Deal, A. G. (1988). *Enabling and empowering families: Principles and* guidelines for practice. Cambridge, MA: Brookline Books.

Eth, S., & Pynoos, R. S. (1985). *Post-traumatic stress disorder in children.* Washington, DC: American Psychiatric Press.

Figley, C. (1999). Compassion fatigue: Toward a new understanding of the costs of caring. In B. Stamm (Ed.), *Secondary traumatic stress: Self-care issues for clinicians, researchers, and educators* (pp. 3–29). Towson, MD: Sidran Press.

Galea, S., Ahern, J., & Resnick, H. A. (2002). Psychological sequelae of the September 11 terrorist attacks in New York City. *New England Journal of Medicine, 346,* 982–987.

Gist, R., & Lubin, B. (Eds.). (1999). *Response to disaster.* Philadelphia: Brunner-Mazel.

Gitterman, A. (2001). Vulnerability, resilience, and social work with groups. In T. B. Kelly, T. Berman-Rossi, & S. Palombo (Eds.), *Group work strategies for strengthening resilience* (pp. 19–33). New York: Hayworth Press.

Gordon, N. S., Farberow, N. L., & Maida, C. A. (1999). *Children and disasters.* Philadelphia: Brunner-Mazel.

Groves, B. M. (2002). *Children who see too much: Lessons from the Child Witness to Violence Project.* Boston: Beacon Press.

Gurwitch, R. H., Sitterle, K. A., Young, B. H., & Pfefferbaum, B. (2002). *The aftermath of terrorism.* In A. M. La Greca, W. K. Silverman, E. M. Vernberg, & M. C. Roberts (Eds.), *Helping children cope with disasters and terrorism* (pp. 327–357). Washington, DC: American Psychological Association.

Harkness, L., & Zador, N. (2001). Treatment of PTSD in families and couples. In J. Wilson, M. J. Friedman, & J. Lindy (Eds.), *Treating psychological trauma and PTSD* (pp. 335–353). New York: Guilford.

Iscoe, I. (1974). Community psychology and the competent community. *American Psychologist, 29,* 607–613.

Itzhaky, H., & York, A. S. (2005). The role of the social worker in the face of terrorism: Israeli community-based experience. *Social Work, 50,* 141–149.

Janoff-Bulman, R. (1985). The aftermath of victimization: Rebuilding shattered assumptions. In C. Figley (Ed.), *Trauma and its wake: V01.1. The study and treatment of post-traumatic stress disorder* (pp. 15–35). New York: Brunner-Mazel.

Joannides, G., Underwood, M., & Kalafat, J. (1986). Families living with cancer: A commitment to life. *Health Progress, 67,* 77–79.

Joshi, P. T., & Lewin, S. M. (2004). Disaster, terrorism, and children. *Psychiatric Annals, 34,* 710–714.

Kalafat, J. & Underwood, M. (1989). *Lifelines.* Dubuque, IA: Kendall-Hunt.

Kalafat, J., Underwood, M., Fiedler, N., & Neigher, W. D. (1990). Divorce workshops: Community education for a high-risk population. *Prevention in Human Services, 7,* 89–107.

Kelly, J. G. (2000). Wellness as an ecological enterprise. In D. Cicchetti, J. Rapapport, J. Sandler, & R. J. Weissberg (Eds.), *The promotion of wellness in children and adolescents* (pp. 101–132). Washington, DC: CWLA Press.

Kelly, T. B., Berman-Rossi, T., & Palombo, S. (Eds.). (2001). *Group work strategies for strengthening resiliency.* New York: Hayworth Press.

Kissane, D. W., & Bloch, S. (1994). Family grief. *British Journal of Psychiatry, 164,* 728–740.

Klein, R. H., & Schermer, V. L. (2000). *Group therapy for psychological trauma.* New York: Guilford.

Knowles, M. S., Swanson, R. A., & Holton, E. F. (2005). *The adult learner: The definitive classic in adult education and human resource development.* New York: Elsevier.

Kumpfer, K. L., & Alvarado, R. (2003). Family-strengthening approaches for the prevention of youth problem behaviors. *American Psychologist, 58,* 457–465.

Layne C., Pynoos R., Saltzman W., Arslangic B., Savjak N., & Popovic T. (2001). Trauma/grief-focused group psychotherapy: School-based postwar intervention with traumatized Bosnian adolescents. *Group Dynamics: Theory, Research, and Practice, 5,* 277–288.

Lieberman, M. A., & Borman, L. D. (1979). Self-help groups for coping with crisis. San Francisco: Jossey-Bass.

Litz, B. T., Gray, M. J., Bryant, R. A., & Adler, A. B. (2002). Early intervention for trauma: Current status and future directions. *Clinical Psychology: Science and Practice, 9,* 112–134.

Mayou, R., Ehlers, A., & Hobbs, M. (2000). Psychological debriefing for road traffic accident victims: Three-year follow-up of a randomised controlled trial. *British Journal of Psychiatry, 176,* 589–593.

Nader, K. (2004). Treating traumatized children and adolescents: Treatment issues, modalities, timing, and methods. In N. Webb (Ed.), *Mass trauma and violence: Helping children and families cope* (pp. 30–76). New York: Guilford.

Nation, M., Crusto, C., Wandersman, A., Kumpfer, K. L., Seybolt, D., Morrisey-Kane, E., & Davino, K. (2003). What works in prevention: Principles of effective programs. *American Psychologist, 58,* 449–456.

National Institute of Mental Health (2002). *Mental health and mass violence: Evidence-based early psychological intervention for victims/survivors of mass violence. A workshop to reach consensus on best practices.* NIH Publication no. 02–5138. Washington, DC: U.S. Government Printing Office.

Neimeyer, R. A., & Levitt, H. M. (2000). What's narrative got to do with it? Construction and coherence in accounts. In J. Harvey & E. Miller (Eds.), *Loss and trauma: General and close relationship perspectives* (pp. 401–411). Philadelphia: Brunner-Routledge.

O'Donnell, D. A., Schwab-Stone, M. E., & Muyeed, A. Z. (2002). Multidimensional resilience in children exposed to community violence. *Child Development, 73,* 1265–1282.

Padgett, D. K. (2002). Social work research on disasters in the aftermath of the September 11 tragedy: Reflections from New York City. *Social Work Research, 26,* 185–193.

Pynoos R. S., Steinberg, A. M., & Wraith, R. A. (1995). A developmental model of childhood traumatic stress. In D. Cicchetti & D. J. Cohen (Eds.), *Manual of developmental psychopathology* (pp. 72–93). New York: Wiley.

Rando, T. (1988) *How to go on living when someone you love dies.* Lexington, MA: Lexington Press.

Rappaport, J. (1981). In praise of paradox: A social policy of empowerment over prevention. *American Journal of Community Psychology, 9,* 1–25.

Reissman, F., & Carroll, D. (1995). *Redefining self-help: Policy and practice.* San Francisco: Jossey-Bass.

Reynolds, G. R., & Kamphaus, R. W. (1992). *Behavior Assessment System for Children* (BASC). Circle Pines, MN: AGS Publishing.

Saltzman, W. R., Layne, C. M., Steinberg, A. M., Arslanagic, B., & Pynoos, R. S. (2003). Developing a culturally and ecologically sound intervention program for youth exposed to war and terrorism. *Child and Adolescent Psychiatric Clinics of North America, 12,* 319–342.

Saltzman, W. R., Layne, C. M., Steinberg, A. M., & Pynoos, R. S. (in press). Trauma/grief-focused group psychotherapy with adolescents. In L. Schein, H. Spitz, G. Burlingham, & P. Muskin (Eds.), *Group approaches for the psychological effects of terrorist disasters.* New York: Hayworth.

Saltzman, W. R., Pynoos, R. S., Layne, C. M., Steinberg, A., & Aisenberg, E. (2001a). A developmental approach to trauma/grief-focused group psychotherapy for youth exposed to community violence. *Journal of Child and Adolescent Group Therapy, 11,* 43–56.

Saltzman, W. R., Pynoos, R. S., Layne, C. M., Steinberg, A., & Aisenberg, E. (2001b). Trauma- and grief-focused intervention for adolescents exposed to

community violence: Results of a school-based screening and group treatment protocol. *Group Dynamics: Theory, Research and Practice, 1,* 291–303.

Shepherd-Levine, S., Underwood, M., & Cernak, M. (2000). *Watermarks: Helping children cope with natural disaster.* Videotape production. Trenton, NJ: New Jersey Department of Health and Human Services.

Shepherd-Levine, S., Underwood, M., Spinazzola, N., & Milani, J. (2003) *Families going on after loss: The story behind the groups.* Videotape production. Trenton, NJ: New Jersey Department of Health and Human Services.

Schlenger, W. E., Caddell, L., Ebert, L., Jordan, B. K., Rourke, K. M., Wilson, D., et al. (2002). Psychological reactions to terrorist attacks: Findings from the National Study of Americans' Reactions to September 11. *Journal of the American Medical Association, 288,* 581–588.

Snyder, C. R., Hoza, B., Pelham, W. E., Rapoff, M., Ware, L., Danovsky, M., et al. (in press). The development and validation of the Children's Hope Scale. *Journal of Pediatric Psychology.*

Snyder, C. R., Sympson, S. C., Ybasco, F. C., Borders, T. F., Babyak, M. A., & Higgins, R. L. (1996). Development and validation of the State Hope Scale. *Journal of Personality and Social Psychology, 2,* 321–335.

Stoiber, K. C., Ribar, R. J., & Waas, G. A. (2004). Enhancing resiliency through multiple family groups. In D. R. Catherall (Ed.), *Handbook of stress, trauma, and the family* (pp. 433–451). New York: Brunner-Routledge.

Terr, L. C. (1989). Treating psychic trauma in children: A preliminary discussion. *Journal of Traumatic Stress, 2,* 3–20.

Underwood, M. M. (2004). A protocol for running groups for complicated bereavement. In B. Buchele & H. Spitz (Eds.), *Protocols for running groups after trauma* (pp. 287–305). New York: American Association for Group Psychotherapy.

———, & Clark, C. (2005). Using metaphor to help children cope with trauma: An example from September 11th. In J. Webber, D. Bass, & R. Yep (Eds.), *Terrorism, trauma, and tragedies: A counselor's guide to preparing and responding* (pp.33–36). Alexandria, VA: American Counseling Association Foundation.

Underwood, M. M., & Dunne-Maxim, K. (1997). *Managing sudden traumatic loss in the schools.* Washington, DC: American Association of Suicidology.

Underwood, M. M., Milani, J., & Spinazzola, N. (2004). *Families GOALs: A training manual.* Verona, NJ: Mental Health Association of New Jersey.

Van den Eynde, J., & Veno, A. (1999) Coping with disastrous events: An empowerment model of community healing. In R. Gist & B. Lubin (Eds.), *Response to disaster* (pp. 167–192). Philadelphia: Brunner-Mazel.

Vernberg, E. M., & Vogel, J. (1993) Interventions with children following disasters. *Journal of Clinical child Psychology, 22,* 485–498

Webb, N. B. (Ed.). (2004). *Mass trauma and violence: Helping families and children cope.* New York: Guilford.

Weingarten, K. (2004). Witnessing the effects of political violence in families: Mechanisms of intergenerational transmission and clinical interventions. *Journal of Marriage and Family Therapy, 30,* 45–59.

Wholey, J. (1979). *Evaluation: Promise and performance.* Washington, DC: Urban Institute.

Worchel, S. (1994). You can go home again: Returning group research to the group context with an eye on developmental issues. *Small Group Research, 25,* 205–223.

Yalom, I. (1995). The theory and practice of group psychotherapy. New York: Basic Books.

22

Cultural Considerations
Caring for Culturally Diverse Communities in the Aftermath of Terrorist Attacks

David Chiriboga

Chaos, loss of control, and health fears are common after catastrophic events.
Engel et al., 2003

This chapter reviews the literature bearing on clinical interventions with diverse communities in the chaotic aftermath of a terrorist attack. In this regard it should be emphasized from the outset that no group is homogeneous with respect to beliefs, values, and psychological characteristics. While health professionals and others speak in terms of broad ethnic, cultural, and geographic categories (e.g., New Yorkers, Mexican Americans, Southerners, African Americans), there obviously are significant intragroup differences. Indeed, in many cases the differences within specific populations of interest are as great as those across groups, and possibly greater. Thus the existence of group differences does not necessarily mean that basic techniques in clinical intervention must vary by group or subgroup. The previous chapters have spelled out in detail the pervasive impact of terrorism and presented information about clinical interventions that has general applicability. For example, those most directly affected by an attack are more likely to experience a greater psychological impact, regardless of their cultural and ethnic group. On the other hand, to the extent that members of specific groups may be more likely to have special vulnerabilities, these vulnerabilities deserve attention.

A second general point, one that is similar to messages in other chapters of this book, is that caring for culturally diverse communities in the aftermath of an attack will be most effective if planning begins before any such attack. As the reader progresses through this chapter, it will become clear that the clinicians who provide interventions in the aftermath of a terrorist attack often face nearly insurmountable difficulties with linguistic, cultural, and possibly legal barriers. Such obstacles can be overcome if the provider establishes an effective working relationship with cultural and religious organizations. The latter often have very effective channels into the community down to the individual level. Since there is evidence that disadvantaged groups, who are likely to include disproportionate numbers of ethnic minorities, are generally the hardest hit by natural as well as intentional disasters (for an extensive review see Norris, 2001), developing intervention strategies that are sensitive and appropriate to cultural differences are a matter of interest.

General Considerations

As documented elsewhere in this book, there is a long history of general disaster and crisis research, going back to Tyhurst's (1957) study of natural disasters, as well as Lindemann's (1944) seminal study of the Coconut Grove disaster. In addition, Bradburn and Caplovitz (1965) conducted two national probability studies with wide age ranges both before and after the assassination of President John F. Kennedy and found a nationwide decline in psychological well-being. Similarly, Three Mile Island, Bosnia, Kosovo, the plight of Asian refugees, and of course the 1995 Oklahoma City bombing and the 2001 Twin Towers attack in New York City have all expanded our knowledge of how diverse populations respond to large-scale crises and terrorism. There is, however, one conspicuous gap in our knowledge base: A review of the literature suggests that the majority of studies focus on the aftermath of an act of terrorism. That is, they have tended to disregard the stress that researchers (e.g., Lazarus, 1966; Chiriboga & Catron, 1991) have for years referred to as the *anticipation period*.

Study of the anticipation period includes an evaluation of perceived or anticipated threat, as well as the value of preparing people for the prospect of future stress. There is some evidence that people vary in how much they worry about future threats at a society level (see, for example, Fiske & Chiriboga, 1990) but very little information about how people from differing ethnic minority backgrounds respond to the general threat of terrorism. In a study by Boscarino, Figley, and Adams (2003) of more than 1,000 New Yorkers a year after the 9/11 attack, Hispanics and African Americans were reported to be more fearful of a future assault. Anticipatory fear and anxiety may be heightened by fact that television and the Internet have made the news of worldwide terrorism much more present in people's lives.

Repeated changes to the threat level, as issued by the Office of Homeland Security, may play into the hands of terrorists by keeping a focus on the potential danger. The continuing threat of terrorism, which varies in intensity and perceived immediacy, may exacerbate the distress of those minorities who have prior experience with traumatic events, even in the absence of an actual act of terrorism. Hence, one of the underlying themes of this chapter is that careful and selective attention to community needs for information and organizational activities before any attack may play an important role in lessening the impact of an act of terrorism.

Another general question that frames any discussion of how members of ethnic and racial groups respond to terrorism concerns their prior experience. At what point, for example, does continued and/or violent acts of discrimination and persecution become the functional equivalent of terrorism? The growing anti-Semitism that has been reported in European countries might be construed as incremental terrorism, and the steady pace of cemetery and synagogue desecration may create feelings that are similar to those of a victim of terrorism. The circumstance of persons living in Palestine or Iraq, in contrast, may be equivalent to chronic terrorism. Furthermore, antagonism against people in the United States who are perceived as being associated with Islamic terrorism or any other terrorist group may create its own trauma. All of these experiences may predispose people to adverse reactions in the context of a discrete act of terrorism. With these thoughts in mind, we review the demographics of ethnic minorities in the United States and basic issues related to mental health.

Ethnic Minority Status and Treatment

The U.S. Census Bureau (2004) has provided estimates for various population groups based on its survey of households conducted in the year 2002. Because the bureau is now including questions that allow responders to endorse not only a fairly extensive array of racial and ethnic categories but also more than one category, it is possible to begin to appreciate in some detail the cultural diversity of the United States. Respondents can now say they are not "Spanish/Hispanic/Latino" or, if they are, they can check off one of four categories. Similarly, for the "race" question, respondents can check any of 15 different categories—all in addition to the "Spanish/Hispanic/Latino" categories.

While providing a more definitive view of ethnic racial mix—multiculturalism—the greater complexity can make information more difficult to interpret. For example, results from the 2002 American Community Survey (U.S. Census Bureau, 2004) indicate there were 33,768,036 individuals living in the United States whose racial identification was solely African American, but this number expands to 35,824,849 if one includes those who see themselves not only as African American but also as a member of one or more other racial groups. Moreover, as shown in table 22.1, 33,175,449 Americans endorsed being African American and were not also classified in the ethnic category of "Spanish/Hispanic/Latino." The point is that what would seem to be a very simple question of who is African American can be ambiguous. This in turn serves to emphasize the idea that one cannot take a person's race or ethnic category for granted.

Table 22.1 also provides estimates of Hispanics by three specific categories and several other groupings. Perhaps the most important information to be gleaned from the table is that 89,302,016 people (total estimated population minus the number who endorsed only the non-Hispanic white category) living in the United States in 2002 were not unambiguously "white." To varying extents these 89+ million people, some 31.8% of the entire population, represent the culturally diverse community addressed in this chapter. To varying extents the standard approach to interventions in the aftermath of a terrorist attack may not be effective with these people.

Before considering strategies for effective interventions in the context of terrorism, it is important to assess what is known about the general clinical and treatment needs of diverse communities. One of the more important themes evident in the clinical literature on minority populations is

that they are generally less likely to utilize mental health services and face more barriers to care than do populations that represent the majority culture (Smedley, Stith, & Nelson, 2003; U.S. Department of Health and Human Services, 2001).

These access barriers have multiple origins, and a great deal of attention has been paid not only to these origins but also to their clinical implications. While it is beyond the scope of this chapter to describe at any level of depth the approaches and skills necessary for clinical interventions with culturally diverse patients and communities, there are numerous excellent texts on the subject (see Bemak, Chung, & Pedersen, 2003; Council of National Psychological Associations for the Advancement of Ethnic Minority Interests, 2003; Dana, 2000; Fukuyama & Sevig, 1999; Palmer, 2002; Paniagua, 2005; Sue, Casas & Manese, 1998; Sue & Sue, 2003; Wehrly, Kenney, & Kenney, 1999). These texts document specific recommendations and issues involved with culturally diverse client populations. The most frequent recommendations include having knowledge of and displaying respect for the client's cultural heritage, providing services in the language of clients who are limited in English proficiency, and understanding how the client's cultural background might affect symptom manifestation, significance, and treatment. The issues underlying

Table 22.1. Data from the 2002 American Community Survey (U.S. Census, 2004), showing numbers of Hispanics and non-Hispanics from various categories

Total U.S. Population (2002)	280,540,330
Hispanic or Latino (any race)	37,872,475
Mexican	23,999,836
Puerto Rican	3,608,309
Cuban	1,357,744
Other Hispanic or Latino	8,906,586
Not Hispanic or Latino	242,667,855
White alone	191,238,314
Black or African American alone	33,175,449
American Indian or Alaska Native alone	1,651,069
Asian alone	11,113,311
Native Hawaiian and Other Pacific Islander alone	331,228
Some other race alone	655,179
Two or more races	4,503,305

these recommendations are complex and far reaching. As one example, the American Psychological Association's (2003) Division 17 guidelines list six principles and 12 guidelines, most of which include multiple subcategories that should be considered when conducting therapy with ethnic minority clients.

The general information provided in clinical texts and guidelines focuses on provider sensitivities as well as language competence. There are, however, a number of specific risk factors related to the minority experience that may facilitate interventions in times of crisis as well as under more normal conditions of care.

Family History in the United States

Generally, first-generation Americans are less acculturated, less assimilated, and less educated and make less use of formal social services. They are also more likely to be uninsured. Hispanics of all generations in fact are far more likely to be uninsured than non-Hispanic whites or African Americans. All of these probabilities occur in varying mixes for any particular client. For example, Cuban Americans are likely—depending on which wave of immigration brought them to the United States—to be better educated than Mexican Americans. On the other hand, in one census-based study of older Cuban Americans, more than 60% reported difficulties in speaking English, compared to 32% of older Mexican Americans who have problems with English. Cuban Americans were also the most likely of all Hispanic groups to live in linguistically isolated households (Mutchler & Brallier, 1999; see also U.S. Census Bureau, 2002). The latter phenomenon, called *linguistic isolation,* is of particular interest to health providers because in times of crisis it may be difficult to reach those who live in linguistic enclaves. When considering how to most effectively work with a community before, during, and after a terrorist attack, clinicians must consider the prevalence of linguistically isolated people in each locality.

Legal Status and Personal History of Immigration

Legal status and history of immigration are related but distinct categories. So-called undocumented aliens number in the millions and are estimated to account for approximately 25% of all immigrants to the United States (Massey & Capoferro, 2004). Coming from a diverse array of nations and countries, they live in an invisible, parallel universe when it comes to ordinary health and human services (Prentice, Pebley & Sastry, 2005; Siddharthan & Alalasundaram, 1993). For such people, participation in any activity they perceive as government sponsored, even something as simple but important as an emergency evacuation may be viewed with alarm due to the increased chance of discovery. The same fears of participation may be found in immediate family members, even if documented and legally present in the country, since they may be torn between leaving an undocumented family member or of being the cause of that person's discovery.

Personal history can lead to the rather mundane anxiety and distress of having to deal with a little-understood bureaucracy once again—a feeling that is easily exacerbated by limited English proficiency. Perhaps more critical is the situation faced by immigrants who arrive as refugees. Usually of low income and from rural areas, they have often encountered traumatic events in the process that led to their becoming refugees. And, while a great deal of attention has been paid to their clinical needs (see, for example, Bemak, Chung, & Pedersen, 2003; Miller & Rasco, 2004), many—if not the majority—have received only minimal clinical attention. As one consequence, refugees are more likely than other immigrants to be suffering from PTSD. Immigrants from Cambodia, Bosnia, and Somalia are particularly likely to exhibit symptoms compatible with the *DSM-IV* classification (American Psychiatric Association, 1994; Bemak & Chung, 2004; Chung & Kagawa-Singer, 1993; Kinzie, Boehnlein, Riley & Sparr, 2002).

Trauma, of course, is not restricted to these groups. For example, Hispanic immigrants from El Salvador and Guatemala frequently present with a history of war-related or other trauma (e.g., Molesky, 1986). Furthermore, Pantin, Schwartz, Prado, Feaster, and Szapocznik (2003) found prior experience with human-induced violence or natural disasters to heighten responses to 9/11 in a nonrandom sample of Hispanic immigrants living in the Miami area—none of whom was directly affected by the attack on the Twin Towers. Generally, it would appear advisable, with clients who have immigrated to the United States or who are members of groups that may have experienced discrimination, for the clinician not only to pay particular attention to obtaining a history of exposure to past trauma but also not to assume that, simply because the trauma occurred several years ago, it has abated in potential influence. There is some evidence that a terrorist attack is likely to exacerbate these problems, and, because many of these experiences involve aspects of terrorism, clients may be especially likely to experience reactivation, intrusive thoughts, and other hallmarks as a result of the current event (e.g., Bemak, Chung, & Pedersen, 2003).

English Fluency Versus Fluency in Other Languages

Fluency in English is probably the most fundamental aspect of acculturation (Chiriboga, 2004). Acculturation essentially refers to a person's knowledge of various aspects of the host culture, including language, what to wear, and when to get to work. Those who are less acculturated are far more likely to encounter barriers to the access of health and human services—obstacles that would almost certainly be greater during a crisis. The barriers may arise in part because so much of our health systems, including interventions designed around the prospect of a terrorist attack, are targeted to those who are proficient in English. For this reason and also because of factors such as the stigma of mental health problems, those who are less acculturated tend to be underutilizers of health care services (Smedley, Stith, & Nelson, 2003).

Social Supports Available Through the Family

The literature generally suggests that ethnic minority families are more likely than non-Hispanic whites to have larger and more closely-knit families and that these families provide a great deal of support during times of stress. On the other hand, the health professional should not assume that the family is always a robust provider of support. There is evidence that such is not always the case. For example, several studies have reported

that Hispanic caregivers exhibit more signs of depression than non-Hispanic whites, African Americans, or Asian Americans (Aranda & Knight, 1997). Further, as a result of the immigration experience, people may be left with a fragmented family that is unable to provide traditional levels of support. Due to work demands and generational differences in family values, older immigrants may also find themselves expecting more from the family than younger members can—or are willing to—provide.

Community Resources

While ethnic minorities, especially those from Hispanic and Asian subgroups, may not be linked into the usual health and human services system, they are often well networked into local community organizations and churches. For African Americans, the church is a particularly effective resource and one that may prove to be invaluable for those involved with interventions in the pre- and post-terrorism periods (e.g., Taylor, Chatters, & Levin, 2004).

Educational Attainment

Aside from persons from Japanese and Chinese backgrounds, ethnic minorities are more likely to manifest comparatively low levels of educational attainment. Immigrant populations, especially those who are older, are especially likely to have received little by way of formal education (e.g., Chiriboga, Black, Aranda, & Markides, 2002). Hence, health providers must ensure that services are provided in the appropriate language, and information and indeed all communication should be tailored to the client's abilities. Possibly the most effective strategy would be to assume that clients have received no more than a grade school education, although this creates the risk of "talking down" to some clients.

Loss of Social Status

While an improvement in status is probably not a matter of concern, those whose status declined in meaningful ways (e.g., physician to janitor) after arriving in the United States may present with increased mental and physical health risks. This issue is more likely to be a factor for the recent immigrant than for longer-term residents (Myers & Rodríguez, 2003).

Stresses Experienced as a Result of the Acculturation Experience

The relocation to a new country may produce what is sometimes referred to as "relocation shock." This disruptive experience seems to last for at most 10 years (Beiser, 1999). However, some evidence indicates that people who are relatively less acculturated—as exemplified by those who have little or no ability in English—may experience more day-to-day stressors and have more symptoms of depression regardless of how long they have lived in the United States (e.g., Chiriboga, Black, Aranda, & Markides, 2002).

In addition to these specific risk factors, there are additional factors that can strongly affect the treatment of ethnic minorities and that are also appropriate to interventions in the wake of a terrorist attack. What follows represents an amalgamation of points raised in various books and articles on the treatment of ethnic minority clients.

Cultural Identity

The health provider should not assume that, simply because clients appear to be from a particular ethnic minority group, this is the group with which they identify. Those whose racial ancestry traces back to Africa but whose immediate past traces to the Dominican Republic, for example, may self-identify as Hispanic Americans and indeed be most fluent in Spanish. Differing generations of ethnic minorities may also have different values and behaviors and self-identify quite differently in terms of ethnic minority group. Making the ad hoc assumption that someone belongs to a particular group may thus trigger inappropriate lines of questioning or unsuitable proposals for action. For example, like many Hispanics, because African Americans often hold deep religious beliefs, religious institutions can not only play an important role in their lives but also provide a vehicle for interventions (e.g., Fukuyama & Sevig, 1999; Taylor, Chatters, & Levin, 2004). However, an African American atheist might be quite insulted if the provider assumed that religion or religious groups should have anything to do with helping that person. Similarly, for geopolitical reasons, some people may prefer the term "Latin American" and would consider the label "Hispanic American" insulting.

The critical factor here is not to assume that, just because someone appears to be of a particular group, that person self-identifies with that group or behaves in ways generally associated with that group (Paniagua, 2005). It is more culturally appropriate, instead, to ask clients how they self-identify in terms of groups and whether they belong to any religious group. Of course, some people may self-identify outside of the presumed reference group and have little contact with the cultural and religious organizations one might expect. If so and if they do have problems as a result of terrorism, they may be difficult to identify and reach.

Place of Birth

More than 33 million residents of the United States were born in other countries, with the majority (more than 17 million) coming from Central and South America and approximately 25% coming from Asia (U.S. Census, 2004). Little or no information is available on their age of entrance into the United States or on their level of acculturation and assimilation. Acculturation, which involves learning the host country's language and also the kinds of behaviors suitable to the host culture, often takes years—even generations—to grow to a level at which the individual is comfortable with a new language and know how to get along in the host society. Indeed, in one epidemiological study of 3,050 Mexican American elders from five states, nearly 47% of whom were born outside the United States, more than 30% did not speak English and more than a third could not read English (Chiriboga, Black, Aranda, & Markides, 2002).

For such immigrant populations, cultural values and beliefs may interfere with mental health interventions. At the least, mental health practitioners involved in pre- and postattack interventions should be sensitive to the interpretations of symptoms made by people of diverse backgrounds. These interpretations are influenced by personal history and cultural background, both of which will also affect decisions on what actions to take (e.g., Engel et al., 2003). For example, mental illness may be viewed as a mark of shame, something that dishonors the family; such a perspective may create a barrier to help seeking and may require strategies such as labeling an intervention as educational or as partnership training rather than therapeutic (e.g., Smedley, Stith, & Nelson, 2003).

The Greater Importance of Gatekeepers

Gatekeepers are usually defined as people who facilitate and negotiate access to various resources. As such, they hold an especially important position in the lives of immigrants and those for whom literacy, education in general, and language create barriers (Myers & Rodríguez, 2003). Gatekeepers can be from organizations (cultural, religious, etc.) or can be individuals (family members or friends). Their presence may be most important when a client lives where there are relatively few people with whom that person shares cultural and linguistic characteristics. On the other hand, in areas where many people with similar backgrounds reside, the need for specific gatekeepers is usually reduced. Examples include the Chinese residents of San Francisco's Chinatown or the Cuban Americans living in Miami, where close to 70% of the residents are of Hispanic origin. Emphasis, however, should be placed on "the usual case": Under emergency conditions such as those associated with a terrorist attack, gatekeepers and other sources of information may be unavailable.

Usual Sources of Care

While people from cultural backgrounds from outside the United States may be more likely than mainstream citizens to seek alternative medical providers, they still are highly likely to seek medical care from physicians. For example, 80% of African American and 78% of Hispanic American beneficiaries of Medicare said they sought help from a specific doctor when necessary (Centers for Medicare and Medicaid Services [CMS], 2002). These percentages are lower than the 91% of white non-Hispanic citizens but still suggest that health providers who provide physical and mental health care in the aftermath of a terrorist attack should develop working relationships and communication systems with primary care physicians. Of particular concern for those charged with clinical interventions, ethnic minorities are often reluctant to seek help for mental health problems (Chen, Chung, Chen, Fang, & Chen, 2003; Leong & Lau, 2001). Hence it would seem critical to educate primary care phy-

sicians with regard to mental health problems in diverse cultural groupings.

Health Literacy

A recent Institute of Medicine (IOM) report estimates that nearly 90 million Americans have problems understanding written (and probably oral, although the research on this topic is less extensive) communications concerning their health (IOM, 2004). Health literacy problems may be found in people who utilize any language: A Spanish-only speaker may have problems comprehending instructions about their health in Spanish. Surprisingly, more than half of those with limited abilities in comprehending health information are Caucasians; in general, those who are poor or elderly, belong to ethnic and racial minorities, and/or have less than a high school education have a higher probability of health illiteracy.

The consequences can be grave: These people have been found to be less likely to use health services, self-report poorer health, and are less knowledgeable about their existing health conditions (IOM, 2004). Such findings raise serious concerns about the efficacy of preattack, periattack, and postattack information and intervention efforts, regardless of the provider's cultural competence. The findings, indeed, highlight the problems of attending to the needs of ethnic and racial minorities, who often present with risk factors for health illiteracy in addition to their minority status: They are more likely to be poor and less educated. Moreover, immigrant populations may also be unfamiliar with the way health services are provided in the United States and may therefore be less effective—for this reason alone, let alone the level of health illiteracy—in seeking help.

Language

Approximately 47,663,000 residents in the United States speak a language other than English at home, and of these, nearly 21 million have problems speaking English (U.S. Census, 2004). As an example, 13,639,423 Hispanics spoke English less than "very well," and the same was true for 7,248,604 Asian and Pacific Islanders. Age differences should be considered because elder members of culturally diverse communities may be particularly needful of help during a crisis but also particularly unlikely to receive help due to language-related problems. Among those aged 65 and over, for example, 2,340,868 individuals were reported in the census to speak English "less than 'very well.'" In addition, as mentioned earlier over 1 million people aged 65 and over live in households where no adult or adolescent is fluent in English.

Although few if any studies have considered the question of whether gatekeeper-enabled families have better access or receive better care for their members, there are numerous anecdotal reports and at least hints in the literature. In one large epidemiological study of Mexican American elders, Chiriboga, Black, Aranda, and Markides (2002) found that, where English was more likely to be spoken at family gatherings, elders also had a lower probability of reporting depressive symptoms. This suggests that, when some members of the extended family are conversant with the host culture, they may have more access to resources. In the case of terrorism, the family may be more effective in providing resources and linking elders (as well as themselves) to more formal resources and may also facilitate any intervention efforts by health providers.

Considering the statistics on English fluency, as well as the great diversity of languages spoken by those who have problems with English and the relatively low numbers of health providers who are bilingual, the task of communicating even in the absence of a terrorist attack is challenging. This is one reason the U.S. Department of Health and Human Services' Office of Minority Health (OMH), established in 1989, has developed 14 standards for what it calls "culturally and linguistically appropriate services," commonly referred to as CLAS (OMH, 2001). If implemented well before a disaster of any sort, these standards should improve the effectiveness of emergency interventions for ethnic minorities.

The CLAS standards actually consist of four mandates that are required of all recipients of federal services, nine guidelines that consist of activities recommended for adoption by programs, and one recommendation that is suggested for consideration by health care programs. Here we briefly review the four mandated standards (Standards 4–7) and three of the guidelines (Standards 1, 11, 12) that seem particularly relevant for the provision of care in the aftermath of terrorism (OMH, pp. 7, 10–13, 17, 18):

a. *Guideline Standard 1.* "Health care organizations should ensure that patients/consumers receive from all staff members effective, understandable, and respectful care that is provided in a manner compatible with their cultural health beliefs and practices and preferred language." This in a nutshell outlines what those who provide mental health services in the aftermath of a disaster should consider. In many ways these things are what any client should expect, but staffing patterns and funding for training often make compliance difficult. The chaotic conditions that can follow a major terrorist incident make a difficult task that much harder. There are, however, steps that can be taken.

b. *Mandated Standard 4.* "Health care organizations must offer and provide language assistance services, including staff and interpreter services, at no cost to each patient/consumer with limited English proficiency at all points of contact, in a timely manner during all hours of operation." This standard is a difficult one to meet even in normal times, and, obviously, in a time of crisis its achievement becomes even more problematic. The likelihood of having trained bilingual (or multilingual) staff available is low, and while the use of telephone interpreter services is recommended, the 9/11 experience indicates that the nation's telephone system is likely to be overloaded during a crisis. One part of the solution is for local and regional intervention services to form partnerships with community-based programs that serve the needs of the various ethnic minority populations. Such community partners can assist in the identification of those who might be at greater risk following an act of terrorism. Whatever the strategy developed for outreach, health providers should recognize that Medicaid and the State Child Health Insurance Program (SCHIP) provide states with matching federal funds to help defray the costs of translational services.

c. *Mandated Standard 5.* "Health care organizations must provide to patients/consumers in their preferred language both verbal offers and written notices informing them of their rights to receive language assistance services." The verbal offer component of this mandate might be satisfied by either tape recordings or—at the most sophisticated levels—by touch screen multimedia computer programs; the latter require neither language nor computer literacy and can provide spoken feedback to clients in the (preprogrammed) language of their choice (Sweeney & Chiriboga, 2003). Regardless, at the organizational level, such information is mandated.

d. *Mandated Standard 6.* "Health care organizations must assure the competence of language assistance provided to limited English proficient patients/consumers by interpreters and bilingual staff. Family and friends should not be used to provide interpretation services (except on request by the patient/consumer)." Clearly meeting this standard—again one that is difficult for organizations to comply with in the best of circumstances—becomes extremely problematic under emergency conditions, especially when the provider may be attempting interventions with people from outside the usual catchment area. The OMH guidelines specifically note that, in emergency situations, the use of telephone interpretation may be the only available recourse.

e. *Mandated Standard 7.* "Health care organizations must make available easily understood patient-related materials and post signage in the languages of the commonly encountered groups and/or groups represented in the service area." For those charged with mental health interventions in the aftermath of a terrorist attack, it might be helpful to develop basic informational packets in all languages likely to be required.

f. *Guideline Standard 11.* "Health care organizations should maintain a current demographic, cultural, and epidemiological profile of the community as well as a needs assessment to accurately plan for and implement services that respond to the cultural and linguistic characteristics of the service area." In other words, providers must be aware of the populations within catchment areas that are likely to have special needs. This allows them to plan for the provision of written and other information in clients' primary languages. One resource for planners is the information that is available at the website of the U.S. Census Bureau, where information on language fluency by county can be plotted in map format. One site of interest

provides tables on a county and state level that detail multiple categories of race and ethnicity. For example, under the category of Asian and Pacific Islander, four separate subcategories are provided (American Community Survey, 2004).

g. *Guideline Standard 12.* "Health care organizations should develop participatory, collaborative partnerships and utilize a variety of formal and informal mechanisms to facilitate community and patient/consumer involvement in designing and implementing CLAS-related activities." In typical bureaucratic language this standard lays out perhaps the most critical element in effective postterrorism interventions: the development of community-provider partnerships. Such partnerships, perhaps with local churches and minority-focused organizations, can identify ethnic minority clients. Community partners could also be trained in preattack actions such as community training and information dissemination; attack phase interventions such as quickly reaching out to isolated members of the community (e.g., those with language barriers); and postattack interventions such as identifying people who exhibit signs of posttraumatic stress, helping to connect them with providers, and providing translation services if necessary.

Considerations Specific to Terrorism

The rapidly evolving literature on terrorism has generally paid only minimal attention to how psychologists should specifically address the needs of ethnic and racial minorities. One exception is a fact sheet (2004) produced by the American Psychological Association's Task Force on Resilience in Response to Terrorism. The task force's recommendations are primarily quite general in nature and overlap substantially with the general clinical literature discussed in the preceding section. Three issues, however, are particularly deserving of attention with respect to terrorism. The first concerns the fact that some members of ethnic minority groups may be more likely to look like the people who have been identified as terrorists and therefore may have a heightened risk of being viewed as terrorists or being attacked. The second concerns a phenomenon referred to by Comas-Díaz and Jacobsen (2001) as "ethnocultural allodynia," which deals with the fact that members of ethnic minority groups are more likely than mainstream patients to present with a history of multiple experiences with bias and discrimination. This history may lead to an unusual sensitivity to situations with even a hint of discrimination. Even without a specific cause, they may feel as though others are identifying them as possible terrorists and therefore feel considerable distress even without a specific cause. And, as noted earlier, immigrants and refugees may have past experiences that can exacerbate responses to terrorism.

The third issue pertains to the significance of the community for ethnic minorities. Citing the work of Clauss-Ehlers (2004), the fact sheet of the American Psychological Association (2004) points out that psychologists who are interested in fostering greater resilience in ethnic minority communities may do well to consider the resilience of the community. By implication, actions that enhance such resilience, including inclusion of community partners in training activities and involvement of local agencies in identification of people at potentially heightened risk of adverse reactions, become particularly important. However, it is also worthy of note that this frequent source of strength may also be a particular vulnerability: Ethnic minority members who may have recently moved, immigrated, or experienced some fragmentation of family and community ties due to circumstances other than relocation may, during a crisis, find themselves without the sources of support upon whom they might normally rely (Organista, Organista, & Kurasaki, 2003; Myers & Rodríguez, 2003).

More discussion of these and related points follows. A key point to keep in mind is that not only may members of ethnic minority communities have special needs but in many cases they may also be quite hard to identify and locate, even if partnerships with organizations and leaders of minority communities are established.

History of Exposure to Traumatic Events

Several chapters in this volume point out that, for those with a history of PTSD, exposure to additional severely traumatic events can reactivate old problems (see also North & Westerhaus, 2003). When dealing with diverse and/or immigrant populations as opposed to the general population, the issue of reactivation becomes a matter of special concern since immigrants and racial or ethnic minorities are more likely to have a history of experiences with discrimination, war-related trauma, internment, and refugee trauma, as well as with the immigration process (e.g., the experiences of the "boat people" from Vietnam), which means that more than the expected proportions have either a history of PTSD or currently active PTSD (Beiser, 1999).

The Invisible Minorities: Vulnerable and Unprotected

As mentioned earlier, people who lack fluency in English often experience serious barriers in terms of access to human services. The group that is potentially most vulnerable consists of *older minorities* who have immigrated to the United States. Among those aged 65 and over, 2,340,868 were reported in the census to speak English "less than 'very well.'" In addition, there were 11,893,572 (4.7% of the population) people aged 5 and over living in what the U.S. Census Bureau (2004) categorizes as "linguistically isolated households," which are households in which no member aged 14 or over either speaks only English or speaks English "very well" if the primary language is not English. Of the latter, 1,279,432 were aged 65 and over. One must consider the barriers faced by those people that do not have family members who can serve as gatekeepers to the English-speaking world.

Even more vulnerable are the *illegal and undocumented* clients, whether younger or older. Although little information about them is readily available, it seems reasonable to assume that such people are less likely to speak English and to have access to English speakers and, further, will feel more reluctant to seek help from formal providers when there is a need. From a clinician's point of view, it is important to note that, pursuant to the Illegal Immigration Reform and Immigrant Responsibility Act of 1996, undocumented aliens qualify only for emergency medical care (see also Siddharthan & Alalasundaram, 1993). Hence reimbursement problems may accrue for any longer-term intervention. A critical point is whether extension of care is required due to the continuation of acute need.

A third group whose access to services may be seriously compromised in the event of a terrorist attack are *homeless people* in general and minority homeless people in particular. As Conroy and Heer (2003) report, Hispanic homeless people are virtually invisible—even to those who study homeless people, since this group often hangs out in locations that are different from those of most homeless people.

A fourth group, *migrant workers,* documented or not, may be invisible due to their frequent movement across county and state lines. Because of this, migrant workers are likely not to be well integrated with other members of the local minority communities. Migrant and undocumented individuals may also be more likely to reside in hard-to-serve rural areas. While more than 90% of Hispanics lived in metropolitan areas in 2000, rural areas have witnessed a dramatic growth: From 1990 to 2000 their number grew from 120% to 416%, depending on the region of the country (Kandel & Cromartie, 2004).

A fifth group at particular risk consists of ethnic and racial minorities who work in relatively menial jobs that pay very low salaries. As de Bocanegra and Brickman (2004) report, a small and nonrepresentative sample of 77 low-income Chinese workers (primarily from New York's garment district) were still suffering economically and frequently in need not only of jobs but assistance with living expenses some 8 months after 9/11. In part their continued problems may have resulted from a historic underutilization of services. Anecdotal evidence also suggests that their low incomes and precarious economic status made this group particularly vulnerable to trauma in the aftermath of the attack since they had relatively fewer options. The vulnerability arising from economic disadvantage is a factor that is generalizable to all groups, but it is more commonly encountered in ethnic minority populations.

Guilt by Association: Clinical Interventions With Those Falsely Identified as Terrorists

There is ample evidence that people from the Middle East, those who follow the Muslim religion, and even those who appear to be from the Arab world may bear a double burden after a terrorist attack. They experience not only the trauma of the attack but also discrimination and anger directed at them by other members of the community. Freyd (2002; see also Ibish, 2003) provides a number of examples of community anger directed at Muslim-appearing adults and children in the aftermath of 9/11. Moreover, Esses, Dovidio, and Hodson (2002) note that America's attitude toward immigration and immigrants may be becoming more negative as a result of 9/11, a factor that may be creating a condition of chronic distress among Muslims and Muslim-appearing people. These examples illustrate the need for preparations and actual interventions now, as opposed to after some future attack has taken place.

Therefore, in the aftermath of a terrorist attack, it would seem unreasonable to assume that health professionals will have adequate resources to provide CLAS-compatible services to all of their potential clients.

Technology and Intervention: A New Frontier

More than ever we now have the capability of disseminating information to a geographically dispersed audience in multiple languages. Indeed, soon after the September 11 attacks, a Committee on Science and Technology for Countering Terrorism (2002) was established, and it subsequently submitted a report detailing in part the potential role of technology. Not all of this role involves the use of unusual and federal resources. Along with newspapers and television, the Internet, CDs, DVDs, and cell phones are potential resources for those charged with preparedness and pre- and postinterventions. Interestingly, cell phones and beepers are disproportionately owned by ethnic and racial minorities in comparison to whites (Katz & Aspden, 1998; Wareham & Levy, 2002), although their Internet usage lags behind that of the mainstream community. Internet usage by Hispanics in the United States is increasing, in part because it is growing in Mexico and other Latin countries (Curry, Contreras, & Kenney, 2004).

The use of multiple media technologies, what is collectively referred to as the information technology (IT) infrastructure, should provide a reasonably effective way to disseminate information from international to national to state and local and finally to the community-member level. Notwithstanding the dependency of these tools on the electrical grid, which may of course be disrupted by acts of terrorism, there are capabilities that can be utilized to rapidly inform members of the diverse and geographically dispersed minority community as well as mainstream Americans.

A vital component of this effort is a more integrated, national system of command, control, communication, and information (C3I). Responsibility for the latter falls under the National Communications System (NCS) and the Government Emergency Telecommunications Service (GETS). At all levels the technology is currently available—but not necessarily implemented—to automatically dial phones (land based as well as cell) with information about appropriate actions to take in the case of an attack—in the language of the call receiver. This type of service therefore has the potential of becoming an invaluable tool for first responders, who must deal with the immediate impact of a catastrophic terrorist attack, since calls in the language of the receiver could be sent not only to individuals but also to agencies that serve minority communities. Indeed, there is evidence that such automated telephone emergency systems can also be used as an information-dissemination tool prior to the emergency (Rich & Conn, 1995). Full implementation of a language translation emergency system, while deemed critical by the Committee on Science and Technology for Countering Terrorism (2002) is still estimated to be perhaps 3 years from deployment. One major drawback is the host of agencies, from federal to local, that not only are involved but also often have competing or conflicting needs.

At the regional and local level, emergency response agencies often maintain and use the basic technologies to warn citizens in a defined area of pending disasters such as floods or hurricanes. For example, Linn County, Iowa, has adapted a geographic information system (GIS), formerly used to map mundane things such as trees and fire hydrants, as part of its metropolitan evacuation plan. With cooperation from the local Red Cross, all of the county's citizens were sent postage-paid cards, with which the citizens supplied information about special needs in case of an emergency evacuation (Linn County is home to a nuclear power plant, whose proximity prompted concerns with evacuation procedures).

By providing information on language problems and identifying other culturally related needs, the procedures implemented in Linn County could readily become part of the larger national programs being developed. The bottom line is that providing the agencies at all levels of government with appropriate information on the necessary and appropriate psychological interventions for its diverse citizenry and also incorporating local minority-oriented religious and secular organizations would be helpful in preevent and immediate-event interventions. This step should be a priority for those who are concerned about psychological interventions with a culturally and ethnically diverse population.

At the level of postattack, the need shifts from informing the population of minorities at risk and learning more about who and where they live to the issue of providing mental health intervention. If location strategies and community partnerships have been developed, communication with community partners and potential patients becomes paramount. Given the great number of potential languages, as well as the fact that the providers may be called to areas outside their own catchment, interpretation becomes an issue. If community partners have undergone training in the ethics and health terminology, they may be an appropriate resource. In addition, it would be advisable to develop collaborations, before the fact, with the telephone services that have historically been used to provide interpretative services in medical settings.

There is evidence that such services are effective, although they may substantially increase the amount of time required for a clinical session (Oviatt & Cohen, 1992). Historically, the AT&T Language Line (http://www.languageline.com) has been the largest provider. While it has already been mentioned that, during an attack, the availability of telephone systems may be temporarily compromised, psychological interventions requiring interpretation (other than alerts and advisories) would generally occur at a time when phone service would generally be restored. It is in this context—the first week following an attack—that clinicians would presumably begin to face an urgent demand for interpretative services. There are several models that might guide those charged with developing intervention services. One example is that developed by the Center for Immigrant Health at New York University School of Medicine. This program is a comprehensive one that includes screening and training (with a 48-hour course on interpretation and a course in medical translation) of potential interpreters, as well as a train-the-trainer program. They have also tested the efficacy of a "remote-simultaneous medical interpreting system."

Planning for the Future

One of the long-term needs is for well-designed research that can guide preattack, attack, and postattack planning that is linguistically and culturally appropriate to a diverse clientele. Clearly, psychological response and intervention with diverse populations has not explicitly been a high priority in disaster planning (Butler, Panzer, & Goldfrank, 2003). At the same time, there is no reason such interventions should not exist. For example, the stated purpose of the Federal Emergency Management Agency (FEMA) is "teaching people how to get through a disaster . . . helping equip local and state emergency preparedness . . . coordinating the federal response to a disaster . . . making disaster assistance available to states, communities, businesses and individuals . . . training emergency managers" (http://www.fema.gov/about/what.shtm). The FEMA webpage also speaks of "the life cycle of disasters" and psychological interventions with vulnerable populations, among whom ethnic minority groupings figure prominently.

Federal and State Responses

There is general agreement at state and federal levels that effective interventions for community health should take place before a terrorist attack occurs. Engel et al. (2003; see also Freedy, Shaw, Jarrell, & Masters, 1992) propose a stepped population-based model of clinical intervention that begins with preattack intervention strategies that include screening for those at heightened risk, as well as general surveillance of how communities are coping at all stages of an attack. At a broader level, a model called the "Haddon matrix" has served as the organizing factor behind a report by the Institute of Medicine's Committee on Responding to the Psychological Consequences of Terrorism (Butler, Panzer, & Goldfrank, 2003). The matrix has often been used in the development of public health interventions and helps planners

think through what is necessary before, during, and after any critical event. Given the greater vulnerability of many ethnic minority groups, especially immigrants and refugees, one value of this model is its readily adaptability with respect to working with these groups.

One key premise of both the matrix and the IOM report is the importance of preparation and of people at all levels working together. In the context of cultural issues, a clear message is that state and local agencies should involve the various cultural communities in the planning phases. These communities can in turn form action groups that can facilitate preevent preparation (for example, by hosting special sessions designed to inform people about what to do in the event of a terrorist attack). This is particularly important in the case of those who speak little or no English and whose specific gatekeepers and/or community supports may be unavailable during the chaotic days and weeks following a terrorist attack (see Table 22.2).

Another benefit of employing the Haddon matrix is that it encourages health professionals to consider responses to terrorism as a process that begins well before an actual terrorist attack and integrates activities across a broad spectrum. On the downside, cultural competence is a broad and challenging task, and, as the IOM report concludes, consideration of the cells of the matrix reveals that "the nation's mental health, public health, medical, and emergency response systems currently are not able to meet the psychological needs that result from terrorism" (Butler et al., 2003, p. 1).

The Haddon matrix focuses on what should be done before an event, in the immediate aftermath of the event, and during the extended postevent phase. These phases overlap completely with the classic stress model (e.g., Lazarus, 1966) and are also similar to models proposed by Kubler-Ross (1969) and Horowitz (1997) as interventions for people who are dealing with extremely distressing events. While the focus of this chapter is more on postevent treatment as it applies to those from diverse cultures, the first two phases also deserve attention. In particular, the IOM report emphasizes the critical importance of prospective activities, including evidence-based research, that will lead to effective preevent activities at every factor level, as well as "psychological first aid" (PFA) interventions that can be applied during the first moments and days following an act of terrorism.

Table 22.2. Haddon matrix for multicultural responses to terrorism

	Significant Factors				
Phases	Federal	State	Local	Health-related Professionals, Workplace, and Religious Organizations	Gatekeepers, Families, and Individuals
Preattack	Develop programs	Disseminate programs to local agencies, religious organizations, programs, and individuals	Implement programs that are CLAS*	Attend training programs that include CLAS	Attend information and training programs and rehearse steps to take
Attack	Limit immediate effect of attack	Limit immediate effect of attack	Take steps to reduce harm	Ensure that immediate needs of ethnic minority members are met	Cooperate with family and local agencies and identify key resources
Postattack	Provide resources	Disseminate information and provide resources	Assist frontline health professionals	Outreach to community members	Identify people in need

*CLAS=culturally and linguistically appropriate service (Office of Minority Health, 2001)

Perhaps the two most relevant findings of the IOM report, in terms of cultural issues, are that the community should be fully represented in preevent planning and that it is important to develop evidence-based training and education programs. The first is valuable because, if carried through, it emphasizes the need to include representatives of ethnic minority groups at every level of planning. Unstated but potentially critical is that the representation should include not only the major ethnic groups but also those that might have special vulnerabilities, including people of the Muslim faith and perhaps refugee groups such as the Cambodians and those from the Slavic areas, who have already been subjected to terrorism and severe deprivation. The role of professional associations such as the American Psychiatric Association and the American Psychological Association are barely mentioned.

The lack of attention to professional organizations is troubling because, as the IOM report and other chapters of this book make clear, there is a paucity of direct information on psychological interventions appropriate to any group exposed to a terrorist attack, let alone those of ethnic and minority communities. Again, underlying both points is the necessity of taking action before any event, rather than after the fact.

On the other hand, the IOM report also pays relatively little attention to the needs of minorities. Furthermore, while its emphasis on the need for an integrated and coordinated system that evolves from the federal level to that of the individual is praiseworthy, it omits what from a cultural perspective might indeed be the most critical—the international level, which, after all, is where the diverse needs of a multicultural world are most clearly seen. Moreover, there is considerable activity at this level. The World Health Organization (WHO), for example, as part of its growing concern with world conflicts, sponsors training in culturally competent responses to terrorism. One training program offers an international diploma in humanitarian assistance during periods of conflict or natural disasters (Mitchell, 2003). Underlying concerns of the WHO are the preparation of people before an untoward event occurs, the maintenance of their training, and the capability of ensuring some continuity of employment for those who are responsible for direct interventions. This concern is mirrored in the IOM report and can help to ensure that identified needs of minorities are kept at the forefront.

The Community Level

In considering how to most effectively develop an infrastructure for interventions with victims of a terrorist attack, proponents of the Haddon matrix and others generally agree that community involvement is essential. This is even more the case when the target populations include ethnic minorities, for the reasons cited earlier. By developing partnerships among its members, the community itself is empowered: Instead of being guided by well-meaning "experts" and authority figures from the dominant culture, the minority groups themselves are enabled to take charge of actions that will result in an enhanced well-being of the community and its individual members.

Primary Care Physicians

Since members of ethnic minority communities—like nearly everyone else—are most likely to turn to primary care physicians for medical assistance, the latter represent an important partner in planning and implementing mental health interventions. Emergency room staff members are also more likely to function in a primary care capacity for ethnic minorities and hence should also be brought in as partners to participate in the planning and implementation stages of programs that address the pre-, peri-, and poststages of a terrorist attack.

Invigorating and Expanding the Role of Community and Religious Organizations

Among certain minority groups, religion and religious organizations may play a vital role in aiding victims of terrorism. For example, because of their historic importance to community life, ministers and church members may be a particularly valuable resource for African Americans (e.g., Taylor, Chatters, & Levin, 2004).

Development of Training Modules

Language-appropriate modules for first responders, clinicians, and community partners would assist in the preattack preparations. Sensitivity to the needs of the minority communities is a difficult goal to achieve not only because of logistic demands but also because of the task of providing multicultural training (e.g., Strous, 2003). Training manuals and workshops associated with them will help all those

involved to better understand their respective roles and responsibilities.

Gatekeepers

Gatekeepers and community facilitators may be unavailable in the event of an attack. To a much greater extent than native-born and highly assimilated individuals, recent immigrants and those who are less acculturated may rely heavily on gatekeepers, who are most often relatives or other members of the informal network, and there is no guarantee that these people will be accessible in the immediate aftermath of a terrorist attack.

At the Level of the Individual

One unresolved issue is the question of whether postattack individual (as well as community) interventions should be tailored to the particular needs of a diverse cultural community or whether the more critical issues involve outreach and information dissemination. Marin (1999) has described steps to take in developing what he calls "culturally appropriate interventions," whose driving assumptions are that (a) behavior is influenced by culture, (b) interventions designed for a specific group will be more readily accepted, and (c) simple adaptations and translations of existing approaches are not sufficient. Significantly, Marin hopes that the targeted group would accept such tailored interventions, but he also acknowledges that it is not known whether interventions that are effective with mainstream Americans would be equally effective with minorities. Clearly there is a need for evidence-based practice in this area. With this in mind, what follows are several areas that deserve attention from clinicians and researchers responsible for planning more culturally competent interventions.

Development of an Effective Screening Tool

In order to identify ethnic minority group members who are at particular risk, we need to include screening tools that effectively identify minority as well as majority Americans (National Institute of Mental Health, 2002; Jang, Kim, & Chiriboga, 2005). A history of traumatic events and/or PTSD, for example, are risk indictors for everyone, but they are likely to be more prevalent among immigrants and refugees and therefore should at least be considered in the development of such a tool.

The Need to Develop Evidence-Based Interventions for Ethnic Minorities

Only recently has evidence begun to surface that some widely accepted strategies for postdisaster care, such as one-on-one recital of traumatic events, may not be appropriate (National Institute of Mental Health, 2002). There are a number of promising avenues to explore in this regard, including approaches that are not heavily dependent on language fluency or health literacy. For example, Shapiro (1999) has conducted a promising approach using eye movement desensitization in the treatment of traumatic memories; one session was found to desensitize memories. Similarly, on the basis of interventions with 110 trauma patients, Larsen reports that a system of memory recall coupled with eye movement tracking may be effective. Moreover, Larsen found that, in the two instances in which interpreters were needed, the intervention remained efficacious (personal communication, June, 2004).

Another intervention with particular promise for ethnic minorities may be the support group. For example, Molesky (1986) has suggested that the use of support groups with members of minority groups may be particularly effective in crises because they may replicate the circumstances of communally oriented life in Central America. However, well-crafted, randomized clinical trials and similar tests have yet to yield definitive statements of best practices for nonminorities, let alone ethnic minorities (National Institute of Mental Health, 2002). In all such efforts, a basic point to bear in mind is that one intervention does not necessarily fit everyone's needs.

Development of Evidence-Based Intervention Manuals

Such manuals should include sections on how to effectively intervene, at all stages of an attack, with ethnic minority segments of the population.

Summing Up

One of the more obvious and immediate needs underlying all future steps is the requirement for well-executed studies of the effectiveness of efforts to develop community partnerships and the determination of how in general to tailor interventions to address the needs of specific cultural groups. This of course is a rather obvious statement, given the daunting lack of evidence-based research even for mainstream Americans.

Conducting research and planning how to better attend to the needs of a diverse population is obviously not the most compelling priority that faces any local, state, or federal organization. There are many challenging and costly tasks to meet as our nation—or any nation—attempts to develop strategies to assist those caught up in the aftermath of terrorism. However, one of the unique aspects of the challenge presented by terrorism is that it affects everyone, from individuals up to the country's leaders. Because of this universal need—for planning, preparation, and actual implementation—and because our efforts in the United States are still in a relatively early stage, there is a window of opportunity to put into place strategies that can at least acquaint mental health practitioners with the basic problems of dealing with people of diverse origins.

In its most basic implementation, the Haddon model suggests that professionals who are operating at each level of the matrix should involve representatives of ethnic minority populations in the decision-making process. These representatives, in turn, should take actions that help not only to disseminate information but also to inform both health professionals and the populations in question about how to get in touch with one another in times of unexpected crises. Implementing such a procedure not only for terrorist events but also for any unexpected disaster, natural or unnatural, will help to ensure that the kinks will be straightened out by the time a real act of terrorism occurs.

Finally, it is perhaps worth pointing out once again that being able to provide linguistically and culturally appropriate care to the victims of terrorism does not necessarily require that one hire health professionals from each and every culture. Certain strategies can be utilized, at least in the short run, to transcend language barriers. Community involvement presents another important strategy, especially if representatives of diverse populations are included in planning or advisory committees. The new technologies that facilitate translation, as well as those that can provide both general and specific client information, constitute a particularly promising avenue for future development. These technologies have the advantage of placing information at the immediate service of the client and the therapist and assisting in triage and general case management. We need to keep in mind that CLAS activities, whether in the context of a terrorist attack or other clinical need, are always framed in the context of recognizing that the bottom line in culturally competent service provision is simply to recognize one's limitations and to respect others.

References

American Community Survey. (2004). *Data Tables 2002*. U.S. Census Bureau. Retrieved January 25, 2006, from http://www.census.gov/acs/www/Products/Profiles/Single/2002/ACS/index.htm

American Psychiatric Association. (1994). *Diagnostic and Statistical Manual of Mental Disorders (DSM-IV,* 4th ed.). Washington, DC: Author.

American Psychological Association. (2003). Guidelines for multicultural counseling proficiency for psychologists: Implications for education and training, research, and clinical practice. *American Psychologist, 58*(5), 377–402.

———. (2004). "Fostering resilience in response to terrorism: For psychologists working with people of color." Fact sheet of the Task Force on Resilience in Response to Terrorism. Washington, DC: Author.

Aranda, M., & Knight, B. (1997). The influence of ethnicity and culture on the caregiver stress and coping process: A sociocultural review and analysis. *Gerontologist, 37,* 342–354.

Beiser, M. (1999). *Strangers at the gate: The "boat people's" first ten years in Canada.* Toronto: Toronto University Press.

Bemak, F., & Chung, R. C.-Y. (2004). Refugees and terrorism: Innovations in clinical practice. In C. E. Stout (Ed.), *The psychology of terrorism, Vol. 2. Clinical aspects and responses* (pp. 1–26). Westport, CT: Praeger.

———, & Pedersen, P. B. (2003). *Counseling refugees: A psychosocial approach to innovative multicultural interventions.* Westport, CT: Greenwood Press.

Boscarino, J. A., Figley, C. R., & Adams, R. E. (2003). Fear of terrorism in New York after the September 11 terrorist attacks: Implications for emergency mental health and preparedness. *International Journal of Emergency Mental Health, 5*(4), 199–209.

Bradburn, N.M., & Caplovitz, D. (1965). *Reports on Happiness: A Pilot Study of Behavior Related to Mental Health.* Chicago: Aldine.

Butler, A. S., Panzer, A. M., & Goldfrank, L. R. (Eds.). (2003). *Preparing for the psychological consequences of terrorism: A public health strategy.* Washington, DC: National Academies Press.

Centers for Medicare and Medicaid Services (CMS). (2002). Program Information on Medicare, Medicaid, SCHIP, and Other Programs of the Centers for Medicare and Medicaid Services. June 2002 Edition. Retrieved February 26, 2006, from http://new.cms.hhs.gov/TheChartSeries/downloads/sec3b_p.pdf.

Chen, H., Chung, H., Chen, T., Fang, L., & Chen, J.-P. (2003). The emotional distress in a community after the terrorist attack on the World Trade Center. *Community Mental Health Journal, 39*(2), 157–165.

Chiriboga, D. A. (2004). Some thoughts on the measurement of acculturation among Mexican American elders. *Hispanic Journal of Behavioral Sciences, 26*(3), 274–292.

———, Black, S.A. Aranda, M. & Markides, K. (2002). Stress and depressive symptoms among Mexican American elderly. *Journal of Gerontology: Psychological Sciences, 57B*(6): P559–568.

———, & Catron, L. S. (Eds.). (1991). *Divorce: Crisis, challenge, or relief?* New York: New York University Press.

Chung, R. C., & Kagawa-Singer, M. (1993). Predictors of psychological distress among southeast Asian refugees. *Social Science and Medicine, 36*(5), 631–639.

Clauss-Ehlers, C. S. (2004). Reinventing resilience: A model of culturally focused resilient adaptation. In C. S. Clauss-Ehlers & M. Weist (Eds.), *Community planning to foster resilience in children* (pp. 27–41). New York: Kluwer Academic/Plenum.

Comas-Díaz, L., & Jacobsen, F. M. (2001). Ethnocultural allodynia. *Journal of Psychotherapy Practice and Research, 10,* 1–6.

Committee on Science and Technology for Countering Terrorism. (2002). *Making the nation safer: The role of science and technology in countering terrorism.* Washington, DC: National Academies Press.

Conroy, S. J., & Heer, D. M. (2003). Hidden Hispanic homelessness in Los Angeles: The "Latino paradox" revisited. *Hispanic Journal of Behavioral Sciences, 25*(4), 530–538.

Council of National Psychological Associations for the Advancement of Ethnic Minority Interests. (2003). *Psychological treatment of ethnic minority populations.* Washington, DC: Association of Black Psychologists.

Curry, J., Contreras, O., & Kenney, M. (2004). The Mexican internet after the boom: Challenges and opportunities. BRIE Working Paper no. 159. Berkeley: Berkeley Roundtable on the International Economy. Retrieved January 25, 2006, from http://brie.berkeley.edu/~briewww/research/WP%20159.pdf

Dana, R. H. (2000). *Handbook of cross-cultural and multicultural personality assessment: LEA series in personality and clinical psychology.* Mahwah, NJ: Erlbaum.

de Bocanegra, H. T. & Brickman, E. (2004). Mental health impact of the World Trade Center attacks on displaced Chinese workers. *Journal of Traumatic Stress, 17*(1): 55–62.

Engel, C. C., Jr., Jaffer, A., Adkins, J., Sheliga, V., Cowan, D., & Katon, W. J. (2003). Population-based health care: A model for restoring community health and productivity following terrorist attack. In R. J., Ursano, C. S. Fullerton, & A. E. Norwood (Eds.), *Terrorism and disaster: Individual and community mental health interventions* (pp. 287–307). New York: Cambridge University Press.

Esses, V. M., Dovidio, J. F., & Hodson, G. (2002). Public attitudes toward immigration in the United States and Canada in response to the September 11, 2001, "attack on America." *Analyses of Social Issues and Public Policy, 2*(1), 69–85.

Fiske, M., & Chiriboga, D. A. (1990). *Change and continuity in adult life.* San Francisco: Jossey-Bass.

Freedy, J. R., Shaw, D. L., Jarrell, M. P., & Masters, C. R. (1992). Toward an understanding of the psychological impact of natural disasters: An application of the conservation resources stress model. *Journal of Traumatic Stress, 5*(3), 441–454.

Freyd, J. J. (2002). In the wake of terrorist attacks, hatred may mask fear. *Analyses of Social Issues and Public Policy, 2*(1), 5–8.

Fukuyama, M. A., & Sevig, T. D. (1999). *Integrating spirituality into multicultural counseling: Multicultural aspects of counseling series 13.* Thousand Oaks, CA: Sage.

Horowitz, M. (1997). *Stress response syndromes: PTSD, grief, and adjustment disorders.* Northvale, NJ: Aronson.

Ibish, I. (2003). Report on hate crimes and discrimination against Arab Americans: The post-September 11 backlash, September 11, 2001–October 11, 2002. Washington, DC: American Arab Anti-Discrimination Committee.

Institute of Medicine. (2004). *Health literacy: A prescription to end confusion.* Washington, DC: National Academies Press.

Jang, Y., Kim, G., & Chiriboga, D. A. (2005). Acculturation and manifestation of depressive symptoms among Korean American older adults. *Journal of Aging and Mental Health, 9*(6): 500–507.

Kandel, W., & Cromartie, J. (2004). New patterns of Hispanic settlement in rural America: Rural development research report number 99. Washington, DC: Economic Research Service, U.S. Department of Agriculture.

Katz, J. E., & Aspden, P. (1998). Theories, data, and potential impacts of mobile communications: A longitudinal analysis of U.S. national surveys. *Technological Forecasting and Social Changes, 57,* 133–156.

Kinzie, J. D., Boehnlein, J. K., Riley, C., & Sparr, L. (2002). The effects of September 11 on traumatized refugees: Reactivation of posttraumatic stress disorder. *Journal of Nervous and Mental Disease, 190*(7), 437–441.

Kubler-Ross, E. (1969). *On death and dying.* New York: Macmillan.

Lazarus, R. S. (1966). *Psychological stress and the coping process.* New York: McGraw-Hill.

Leong, F. T. L., & Lau, S. L. (2001). Barriers to providing effective mental health services to Asian Americans. *Mental Health Services Research, 3,* 201–214.

Lindemann, E. (1944). Symptomatology and management of acute grief. *American Journal of Psychiatry, 101,* 141–148.

Marin, G. (1999). Subjective culture in health interventions. In J. Adamopoulis & Y. Kashima (Eds.), *Social psychology and cultural context* (pp. 139–150). Thousand Oaks, CA: Sage.

Massey, D. S., & Capoferro, C. (2004). Measuring undocumented immigration. *International Migration Review, 38*(3), 1075–1102.

Miller, K. E., & Rasco, L. M. (Eds.). (2004). Mental health of refugees: Ecological approaches to healing and adaptation. Mahwah, NJ: Erlbaum.

Mitchell, J. 2003. The new humanitarianism: Challenges for the emergency health sector to improve learning and competency. *Health Emergencies, 16,* 1–16.

Molesky, J. (1986). Pathology of Central American refugees. *Migration World 14*(4), 19–23.

Mutchler, J. E., & Brallier, S. (1999). English language proficiency among older Hispanics in the United States. *Gerontologist, 39*(3), 310–319.

Myers, H. F., & Rodríguez, N. (2003). Acculturation and physical health in racial and ethnic minorities. In K. M. Chun, P. B. Organista, & G. Marin (Eds.), *Acculturation: Advances in theory, measurement, and applied research* (pp. 163–185). Washington, DC: American Psychological Association.

National Institute of Mental Health. (2002). Mental health and mass violence: Evidence-based early psychological intervention for victims/survivors of mass violence: A workshop to reach consensus on best practices. NIH Publication no. 02–5138. Washington, DC: U.S. Government Printing Office.

Norris, F. (2001). *50,000 disaster victims speak: An empirical review of the empirical literature, 1981–2001.* Washington, DC: National Center for PTSD and the Center for Mental Health Services.

North, C. S., & Westerhaus, E. T. (2003). Applications from previous disaster research to guide mental health interventions after the September 11 attacks. In R. J. Ursano, C. S. Fullerton, & A.E. Norwood (Eds.), *Terrorism and disaster: Individual and community mental health interventions* (pp. 93–106). New York: Cambridge University Press.

Office of Minority Health. (2001). National standards for culturally and linguistically appropriate services in health care: Final report. Washington, DC: U.S. Department of Health and Human Services. Retrieved February 26, 2006, from http://www .hablamosjuntos.org/signage/PDF/omh.pdf.

Organista, P. B., Organista, K. C., & Kurasaki, K. (2003). The relationship between acculturation and ethnic minority mental health. In K. M. Chun, P. B. Organista, & G. Marin (Eds.), *Acculturation: Advances in theory, measurement, and applied research* (pp. 139–161). Washington, DC: American Psychological Association.

Oviatt, S. K., & Cohen, P. R. (1992). Spoken language in interpreted telephone dialogues. *Computer Speech and Language, 6,* 277–302.

Palmer, S. (Ed.). (2002). *Multicultural counseling: A reader.* Thousand Oaks, CA: Sage.

Paniagua, F. A. (2005). *Assessing and treating culturally diverse clients: A practical guide.* 3d ed. Multicultural Aspects of Counseling Series 4. Thousand Oaks, CA: Sage.

Pantin, H. M., Schwartz, S. J., Prado, G., Feaster, F. J., & Szapocznik, J. (2003). Posttraumatic stress disorder syndromes in Hispanic immigrants after the September 11th attacks: Severity and relationship to previous traumatic exposure. *Hispanic Journal of Behavioral Sciences, 25*(1), 56–72.

Prentice, J. C., Pebley, A. R., & Sastry, N. (2005). Immigration status and health insurance coverage: Who gains? Who loses? *American Journal of Public Health, 95*(1), 109–116.

Rich, R. C., & Conn, W. D. (1995). Using automated emergency notification systems to inform the public: A field experiment. *Risk Analysis, 15*(1), 23–28.

Shapiro, F. (1999). Efficacy of the eye movement desensitization procedure in the treatment of traumatic memories. In M. J. Horowitz (Ed.), *Essential papers on posttraumatic stress disorder* (pp. 433–457). New York: New York University Press.

Siddharthan, K., & Alalasundaram, S. (1993). Undocumented aliens and uncompensated care: Whose responsibility? *American Journal of Public Health, 83,* 410–412.

Smedley, B. D., Stith, A. Y., & Nelson, A. R. (Eds.). (2003). *Unequal treatment: Confronting racial and ethnic disparities in health care.* Washington, DC: National Academies Press.

Strous, M. (2003). *Racial sensitivity and multicultural training.* Westport, CT: Praeger.

Sue, D. W., Casas, J. M., & Manese, J. E. (1998). *Multicultural aspects of counseling: Multicultural aspects of counseling series 11.* Thousand Oaks, CA: Sage.

Sue, D. W., & Sue, D. (2003). *Counseling the culturally diverse: Theory and practice* (4th ed.). New York: Wiley.

Sweeney, M. A., & Chiriboga, D. A. (2003). Evaluating the effectiveness of a multimedia program on home safety. *Gerontologist, 43*(3), 325–334.

Taylor, R. J., Chatters, L. M., & Levin, J. (2004). *Religion in the lives of African Americans: Social, psychological, and health perspectives.* Irvine, CA: Sage.

Tyhurst, J. S. (1957). Psychological and social aspects of civilian disaster. *Canadian Medical Association Journal, 76,* 385–393.

U.S. Census Bureau. (2002). Census 2000 summary file 3, matrices, P19, P20, PCT13, and PCT14. Retrieved January 26, 2006, from http://factfinder .census.gov/servlet/QTTable?_bm=y&-geo_ id=01000US&-qr_name=DEC_2000_SF3_U_ QTP17&-ds_name=DEC_2000_SF3_U&-_lang =en&-_sse=on

———. (2004). American community survey profile 2002. Retrieved January 26, 2006, from http:// www.census.gov/acs/www/Products/Profiles/Sin gle/2002/ACS/Tabular/010/01000US1.htm

U.S. Department of Health and Human Services. (2001). *Mental health: Culture, race, and ethnicity— a supplement to mental health: A report of the surgeon general (SMA01–3613).* Rockville, MD: U.S. Department of Health and Human Services, Substance Abuse and Mental Health Services Administration, Center for Mental Health Services, National Institutes of Health, National Institute of Mental Health. Retrieved January 26, 2006, from http://www.mentalhealth.samhsa.gov/ publications/Publications_browse.asp?ID=168& Topic=Surgeon+General+Reports

Wareham, J., & Levy, A. (2002). Who will be the adopters of 3G mobile computing devices? A probit estimation of mobile telecom diffusion. *Journal of Organizational Computing and Electronic Commerce, 12*(2), 161–174.

Wehrly, B., Kenney, K. R., & Kenney, M. E. (1999). *Counseling multiracial families: Multicultural aspects of counseling series 12.* Thousand Oaks, CA: Sage.

23

The Psychological Consequences of Terrorist Alerts

Rose McDermott
Philip G. Zimbardo

Why, of course, the people don't want war. . . . That is understood. But, after all, it is the leaders of the country who determine the policy, and it is always a simple matter to drag the people along, whether it is a democracy, or a fascist dictatorship, or a parliament, or a communist dictatorship. Voice or no voice, the people can always be brought to the bidding of the leaders. That is easy. All you have to do is tell them they are being attacked and denounce the peacemakers for lack of patriotism and exposing the country to danger. It works the same in any country.
Hermann Goering, during his Nuremberg war crimes trial

On April 18, 1775, patriot Paul Revere rode his horse on his famous "midnight ride" from Boston harbor toward Lexington, warning local colonial leaders along the way that the British—the redcoats—were coming. He urged them to take up arms to oppose their tyrannical rulers. When the British arrived the next day, they were defeated at Concord by the colonial militia, and America's Revolutionary War had its auspicious beginning.

Revere's warning was effective for four reasons: (1) He was known to be a highly credible communicator, both expert and trustworthy; (2) his alarm was focused on a specific anticipated event; (3) it was designed to motivate citizens to act; and (4) it called for a concrete set of actions. Moreover, the people who heard Revere's warning were primed to accept it; they believed that the redcoats represented an imminent threat. This Paul Revere paradigm for the successful dissemination of public alarms is supported by contemporary psychological research. To be optimally effective, such distress signals should arouse only a moderate level of motivation—too little fails to energize action and too much creates emotional overload and competing, distracting behaviors.

Moreover, the warning notice must be based on reliable evidence and presented clearly by trust-worthy sources about specific dangers or threats that may be dealt with by taking some recommended action. If the threat is likely to persist over an extended period of time, debriefing after each danger signal is essential to correct misinformation, modify faulty recommendations, reinforce citizens for heeding the message, and reassure them of the value of their collaborative efforts. Finally, if the threat does not materialize, a reputable authority must explain why and then also lower or remove the alert. Experimenters working with volunteers in institutional and medical research are required to inform and debrief their subjects; a democratic government should follow similar procedures of ethical behavior toward its constituency.

We acknowledge that such debriefing can incur a substantial security cost. However, one of the real, if inadvertent, political advantages of the terror alert system is to direct increased funding to first responders at a time when their resources are particularly constrained, given that many of these officials are currently serving abroad as part of the National Guard. Unlike alerts, which require a single credible source, locally specific debriefing can prove adequate to ameliorate the perception of threat and its concomitant negative psychological sequelae. To the extent that state and local officials

357

feel their credibility depends on getting their message out before national leaders, such responders may also serve a dual purpose in aiding with appropriate, timely, and geographically specific debriefing. Using first responders to help with debriefing can help defray costs that will accrue to these forces nonetheless and help alleviate the debriefing burden that falls on federal officials. Furthermore, adequate debriefing serves to make citizens feel included in the process of their own defense in ways that reinforce the democratic process; in this way, the additional cost of debriefing, however allocated and directed, can be justified on normative grounds.

One of the important ways in which the current color-coded system diverges from the more effective Revere paradigm is that, in reality, only two real colors exist. A five-stage scheme may have been chosen to produce an agile, specific system (Cohen & Shapiro, 2005), but no one foresaw how this strategy would play out in practice. Red means that the United States is under attack, so red is not in effect an alert but rather an immediate warning of an ongoing event that should be obvious to all. And because no politician appears willing to lower the alert below yellow for fear that an attack will be staged during a period of ostensible calm, only yellow and orange remain actually viable colors. Such a restrictive range hardly seems effective, efficient, or useful for informing people about the level of threat they face.

This chapter presents a theoretically informed critique of the current system of terrorist alarms. Terrorist alerts produce both political and psychological effects. Politically, terrorist warnings mobilize first responders as well as the public to increased vigilance, for example. However, while ostensibly designed to improve the effectiveness of homeland defense, terrorist alerts also result in various negative outcomes. In this chapter we concentrate on three such specific problems. First, raising—as well as lowering—terrorist alarms produces negative public mental health outcomes and increases depression and posttraumatic stress disorder (PTSD) in the population at large. Second, this system encourages unthinking support for standing, charismatic leadership through a combination of heightened in-group bias and mortality salience. Last, the current system of terrorist alerts poses a threat to the diverse political culture on which our current governmental system rests.

We begin with a brief history of the use and implementation of the color-coded scheme. Next, we present evidence summarizing the counterproductive impact of this system on the national state of mental health. In short, we argue that the impact of this system does the terrorists' work for them by inducing a destructive degree of anxiety, depression, and paralysis in the population at large. Then we combine two theoretical models, social identity theory and terror management theory, both drawn from social psychology, to help explain how the current system encourages support for standing, charismatic leadership. We then discuss the reason that government leaders may have political and strategic incentives to continue to employ the current system despite the widespread mental health damage it incurs. Next we draw on these earlier arguments to explain how and why the current system poses threats to democratic values we should cherish. Finally, we offer some suggestions for how to develop a more effective and less destructive terrorist alert system.

Implementation and Use of the Current System

Terrorism is not about war in any traditional sense of destroying the material resources of an enemy nation and taking over that country. Rather, terrorism is fundamentally about psychology. It is about taking strategic actions that incite terror and fright in civilian populations. One goal of some terrorists is to make ordinary people feel vulnerable, anxious, confused, uncertain, and helpless. Ultimately, when terrorism works, citizens feel hopeless and lose trust in their leaders to guarantee the fundamentals of existence—safety and security. This is one of the reasons governments need to work hard to preserve their basic values as they seek to make their populations more physically secure. Terrorism is about imagining the monster under our beds or lurking in dark closets—the faceless, omnipotent enemy who might be our friend, our neighbor, or some horrible creature of our imagination. It has no one place, time, space, or face. The power of terrorism lies precisely in its pervasive ambiguity and in its invasion of our minds.

Obviously, a difference exists between terror as a category of actions and terror as a systematic political strategy. The appropriate categorization depends on who undertakes a particular action for what purpose. As a result, the target of terror alerts can vary between two distinct audiences: (1) the citizens of the United States who remain at risk; and (2) the terrorists themselves and what they can learn about domestic intentions from watching reactions to their threat. In this chapter we examine both effects.

In particular, we argue that terror alerts can increase the salience of the threat in ways that raise negative public mental health outcomes without a commensurate increase in public safety as a result. Reactions to increased feelings of personal vulnerability vary considerably, from stimulating phobias, to triggering unresolved childhood conflicts, to prolonging stress reactions, to blindly obeying powerful leaders, to arousing intense feelings of fear and anger. Fear can make people more anxious and vigilant, motivating them to seek out more information (Gray, 1982, 1987).

Anger is another form of displaced emotion that arises from feeling helpless or vulnerable. It can represent a turning out of intense and concealed feelings of weakness. Prejudice against out-groups is one consequence of such strong negative feelings, which can prove particularly problematic when a particular ethnic group is targeted and held accountable for the acts of unrelated others. In addition, negative emotions can lead to an increased readiness to attack "safe" targets, such as marginalized peoples in our nation or even family members. Indeed, evidence suggests that angry people support more punitive public policy choices. And, importantly, angry people also appear more optimistic in their judgments about the risk of future events (Lerner & Keltner, 2000).

Human nature, or at least traditional male human nature, seems to abhor feelings of personal weakness and uncertainty, seeking instead to ally one's identity with those manifesting strength and conviction. In times of crisis, people want to support leaders who are bold, single-minded, aggressive, and even arrogant. Those who supported Hitler and thus felt the shame and humiliation foisted upon Germany following its defeat at the end of World War I can be seen as succumbing to this temptation. In the face of ambiguous vulnerability, people want leaders to identify the "enemy" for them, to give it a name, a face, and a location so that the public can channel their collective hatred and unleash the strength of the military on a readily winnable war against that evil, although weak, enemy.

The irony, of course, is that terrorists are also often motivated to attack because they perceive themselves to be too weak to engage in a full frontal military assault against their perceived enemies. Yet once they attack, they create their mirror image: a targeted population bent on the destruction of the terrorists as well. The psychology of such a strategy at first seems ill formed, until analysts focus on the often hidden, secondary benefits of such a policy. Terrorist leaders find recruits in the losses their cause sustains, just as leaders in a targeted nation can manipulate the very real psychology of fear and anger perpetuated by the terrorists for their own domestic political purposes, as the Goering quote indicates. This transferential power lock deserves greater explanation and attention if efforts to break it are to succeed.

Violations of Effective Alarm Principles

All of the basic principles embodied in the Revere paradigm were systematically violated in the design and delivery of the first six terrorist alarms issued by U.S. government officials to warn the public of imminent terrorist dangers after September 11, 2001. Different communicators, alleged to have reliable information from "credible" yet unnamed sources, warned of an imminent attack by terrorists somewhere, sometime soon, in the United States or elsewhere in the world, against its offices or agencies. These warnings worked to create high levels of citizen fear, which over time morphed into generalized anxiety for many. There were no concrete actions that citizens could take other than to remain on alert and keep their eyes open. This vague recommendation was termed "BOLO" for "Be on the lookout." This initial message, reiterated endlessly but emanating from a wide variety of different official and media sources, was then elaborated by various "expert" commentators. The psychological situation worsened when cognitive-emotional dissonance was induced by the government's collateral message to "go about your business as usual."

It is psychologically impossible to remain both hypervigilant and to go about your business as usual at the same time. How was it possible to go about our normal business after having declared that the nation was under potential terrorist threat and that our personal safety was about to be violated once again as it was on 9/11? The resulting sense of confusion spills over into feelings of helplessness and results in suboptimal information processing, which in the event of a real attack would leave people less able to cope effectively.

But then there was none! Not a single terrorist attack on U.S. soil for the past 3 years. Where are the alleged thousands of terrorists inhabiting cells in our country? And where was the debriefing by our authorities to explain why nothing happened? Had U.S. defenses proved invulnerable? Had attacks been thwarted? Were the terrorists merely waiting until the vigilance passed and vulnerability increased? Explanations were nowhere in sight or sound. The high alert and its high anxiety induction just silently evaporated until another month or two went by, when the next call to alarm was sounded again and again. We all know from the classic story of the boy who cried wolf that, after only three false alarms, people cease to take seriously the validity of previously credible messages. Indeed, they come to dismiss such warnings fairly quickly over time because they prove to be inaccurate; when warning comes without anything happening afterward, people lose faith in the alert system itself.

Therefore, habituation effects set in, and people cease to take such notices of danger seriously, as calls to action, after the first three or four times. Indeed, providing immediate and accurate feedback and debriefing after a failed warning serves to prevent such habituation effects. Once people know why a false alert was issued, they can learn from the event. New information can help people to better recognize real threats, while knowing which potential ones they might safely ignore. Such knowledge helps people assimilate threats in constructive ways that do not result in their feeling too overwhelmed to do anything at all, in which case they must either ignore the alert or remain hypervigilant and anxious all of the time.

Indeed, after six no-consequence alarms, many Americans became desensitized to the need to be on high alert—yet still to lead normal lives. Moreover, with no specific information that taught

people what to be on the lookout for, it became "normal" to be anxiously dreading the worst, given the lesson of the first horrific attacks on the World Trade Center and the Pentagon, but being able to do nothing to prevent it. This situation produces the ironic and seemingly conflictual worst of all conundrums: People remain too inured to report suspicious events and individuals but too anxious to return to life as normal.

And Then There Were Seven

Something happened between the last of the earliest unmarked six-pack of terrorist warnings and the later institution of the newly framed color-coded alert that seemed at first to fit the psychologically effective Revere paradigm. It was clearly presented by one communicator, Tom Ridge, the head of Homeland Security, and it amplified the reliability of his informant by indicating that it was detected from multiple intelligence sources. It identified the terrorist targets as "soft"—U.S. homes and hotels—which, of course, targets everybody. In the next days, the target list expanded to include airlines and other symbolic and strategic venues. The anticipated terrorist weapons escalated to the unthinkable: "weapons of mass destruction"—chemical, biological, and radiological "dirty bombs." With that much detail on the input side, the Homeland Security head then added a shopping list of concrete actions that Americans should take on the output side to be prepared for an all-out attack from any of the reported thousand terrorists operating on U.S. soil and preparing to use these weapons of mass destruction against innocent civilians.

Experts warned U.S. citizens over and over in all of the media outlets to gas up their cars in case of emergency evacuation, store emergency supplies, and seal themselves in their homes using plastic sheeting and duct tape. Specific warnings were put up on the website of the Department of Homeland Security to aid in general emergency preparedness for the nation. For example, in the worst-case scenario of a neighborhood nuclear blast, citizens were warned to take cover, assess the situation, and limit their exposure to radiation. To make sure the message appeared on the nation's radar screen, after the mind-dulling previous six false alarms, the Orange Alert was sounded, and local, state, and federal forces swung into defensive action. At last, it seemed as though American citizens had been given a concrete set of actions they could take to protect themselves, which seemed better than just sitting idly by, waiting for inevitable death and destruction.

However, then it all began to unravel, as experts asserted that we could suffocate ourselves by sealing off the ventilation to our houses. We learned that some of the "reliable" sources of information were hoaxes. And, again, there was no debriefing from the government as to why the attacks did not occur or what had been done to prevent them. Instead, the Orange Alert stayed in effect for weeks while the Department of Homeland Security continued a nationwide campaign to promote emergency preparedness, fashioned after the programs of the Federal Emergency Management Administration's natural disaster readiness programs.

Five more color-coded terror alerts followed in the wake of the seventh. The one just before the 2004 presidential election appeared the most threatening because it predicted attacks on major financial centers and government buildings, which presented the potential prospect of interrupting the electoral process itself. The credible source for this alarm was a CD found in a terrorist's computer, which subsequently proved to be more than 3 years old; indeed, this information might well have been research conducted before the attacks on the World Trade Center occurred. But even when the age of the source was discovered, the high alert stayed in place for several months, throughout the electoral campaign and the voting itself, under the reasonable argument that it is not unusual for terrorists to plan their attacks far in advance.

A cell was in fact broken up in London a few days after the last orange alert. The information that led to the warning helped break it up. That is in fact how the alert system should work. What remains interesting in this case is the reason the danger signal stayed in place for so long after the cell was disrupted if such action provided the original reason for the alert.

Public Mental Health Outcomes

Mismanaged alarm procedures do the terrorists' work for them. If the goal of at least some terrorists is to instill fear and anxiety in the hearts and minds of civilians, they will not need to engage in any actual attacks as long as the target government acts to keep the population continually fearful. This is what the current system of color-coded terror alerts accomplishes in effect if not in intent. Mismanaged and misplaced warnings distress people well beyond a realistic nationwide risk level for any new terrorist attack, and they force the government to spend billions of dollars in combating potential incipient threats. These danger signals are creating a pretraumatic stress syndrome among Americans that gets reinforced and deepened with each new alert, especially among those with more fragile psyches.

One possibility to consider is that terrorists, seeing the frenzy caused by the first alarms, learned to intentionally put out misinformation on channels that they know or assume are monitored by U.S. intelligence. That "chatter," detected by U.S. intelligence services, stirs up the desired national turmoil and wastes a good deal of money in heightened security—without terrorists' ever having to engage in actual attacks. In fact, terror alarms reinforce a public willingness to spend huge sums of money on military defense and homeland security efforts, none of which have actually been shown to have made the American public more secure in any real way. Indeed, members of al-Queda, many of whom were originally schooled in the Afghan war against the Soviets, may in fact recall that part of the U.S. strategy in the Cold War was to force the Soviets to spend themselves into self-destruction without ever having to fight the other superpower directly. This lesson may not have been lost on those who saw one superpower decline precipitously, at least in part, because of excessive military spending.

Another conjecture concerns the unintended consequences of these many false alarms and perhaps some intended ones as well. Given the absence of actual terrorist attacks in this country since 9/11, as compared with Israel, for example, where many attacks have actually taken place, these warnings have worked to sustain a heightened sense of anxiety and confusion. In Israel, where specific warnings, similar to weather reports, are given on the radio, more than 300 Israelis have been killed, and more than 4,000 more have been wounded in suicide bombings since the start of the intifada in 2000 (see Chapter 13 in this volume). Between November of 2000 and May of 2004, 147 successful and 376 foiled suicide attacks were carried out in Israel. This constitutes less than 5% of the total number of attacks against Israeli targets in that time but represents the majority of those inside the state of Israel proper. To combat this threat, Israel spends about 8.75% of its gross domestic product on defense, which was more than $8.97 billion in 2002 (Cordesman, 2005).

Moreover, these alerts also create a climate of hostility and danger that encourages political disengagement. People are more willing to accept both restrictions on their personal freedoms in the form of legislation like the Patriot Act and violent actions against others, such as those that were directed at the prisoners in Abu Ghraib. Our argument is not that the prison guards at Abu Ghraib did their dirty deeds in response to fears of terrorism. Rather, President Bush has said that his goal is to keep the terrorists contained abroad so that they will not strike here at home. Furthermore, once afraid, people become more willing to accept punitive action against others; this tendency may become heightened if they believe such steps will also help prevent violence against them.

How exactly do these terror alarms do the terrorists' work for them? Two strands of evidence suggest both the tremendous and continuing toll of the terrorist attacks and their aftermath on the health of the American public. First, a number of studies indicate the enduring psychological impact of terrorism in Americans' psychological responses to the attacks on September 11, 2001. Second, additional evidence suggests the powerful impact of announcements of changes in the National Terror Alert System of the Department of Homeland Security on a large population of stable, largely married, well-trained first responders who work for Con Edison in New York City and have been systematically followed since the original attacks.

Several studies indicate the high and enduring level of psychological trauma following the 9/11 attacks in New York and elsewhere. In a random telephone survey, Galea et al. (2002) found that, among Manhattan residents, 8% reported symptoms that met the official diagnosis for posttraumatic stress disorder (PTSD), and 10% reported depressive symptoms in the months following the attacks on the World Trade Center. The closer a person lived to New York, the higher the rates of PTSD. In the area closest to the attacks, rates of PTSD ran as high as 20%. The vicarious nature of the impact of the terrorist attacks is revealed by the fact that most of those who reported PTSD or depressive symptoms had not been at the World Trade Center at the time of the attack, nor had they themselves ever been in any personal danger from the assault. In addition, those reporting symptoms were not more likely to be related to one of the victims of the violence.

Outside of New York City, the story remains similar. In a random-digit dial telephone survey of a representative sample of the United States, more than 40% reported at least one of five "substantial stress symptoms," and 90% reported low levels of stress symptoms (Schuster et al., 2001). Not surprisingly, those closer to New York City reported the highest rates overall, but many people who lived at a great distance from the terrorist attack venue reported high levels of stress symptoms as well.

In a very large sample of 2,729 U.S. residents living entirely outside New York City, Silver, Holman, McIntosh, Poulin, and Gil-Rivas (2002) found that 17% reported PTSD symptoms in the first 2 months after 9/11, and about 6% still reported symptoms more than 6 months later. The highest levels of stress were found among women, those were who maritally separated, those with preexisting medical or psychological health problems, and those who had stopped active coping efforts early in the aftermath of the attacks. Spiegel et al. (2002) also reported that the highest levels of distress were found among those with inadequate social support and maladaptive coping strategies. Such strategies included self-blame, substance abuse, and emotional suppression. Schuster et al. (2001) studied children's reactions by interviewing their parents and found that more than a third of parents reported that their children demonstrated at least one of five stress reactions, and more than half reported that their children worried about their own safety or that of loved ones.

Reporting similar findings in a sample of 1,142, Johll & Brant (2002) also found that women reported more stress. Interestingly, in this study, the authors found that those residing in New York turned more to social support and active problem solving in the wake of the attacks than did other people who lived farther away from the tragedy. One potential explanation for this finding derives from Schuster et al. (2001), who have reported a positive correlation between television exposure and stress reactions. Galea et al. (2002) have also found that people who lived farther away from the attacks, not surprisingly, relied more on television, radio, and the Internet to learn about what happened. They too found a positive correlation between the degree of media exposure and stress symptoms.

However, these effects might easily have resulted simply from the attacks themselves. What evidence do we have that the terror alert system exacerbated or prolonged the psychological effects triggered by the attacks? The most convincing evidence comes from a Cornell medical school study of 1,924 New York City Con Edison disaster relief workers, a sample that represents a remarkably stable population. All of the subjects are employed and trained to respond to crises in an effective and efficient manner. Most of them are married. Yet researchers at Cornell University's Weill Medical College found that changes in the color-coded alert were linked with increased levels of psychological distress, even among those who were already upset as a result of their direct contact with the World Trade Center site after 9/11. These relief workers showed significant increases in rates of physiological arousal, general and phobic anxiety, depression, and other PTSD symptoms when the alert code shifted from yellow to orange, which occurred on the third and fourth color-coded alerts on March 17 and May 20. Curiously, these symptoms were elevated again when these warning were lowered (Kramer, Brown, Spielman, Goisan, & Rothrock, 2004). In all likelihood, this means that calling attention to the danger signals proved sufficient to trigger strong negative emotional reactions, even among a sample of men who are trained relief workers.

Social Identity and Terror Management

Why should terror alerts increase levels of psychological distress? What other impact might such alarms have on the general public? Drawing on two theoretical models from social psychology, we argue that they serve to enhance social identity in-group biases while simultaneously heightening the salience of mortality for the targets of terrorist acts. These effects combine to simultaneously exacerbate symptoms of psychological distress and increase support for the current leadership.

Social identity theory (Tajfel & Turner, 1986) draws on the basic human tendency to engage in social categorization to explain how people become motivated to increase their sense of self-esteem through their sense of belonging to a group of similar others. This in-group identification leads to a bias toward those who are part of the in-group and against those who are not part of the group, the so-called out-group. One of the most important consequences of social identity theory lies in the insight that people want to see themselves and their own group members as being superior to excluded others on whatever relevant, albeit potentially arbitrary, dimension upon which group inclusion is assessed. In particular, when allocating resources across groups, individuals appear prone to give more to members of their own group and less to outsiders. This pattern of distribution persists even when people do not personally benefit from this system of allocation and even when doing so proves personally disadvantageous (Turner, Brown, & Tajfel, 1979). People allocate resources in this way not simply to provide an advantage for the in-group but also to create an explicit relative advantage for the in-group over the out-group (Tajfel, Billing, Bundy, & Flament, 1971). From this perspective, terrorist attacks—or the threat of them—would simultaneously increase in-group identification among Americans, with consequent rally-round-the-flag support for the country's leadership, and simultaneous out-group denigration or hatred of foreign groups perceived to be responsible for the violent acts.

The in-group bias posited by social identity theory becomes enhanced through the mechanism of terror management theory (Pyszczynski, Solomon, & Greenberg, 2003) and its validating research, which shows that human behavior is significantly affected by anything that makes people aware of their own potential death or sensitizes them to their mortality. Death-related thoughts affect everyone at conscious and nonconscious levels and channel people to express long-standing values and "increased need for safety and psychological security that this horrible reminder of our vulnerability has awakened in us all" (Pyszczynski et al., 2003, p. 112).

Terror management theory has demonstrated that reminding people of their mortality affects their evaluations of others. When mortality is made salient, people find others who conform to their own worldview to be more attractive, while judging those who threaten their worldview to be less so (Greenberg et al., 1990). In particular, subjects evaluate those who praise their cultural worldview especially positively and assess those who criticize it especially negatively. In addition, mortality salience makes people seek out cognitive consistency as well. When their death is made salient, people show an increased preference for seeking out information supporting their decisions as opposed to information that conflicts with it (Jonas, Greenberg, & Frey, 2003). Indeed, morality salience increases stereotypic thinking and induces preferences for stereotype-confirming individuals (Schimel et al., 1999).

This bias has been explored in explicitly political contexts as well. Mortality salience increases people's preference for charismatic political candidates and decreases inclination for relationship-oriented political candidates (Cohen, Solomon, Maxfield, Pyszczynski, & Greenberg, 2004). This so-called fatal attraction clearly demonstrates the impact of mortality salience on the evaluation of political leaders as a function of their leadership style. In a test of this hypothesis specifically designed to examine people's reactions to George Bush and the mortality salience induced by the terrorist attacks of 9/11, Landau et al. (2004) found that heightened concerns about mortality intensified Bush's appeal. In particular, reminding people of their mortality increased support for Bush and his counterterrorism policy. Subliminal exposure to reminders of 9/11 not surprisingly brought mortality-related thoughts closer to consciousness, and this too increased support for him. Mortality salience led subjects to become more favorable toward Bush and more likely to vote for him, while making them less predisposed toward John Kerry and less likely to vote for him.

Such a bias extends to other behaviors as well. Subjects whose mortality is made salient show increased aggression toward those who threaten their worldview. In a clever experiment, McGregor et al. (1998) showed that subjects forced others who threatened their worldview to consume a much larger amount of hot sauce. However, such aggression appeared confined to those who jeopardized the subjects' worldview; they did not force others who had made them drink an unpleasant tasting juice to eat more hot sauce. Interestingly, when subjects were allowed to express their hostility openly toward the critical target, greater aggression was eliminated.

This evaluation extends to reward and punishment as well. When mortality was made salient to subjects prior to decision making, they proved much more likely to reward a hero who upheld their cultural values, while recommending especially harsh sentences for those who violated those values (Rosenblatt et al., 1989). The authors have demonstrated that these effects do not result simply from greater physiological arousal or heightened self-awareness.

Researchers have also tied terror management theory to social identity theory by demonstrating that making people aware of their death increases intergroup bias in minimal groups (Harmon-Jones, Greenberg, Solomon, & Simon, 1996). Taken together, this research suggests that reminders of death serve to increase both in-group bias and out-group derogation. In short, mortality salience increases support for and decreases criticism of standing, charismatic leadership.

Strategic and Political Manipulations of Alarms

Why would a government create and maintain such an ineffective and psychologically damaging alarm system? Here, when we argue that the alarm system remains ineffective, we mean that it seems inadequate for motivating appropriate citizen action; the system may nonetheless serve as an effective deterrent or political tool. One explanation for this ostensible conundrum posits that, although politicians may be aware that the current system is neither ideal nor as effective as they might like, it serves important and legitimate subsidiary political goals. In particular, while not necessarily efficient, the current system is not useless in effecting first responder mobilization goals. Indeed, first responders may support this system because it provides them with desperately needed additional funding to meet their newly increased responsibilities. In addition, the system offers a kind of political cover electorally. No one wants to be caught under attack without having issued a warning first. How long the system will remain in place under this interpretation depends on how long it serves this purpose. Should another major act of violence occur and should the current system fail to provide adequate warning, politicians will no doubt be forced to revisit its effectiveness.

An alternate hypothesis for the current system that bears examination suggests that leaders strive to manipulate public opinion through the strategic use of fear and anger in order to gain political power and advantage. As the Goering quote suggests, if leaders want or need backing for a particular campaign that is likely to be unpopular or expensive in lives and material, such as a war, or restrictions on civil liberties, then the effective use of anger, threat, and fear can work to enhance public support. In this way, a terrorism alarm system can simultaneously serve as both a political and a strategic tool.

Evidence in support of this argument comes from Willer (2004, p. 1), who tracked the 26 times that the government issued a terror alert between February 2001 and May 2004. He matched these to 131 Gallup public opinion polls conducted during that same period. Using a time-series regression analysis, Willer examined the relationship between the warnings and the president's approval ratings. He found that, on average, each alert resulted in a 2.75 point increase in Bush's approval rating in the week following the alert. Significantly, this approval extended to increased support for the president's handling of the economy, an issue largely irrelevant to the war on terrorism. This finding demonstrates a substantial halo effect surrounding Bush following terror warnings, most likely because they increase mortality salience.

This process of enhanced support for the president and his policies can happen through several specific psychological mechanisms triggered by an alert system that simultaneously serves to enhance a person's sense of identification with the nation-group, while making one's mortality increasingly salient. First, fear motivates people to become more vigilant and to seek out more information, and mortality salience induces a preferential search for confirmatory evidence; in other words, fear gets people's attention. However, high levels of fear can also prove distracting, so while leaders garner people's attention, they do not necessarily gain their fully critically engaged attention. People are scared of dying, and, in the midst of that fear, they look to their leaders to provide a solution that is consistent with their preexisting worldview, which maintains that the in-group is good and the out-group is bad and threatening.

Second, attacks such as those on 9/11 can generate anger, and anger makes people much more supportive of punitive public policy choices (Lerner & Keltner, 2000; Gault & Sabini, 2000). Third, anger leads to more optimistic judgments; a government that encourages a population to be angry increases the likelihood that the public will remain supportive of and optimistic about the likelihood of success in punitive acts, such as war (Lerner & Keltner, 2000). Believing they will prevail, in turn, may render a public more willing to bear the cost of the effort. In addition, the extent to which leaders themselves share the emotional reaction of the public, they too may be affected in their decision-making abilities. Not only may angry leaders be inclined to be overoptimistic in their estimates of the probability of their own success, but anger also hinders creative decision making more broadly (Keinan, 1987; Forgas, 1992).

In this way, the larger problem with the current alert system lies not only in its negative public mental health outcomes. Rather, an alarm system that encourages unthinking and uncritical support for standing, charismatic leadership poses a far greater risk to the diversity of political culture. When people stop questioning the public policies of their government and react with knee-jerk support, democracy itself becomes threatened. Americans want to feel safe, but they also want to support the basic ideals of justice, equality, and equal representation. Public policy agendas that manage to circumvent critical consultation on important issues of security pose a threat to the maintenance of a diverse political culture, whereby distinct voices and interest groups receive equal treatment before the law.

Action Conclusions

There are at least two important limitations to the current color-coded terror alert system. First, warnings should be issued by a single credible source based on specific information. To the extent possible, people should be told where and when the threat is most likely to occur and how long the risk will last. After the time has passed, people should be debriefed and told whether an attack was preempted or whether and how the information that incorrectly predicted a threat was flawed and what steps will be taken to prevent such mistakes in the future. Only through such a system can people remain attentive in ways that might prove effective in thwarting potential attacks without falling into paralyzing depression or anxiety.

Obviously, the most difficult aspects of instituting such a system lie in conflicting political incentives. While it may be best for citizen awareness and anxiety to have a single credible source of terrorist threats, many state and local officials have strong incentives to get the message out first; recall the political fracas that occurred when the governor of California issued a specific alert about the threat to bridges in the Bay Area; federal officials felt that making such an announcement was irresponsible, but the governor was unwilling to take the political risk of not issuing an alert should a subsequent attack occur. Indeed, while the government has in fact hardened important sites such as bridges, not much of this preparation has been made public. The federal perception is that making known the extent of our protective measures with regard to critical infrastructures provides an incentive for terrorists to hit softer targets. According to this logic, it is better for terrorists to hit a protected critical infrastructure than to concentrate on unprotected civilian targets such as malls (Cohen & Shapiro, 2005). Thus, the federal government opposes announcing specific threats to hardened targets such as bridges, which remain easier to protect than softer targets, which terrorist might choose if they believed that everyone was watching their first target, making success less likely.

Yet local leaders feel their credibility depends on being the ones to issue local warnings, and their political incentives do not always align with a single source model. New alert models must remain aware of the perceived political needs of local leaders. One possibility is to have a single national source for information on terrorist threats, followed closely by local reports on specific area threats. However, such a strategy would require close and trusting relationships between federal and local leaders, which may prove challenging in reality, especially under conditions of threat and time pressure.

Second, for alerts to prove effective in actually reducing the risk of harm, they need to be specifically tied to actual behaviors. A heightened alert must mean more than merely increased vigilance, or it will result in nothing more than increased anxiety, depression, and hopelessness in the general population. Intensified alerts should come with specific, concrete, realistic actions for people to take to reduce the threat or protect themselves and their families from harm should the threat materialize. Such actions can include lessons about what people should look for and what kinds of suspicious actions or people should be reported to which authorities. Clearly, trade-offs exist in educating people about the best way to notice terrorist threats. Some of the realistic things that governments may want people to do, such as spy on their neighbors, are not so nice and certainly run contrary to an established culture of individual rights and freedom.

Further, having the government name particular groups as likely targets for suspicion, such as Muslims or people of Middle Eastern descent, can produce adverse consequences, such as the lynching of innocents. Such warnings might indeed create greater violence in reaction than any real threat may pose. As a result, government officials need to think carefully about how to educate the public about the specific ways in which they need to remain alert to threat. Indeed, one of the functions of heightened airport scrutiny, intentional or otherwise, is merely to keep people aware that the threat is real: Vigilance remains necessary; risk exists everywhere; and bad things can happen despite the best of intentions and preparations. The unconscious message is that the government is trying its best and doing all it can do to protect its citizens, so if something goes wrong, it is the fault of the perpetrators, not the defenders.

Alerts should be targeted geographically as much as possible, so that those who are outside the greatest risk zone need not worry unnecessarily. In addition, some warnings, especially those that remain vague in intent, should be issued only to first responders and other trained personnel. Oftentimes, alerting the general public serves no useful purpose but increases psychological distress for no practical reason. Raising alert levels may be useful for particular security personnel and other first responders to take specific actions, including raising force levels, but it may only cause confusion and anxiety on the part of the general public. Authorities should utilize the opportunities provided by first responders to support both preparedness and response in natural environments such as hospitals, police stations, and fire departments. In addition, for government communication to improve, authorities should understand the critical role that the nation's health care system should play, including primary care providers, psychologists, and social workers (Heldring, 2004). Doctors remain trusted, credible sources in the eyes of most people and often provide the first contact for those who are injured in attacks.

Even assuming no manipulative political intent, conscious or coincidental, there needs to be a serious reexamination of how to best construct future terrorist alarms, guide their optimal utilization, and, when they do not materialize, explain the reason to the public. Of course, we are all relieved when the alarms prove false, but when repeated over time they may serve only to induce a kind of psychic numbing, lulling us to sleep and leaving us unprepared to act constructively and effectively if and when the wolf actually does come to the door.

There are terrorists who are indeed dangerous and who hate some of what the United States stands for in their eyes. They will try to attack the country in various ways, including suicide bombings. Security and preparedness are essential components in countering terrorism. In particular, advice about how to prevent public overreaction and promote citizen cooperation when in dangerous situations, where mass hysteria can kill, as in bombings, are necessary. Further, honesty, transparency, and accountability on the part of leaders is essential if terrorist alarms are to be taken seriously in the future.

Currently, the government does not seem to be using the best scientific advice available on how to construct terror warnings or how to educate the public in this new threat. Managing human-made disasters requires models that are different from those that have traditionally been used to handle natural disasters. In fighting terrorism, strategists need to think like terrorists in order to select and protect likely targets. The United States ought to reassess its full-coverage security of venues that are unlikely to ever be considered targets by terrorists. Security focus should be placed on higher probability targets, including limited municipal resources (e.g., water supplies), symbolic, sentimental targets (e.g., Disneyland), places with potential for major urban disruptions that can never have comprehensive security checks (e.g., urban subways), or school buses.

High levels of sustained stress in many citizens of all ages can have a greater long-term destructive impact on the nation than the consequences of any single terrorist attack. Emergency preparedness for any form of terrorist assault would benefit from a wider appreciation of the mental health implica-

tions and essential features of the psychology and rationality of terrorism, as well as from less political involvement and manipulation. Further, the general public should remain aware of the threats to diverse political culture and a genuinely representative democratic government posed by appeals to in-group superiority, out-group prejudice and denigration, and death threat reminders, which all combine to generate uncritical support for the standing leadership and punitive public policy choices.

Responses to the Terrorist Threat

Terrorists remain effective at getting attention on the international stage. This is indeed part of the reason they engage in campaigns of wanton fear and destruction, and they will continue to do so as long as they have unresolved grievances. To the extent that Western governments, including the United States, want to wage a truly effective war on terrorism, they need to begin to understand and grapple with some of the psychological and strategic motivations of terrorists. Military action alone is unlikely to suffice as an adequate response to terrorist action and activity. In this, Buddhists are not alone in their belief that violence begets violence. Recent studies appear to validate the intuition that military action against terrorists only increase aggressive responses and reprisals. In one time-series analysis, for example, Enders & Sandler (1993) found that, 20 years after a retaliatory raid against Libya in 1986, terrorist attacks against the United States from this region were still increasing. Silke (2004) notes similar patterns in his review of the impact of military action on subsequent terrorist activities.

Terrorists are neither crazy nor irrational, even when their actions are evil. All of the recent accounts make it evident that terrorists do not fit any mentally pathological profile. A 2003 survey by Horgan has found no empirical support for the notion of a terrorist "personality." The National Research Council has reported that "There is no single or typical mentality—much less a specific pathology—of terrorists" (Smelser & Mitchell, 2002, p. 3). Indeed, one woman who spent years studying Palestinian terrorists argues that "What is frightening is not the abnormality of those who carry out the suicide attacks, but their sheer normality" (as quoted in Silke, 2003). This finding is strikingly reminiscent of Hannah Arendt's similar conclusion in her analysis of Nazi henchman Adolf Eichmann, who appeared terrifyingly normal; the banality of his evil seemed the most frightening aspect of his personality.

Indeed, the only systematic attribute that behavioral researchers have found associated with terrorists is a propensity toward rage (Plous & Zimbardo, 2004). Moreover, this factor may simply be a function of the larger demographic reality that most terrorists are males between the ages of 15 and 30, the group that is most likely to commit violent crimes in general, regardless of place or motivation (Daly & Wilson, 1988). Upon reflection, it should make sense that effective terrorists cannot be crazy even if their intentions are malevolent. Successful terrorist action requires patience, problem-solving skills, and the ability to work efficiently in groups, all traits that run counter to the existence of systematic mental illness.

We contend that more effective responses to terrorist threats would encompass a two-track policy. First, to the extent that domestic governments use terrorist threats for their own domestic political purposes, they should realize that such strategies reduce the prospects for achieving an effective dialogue with their population, as well as with their enemies, and accomplish the terrorists' work by effectively debilitating the target population with fear and other forms of mental disorder and distress (Zimbardo, 2001a, 2001b, 2003). After all, the widespread public perception that alerts can be manipulated for political reasons undermines their very credibility. Indeed, this manipulation is not lost on people. *Time* magazine reported in its August 6, 2004, poll that fully 38% of Americans think that the alerts might be manipulated for political reasons (Tumulty, 2004).

Second, when realistic terrorist threats confront American citizens, warnings should be credible, specific, timely, and designed to motivate people to take particular reasonable actions to protect themselves and others. When such threats do not materialize, effective debriefing should explain how and why the threat was either misplaced or averted. Open and honest dialogue about realistic threats can help to preserve democratic values concerning effective representation. With this plan of attack, greater safety and security could be achieved with more effectiveness, less cost, and less anxiety.

Addendum

In an investigative report dated October 12, 2005, MSNBC commentator Keith Olberman analyzed the recent threats against the New York City subway system in light of previous terror alerts. He documented 13 cases between May 2002 and October 2005 in which a significant political downturn by the Bush administration was immediately followed by a terror warning within a matter of days. These coincidences included John Kerry's nomination as the Democratic candidate for president, followed 2 days later by a jump in the color-coded system to orange, based on a threat against financial centers in New York, New Jersey, and Washington that turned out to be 4 years old. Similar threats against the New York City subway were issued in the wake of some of Bush's lowest public opinion poll numbers ever, following the administration's debacle in response to Hurricane Katrina's flooding of New Orleans, renewed violence and political opposition in Iraq, and questioning by the grand jury of Karl Rove's participation in outing CIA agent Valerie Plame to *New York Times* reporter Judith Miller.

Significantly, even former head of Homeland Security Tom Ridge publicly questioned the timing of such alerts in view of the classified information he received: "More often than not we were the least inclined to raise it. Sometimes we disagreed with the intelligence assessment. Sometimes we thought even if the intelligence was good, you don't necessarily put the country on [alert]. . . . There were times when some people were really aggressive about raising it, and we said 'for that?'" Although correlation between events does not necessarily signify or document causation, the pattern of events remains striking, especially in light of the concerns raised in this chapter about the negative impact of such alerts on public health. In his report, Keith Olberman concluded by asking, "if merely a reasonable case can be made that any of these juxtapositions of events are more than just coincidences, it underscores the need for questions to be asked in this country—questions about what is prudence, and what is fear-mongering; questions about which is the threat of death by terror, and which is the terror of threat" (cited at http://www.msnbc.msn.com/id/6210240/).

Acknowledgments. We would like to thank Jacob Shapiro for his helpful comments and suggestions. We would also like to thank the participants of the Dartmouth seminar, especially Carol Bohmer, Stephen Brooks, Richard Ned Lebow, Jennifer Lind, Roger Masters, Anne Sa'adah, Allan Stam, Ben Valentino, Christianne Hardy Wohlforth, and William Wohlforth, for lively discussion and extremely helpful suggestions on the previous version of this chapter.

References

Cohen, D., & Shapiro, J. (2005). Going to red: The failure of the Homeland Security Advisory System. Unpublished manuscript, Stanford University.

Cohen, F., Solomon, S., Maxfield, M., Pyszczynski, T., & Greenberg, J. (2004). Fatal attraction: The effects of mortality salience on evaluations of charismatic, task-oriented, and relationship-oriented leaders. *Psychological Science, 15*(12), 846–851.

Cordesman, A., with Moravitz, J. (2005). The course of the conflict in Israel proper. Unpublished manuscript, Center for Strategic and International Studies, Washington, DC.

Daly, M., & Wilson, M. (1988). *Homicide.* New York: A. de Gruyter.

Enders, W., & Sandler, T. (1993). The effectiveness of antiterrorism policies: A vector-autoregression-intervention analysis. *American Political Science Review, 87*(4), 829–844.

Forgas, J. (1992). Affect in social judgments and decisions: A multi-process model. *Advances in Experimental Social Psychology, 25,* 227–275.

Galea, S., Ahern, J., Resnick, H., Kilpatrick, D., Bucuvalas, M., Gold, J., et al. (2002). Psychological sequelae of the September 11 terrorist attacks in New York City. *New England Journal of Medicine, 346,* 982–987.

Gault, B., & Sabini, J. (2000). The role of empathy, anger, and gender in predicting attitudes toward punitive, reparative, and preventive public policies. *Cognition and Emotion, 14*(4), 495–520.

Greenberg, J., Pyszczynski, T., Solomon, S., Rosenblatt, A., et al. (1990). Evidence for terror management II: The effects of mortality salience on reactions to those who threaten or bolster the cultural worldview. *Journal of Personality and Social Psychology, 58*(2), 308–318.

Gray, J. (1982). *The neuropsychology of anxiety: An enquiry into the functions of the septo-hippocampal system.* New York: Clarendon/Oxford University Press.

Gray, J. (1987). *The psychology of fear and stress.* 2d ed. New York: Cambridge University Press.

Harmon-Jones, E., Greenberg, J., Solomon, S., & Simon, L. (1996). The effects of mortality salience on intergroup bias between minimal groups. *European Journal of Social Psychology, 26*(4), 677–681.

Heldring, M. (2004). Talking to the public about terrorism: Promoting health and resilience. *Families, Systems, and Health, 22*(1), 67–71.

Horgan, J. (2003). Introduction. In Andrew Silke (Ed.), *Terrorists, victims, and society: Psychological perspectives on terrorism and its consequences,* (pp. 3–27). New York: Wiley.

Johll, M., & Brant, C. (2002, August). Coping with a traumatic life experience. Paper presented at congressional briefing, Washington, DC.

Jonas, E., Greenberg, J., & Frey, D. (2003). Connecting terror management and dissonance theory: Evidence that mortality salience increases the preference for supporting information after decisions. *Personality and Social Psychology Bulletin, 29*(9), 1181–1189.

Keinan, G. (1987). Decision under stress: Scanning of alternatives under controllable and uncontrollable circumstances. *Journal of Personality and Social Psychology, 52*(3), 639–644.

Kramer, M., Brown, A., Spielman, L., Goisan, C., & Rothrock, M. (2004). Psychological reactions to the national terror-alert system. Poster session no. 4227. Presentation to the American Psychological Association.

Landau, M., Solomon, S., Greenberg, J., Cohen, F., Pyszczynski, T., Arndt, J., et al. (2004). Deliver us from evil: The effects of mortality salience and reminders of 9/11 on support for President George W. Bush. *Personality and Social Psychology Bulletin, 30*(9), 1136–1150.

Lerner, J., & Keltner, D. (2000). Beyond valence: Toward a model of emotion-specific influences on judgment and choice. *Cognition and Emotion, 14*(4), 473–493.

McGregor, H., Lieberman, J., Greenberg, J., Solomon, S., Arndt, J., Simon, L., et al. (1998). Terror management and aggression: Evidence that mortality salience motivates aggression against worldview-threatening others. *Journal of Personality and Social Psychology, 74*(3), 590–605.

Plous, S., & Zimbardo, P. (2004). How social science can reduce terrorism. *Chronicle of Higher Education, 51*(3), p. B9.

Pyszczynski, T., Solomon, S., & Greenberg, J. (2003). *In the wake of 9/11: The psychology of terror.* Washington, DC: American Psychological Association.

Rosenblatt, A., Greenberg, J., Solomon, S., Pyszczynski, T., et al. (1989). Evidence for terror management theory I: The effects of mortality salience on reactions to those who violate or uphold cultural values. *Journal of Personality and Social Psychology, 57*(4), 681–690.

Schimel, J., Simon, L., Greenberg, J., Pyszczynski, T., Solomon, S., Waxonsky, J., et al. (1999). Stereotypes and terror management: Evidence that mortality salience enhances stereotypic thinking and preferences. *Journal of Personality and Social Psychology, 77*(5), 905–926.

Schuster, M., Stein, B., Jaycox, L., Collins, R., Marshall, G., Elliott, M., et al. (2001). A national survey of stress reactions after the September 11, 2001, terrorist attacks. *New England Journal of Medicine, 345,* 1507–1512.

Silke, A. (2003). Ultimate outrage. *The Times of London.*
———. (2004). Terrorism, 9/11, and psychology. *Psychologist, 17,* 518–521.

Silver, R., Holman, A., McIntosh, D., Poulin, M., & Gil-Rivas, V. (2002). Nationwide longitudinal study of psychological reactions to September 11. *Journal of the American Medical Association, 288,* 1235–1244.

Smelser, N. J., & Mitchell, F. (Eds.). (2002). *Terrorism: Perspectives from the behavioral and social sciences.* Panel on Behavioral, Social, and Institutional Issues, Committee on Science and Technology for Countering Terrorism, Center for Social and Economic Studies, National Research Council. Washington, D.C.: National Academies Press.

Spiegel, D., Butler, L., Azarow, J., Koopman, C., DiMiceli, S., & McCaslin, S. (2002, August).

Distress and coping after the terrorist attacks: Preliminary survey results. Paper presented at the American Psychological Association annual meeting, Chicago.

Tajfel, H., Billing, M., Bundy, R., & Flament, C. (1971). Social categorization and intergroup behavior. *European Journal of Social Psychology, 1*(2), 149–178.

Tajfel, H., & Turner, J. (1986). The social identity theory of intergroup behavior. In S. Worchel & W. Austin (Eds.), *Psychology of Intergroup Relations* (pp. 7–24). Chicago: Nelson-Hall.

Tumulty, Karen. (August 16, 2004). Hijacking the Campaign. *Time Magazine.*

Turner, J., Brown, R., & Tajfel, H. (1979). Social comparison and group interest in ingroup favoritism. *European Journal of Social Psychology, 9*(2), 187–204.

Willer, R. (2004). The effects of government-issued terror warnings on presidential approval ratings. *Current Research in Social Psychology, 10*(1), 1. Retrieved January 27, 2006, from http://www.uiowa.edu/~grpproc/crisp/crisp.html

Zimbardo, P. (2001a, November 4). Mind games: Don't play on terrorists' turf. *San Francisco Chronicle,* C6.
———. (2001b, December 30). Psychology of terrorism: Mind games, mind healing. *San Francisco Chronicle,* D6.
———. (2003). Phantom menace: Is Washington terrorizing us more than Al-Queda? *Psychology Today, 36,* 34–36.

V

Prevention and Psychological Problems in Reaction to Acts of Terrorism

24

Defusing the Terrorism of Terror

A. J. W. Taylor

The study of terrorism—the ideology, recruitment, training, financial, and organizational base of any faction seeking to change the balance of power—is fraught with difficulties of an intellectual, professional, and political kind (Silke, 2003, pp. xv–xxi). Intellectually, the topic has more than the usual insecurity of applied research in which the occurrence of events and the extent of their consequences are not under the researchers' control. Professionally there are few attested protocols for researchers to adopt, and governments are more inclined to move swiftly to retaliate against terrorists than to promote studies of the complex causes of terrorism and to apply the remedies.

In taking such peremptory action, governments have the support of Stahelski (2004), a specialist in the operation of extremist cults who recommends the "elimination" of terrorist leaders, "aggressively disrupting" the training camps, and "aggressively pursuing and eliminating" the funding sources of the fundamentalist religious schools that provide malleable recruits for terrorist training schools. He has described the terrorists as dispossessed and social misfits who emanate primarily "from dysfunctional families where the father is absent, estranged, or economically or politically impotent," and he has reported that recruits are captured by the "seductive charm" of charismatic leaders, who, in return for absolute compliance in a well-designed conditioning program, provide ready answers to "life's perplexing questions."[1]

However, in her study of gross violators of human rights, which might also have a bearing on terrorists, Smeulers (2002) has drawn on the social psychological laboratory studies of Milgram (1969) and Zimbardo (Haney, Banks, & Zimbardo, 1973) and the fieldwork of Gibson and Haritos-Fatouros (1986) to make the chilling comment that most perpetrators are ordinary people and that within specific circumstances anyone might become a perpetrator. She goes on to report the residual traces of humanity remaining in some killers on particular assignments that caused them such revulsion as to make them quit.

In their retaliatory moves against terrorists, governments are known to fudge the matter of human rights, avoid due process of law, and use dubious tactics to achieve the results they desire—sometimes at the expense of scapegoats. In fact, a detached observer would find it difficult sometimes to differentiate between the opposing parties on moral grounds because governments have sponsored the terrorist groups they now oppose, and their own agencies have operated in ways not unlike those of terrorists whom they revile (cf. Meldrum, 2002, p. 79).[2] Sluka (2000, p. 6) has given specific examples of this double standard of morality, citing Rummell's conservative estimate of some 170 million victims of such government action in the first 88 years of the twentieth century, with nearly the same number afterward from the "government-inspired genocides and starvations" in Bosnia, Rwanda, Somalia, Sudan, and elsewhere.[3] Sluka (2000, p. 15) then follows E. V. Walter in describing the functions of such government-promoted death squads as maintaining order and counteracting "fissiparous tendencies" by inhibiting resistance, preventing change, and maintaining the political status quo of the ruling elite. Somewhat dryly, he follows Chomsky and Herman in describing state-sponsored terrorism as "wholesale" and that of its assailants as "retail" (Sluka, 2002, p.1).

Aside from such contentious moral issues, there are questions about the kind of protective measures societies should adopt against terrorism and at what psychological and economic cost. In the United States, the intelligence agencies that were found incompetent for the way they handled the warnings preceding the 9/11 al-Qaeda attacks on the World Trade Center and the Pentagon have quadrupled, intensified, and prolonged their precautionary systems, regardless of the negative economic and emotional effects of creating and maintaining a high state of vigilance (see McDermott & Zimbardo, Chapter 23, this volume). Then the gross disparity between the expenditure of resources to deal with the comparatively few violent deaths from "external" agents as compared with fatalities from other causes must also come into consideration. Wallace and Pritchard (2004), for example, pointed out that, in 2000, grave as the losses of nearly 3,000 "external" deaths through terrorism were in the United States, those occurring "internally" from road deaths, suicide, and homicide were about 30 times greater, but the allocation of resources was far from equitable. The International Federation of Red Cross and Red Crescent Societies (IFRC&RCS, 2005, p.131) made a similar point about the neglect of chronic disease and many long-standing conflicts.[4]

Regarding the emotional effects of terrorist attacks, the pioneer disaster researcher Russell Dynes (2003) attempts to reduce the hyperarousal by comparing the immediate effects of the terrorist attacks of September 11, 2001, in New York with those from the British bombing of Hamburg in July 1943 and the United States' atomic bombing of Hiroshima in August 1945 (to say nothing of Nagasaki 10 days later). He shows that these attacks by the Allies in World War II caused far more death and destruction than al-Qaeda in September 2001, and that, in those cities the clearance, reconstruction, and recovery proceeded apace without much outside help. Then, after lamenting the "new class of experts of terrorism and security identified by their mastery of Machiavelli," Dynes goes on to praise "the willingness [of those ready at the organizational level] to overturn or by-pass experience since the situation to be faced has novel elements requiring ingenuity" and to warn against the apparent centralization of problem solving and decision making that seemed to be emerging in the newly created U.S. Department of Homeland Security.

In synchrony with the United States after 9/11, many countries throughout the world tightened their security screens against potential terrorists. In the antipodes Australia already had a strict policy against asylum seekers that led to riots, self-mutilation, and suicides in detention camps. In a dramatic move on August 29, 2001, it had also blocked the arrival of 460 Afghan fugitives from an overloaded vessel, the *Tampa,* and transferred them to the remote Nauru Island some 4,000 kilometers northeast of Sydney. Following 9/11, the Australian Government (2004, Ch. 7) made a number of bilateral counter-terrorism arrangements with countries throughout South-East Asi, and it reinforced those measures after 83 Australians were among the 203 killed by the al-Qaeda bombing of two nightclubs in Bali on October 12, 2002.

In New Zealand, the government held a high-level conference (*World Terrorism and Political Violence: Implications for New Zealand,* 2002) and took precautionary measures to hunt terrorists abroad—without going beyond the scope of the United Nations (Smith, 2003). However, it caused widespread consternation by holding a refuge seeker (Ahmed Zaoui) in solitary confinement for 10 months in Kafkaesque fashion without legal charges being brought, until his mental condition so deteriorated that the Department of Corrections was obliged to transfer him to less restrictive quarters. The man was a reputable academic and cleric who in 1991 had been elected to the first democratic government of Algeria. The military there responded with an iron fist by torturing and killing thousands of civilians. Zaoui escaped to seek sanctuary and elicit support in Europe, Africa, and Southeast Asia before making his way further South in December 2002. The New Zealand Refugee Status Appeals Authority conceded the merits of his case (cf. Zaoui, 2004), but at the time of this writing he remains in an anomalous legal position—although thanks to the New Zealand Supreme Court he is being held under far less restrictive conditions than the Crown would impose.

Currently in the United States, as in the McCarthy era of the 1950s, the administration is known to suspect the loyalty and political allegiance of potential researchers and to challenge their motivation (cf. http//:www.counterpunch.org/dprice2 .html). It has brought indirect and subtle pressure to bear on communities in which investigators live and put their personal safety and that of their families at risk. Such extraneous pressures could not but have compromised the intellectual and emotional detachment of all but a handful of hardy souls who pursue terrorism as a topic of behavioral research.

Obviously the continuing high level of public concern about terrorists and terrorism needs to abate before field-workers can safely bring the subject more into the mainstream for proper scrutiny.[5] Conceivably researchers who collect data in the classroom or laboratory might find themselves under less extraneous pressure than their colleagues in the field, but their findings might be too simplistic for immediate application to the infinitely more complex problems people face in the real world. For example, Pyszczynski, Solomon, and Greenberg (2003) worked with student volunteers in contrived studies of conflict in the safety of a laboratory to generate a plausible Terror Management Theory—derived from Becker's (1971) earlier focus on the existential meaning of death—and they offered it as a partial explanation for the psychological after-effects of 9/11 on the general population. However, as DeLisle (2003) has said, the direct extrapolation of such a laboratory finding from a sample of students to the consequences of terrorists operating in situations of international political conflict is open to question.

Regrettably, too many clinicians abandon their responsibility for conducting research once they have qualified, and too many of the remainder adopt ad hoc procedures and questionnaires for quick investigations without heeding the advice of stalwarts such as Raphael, Lundin, and Weisaeth (1989). It is true that field-workers contemplating research after disasters will have to overcome particular obstacles concerning methodology, methods, design, logistics, and funding—as well as the appropriate time to launch their studies.[6] However, it seems that 9/11 gave the National Institute of Health, the U.S. Department of Veterans Affairs, and the National Center for Posttraumatic Stress Disorders the necessary impetus to address some of these issues, because they combined in 2004 to launch the first of a series of four annual conferences on innovative trends in trauma research methods.

However, it remains that any plausible findings from empirical research on highly sensitive public issues such as terrorism deserve consideration.[7] Toward that end, the rest of this chapter focuses on the definition and origins of terrorism, its changing appraisal, and frontline responses. It construes terrorism as a kind of disaster, presents a classification of disasters, explains their various phases, discusses victims/casualties and their psychological needs, phasic community reactions, cross-cultural features, and the importance of belief and value systems in effecting the recovery of casualties.

Terrorism is a complex phenomenon that needs to be put into a disciplinary framework before it can properly be understood, defused, and remedied. The understanding will generate less anxiety, the defusing will lead to a more rational appraisal of causative factors, and the remedies will be other than those of counterattack, retribution, and deterrence.

Definitions and Origins

According to the *Oxford English Dictionary* (1999), the word "terrorism," which is defined as the "unlawful use of force by militant organizations for economic, ideological, political, and religious purposes," is of comparatively recent origin. It was attributed first to the Jacobins and their agents in the French Revolution for the cruel manner in which they kept people in "implicit subjection by a merciless severity." Subsequently it was the method used by clandestine groups or expatriate organizations "aiming to coerce an established government by acts of violence against it or its subjects." More recently, the advance of technology and weaponry and the creation of international networks enabled small coteries of committed and highly skilled operatives to target economic and political systems with greater destructive effect than before.

However, the capacity of militants to create terror can be traced back to earlier times, and it has even been thought the last of different devastating events in the chain of human survival. For example, paleoarcheologist David Keys (1999) took a macroscopic, longitudinal, and interdisciplinary approach with more than 50 academic specialists and authorities in more than 20 disciplines, and he produced a compelling argument for a volcanic eruption about 535 or 536 A.D. that caused the worldwide collapse of major civilizations. His thesis is that a massive explosion in the Indonesian archipelago brought about a severe climatic change, followed by food shortages that caused a virulent plague to spread in North African and Mediterranean countries, and finally led invaders from the north and east of Asia to extend their boundaries into the Balkans and Europe in a fight for political and religious survival.[8]

With the detachment that such historical scholarship affords, one could also state that *social* eruptions without geophysical inducement also have the potential for bringing about significant social change (cf. Sjoberg, 1962). Bankoff (2003, p. 20) says as much, commenting that disasters can be significant catalysts of change in their own right, "triggering needed adaptations in human behavior and modification to structures, and even contributing to the overthrow of civilizations at times." In short, as the Chinese calligrapher makes clear, the pictograph brush strokes of the character for "stress" combine the two words "crisis" and "opportunity."

In fact, Bankoff (2003, p. 23), an anthropologist, takes the holistic approach to disasters, regarding them as "embedded in the daily human condition . . . in terms of a seamless web of relations that link society to environment and culture." In his seminal article, he advances the ecological concept of community life as the dynamic interaction between people and their environments, and he goes on to say that disasters "are only one more impermanent and irregular component of a threat to general human physical and psychological security represented by health problems, malnutrition, unor underemployment, income deficit, illiteracy, substance abuse and endemic violence." Quite thoughtfully, he also distinguishes between communities with "layered resilience" that have many coping practices and those with fewer that are inherently vulnerable.

The Changing Appraisal

Regardless of the causes and consequences of terrorism, a combined North Atlantic Treaty Organization (NATO) and Russian military workshop has acknowledged terrorism to be "a fundamental method of waging social and psychological warfare" (Wessely & Krasnov, 2002). It recognized that civilians were having to live with the prospect of encountering terrorism, and thought it some consolation that communities and their systems were usually the targets rather than individuals.[9] The workshop commented that civilians could be expected to respond with resilience and cohesion rather than panic, especially if they had confidence in the information given by the authorities and the news media. Nevertheless, it warned that both military personnel and civilians could have similar apprehensions about the biological, chemical, and explosive methods that terrorists now use, expressing confidence that the majority would recover quickly, leaving the remainder liable to present psychological problems leading to personality change and mental illness.

Still focusing on the techniques adopted by terrorists, O'Brien and Nusbaum (2002) speak of the "David and Goliath" disparity between the resources of personnel, weaponry, economic resources, and political power of the terrorists and their quarry, and they refer to it as "asymmetrical terrorism." Homer-Dixon (2002, n.p.) draws much the same distinction, but he coined the term "complex terrorism" to emphasize the "growing technological capacity of small groups and individuals to destroy things and people, and . . . the increasing vulnerability of our economic and technological systems to carefully aimed attacks." Of the two terms, complex terrorism is preferred because, of the two conceptualizations, it can more easily be broadened to encompass the other.

Even though the inclusion of such systems as a target of terrorism might be new, economic factors have frequently been a source of massive discontent in the development of many countries. In 1995 IFRC&RCS were concerned about the "*disaster inducement work"* (italics added) of powerful, self-promoting economic and political groups (IFRC&RCS, 1995, p. 52). With clarity and forceful expression, Korten (1996) points to the vulnerability of complex socioeconomic global systems with monolithic and monopolistic conglomerates that centralize decision making at the expense of smaller, independent units of production, distribution, and exchange. In particular, his argument is that, for the sake of maximizing their own profits, the most powerful and affluent strata of society had destroyed the concept of work for the sustainability of individuals and their local communities. Indeed, in 1998 the IFRC&RCS described the increasing alienation, degradation, famine, and poverty of people who were most vulnerable to major adversity. It went on to define disasters as "exceptional events which suddenly kill or injure large numbers of people or cause major economic losses" (IFRC&RCS, 1998, p.12), and it identified areas of "socioeconomic dislocation" in its map of relief operations (IFRC&RCS, 1998, p. 188).

In his introduction to that same volume (IFRC&RCS, 1998, p. 8), the secretary-general of the IFRC&RCS went so far as to declare that, as "economic globalization becomes a reality, and as the debate surrounding the role of civil society evolves, opportunities are presenting themselves to governments and to other forms of civil action, to reduce risk and plan for a safer future."[10] Then, immediately after September 11, from within the camp of international economists, none other than James D. Wolfenson, president of the World Bank, reiterated his concern that poverty and inequality were at the root of global ills that generate terrorism (Sullivan, 2002). In January 2001 the World Economic Forum even made terrorism the theme of its annual conference, and among its galaxy of speakers Kofi Annan, secretary-general of the United Nations, appealed for the adoption of an outlook of global citizenship with humanitarian as well as economic concerns to overcome "the fragility of globalization" (2002). His subsequent High-Level Panel on Threats, Challenges, and Change (2004, p. 2) went so far as to say that "combating poverty will not only save millions of lives but also strengthen states' capacity to combat terrorism, organized crime and proliferation."[11]

Were the disastrous effects of microeconomic factors also to be taken into account, it would be a moot point as to whether, except for the terrible loss of life from the exploding aircraft on 9/11, the machinations of incalculable magnitude perpetrated by white-collar fraudsters that have surfaced in many parts of the world might not be as destructive in their effects as the activity of terrorists attacking the macroeconomic system.[12] The managerial depredations affected the livelihood of millions of employees, in many instances wiping out their pension funds and jeopardizing the security of many investors. The reputable billionaire investors Warren Buffett and Charlie Munger, no less, are quoted as saying that they were disgusted by the way in which "in the last few years...shareholders have suffered billions in losses while the CEOs, promoters, and other higher-ups who fathered these *disasters* [italics added] have walked away with extraordinary wealth" (Reuters, March 3, 2002). Indeed, there are so many malefactors that the U.S. Department of Justice (2001) has provided a resource handbook for their victims (with an appendix that just might give other people the wrong idea about crimes they might perpetrate). Now the seemingly invincible auditors who earned more from advising their avaricious clients about their business methods than from auditing company books are attracting the attention of regulatory agencies and professional bodies—and the extent of their malfeasance when fully revealed might also come to be regarded as disastrous.

Frontline Response

Turning from the scope of terrorism to its enactment, records show that in 2001 there were 355 international terrorist attacks, with 198 in 2002 and 208 in 2003 (Patterns of Global Terrorism, 2004).[13] In addition, there were 33 in 2003 that were recorded as "nonsignificant" because they did not result in loss of life, serious injury, or major property damage (Chronology of nonsignificant international terrorist incidents, 2003). The attacks took place on every continent but Australia and Antarctica, and, leaving aside any others that might have been instigated by governments for whatever reason, there is no doubt that the major attacks were those perpetrated by al-Qaeda in the United States on September 11, 2001—they attracted the greatest attention of the authorities, behavioral scientists, and the general population worldwide in the hope of learning from the United States' experience.

For the record, the leading agencies in the United States responded with emergency trauma teams (cf. American Red Cross, 2002; Figley, Figley, & Norman, 2002). Clinical authorities updated their websites with information for health professionals about the possible consequences of traumatic stress, and others gave advice to the general population about the services available for those in need.[14] Providers began to appraise their interventions, and a number of epidemiologists started a flow of papers based on their sample-surveys of the general population of the whole country as well as those that were at greater risk in New York. Yet to be undertaken are psychological studies of the estimated 25,000 survivors who evacuated the twin towers of the World Training Center in orderly fashion despite the chaos in which they found themselves. The National Institute of Standards and Technology, (NIST) (2004) compiled an extensive dossier of over 10,000 pages of findings from stratified groups of hundreds of survivors about the architectural and operational aspects of the evacuation procedures, among which there should be some clues about the psychological reactions of evacuees to encourage behavioural scientists to go further. The initial account of blind Michael Hingston making his way down safely from the 78th floor with his guide dog would also make a good start (*Guide Dog News,* 2001).

Here the importance of agencies coming together with community leaders in order to reinforce working relationships, improve performance, and convert anxieties into acceptable fears has to be acknowledged. The first of these meetings to discuss the September 11, 2001, terrorist attacks was held just 3 months later on December 9–11 (Jackson et al., 2002, p. 89). Understandably, because of the imminent threat of further terrorist activity, the conference focused on the firsthand experiences of the emergency responders regarding the performance, availability, and adequacy of their personal protective clothing and equipment as they responded to the incidents. However, with 450 of their colleagues having perished on duty, the large scale of the operation, the communication and command strategies rendered ineffective, and the range and duration of unfamiliar and demanding tasks, it was inevitable that other topics did not escape mention.[15] Among these were the removal of decayed bodies and parts, methods of protecting the crime scene, and ways of coping with the

massive influx of skilled and unskilled volunteers day after day.

Early in 2003 such a conference was held in Washington, DC (Leading during times of trouble: A roundtable discussion of recent terror events, 2003), to the evident satisfaction of all of the participants. They shared their insecurities, spoke of their under- and overreactions—including those to the 17,000 reports of anthrax deposits in the postal system—and the need to have the news media on one's side (cf. Taylor, 2006a). The role of the news media certainly warranted attention, because the New Yorkers directly exposed to the 9/11 attacks on the World Trade Center who also viewed the televised images of that event more than seven times, were found to be more likely to suffer posttraumatic stress disorders (PTSD) and/ or depression than a control group (Ahern et al., 2002). Another study found that 10% of a widespread group had developed PTSD by proxy from witnessing the graphic and persistent portrayal of the tragedy on television (Schuster et al., 2001). The latter was consistent with the findings of an earlier study after the Oklahoma City bombing (cited by Hamblen & Slone, 2002).

On the same theme, when appearing live on New Zealand television as a commentator 2 days after the September 11 tragedy, I felt obliged to question a television reporter about the wisdom of the nonstop exposure that her channel was giving to the event. She replied that it was important for the news media to make an indelible impression on the minds of its viewers. However, neither she nor her program producer had considered the negative effects on viewers witnessing the constant repetition of the plane striking the second tower and of people plunging to their deaths to avoid being burned alive, nor of their responsibility for causing such vicarious traumatic reactions. In fact the experience left many children in a state of anxiety, and was sufficiently disruptive to leave adults in no condition to begin thinking rationally of the causes and the consequences of the events.

A few months later, after the unprecedented news coverage of the war in Iraq, Mark Reinecke of Northwestern University Medical School provided a fact sheet of advice to help viewers who were "battling war-induced stress" (retrieved March 29, 2003, from http://www.msnbc.com/news/892080 .asp?0q12=c8p&cp1=1). But unlike the group of psychoanalysts after the 1985 earthquake in

Mexico, no one seems to have been invited to appear before radio and television audiences on government and commercially run stations to give advice and reassurance (Palacios et al., 1986).

However, in an initial overview of the research findings on populations after 9/11, Hamblen and Slone (2002, n.p.) reported that, in common with reactions to other kinds of disasters, the initial rates of distress and posttraumatic symptoms were high:

> Ultimately reducing the risk of traumatic stress reactions is best accomplished by abolishing trauma in the first place by preventing war, terrorism, and other traumatic stressors. The next best approach is to foster resilience and bolster support so that individuals have better coping capacity prior to and during traumatic stress. The third best option is early detection and treatment of traumatized individuals to prevent a prolonged stress response.

To follow that prescription, the immediate job of those who provide psychological first aid after disasters is to give the necessary encouragement and support to casualties to help them regain their stability. In addition, it requires social scientists to help communities restore the essentials and get back into operation rather than try immediately to address the endemic causes of, say, terrorism, Islamophobia, or anti-Semitism which currently grip the world (cf. Annan, 2004). Nonetheless, should people be intrigued by the possibility of trying to effect an improvement, they might consider the New Rules Project (2004) proposed by the Institute for Local Self-reliance, which calls upon communities and regions to be viewed not only as places of residence, recreation, and retail but also as places that nurture active and informed citizens with the skills and productive capacity to generate real wealth and the authority to govern their own lives. To be sure, cultural, ideological, philosophical, political, and religious differences need to be brought into consideration at some

stage in the recovery process, and psychologists should play their part in the proceedings.

Phases of Disaster

The appropriate kind of intervention suggested for different stages of after-effects caused by disasters brings to mind Drabek's monumental task (1986) in scanning more than 1,000 published reports of all kinds of catastrophes in a search for their essential components. Eventually he identified and named four major phases of disasters—preparedness, response, recovery, and mitigation—each of which he subdivided and related to the individual, group, organization, community, society, and nation (see Table 24.1).[16] Then he suggested priorities that others might take up (i.e., automated information retrieval systems, taxonomies of disaster events and response systems, access to comparative international databases, linking theory of human behavior with practice, increased practitioner/researcher interaction, and the mental health needs of the first responders to a disaster scene).

This chapter does no more than applaud Drabek's diligence and perspicacity while (a) endorsing the need for a classification of disasters and of potential casualties and (b) extending his concern for the postdisaster mental health needs of emergency workers to a wider range of people adversely affected.

Classification of Disasters

Classification is at the heart of every intellectual, empirical, and pragmatic endeavor. Paradoxically it helps researchers to establish the boundaries of a given topic and separates a subject into manageable parts for closer scrutiny. In disaster work it is a prerequisite for assessing the adequacy of resources to meet clinical and organizational emergencies. However, before we consider any classification scheme, three warnings need to be given. The first is

Table 24.1. Phasic responses to disasters

Preparedness	Response	Recovery	Mitigation
Planning	Preimpact mobilization	Restoration	Hazard perceptions
Warning	Postimpact emergency action	Reconstruction	Consequent adjustment

that some people are inclined doggedly to seek either the general factors or the unique, like the contentious medieval scholars who had insufficient flexibility of mind either to clump or to split the components according to the pattern of material presented (Schachner, 1962, pp. 19–24). The second is that some people are either prehistoric iconoclasts or scatterbrained individuals who deny the value of classification altogether: At best both extremes approach each situation de novo and at worst do not learn from their own experience, much less from others. The third is that the process of classification can be a seductive diversion for those who admire elegance at the expense of utility and use it as a protective shield to avoid practical involvement in the problems of the real world.

For my part, I developed a framework for disasters and victims after the Mount Erebus plane crash in Antarctica in November 1979, in which all 237 passengers and 20 crew were killed (Taylor & Frazer, 1981, p. 72; 1982), simply because I wanted to bring together the many reports scattered throughout professional journals about various groups of people that had been involved in different types of disaster. At the time the existing reports fell short of elaborating the category of human disasters as distinct from the natural or the industrial. However, I soon found that the previous studies could be sorted into the three relatively distinct categories and then be cross-matched with earth, air, fire, liquid, or biological components—despite the occasional disaster with multiple compounding features, such as that from a dam failure dislocating a poor community, followed by the methyl mercury contaminating its water supply, and finally the widespread theft of

Table 24.2. Matrix of disasters

	Natural	Industrial Technological	Human Reactors
Earth	Avalanches Earthquakes	Dam failures Ecological neglect	Ecological irresponsibility Motor vehicle and train accidents
	Erosions Eruptions Meteorite crashes Mudflows Toxic mineral deposits	Landslides Outerspace debris Radioactive substances Toxic waste disposal	
Air	Blizzards Tornadoes Dust storms	Acid rain Chemical pollution Explosions, surface and underground	Aircraft accidents Hijackings Spacecraft accidents
	Hurricanes Meteorite and planetary shifts Thermal shifts	Radioactive clouds and soot Urban smog	
Fire	Lightning damage Spontaneous combustion	Boiling liquid Expanding vapor accidents Electrical fires Hazardous chemicals	Arson
Liquid	Droughts Floods Storms Tsunamis	Effluent contamination Oil spills Waste disposal	Maritime accidents River tragedies
Biological Elements	Endemic diseases Epidemics Famine	Design flaws Equipment problems Illicit manufacture and use of explosives and poisons	Complex terrorism Corporate Criminal extortion via viruses and poisons
	Overpopulation Plague Pestilence		Guerilla warfare Hostage taking Sports crowd violance Warfare

its precious savings by devious landowners who operated the company store (Erikson, 1994).

Then, following Drabek, it became possible to compare the studies according to both the particular phase in which they were conducted and the specific effects on any particular sample of the population on which they were based (Table 24.2).

Victims, Casualties, and Their Psychological Needs

Turning from the classification of catastrophes to a corresponding classification of victims and casualties, according to the *New Shorter Oxford Dictionary,* the word "victim" first appeared in print in the Rhemish translation of the Bible in 1592, and it came into general currency in the seventeenth century to describe living creatures that were sacrificed to the deities. After that the noun was generalized to describe "any person put to death, subjected to torture or suffering, or property loss, through cruel or oppressive treatment or a destructive agency."

The classification of victims began to serve a purpose other than the religious in the Napoleonic wars, when frontline medical staff introduced a triage system for sorting surgical casualties into four groups according to the critical nature of their injuries (http://en.wikipedia.org/wiki/Triage). More recently, medical and social scientists have come to classify casualties by the magnitude of the external social chaos, the spread of disruptive effects, the extent of personal injuries sustained, sickness, bereavement, property loss, physical and emotional vulnerability, and the reserves of resilience that individuals and their groups have for coping with adversity. Then finally, perhaps in an attempt to assert its nonpolitical organizational stance in making help available to everyone, the IFRC&RCS defined victims more simply as people with basic needs for survival (*DHA News,* 1994, pp. 60–61).

Again, any such classification schema needs to be used with care because labeling people instantly as victims can create secondary problems for both the labeled and the labelers. In the labeled it can induce feelings of hopelessness and discouragement that make them succumb more easily to adversity and keep them in a state of perpetual dependence on the clinical and social services that their community might provide. In the labelers it can induce feelings of dominance and indis-

pensability that make for difficulty in bringing closure to professional relationships. Not that the "helpers" should be encouraged to go the other extreme and adopt a buccaneer gung-ho attitude to obscure the potential pathological consequences of suffering, but they should be prepared to accept a time-limited role in the compassionate application of the appropriate skills for which they have been trained.[17]

For such reasons and except for those that have either died from the calamity or suffered irrevocably in some other equally significant way, the term "casualty" is to be preferred for those whose lives have been affected adversely by exposure to catastrophe. Explicitly the term implies the membership of a provisional rather than a permanent category. It applies to people that have survived the initial impact of a life-threatening event of some magnitude, but it encourages self-reliance and is consistent with the thought that, no matter what has happened, it is better to live in hope than to die in despair. It is consistent with the adaptation of Nietzsche's saying—"that which does not kill me [can make] me strong"—thereby fostering hope for recovery through the positive power of the *placebo effect* and at the same time negating the stultifying power of its counterpart, the *nocebo effect.*

Both of such polar opposites deserve consideration because, at present, clinicians and researchers, unlike managers and educators (cf. accel/TEAM, 2005), tend either to denigrate or trivialize the placebo for being subjective and beyond the realm of science, and they ignore the nocebo completely. Rarely do they comment on the fact that their own optimism and pessimism toward other people operate as self-fulfilling prophecies to bring about their expectations. They are not likely to change their stance until they can (a) accept that one of their functions is to reinforce the natural powers of recovery of those seeking their help, rather than to be held entirely responsible for any more identifiable remedial intervention, and (b) not feel ashamed or embarrassed to promote research into the recuperative powers of the mind.

The definition of the placebo ("I will please") harks back to the use of the word by Chaucer in 1386 when describing "a flatterer, sycophant, parasite" (*Oxford English Dictionary* [OED] Online, 2005). In 1811 the word was recorded as "an epithet given to any medicine adapted more to please than benefit...a substance or procedure which a patient accepts as a medicine or therapy but which has no specific therapeutic activity for his condition or is prescribed in the belief that it has no such activity." Today, clinicians are thought not inclined to foster the practice, despite the gradually accumulating evidence of its efficacy, because of the risk to their reputations as biomedical scientists (Benson & Stark, 1996, Chapters 1–3; Carroll, 2005). However, far from feeling intellectually embarrassed by having fostered any inherent recuperative powers, healers invoking the placebo should be pleased to think that they have developed their skills sufficiently to promote its application. They might then promote studies of its efficacy.

The nocebo effect ("I will harm") is not so well known as the placebo, and its definition appears only as "Draft entry December 2003" in the OED Online as the "detrimental effect on health produced by psychological or psychosomatic factors such as negative expectations of treatment or prognosis, cultural beliefs about illness, personality traits, etc." Even fewer studies have been undertaken of the nocebo that of its opposite (cf. Carroll, 2002). However, there are many everyday examples of the harmful effects induced by noxious parents and work supervisors, to say nothing of certain anachronistic cultural prohibitions to affirm the significance of the concept. They are something that potential helpers should try to obviate.

The maximizing of the placebo and the minimizing of the nocebo have elements in common with the processes of the therapist showing "absolute positive regard" emphasized by the Rogerian therapists, of "establishing rapport" on first acquaintance (usually mentioned without elaboration in professional training courses), of monitoring the two-way transference effects in psychoanalytic treatments (cf. Wilson & Lindy, 1994), and of portraying the cardinal virtues of conveying "emotional warmth, empathy, and congruence" to clients (cf. Patterson, 1989/2000). But the intent is to encourage those in need to draw initially on their own resources and then for the helper to join in, rather than for the helper to play a more active part right away.

Fostering self-help, once any threats to life and limb are reduced, also requires health professionals not to give undue attention immediately to any particular psychological symptoms that casualties might report or to signs they might themselves observe, but to allow casualties a few days grace in which they might begin to use their inner strength

and regain composure. Within the limits of common sense, the time for them to register features of psychopathology comes later, should casualties find intrusive thoughts, avoidance behavior, and state of high arousal beginning seriously to interfere with their everyday lives (cf. Young, Ford, Ruzek, Friedman, & Gusman, 1998; Raphael, 2000). Doing so would not put the casualties unduly at risk because, as the World Health Organization (WHO) (2003, p. 4) has stated:

> Most acute mental health problems during the acute emergency phase are best managed without medication following the principles of "psychological first-aid" (i.e., listen, convey compassion, assess needs, ensure basic physical needs are met, do not force talking, provide or mobilize company from preferably family or significant others, encourage but do not force social support, protect from further harm).

These procedures can be supported with programs of stress reduction in which stimulants are avoided, exercise is encouraged, social supports are utilized, and life styles are reexamined (Davis, Eshelman, and McKay, 1995; WHO, 1997).

However, no matter how prestigious the authority recommending treatments, health professionals themselves will still be held accountable for the potency and impotency of their interventions, and for that reason they and their organizations will have to address the difficult question of designing appropriate procedures for evaluating the quality of their work.[18] Novices can derive benefit from the reassurance of Norris et al. (2001) and Norris, Friedman, and Watson (2002), who maintain that disasters rarely engender severe, lasting, and pervasive effects unless the damage to property is extreme and widespread, financial problems for the community are serious and ongoing, or the disaster is caused by human carelessness or intent, with a high prevalence of trauma in the form of injuries, threats to life, and actual loss of life. Yet those authors make no mention of casualties gaining benefit psychologically from surviving catastrophic experience (cf. Tedeschi, Park, and Calhoun, 1998). In fact, and without going quite so far as to say with Samuel Johnson that "when a man knows he is to be hanged in a fortnight, it concentrates his mind wonderfully," there is truth in the saying that the awareness of death causes a reexamination of value systems (Ursano, Tzu-Cheg, & Fullerton, 1992).

Despite the embarrassment that the bare mention of human values might cause some behavioral scientists, value systems give a sense of meaning and purpose to life that becomes only too apparent after they have been fractured by emergencies and disasters. People who are hesitant to acknowledge such subjective factors might be persuaded (a) by the idea that human beings could be construed somewhat like computers, in that they too need a comparable basic DOS, Windows 95, 98, 2000xp, or Linux operating system; and (b) by the realization that the WHO's definition of health does not reflect merely the absence of disease or infirmity but also the state of complete mental, physical, and social well-being (WHO, 1997). They might also go further to reflect on the additional spiritual dimension of *te kaha wairua,* which, together with *te kaha hinengaro, te kaha tinana,* and *te kaha whanau,* constitutes the traditional Maori fourfold concept of spiritual, mental, physical, and sociocultural health (Durie, 1985).[19] Finally, they might appraise the physiological underpinnings of religious belief (cf. Benson and Stark, 1996, Chapter 8) and consider W. R. Miller's (1999) integration of spiritual and psychological treatments in a book published by the American Psychological Association (APA), no less.

Spirituality is a term that covers religious attitudes, experiential dimensions, existential well-being, paranormal beliefs, and religious practices (McDonald, 2000). It offers a sense of meaning and purpose in life and sets a framework for personal conduct and group relationships that can at least withstand scrutiny. It is of particular relevance in the recovery period after disasters, when casualties search for explanations of events, as I elaborate later with an example from the Cook Islands after a devastating cyclone (Taylor, 2001). Nevertheless, its incorporation into recovery plans presents a challenge for health professionals—not all of whom will be emotionally or intellectually willing to consider the metaphysician-scientist-practitioner model that O'Donohue (1989) advanced. Beit-Hallami and Argyle (1997) attempted valiantly to bridge the academic divide, but with a touch of resignation Argyle (2002) was forced to conclude that perhaps the best psychology can hope for is to study the causes, correlates, and effects of religion but not to explain it.[20]

Despite the intellectual difficulties, Loewenthal (2001, pp. 82–83), a leading British authority on test construction, has used prayer as one of four topics to illustrate the application of psychometric techniques, and the *Journal of Community Psychology* has devoted two special volumes to the subject (Kloos & Moore, 2000, 2001). Then, after 9/11, the APA went so far as to advise its clinical members to respond to disasters by recognizing professional challenges, attending to self-care strategies that included their own spiritual needs, adopting professional support, and enhancing their commitment to those in need (cf. http://www.apa.org/practice/practitionerhelp.html [retrieved January 31, 2006]). Subsequently, the APA commissioned a book by Pyszczynski, Solomon, and Greenberg (2003), in which the authors elaborate on Ernest Becker's *Denial of Death* (1973) when applying their "Terror Management Theory" (TMT) to post-9/11 reactions. TMT proposes that innate anxiety about annihilation combined with the inevitability of death creates a basis for terror for the adversaries on both sides and that it can be reduced only by addressing the causes of fundamentalism.

However, at the more immediate interactive level with casualties after a disaster, I have found it helpful to create six somewhat distinct categories according to their kind of involvement they had in the event (Table 24.3)—while accepting that the blurring of categories might occur when some people fall into more than one grouping. Not all of those in any particular category will necessarily require the same kind of intervention because their needs will depend on their personal perceptions of particular traumatic events, their unfinished business from previous events, their current state of mental and physical health, their mental resilience, and the adequacy of their support systems. A few casualties might also find that the disaster experience has exacerbated dormant emotional problems that now demand more intense attention than psychological first aid provides, but at least the categories provide a starting point for health professionals who are concerned about appraising the diversity of perceptions and psychological problems of people affected by all kinds of disasters (cf. Office for Victims of Crime, 2000; 2001).

With these provisos, the primary casualties are those who suffer directly from a catastrophe. Many do not survive, but those who do might develop symptoms ranging from the mild to the severe that can be instant, delayed, transient, or chronic. They have to reassemble their shattered lives sufficiently

Table 24.3. Classification of victims and casualties

1. Those who are adversely affected at the epicenter of a disaster
2. Their families and close friends
3. The emergency workers and those whose jobs oblige them to become directly involved in the rescue and recovery operations
4. The grieving community that identifies with those who are suffering
5. The psychologically troubled whose reactions are exacerbated; troublemakers who are inclined to exploit the situation and use it to their own advantage
6. Various other people who are adversely affected

to satisfy their basic needs for shelter, food and drink, belonging and security, while leaving aside their needs for self-esteem and self-actualization until the semblance of normality returns (cf. Maslow, 1987). Like everyone who suffers acutely, they will be faced with rebuilding their perception of the world in a way that restores meaning and purpose to their lives (Bracken, 2002). Eventually some will find that they have been strengthened by their experience of adversity.

The secondary casualties are the family members and close friends of the primary group who develop symptoms vicariously, sometimes with a greater intensity than those more directly involved. Depending on the intensity of their personal attachments and extent of loss, they will need time, opportunity, and encouragement to grieve and express a mixture of feelings that include anger, distress, guilt, and despair at their loss before they can pick up the threads of life again (cf. Young, 2001, Chapter 5). Their reactions are likely to be prolonged if delays occur in the identification of their loved ones, which makes it difficult to bring closure to a fatal episode to fulfill their cultural and religious obligations.[21] However, the careful identification of the dead makes delays inevitable, and the Pan American Health Organization and the World Health Organization (2004) warn against the greater psychological harm caused to relatives and their communities by speedy and anonymous mass burials or cremations: they are also at pains to explode the myth that hasty mass burials are necessary to prevent disease from spreading—except in regions where disease is endemic or where the fresh water supply is endangered. However, the warnings

seem not to have been heeded in Banda Aceh after the devastating tsunami came ashore on 26th December 2004 (IFRC&RCS, 2005, p.87).

The tertiary casualties are the workers in all types of agencies who succumb during the course of their postimpact assignments. If once they were described as the "hidden victims" of disaster, today they are recognized more openly as being vulnerable to occupational fatigue and stress reaction. Fatigue arises from the impulse of workers after a disaster not to impose a daily routine of a reasonable length that allows them sufficient time between shifts for rest and recovery. Stress arises from the substantial imbalance between demands that are made and the ability of individuals to respond with the organizational support available.

To their own detriment, emergency workers sometimes identify too closely with the primary victims and lose their objectivity (Asken, 1993), particularly if they are engaged in gruesome and prolonged body-recovery work and if their colleagues are among the dead.[22] In such circumstances many of the firefighters in the immediate aftermath of 9/11 were said to have broken ranks, disobeyed orders, and acted impulsively (McKinsey Report, 2002), rushing up the towers in a way that has been likened to "Pickett's charge" of futility, which occurred in the U.S. Civil War (Massey, 2002). In states of sustained high arousal many resisted the attempts of management to get them to moderate their hours of duty and change their strategic priorities (Eisner, 2002).

Consequently, emergency workers should be encouraged to develop emotional shields for the duration of their assignments and to undergo occupational debriefing afterward to help them regain their composure and their resilience for living—otherwise they might become case hardened and burned out.[23] I raise this point because many of the emergency personnel who collected parts of 257 victims in 347 bags after the crash of an airliner were found to have made spontaneous conceptual transformations to help them deal with the immediate horror of the job, but afterward they expressed the need to restore the reality of the assignment.[24] Initially when working, they found themselves regarding the body parts as broken dolls, tailor's dummies, waxworks, meat from a slaughterhouse, medical specimens, jigsaw puzzles, and scientific problems to be solved, but when off duty they reflected on the human side of the work. Consistent with van Der Kolk's conceptualization some years later (1996), the creation and adoption of such personal cognitive defenses helped to prevent traumatically disturbing images from being fixed in the nondeclarative part of memory and gradually made them available for processing, absorption, and availability in the declarative part.

Following the same plane crash, an interest was taken in the design and operation of mortuaries and embalming facilities, and changes were recommended that might be beneficial to the operatives, as well as the families of the deceased who identify their loved ones (Taylor, 1984, 1987). Research was also undertaken with students of health science and medicine to assess their reactions to the cadaver work they did in their training and to minimize any emotional impact (Hancock, Williams, & Taylor, 1998; Hancock, Williams, Taylor, & Dawson, 2004).[25]

Yet to come into consideration are the trainee mental health service providers who might need to witness brain prosections and postmortems in their training to help them to prepare for on-the-scene disaster fatalities they might encounter later on.[26] Reports of the reactions of the health care workers who conducted body recovery operations at the World Trade Center have yet to come to light, but the early indications of the 10 uniformed staff that worked at the Pentagon are that medical training and clinical exposure were perceived as "somewhat protective by some but did not seem to prevent vulnerability to the emotional impact of their experiences" (Keller & Bobo, 2002, p. 8).

Apart from preparation for working near disaster sites, the normal professional training and experience of health professionals does not prepare them for the transient trauma recovery work of the kind to which Knop (2001) and Gold and Faust (2002) have drawn attention. For example, the conventional courtesies of professional referral for specific appointments to the security of consulting rooms do not apply in emergency situations. To the contrary, providers of psychological first aid have to be prepared to adapt their schedules, procedures, and interventions to the prevailing circumstances. They might have to work in makeshift quarters, reach out to find clients, make arrangements as appropriate for the management and care of anyone showing a warning cluster of psychological signs, provide simple, informative handouts for follow-up purposes should help be required later, and impose reasonable limits on their own daily schedules of work.

The quaternary group of casualties might be symptom free except for their behavioral excess. It consists of the well-intentioned but emotionally labile people in the community at large who identify with the primary victims and act inappropriately themselves. It includes those who display what has been called the "cornucopia syndrome" from opening their pantries and their hearts with goodwill but little imagination to impose burdens of perishable food, unsuitable clothing, and offers of hospitality on unwilling recipients.[27] These are the people for whom the term "compassion fatigue" was originally coined because they could not sustain for long the additional burden their emotions obliged them to carry—plus the fact that any constantly accumulating and evolving trauma scene makes more demands than anyone can possibly meet.[28] The category includes those that converge on disaster sites, like the estimated 10,000–15,000 volunteers who turned up daily at the World Trade Center to help in the recovery of victims, most of whom complicated the operations (Rick Shivar, External Affairs Directorate, U.S. Federal Emergency Management Agency, live video conference, March 14, 2002). So many firefighters were said to have arrived uninvited from neighboring counties and even from other countries that a special "maverick holding pen" was proposed for the coordination, management, and deployment of all kinds of volunteers until they were needed (Ludwig, 2002).

The same quaternary, or fourth, group includes the citizens who in 1981 hammered on the door of a mortuary in Rome, demanding to see the corpse of a 7-year-old boy that had died tragically after slipping down a pothole (*Paese Sera,* July 18, 1981). Thanks to the power of nonstop overnight television coverage of the scene, the viewers had identified emotionally with the boy's family as the emergency services made futile attempts to recover the boy alive. But the news reporters, who had created and sustained the high level of excitement, stopped short of releasing the pressure and helping viewers to regain their composure. Instead, they left them to make intrusive claims at the mortuary on the basis of their newly acquired quasi-family connections.

The quinternary, or fifth, group of disaster casualties consists of the troubled and the troublesome with pathological proclivities that, in times of phantasmagoria, lose their self-control. The troubled give free rein to their fantasies by indulging in voyeuristic activities, collecting pictures of body parts, and even expressing necrophilic desires. Some of them pretend to have been involved in any well-publicized disaster, either to play on the sympathy of donors or to seek notoriety. It is a moot point whether this category might include the "disasterotropic," who chase tornadoes, tsunamis, and volcanic activity to satisfy desires other than the scientific, or the surge of tourists with ghoulish tastes that visit the sites of devastation—such as those for whom the government of Honduras made provision after Hurricane Mitch in 1998 or those for whom a Ukraine tourist agency is now promoting visits to the site of the leaking radioactive power station at Chernobyl.

The troublesome are those who in times of social chaos go on the rampage to loot, plunder, and riot. Their more calculating and sophisticated counterparts with greater impulse control perpetrate insurance fraud, and hoaxers have to be taken seriously.[29] Sundry reports in the news media showed that after 9/11 thieves tried to steal gold from the vaults in the rubble, a photographer distributed a picture he claimed to be of one of the planes a few moments before the impact, a few people in different parts of the United States made dramatic—but fraudulent—appeals for relief, with some posting names of missing people fraudulently on the official website. Another matter in Canada dreamed up the story of five terrorists crossing the border to divert attention from his own criminal activities.[30] At the higher end of the scale of criminality, one of the firms with offices in the World Trade Center came under suspicion with regard to about $105 million of investment funds that went missing with a financier soon after the catastrophe, and some 2 years after the event the Empire State Development Corporation reported that it had been obliged to recover $1.2 million in payments from 66 companies that had claimed emergency grants. Hoaxers in the United States and elsewhere caused bomb scares at many airports, and in many countries they caused widespread fear and disruption by distributing white powder resembling anthrax.[31]

In this connection the point could be made again that good clinicians exude acceptance, empathy, and absolute positive regard toward their clients and patients. Rarely do they operate otherwise, unless they are burned out. And rarely do they consider malingering as a differential diagnosis "in those situations in which financial remuneration, benefit eligibility, or forensic determination play a role" (American Psychiatric Association, 2000, pp. 467, 471). However, in trauma work, especially when substantial economic and psychological benefits are to be gained, such a differential diagnosis should not be entirely overlooked (Taylor, 2003a).

The final category is for the miscellaneous group of casualties that has a diverse array of associations with disasters that present problems with which they have difficulty in coping. It includes those that, but for chance, would themselves have been primary victims and who constantly torment themselves with questions as to why they were saved from fatality. It also includes those who in all innocence had persuaded their friends and acquaintances to go into a situation that subsequently became disastrous, as well as those who believe that in some way—by their activity or inactivity—they have brought about a given disaster. It includes trauma workers and researchers, who in their postdisaster work are sometimes unaware of the insidious effects of the strain and fatigue upon themselves. Moreover, unlike the compassion fatigue prevention service that the Green Cross now provides for trauma teams (http://www.greencross.org), they had neither personal nor professional networks available to support them (Gentry, 2002). A glaring example is that of a first-line responder of an international aid agency I encountered on a disaster scene who was quite dysfunctional after spending years of travail in battle-torn Angola, Burundi, Cambodia, Cyprus, Kosovo, Laos, Liberia, Serbia, Somalia, and Vietnam. All he could do to gain respite was to express cynicism, indulge his interest in the history of conflict in the region wherever he found himself, and smoke like a chimney. I was not at all surprised to learn that he resigned soon after we met.

The classification systems for disasters and casualties can be combined conveniently and applied to the study of any given catastrophe and its human effects (Figure 24.1). First, the elements, factors, and phases of a disaster can be located in three-dimensional space, and then the corresponding features of the casualties can be compacted into the form of a smaller cube and placed in the precise disaster location. Then, with several disaster studies so placed, it is possible to have a comprehensive grasp of different types of disasters and of different types of casualties.

Phasic Community Reactions

Before considering some applications of the model, it is necessary to mention the sequence of community reactions that typically occur after any catastrophe. These tend to overlay any clinical symptoms that individuals might describe and color the responses a community might make to any plans for rescue and recovery work. The sequence begins with the *heroic* period, which occurs immediately after the impact of any disaster, in which the community excels in attending to the needs of its members long before outside aid can be brought in (Young et al., 1998, pp. 17–19). However, in view of the mounting apprehension and anxiety about pending terrorist threats and the fear generated by the hypersensitive precautions taken by the authorities to safeguard the commu-

nity, a case can be made for restoring the earlier stages of warning, threat, and impact that Powell, Rayner, and Finesinger published originally in 1953 (cited by Cisin & Clark, 1962). Potentially each of such stages has anxiety-producing features that are worthy of detailed consideration, and with the present and prolonged imposition of widespread national and international security measures, there would be no shortage of subjects with whom they could be explored.

After the heroic period follows the *honeymoon* of supreme optimism, in which the community enjoys being the center of worldwide attention, with promises of support coming from all quarters to help to restore the status quo. After about 3 weeks *disillusionment* sets in, when these promises have not all been fulfilled, some are found to be conditional, the donations received are neither readily nor evenly dispensed, internal dissensions arise, and the future looks bleak. Finally, after many months the *restabilization* phase occurs, in which recovery plans begin to bear fruit, signs of reconstruction are seen, the community restructures itself, some evacuees return home to the disaster zone, commemoration days are established, memorials are erected, and the catastrophe is incorporated into the cultural life of the community.

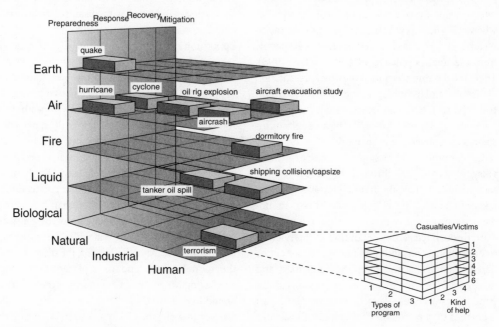

Figure 24.1. A conceptual model to integrate disaster studies.

Cross-Cultural Considerations

Mention of the cultural life of a devastated community brings to mind the need for clinicians and researchers to attend to cross-cultural factors whether they are working either in a multicultural community at home (see Mollica, Wyshak, & Lavelle, 1987) or in a community abroad where the attitudes, beliefs, customs, and language differ markedly from theirs (DeVries, 1996, Chapter 17; Lindner, 2001). In particular they have to be satisfied that their specific clinical concepts, methods of assessment, and treatments are appropriate for the ethnic groups and the settings in which they are to be applied (Marsella, Friedman, Gerrity, & Scurfield, 1996; Culbertson, 1997; Waxler-Morrison, Richardson, Anderson, & Chambers, 2001). Finally, following the development of cultural anthropology and cross-cultural psychiatry since the 1930s, trauma clinicians concerned with the dissonance of systems, as well as the psychopathology of individuals and groups, will need to regard cultures as dynamic entities and anticipate the possible consequences of any intervention they propose or changes they might feel obliged to recommend.

On such matters three fairly recent assignments in different countries in the South Pacific yielded a few clinical features worthy of special mention (Taylor, 2003b). The first occurred in Manihiki, a remote island in the Cook group, near the equator, where a 30-meter cyclonic wave swept over the 5-meter-high island and caused the loss of 20 people from the total population of 680 (Taylor, 1998). There the discourse included the open presentation of dreams and prophecies, and it was often embellished with tales and legends from the past (cf. Luomala, 1984, pp. 876–879). In a couple of instances the conventional "memory-evocation" technique for trauma reduction was enriched when villagers led the way through the rubble of their settlement to retrace the frantic journeys they had taken to reach "higher" ground. There, in immediate virtual reality in situ instead of long afterward through recall of detail during an interview in a conventional consulting room, they reentered the derelict homes that had given them sanctuary and now evoked tearful memories of previous occupants, organizations, possessions, and long-past events. As they spoke, they reexamined the actions they had taken for self-preservation during the maelstrom, expressing regret for not having been

able to persuade more of the bewildered community to tag along with them, praising the heroic deeds of their stalwart rescuers, and being critical of those who were unprepared and had chosen to ignore the weather reports or who had behaved badly by taking to alcohol or looting unoccupied premises.

However, the clergy of all four of the recognized Christian denominations (i.e., the Cook Island Christian Church, the Latter Day Saints, Roman Catholics, and the Seventh Day Adventists) hammered home Old Testament admonitions in their daily community services and obliged the survivors to search their souls and seek redemption for their moral transgressions, which had brought the cyclone on them as a punishment. At a time when their congregation was grieving and struggling to regain enough courage to continue with life, they made no reference to the teachings of the loving God of the Gospels. Only a few of the villagers were heard to question the validity of the religious intervention, despite the fact that their island lay in the seasonal path of hurricanes and that the devout and innocent were among the affected.

In response to their direct inquiries about my personal position on the matter, I could only say that, in all honesty, for me there were other more compelling explanations—such as El Niño and global warming—than the religious to account for the cyclone. But later, with distance, detachment, and access to theologians and libraries, I took the opportunity to reflect on the origins of different religious explanations for adversity before trying to resolve the issue—at least to my own satisfaction (Taylor, 1999). The problem seemed to be that the Cook Island pastors were faithfully repeating the fundamentalist doctrines of the early nineteenth-century missionaries to account for adversity, without regard for later theological interpretations as well as developments in science. To them, as Keys (1999, p. 67) wrote in another connection, it was as if "the broad outline of human history was seen as a divinely preordained chronological structure which one day would end with the resurrection of the dead, the Day of Judgment, the dissolution of the mortal world, and its replacement with an everlasting Kingdom of God in which the righteous would live forever."

Fortunately, the Christian clergy in Tuvalu, the place of the second South Pacific assignment, took a more liberal stand after a dormitory fire in which the house mother and 19 schoolgirls lost their lives. They asserted that fire was not an act of God, a *Kole fakasola,* but a pure accident, a *fakalavalava* (Taylor, 2000). They further asserted that any behavioral reactions of the bereaved were within the normal range to be expected, rather than a sign of madness, a *fakavalevale.* In offering such explanations they used the supportive strength of the scriptures and of their culture to help the bereaved come to terms with the tragedy.

The clergy also conducted a moving *matafaga* dawn service at which the congregation gathered in the darkness and took turns spontaneously sharing their grief until the rising sun streamed through the building as if to give them enough hope to face the new day. It was a remarkable ceremony that could only have been therapeutic to the overburdened. At the other end of the scale of sensitivity but no less helpful in stress reduction were the fervor and excitement of the regular drumming and dancing competitions that took place between the villages—the people needed no encouragement to use physical exercise to reduce their stress.

However, because Tuvaluans of all ages spoke about the existence of ghosts and evil spirits associated with the dead, it seemed appropriate to ask the clergy what they could do to exorcise the malevolence. There was talk of abandoning the school at which the victims were buried—and, had that happened, there would have been serious repercussions because there was only the one post-primary school in the remote island chain. The brighter students would have lost the opportunity to compete for higher education abroad, their job prospects would have been adversely affected, and they would have had more of a struggle to provide security for their parents in old age as their culture required.[32]

To their credit, the clergy in Tuvalu responded positively in their sermons and pastoral work by putting the malevolent spirits into theological context. One minister, at the behest of school-children that swore they heard the voices of ghosts over the grave, even appealed directly to the spirits of the deceased to rest in peace and not to trouble their friends who were grieving. About the same time, several students were seen sitting by the common grave and talking to their companions that had died. Their evident need to feel able to approach the grave rather than to shrink away from it was borne in mind later by the designers of

a memorial for the site. A year after the event there was far less talk of ghosts and spirits to be heard than there had been around the time of the tragedy. A gala recreation day was held to commemorate the first anniversary of the tragedy to which relatives of the deceased from far-flung islands were welcomed. Moreover, by then the number of students at the school had increased rather than decreased, as initially had been feared.

As to be expected, the schoolgirls who escaped the blazing dormitory had symptoms of avoidance, intrusive imagery, episodes of reliving the experience, and sleep disturbance. They had very mixed feelings about having survived while their friends in the same dormitory had been burned alive. The others, like many adolescents, were reflective but less expressive. At the time of the fire they had rushed to the scene, having been aroused by the alarm given by the staff and the noise of the burning timbers, and they formed a bucket brigade with their teachers to bring water from the ocean nearby until the fire raced beyond control. Thereafter they remained as silent sentinels, watching at a safe distance from the site until the fire died away and the staff could protect the burned bodies from marauding dogs. They crept back to bed for a troublesome few hours and returned the next morning to witness the recovery of the unidentifiable charred remains of their friends. Some of the senior pupils took part in wrapping the dead in woven-flax sleeping mats before the coffins were made, and a few acted as pallbearers later at the funeral service in the evening.

The active participation seemed to help many of the school pupils come to terms with the trauma of the event—much as Milne (1979) had found with the survivors of Cyclone Tracy and as Hoiberg and McCaughey (1982, p. 25) found with injured sailors after a collision between ships at sea. They remained on the spot with their group, and they stayed together either in their own homes or with their extended families on the capital island, Funafuti, for about 4 weeks while their school was closed. The continuing association gave them an opportunity to restore their emotional security with the group with which they had undergone the traumatic experience, while remaining in the supportive fold of their immediate and extended families.

To a European, it was interesting that the whole community rather than specific nuclear families were grieving. This was because, under the Polynesian kinship system, relatives of the same generation as the parents were regarded culturally as parents, no matter how biologically distant their personal position in the extended lineage (Danielsson, 1956, p. 89). Similarly, relatives of the same generation as the grandparents were all grandparents, and cousins were as brothers and sisters. The interweaving of family relationships made for a more extensive sharing of grief in the postimpact phase than would be the case in Western societies, but it also made for closer support in the recovery period.

In Fiji, the third assignment was to assess the reactions of parliamentarians taken hostage by terrorists once they had been released (Taylor, Nailatikau, and Walkey, 2002). Following McDuff (1992, Abstr.), the plan was to "create a healing social environment immediately after release . . . that encourage[s] strong cohesiveness . . . isolates the victims from external groups, promotes abreaction, and provides an opportunity for rest and replenishment . . . restore[s] a sense of power to the victims and . . . reduce[s] their feelings of isolation and helplessness and of being dominated by the terrorists." The task was also to monitor the hostages' emotional reactions to the critical event (Frederick, 1987), to look for signs of the adverse emotional attachments that sometimes develop between captors and captives (Strentz, 1979; Turner, 1985), and to offer whatever assistance seemed appropriate.[33]

However, because the coup was unresolved and continuing, it was difficult to gain access to the hostages still in custody. Those that had been released early were difficult to locate because they had scattered to the four winds—some had gone into hiding, and others had gone abroad. Consequently, approaches were made to the families of the hostages still in custody to let them know what provisions had been made for the reception of their loved ones and to ask whether they would pass on information in their letters to help them sustain their resistance to captivity.

Like some of the released hostages, the families were difficult to locate. For reasons of personal security a few had made a point of constantly shifting their whereabouts. Those that stayed put had reinforced the fences around their homes and taken extra precautions to have relatives and friends keep a watchful eye on unknown visitors.

Although their partners had been taken prisoner, for self-protection some of the families had made themselves prisoners in their own homes. During interviews with the families, the reactions of the first few were so extreme that the clinical program was extended to include them.

In the event, 10 former hostages and 31 key family members were interviewed in depth (together with two of the families of the coup leaders), their clinical needs were assessed, and they completed clinical questionnaires. They were given advice to help them put their suffering into better context, with prescriptions for minimal dosages of medication where necessary to reduce anxiety and induce routines of sleep.

But it was most noticeable that all of the respondents, whether Christian, Hindu, or Muslim, used sacred texts and phrases to cope with the continuing saga of intimidation, threats, and the extreme uncertainty of their situations. The personal benefit the believers derived from their faith, and their readiness to expound the tenet, contrasted sharply with the experience derived from trauma groups encountered in European countries, in which belief systems are rarely discussed.[34] The difference led to reflections about the importance of belief and value systems in helping casualties to retain their hold on life (Taylor, 2001).

Belief and Value Systems

Yet the propensity of some believers to perpetrate violence in the name of religion calls for serious consideration, as also does the evangelical zeal of those claiming religious authority for predicting the inevitability of Armageddon unless mankind becomes converted to Christianity (cf. http://en.wikipedia.org/wiki/Armageddon). From such evidence, those hoping to seek peaceful coexistence through formalized religion would be doomed to disappointment unless they had the strength to make more of a humanistic than a political interpretation of religious teachings. In a condemnation of this proposition, Sells (1996) has detailed the attempts that were made in Bosnia to cloak a basic ethnic war with religious overtones to justify the atrocities perpetrated there. Ignatieff (1998) has done the same for Afghanistan, and Read (2001) has gone further back to make a critical reappraisal of the complex motivations of the Crusaders.

It follows that religious explanations for disasters merit further debate. However, they are much neglected by psychologists, with authorities such as Beit-Hallahmi and Argyle (1997) making no mention of them in their most comprehensive appraisal of religious behavior, beliefs, and experience. Perhaps the different explanations for disaster simply reflect the prevailing educational, experiential, and intellectual climate of the times in which they were originally made. They could be construed as having the function of myths—defined by McLeish (1996, p. v) as providing "the continuum of identity which allows the community to make sense of everything it experiences or thinks"—except that they are based on either supernatural belief or direct evidence, and sometimes a mixture of both. The first is drawn either from superstition or scripture, the second from observation and verification, and the third from an amalgam when either kind of explanation alone is insufficient to account for the facts as observed.

In due course it might be possible to complete the Fiji hostage study, with the former hostages providing responses perhaps of a less reactive but of a more reflective kind—and from the evidence of Engdahl, Harkness, Eberly, Page, and Bielinski (1993), who interviewed former hostages after a minimum period of 20 years had elapsed since their release, any delay might not be too problematic. However, as a first step toward addressing the wrongs in all such situations, it seemed that justice should be construed formally as a basic human need to merit a place in the familiar hierarchy of the kind that Maslow espoused (Taylor, 2003c, 2006b). Maslow (1987, p. xxv) himself warned of the consequences of injustice, and he described justice as "*almost* a basic need," placing it with fairness, honesty, and orderliness in a cluster as being a precondition for their fulfillment (Maslow, 1987, p. 22). The suggestion is that, in light of the many recent violations of human rights, if Maslow were alive today, he might bring justice more firmly into his model of human motivation.

Overview

Collectively, the studies concluding this chapter will point to the amalgamation of constitutional, cultural, economic, historical, political, psychological, religious, social, and sociological tensions that lie behind many kinds of human disasters. The proposition is that some of the tensions might also be found behind terrorism, and for that reason behavioral scientists should develop a healthy respect for a general systems theory is receptive to contributions from different fields. It would require researchers to resist the competitive trend for supremacy between the different disciplines on which they have been brought up and, like Bertalanaffy (1951) and J. G. Miller (1990), be open to the thought that the disparate findings from studies of cells, microorganisms, organs, organisms, groups, organizations, communities, and beyond might ultimately be integrated as equally vital components of a vibrant whole.

The fresh epistemological approach would revive the Baconian commitment to the integration of knowledge rather than its fragmentation (Colverson, 1989). It could begin with a reconsideration of the reformulation of Kuhn's (1970) fundamentals to highlight the conceptual changes that have occurred in the history of science. Then it could lead to an indulgence in Hellemans and Bunch's (1988) assembly of historical facts from diverse fields of scientific endeavor that strings the major contributions of science together with regard more to their significance than to their disciplinary source.

The challenge is for behavioral scientists to entertain such a theory, be open to contributions from different academic disciplines about the causes and the consequences of terrorism, and consider whether the outcome might help them to unravel more of the complexities of the problems they face. To do otherwise, ignore the available leads, and continue simply to endorse ruthless policies of deterrence and retribution, would be foolhardy in the extreme.

Notes

1. The five-stage process that Stahelski describes (i.e., stripping away all other group memberships, as well as each recruit's personal identity and that of enemies, identifying enemies as subhuman and evil) closely resembles those adopted by military boot camps in converting raw recruits into fighters.

2. The immorality of the end justifying the means is compounded when, in a process termed "rendition," for the purpose of interrogation, governments place suspected terrorists outside the boundaries covered by the Geneva Convention relative to the protection of

civilians (1949), the Geneva Convention relative to the treatment of prisoners of war (1949), the UN minimum standard rules for the treatment of prisoners (1977), and the Convention against torture and other cruel and degrading treatment or punishment (1984).

3. Currently, government-sponsored attacks on sectors of their civilian population and the lack of progress in providing basic essentials for human development are matters of great concern to the secretary-general of the United Nations (Annan, 2005). He affirms that, while "poverty and denial of human rights may not be said to 'cause' civil war, terrorism or organized crime, they all greatly increase the risk of instability and violence" (Annan, 2005, sec. 1, para. 16).

4. See the series of articles on chronic disease prevention in "resource-poor" nations that Richard Horton (2005) introduced in his editorial in *The Lancet*.

5. The level of interest of the population at large is such that a Google search on "terrorism" made on December 23, 2003, brought a response of "about 7,830,000" items, and a similar search specifically on 9/11 brought more than 12,000,000.

6. This point occurred to me in Beijing during the student protests in 1989, when demonstrations in Tienanmen Square and on the main streets ranged from the passive to the militant and involved hundreds of thousands of people (Taylor, 1992).

7. A summary shows no less than 240 of such studies of Americans' responses to 9/11 have been reported. Retrieved January 30, 2006, from http://ps .psychiatryonline.org/cgi/search?andorexactfulltext =and&resourcetype=1&disp_type=&sortspec= relevance&author1=&fulltext=september+11& pubdate_year=&volume=&firstpage.

8. However, the thesis has been criticized for its "suppositional flow charts" (Browne, 1999) and for vaulting "blithely . . . where the academics stumble on interpretative doubts and methodological provisions" (James, 1999, p. 698).

9. The assurance brings cold comfort to those that might already agree with Thomas Hobbes's (1588–1679) melancholy appraisal that continual fear and the dangers of violent death make life "solitary, poor, nasty, brutish, and short."

10. It is a sobering thought that a few reviled terrorists became revered as "statespersons" because of the reforms they brought about once they gained political power, although others simply redressed the balance of oppression against their enemies in a continuing seesaw of action and reaction that ceased only when bankruptcy, exhaustion, or common sense prevailed (cf. Abramowitz, 1946: Mandela, 1995).

11. However, the secretary general's call for the United Nations to agree on a definition of terrorism is interesting (Annan, 2004, paragraphs 84, 91) because

he would go beyond the *Oxford English Dictionary*'s online definition of terrorism as "a policy intended to strike with terror those against whom it is adopted" to seek extra protection for civilians and non-combatants.

12. Consider, for example, the debacles of the Bank of Credit and Commerce International, the Barings Bank, and the insider trading at Lloyds in the UK, of Elf Acquitaine in France, LG Card in Korea, Akold in the Netherlands, the Parmalat Corporation in Italy, the Allied Irish Bank, Andersons, Enron Energy, Xerox, Worldcom, Merrill Lynch, and a number of big investment banks in the United States, and of Ariadne, Reid Murray, and the HIH Insurance Company in Australia—to say nothing of the celebrated cases of JBL, Equity Corporation, and Ansett NZ, plus many other large companies that sailed close to the wind in the heady days of global free-market deregulation. Certainly the revelations of the indefatigable campaigner Lincoln Steffens (1931) against local government corruption in the United States at the turn of the last century have almost passed into oblivion.

13. Although the 2003 figure was subsequently found to be inaccurate (*New York Times*, June 11, 2004) and the official record does not include the domestic activities of animal rights supporters (cf. Notebook, 2004), the presentation here simply reflects the overall magnitude of terrorist incidents.

14. The fact sheets prepared by the American Red Cross stand out for the sensible advice they present, together with those on the websites of major professional organizations and clinical service providers. Benevolent websites such as those of David Baldwin (http://www.trauma-pages.com/pg5.htm) and Hope Morrow have increased their materials on terrorism substantially (http://home.earthlink.net/~hopefull/ home/home_contents.htm), and sages such as George Doherty (http://www.rmrinstitute.org/mhm131d7.html) and Ken Pope (http://kspope.com/index.php) offer regular commentaries on the topic.

15. With discoveries of duplication, mistaken death reports, and fraudulent claims, the official notification of the number killed dropped from 6,700 in the first harrowing weeks to 2,801 by the first anniversary and to 2,752 just after the second. A far greater number of people were seriously injured.

16. The phases of which, for convenience of recall, some users have changed to the four Rs—Readiness, Response, Recovery, and Reduction.

17. As Fritz and Mathewson (1957, Chapter 3) pointed out long ago, those offering to help should also question their motives to ensure that they have their need for "convergence" under control when moving to disasters sites. According to skeptics Gist and Devilly (2002, p. 741), reports from New York City after the

Word Trade Center attacks indicated that "more than 9000 purveyors of debriefing and other popularised interventions...swarmed there, advocating intervention for any person even remotely connected with the tragedy."

18. Clinicians grappling with the problem will benefit from the 2004 reprint of Helen Sergent's perceptive 1961 article on the epistemological and methodological issues involved. However, there might also be difficult ethical questions to be faced—as in the case of Ahmed Zaoui, the man held without charge on suspicion of being a terrorist, when his mental state was found to be so fragile that, in order to encourage the placebo response, it was decided not to share the professional opinion with him directly as had been promised when establishing rapport but to disclose it in full to his lawyers.

19. Here I might add that the WHO considered including a fourth dimension of spiritual values, but it was unable to persuade its vast assemblage of member countries that the purpose was not to endorse pagan worship: Other objectors might not have wished to be thought of sponsoring either the "Armageddon cult" (cf. Geering, 1986) or "the hidden dangers of fundamentalism" (Woodall, 2006). Nonetheless, the Public Health Advisory Committee to the New Zealand Minister of Health (2004, p. 8) made a stand by defining "health" broadly as including "physical, mental, emotional, family/whanau, community and spiritual well-being."

20. Strong tendrils also came from the theological side to integrate religion, mental health, and psychology. Long ago the clergy reached across a field that came to be known as pastoral psychology and now has several journals (e.g., *Mental Health, Religion and Culture, Psychology and Christianity, Psychology and Judaism, Psychology and Theology, Religion and Health*). Whether or not in response, the American Psychological Association created Division 36, Psychology of Religion, to explore the common ground between the two academic and professional disciplines.

21. Even in the very best of forensic and mortuary facilities in New York, a year after September 11, only 1,439 (51%) of the victims had been identified from the 292 bodies and 19,932 body parts that had been recovered at the World Trade Center site (Chen, 2002). When the operation was brought to a close 3 and a half years after the attack, 1,592 (58%) had been identified, and the authorities conceded that they had "hit the limits of science" (Lipton, 2005).

22. In the same way, psychotherapists are prone to succumb to "countertransference" effects with their clients unless they take standard precautions with clinical supervisors or co-counselors that help them to retain their objectivity.

23. Although the actual therapeutic benefits of such debriefings are still debated (cf. Gist & Woodall, 1998, versus Everly & Mitchell, 2000), a consensus is emerging that some form of psychological first aid is of value in helping people to cope with the trauma (Australasian Critical Incident Stress Association, 1999; Litz & Gray, 2002).

24. The emergency personnel were New Zealand rescue climbers, Antarctic field staff, police victim identification personnel, U.S. Navy chaplains, medical staff, photographers, and helicopter crews that collected dismembered bodies, as well as the regular medical staff of the mortuary at the Auckland Medical School as augmented with forensic dentists, funeral directors, embalmers, and additional police.

25. However, the basic explanations behind the transient reactions have yet to be elicited, and it could be that confrontation with the notion of personal death as reported in the Terror Management Theory may be worth considering.

26. The deficit can be rectified through well-planned seminars arranged by departments of pathology at medical schools and funeral directors—taking care that no participators have necrophilic needs.

27. The most lurid of these was the donation of "adult sex toys" to a Red Cross chapter in New Zealand after a flood had caused such devastation that enhancing sexual performance was not in the forefront of the minds of the casualties.

28. In the Christmas season of 2003, for example, simultaneous public appeals were made for victims and casualties on all sides in Afghanistan, Iraq, Israel, and Palestine; for victims of HIV and AIDS in Africa; for victims of a natural gas explosion in China, mud slides in California, an enormous earthquake in Iran; and for the abandoned boat refugees in confinement on the Pacific Island of Nauru, plus those affected locally by an avalanche, bush fires, mountain-climbing accidents, a plane crash, and road traffic accidents. Attention was also drawn to an outbreak of bovine spongiform encephalopathy (BSE)—"mad cow disease"—in the United States that might have similar consequences to those that occurred in Britain 2 years before. People who are bombarded with such a variety of concerns might do well to adopt the prayer of Alcoholics Anonymous for the serenity to accept the things they cannot change, the courage to change the things they can, and the wisdom to know the difference.

29. However, when the statistics become available, the actual number of crimes committed in New York immediately after 9/11 might possibly be lower than normal, because criminals might have either been distracted by the enormity of the events, deterred by the heightened police presence, or undetected because the police had to give higher priority to other matters.

30. In the USA United States some 17,000 "anthrax incidents" were reported in the first 12 months of the scare that closed the postal service for at least 4 hours (Leading During Times of Trouble, Biosecurity & Bioterrorism, 2003), and some 2,500 anthrax scares were reported in Australia (McKinnon, 2002). The odd frivolous remark by aircraft passengers in New Zealand and elsewhere about carrying weapons is known to have had immediate and serious repercussions.

31. The epidemiologist Leonard Horowitz (2004) went so far as to posit a relationship between the "petro-chemical pharmaceutical cartel" and the political bureaucracy in engineering the anthrax scare.

32. The problem could not have been anticipated, otherwise the local authorities would have acted swiftly to bury the bodies as planned in the nearby cemetery without waiting for the official party of politicians to arrive from the island capital. However, putrefaction from the tropical heat made it imperative for the burials to be on the school-site.

33. There is now evidence of a complementary relationship—tentatively named the Jolo syndrome after the remote jungle islands in the Philippines—in which the positive attachment of the rebels to the captives was so strong that two of their French hostages feared they might never be released (Reuters, September 22, 2000). Positive reciprocal relationships are known to sometimes develop between guards and prisoners and between prisoners and their visitors, but they are not so incomprehensible as to warrant a special name.

34. An exception was made by the U.S. Department of Justice (2000, recommendation 4) after the Oklahoma bombing because of the need to address "diverse needs, beliefs, and lifestyles of all affected victims." However, the manual for clergy and congregations it subsequently sponsored (Delaplane & Delaplane, 2002) made no mention of meeting the needs of religions other than those of Christians and Jews.

References

Abramowitz, I. (Ed.). (1946). *The great prisoners: The first anthology of literature written in prison.* New York: Dutton.

accel/TEAM. (2005). Employee motivation, the organizational environment, and productivity. Retrieved January 29, 2006, from http://www.accel-team.com/.

Ahern, J., Galea, S., Resnick, H., Kilpatrick, D., Bucuvalas, M., Gold, J., et al. (2002). Television images and psychological symptoms after the September 11 terrorist attack. *Psychiatry, 65*(4), 289–300.

American Psychiatric Association. (2000). *Diagnostic and statistical manual of mental disorders (DSM-IV-TR)* (4th ed.). Washington, DC: Author.

American Red Cross. (2002). Terrorism: Preparing for the unexpected. Retrieved January 29, 2006, from http://www.redcross.org/services/disaster/0,1082,0_589_,00.html.

Annan, K. (2002). In address to World Economic Forum, Secretary-General says globalization must work for all. Retrieved January 29, 2006, from www.un.org/News/dh/latest/address_2001.htm

———. (2004). The brotherhood of man. Inaugural Robert Burns Memorial Lecture. Retrieved January 29, 2006, from http://www.un.org/News/Press/docs/2004/sgsm9112.doc.htm

———. (2005). In larger freedom: Toward development, security, and human rights for all. Report of the secretary-general. Retrieved January 29, 2006, from http://www.un.org/largerfreedom/contents.htm

Argyle, M. (2002). State of the art: Religion. *Psychologist, 15*(1), 22–26.

Asken, M. J. (1993, June). Fire psychology: Post-call visits to victims. *Firehouse,* 100.

Australasian Critical Incident Stress Association. (1999). Guidelines for good practice for emergency responder groups in relation to early intervention after trauma and critical incidents. Glenelg Declaration. Retrieved January 29, 2006, from http://www.ctsn-rcst.ca/glenelg.html.

Australian Government. (2004). *Transnational terrorism: The threat to Australia.* Canberra: Australian Department of Foreign Affairs and Trade.

Bankoff, G. (2003). Vulnerability as a measure of change in society. *International Journal of Mass Emergencies and Disasters, 21*(2), 5–30.

Becker, E. (1971). *The birth and death of meaning: An interdisciplinary perspective on the problem of man.* New York: Free Press.

———. (1973). *The denial of death.* New York: Free Press.

Beit-Hallahmi, B., & Argyle, M. (1997). *Religious behaviour, belief, and experience.* London: Routledge.

Benson, H., & Stark, M. (1996). *Timeless healing: The power and biology of religious belief.* London: Simon & Schuster.

Bertalanaffy, von L. (1951). Problems of general system theory. *Human Biology, 23,* 302–311.

Bracken, P. (2002). *Trauma: Culture, meaning, and philosophy.* London: Whurr.

Browne, M. W. (1999, February 27). A review of the book *Catastrophe: A quest for the origins of the modern world. New York Times Book Review,* 30.

Carroll, R. T. (2002). The nocebo effect. *The Skeptic's dictionary*. Retrieved March 26, 2005, from http://skepdic.com/nocebo.html.

————. (2005). The placebo effect. *The Skeptic's dictionary*. Retrieved January 29, 2005 from http://skepdic.com/placebo.html

Chen, D. W. (2002, December 1). New test for 9/11 IDs is moving much slower than scientists had hoped. *New York Times*.

Chronology of nonsignificant international terrorist incidents. (2003). Rev. June 6, 2004. Retrieved June 30, 2004, from http://www.state.gov/s/ct/rls/fs/2004/33786pf.htm.

Cisin, I. H., & Clark, W. B. (1962). The methodological challenge of disaster research. In G. W. Baker & D. W. Chapman (Eds.), *Man and society in disaster* (pp. 23–49). New York: Basic Books.

Colverson, T. (Ed.). (1989). *The roots of modern environmentalism*. London: Routledge.

Convention against torture and other cruel and degrading treatment or punishment. (1984). Geneva: Office of the High Commissioner for Human Rights. Retrieved May 22, 2004, from http://www.unchr.ch//html/menu3/b/h_cat39.htm.

Culbertson, P. L. (Ed.) (1997). *Counselling issues and South Pacific communities*. Auckland, New Zealand: Accent.

Danielsson, B. (1956). *Love in the South Seas*. London: Allen & Unwin.

Davis, M., Eshelman, E. R., & McKay, M. (1995). *The relaxation and stress reduction workbook* (4th ed.). Oakland, CA: New Harbinger.

Delaplane, D., & Delaplane, A. (2002). Victims of child abuse, domestic violence, elder abuse, rape, robbery, assault, and violent death: A manual for clergy and congregations. Washington, DC: U.S. Department of Justice.

DeLisle, L. (2003). Review of the book *In the wake of 9/11: The psychology of terror. American Journal of Psychiatry, 160*(5), 1019.

DeVries, K. M. W. (1996). Trauma in cultural perspective. In B. A. van Der Kolk, A. C. McFarlane, & L. Weisaeth (Eds.), *Traumatic stress: The effects of overwhelming experience on mind, body, and society* (pp. 398–411). New York: Guilford.

DHA News: 1993 in review. (1994). Special edition (7).

Drabek, T. (1986). *Human responses to disaster: An inventory of sociological findings*. New York: Springer.

Durie, M. (1985). The Maori concept of health. *Social Science and Medicine, 20*(5), 483–486.

Dynes, R. R. (2003). Finding order in disorder: Continuities in the 9/11 response. *International Journal of Mass Emergencies and Disasters, 21*(3),

9–23. Eisner, H. (2002). FDNY at Ground Zero. *Firehouse, 27*(5), 32–37.

Engdahl, B. E., Harkness, A. R., Eberly, R. E., Page, W. E., & Bielinski, J. (1993). Structural models of captivity trauma, resilience, and trauma response among former prisoners of war 20 to 40 years after release. *Social Psychiatry and Psychiatric Epidemiology, 28*, 109–115.

Erikson, K. (1994). *A new species of trouble: Explorations in disaster, trauma, and community*. New York: Norton.

Everly, G. S., & Mitchell, J. T. (2000). The debriefing "controversy" and crisis intervention: A review of lexical and substantive issues. *International Journal of Emergency Mental Health, 2*(4), 211–225.

Figley, C. R., Figley, K. R., & Norman, J. (2002). Tuesday morning, September 11, 2001: The Green Cross Projects' role as a case study in community-based traumatology services. In S. N. Gold & J. Faust (Eds.), *Trauma practice in the wake of September 11, 2001* (pp. 13–36). New York: Haworth.

Frederick, C. J. (1987). Psychic trauma in victims of crime and terrorism. In A. Baum, C. J. Frederick, I. H. Frieze, E. S. Shneidman, & C. B. Wortman (Eds.), *Cataclysms, crises, and catastrophes: Psychology in action* (pp. 59–108). Washington, DC: American Psychological Society.

Fritz, C. E., & Mathewson, J. H. (1957) *Convergence behavior in disasters: Problems in social control*. Publication no. 476. Washington, DC: National Academy of Sciences, National Research Council.

Geering, L. (1986). *Encounter with evil*. Wellington, New Zealand: St. Andrew's Trust for the Study of Religion and Society.

Geneva Convention relative to the protection of civilian persons in time of war. (1949). Geneva: United Nations.

Geneva Convention relative to the treatment of prisoners of war. (1949). Geneva: United Nations.

Gentry, J. E. (2002). Compassion fatigue: A crucible of transformation. In S. N. Gold & J. Faust (Eds.), *Trauma practice in the wake of September 11, 2001* (pp. 37–61). New York: Haworth.

Gibson, J. T., & Haritos-Fatouros, M. (1986, November). The education of a torturer. *Psychology Today*, 50–58.

Gist, R., & Devilly, G. J. (2002, September 7). Post-trauma debriefing: The road too frequently traveled. Letter to *Lancet, 360*, 741–742.

Gist, R., & Woodall, J. (1998). Social science versus social movements: The origins and natural history of debriefing. *Australasian Journal of Disaster and Trauma Studies, 1*. Retrieved

January 26, 2006, from http://www.massey.ac.nz/
~trauma/issues/1998–1/gist1.htm.

Gold, S. N., & Faust, J. (Eds.). (2002). *Trauma practice in the wake of September 11, 2001.* New York: Haworth.

Guide Dog News. (2001). The path to safety: A survivor of the World Trade Centre tragedy tells his story. Fall. Retrieved February 9, 2004, from http://www.guidedogs.com/news-Hingston.html.

Hamblen, J. (2002). What are the traumatic effects of terrorism? National Center for Post-Traumatic Stress Disorder, Department of Veterans Affairs. Retrieved June 1, 2002, from http://www.ncptsd.org/facts/disasters/fs-terrorism.html.

Hancock, D. F., Williams, M. M., & Taylor, A. J. W. (1998). Psychological impact of cadavers and prosections on physiotherapy and occupational therapy students. *Australian Journal of Physiotherapy, 44*(4), 247–255.

———, & Dawson, B. (2004). Impact of dissection on medical students. *New Zealand Journal of Psychology, 33*(1), 17–25.

Haney, C., Banks, C., & Zimbardo, P. (1973). Interpersonal dynamics in a simulated prison. *International Journal of Criminology and Penology, 1,* 69–97.

Hellemans, A., & Bunch, B. (1988). *The timetables of science: A chronology of the most important people and events in the history of science.* New York: Simon & Schuster.

High-level Panel on Threats, Challenges, and Change. (2004). A more secure world: Our shared responsibility. New York: United Nations. Retrieved February 10, 2006, from http://www.un.org/secureworld.

Hoiberg, A., & McCaughey, B. G. (1982). Collision at sea: The traumatic aftereffects. Report 81/39. San Diego: Naval Medical Research & Development Command.

Homer-Dixon, T. (2002). The rise of complex terrorism. *Foreign Policy: The Magazine of Global Politics, Economics, and Ideas.* Retrieved February 6, 2002, from http://www.foreignpolicy.com/issue_jan feb_2002/homer-dixon.html.

Horowitz, L. G. (2001). The CIA's role in the anthrax mailings: Could our spies be agents for military-industrial sabotage, terrorism, and even population control? A special report for simultaneous publication in *The Spectrum* and *Media Bypass.* Retrieved March 9, 2006, from http://www.tetra hedron.org/articles/anthrax/anthrax_espionage .html.

Horton, R. (2005). The neglected epidemic of chronic disease. *The Lancet, 366*(9496), 1514.

Ignatieff, M. (1998). *The warrior's honor: Ethnic war and the modern conscience.* London: Chatto & Windus.

International Federation of Red Cross and Red Crescent Societies. (1995). *World disasters report 1994.* New York: Oxford University Press.

———. (1998). *World disasters report 1998.* Oxford University Press.

———. (2005). *World disasters report 2004: Focus on information in disasters.* Geneva.

Jackson, B. A., Peterson, D. J., Bartis, J. T., LaTourette, T., Brahmakulam, I., Houser, A., & Sollinger, J. (2002). *Responding to acts of terrorism: Conference proceedings.* Washington, DC: RAND/NIOSH.

James, N. (1999). A review of the book *Catastrophe: A quest for the origins of the modern world. Antiquity, 73*(281), 698.

Keller, R. T., & Bobo, W. V. (2002). Handling human remains following the terrorist attack on the Pentagon: Experiences of 10 uniformed health care workers. *Military Medicine, 167*(Suppl.), 4–8.

Keys, D. (1999). *Catastrophe: An investigation into the origins of the modern world.* London: Century.

Kloos, B., & Moore, T. (Eds.). (2000). Special issue: Spirituality, religion, and community psychology. *Journal of Community Psychology, 28,* 2.

———. (Eds.). (2001). Spirituality, religion, and community psychology: Resources, pathways, perspectives. Special issue: Part 2. *Journal of Community Psychology, 29,* 5.

Knop, J. (2001). Ground Zero, almost. *Traumatology, 7*(4), 161–166. Retrieved January 29, 2006, from http://www.fsu.edu/%7etrauma/v7/GroundZero Almost.pdf.

Korten, D. C. (1996). *When corporations rule the world.* West Hartford, CT: Kumarian Press.

Kuhn, T. S. (1970). *The structure of scientific revolutions* (2d ed.). Chicago: University of Chicago Press.

Leading during times of trouble: A roundtable discussion of recent terror events. (2003, June). *Biosecurity and bioterrorism: Biodefense strategy, practice, and science, 1*(2), 67–75. Retrieved February 10, 2006, from http://www.liebertonline.com/doi/pdf/ 10.1089/153871303766275736?cookieSet=1.

Lindner, E. G. (2001). Humiliation—trauma that has been overlooked: An analysis based on fieldwork in Germany, Rwanda/Burundi, and Somalia, *Traumatology 7*(1), 43–68.

Lipton, W. (2005, April 3). At limits of science, 9/11 ID effort comes to end. *New York Times.*

Litz, B., & Gray, M. (2002). *Early intervention for trauma: Current status and future directions.* Washington, DC: National Center for PTSD.

Loewenthal, K. M. (2001). *An introduction to psychological tests and scales* (2d ed.). Philadelphia: Psychology Press.

Ludwig, G. (2002, January). Were you one of the thousands who responded to New York? *Firehouse, 1,* 26.

Luomala, K. (1984). Polynesian mythology. In M. Leach & J. Fried (Eds.), *Funk and Wagnall's standard dictionary of folklore mythology and legend* (pp. 876–879). San Francisco: Harper.

Mandela, N. (1995). *Long walk to freedom.* London: Abacus.

Marsella, A. J., Friedman, M. J., Gerrity, E. T., & Scurfield, R. M. (Eds.). (1996). *Ethnocultural aspects of posttraumatic stress disorder: Issues, research, and clinical applications.* Washington DC: American Psychological Association.

Maslow, A. H. (1987). *Motivation and personality* (3d rev. ed.). New York: Harper & Row.

Massey, C. S. D. (2002). Ten days at Ground Zero. *Firehouse, 27*(4), 122–141.

McDonald, D. A. (2000). Spirituality: Description, measurement, and relation to the five-factor model of personality. *Journal of Personality, 68*(1), 153–197.

McDuff, D. R. (1992). Social issues in the management of released hostages. Abstract. *Hospital and Community Psychiatry, 43*(8), 825–828.

McKinsey Report: Increasing FDNY's preparedness. (2002). New York: New York City Fire Department.

McLeish, K. (1996). *Myth: Myths and legends of the world explored.* London: Bloomsbury.

Meldrum, L. (2002). September 11 and its impact around the globe. In S. N. Gold & J. Faust (Eds.), *Trauma practice in the wake of September 11, 2001* (pp. 63–81). New York: Haworth.

Milgram, S. (1969). *Obedience to authority.* New York: Harper.

Miller, J. G. (1990). Applications of living systems theory to life in space. In A. A. Harrison, Y. A. Clearwater, & C. P. McKay (Eds.), *From Antarctica to outer space: Life in isolation and confinement* (pp. 177–198). New York: Springer.

Miller, W. R. (Ed.). (1999). *Integrating spirituality into treatment.* Washington, DC: American Psychological Association.

Milne, G. (1979). Cyclone Tracy: Psychological and social consequences. In J. L. Reid (Ed.), *Planning for people in natural disaster* (pp. 116–123). Queensland, New Zealand: University Press.

Mollica, R. F., Wyshak, K., & Lavelle, J. (1987). The psychosocial impact of war trauma on Southeast Asian refugees. *American Journal of Psychiatry, 144*(12), 1567–1572.

National Institute of Standards and Technology. (2004). Executive summary. Extracted from *NIST NCSTAR 1 (draft) Federal building and fire safety investigation of the World Trade Center disaster. Final report of the National Construction Safety Team on the collapses of the World Trade Center towers (draft).* Retrieved February 28, 2006, from http://wtc.nist.gov.pubs/NCSTAR1Executivesummary.pdf.

New Rules Project, The. (2004). Institute for Local Self-reliance. Retrieved January 29, 2006, from http://www.newrules.org/.

Norris, F. H., Friedman, M. J., & Watson, P. J. (2002). 60,000 disaster victims speak: Part 2. Summary and implications of disaster mental health research. *Psychiatry, 65*(3), 240–260.

————, Byrne, C. M., Díaz, E., & Kaniasty, K. (2001). 60,000 disaster victims speak: Part 1. An empirical view of the empirical literature, 1981–2001. *Psychiatry, 65*(3), 207–239.

Notebook. (2004, July 5). The British terror invasion: RIP. Bio-MedNet, 1995–2004. *Scientist, 18*(13), 13.

O'Brien, K., & Nusbaum, J. (2002). Intelligence gathering on asymmetrical threats: Parts 1 and 2. In *World terrorism and political violence: Implications for New Zealand and the South Pacific* (pp. 109–122). Wellington, New Zealand: Victoria University.

O'Donohue, W. (1989). The (even) bolder model. *American Psychologist, 44*(12), 1460–1468.

Office for Victims of Crime. (2000). *Responding to terrorism victims: Oklahoma City and beyond.* Washington, DC: U.S. Department of Justice Programs.

————. (2001). *OVC Handbook for coping after terrorism.* Washington, DC: U.S. Department of Justice Programs.

Oxford English Dictionary Online. (2005). Retrieved March 2, 2006, from http://dictionary.oed.com/entrance.dtl.

Palacios, A., Cueli, J., Camacho, J., Clérica, R., Ceuevas, P., Ayala, J., et al. (1986). *International Review of Psychoanalysis, 13,* 279–293.

Pan American Health Organization and World Health Organization. (2004). *Management of dead bodies in disaster situations.* Washington, DC: Author.

Patterns of global terrorism. (2004). U.S. Department of State. Retrieved January 29, 2006, from http://www.state.gov/s/ct/rls/pgtrpt/2003/33771.htm.

Patterson, C. H. (1989/2000). Foundations for a systematic eclectic psychotherapy. Retrieved April, 2, 2005, from http://www.sageofashville.com/pub_download

Public Health Advisory Committee. (2004). The health of people and communities: Report to the Minister of Health. Wellington, New Zealand: Ministry of Health.

Pyszczynski, T., Solomon, S., & Greenberg, J. (2003). *In the wake of 9/11: The psychology of terror.*

Washington, DC: American Psychological Association.

Raphael, B. (2000). *Disaster mental health handbook: An educational resource for health professionals involved in disaster management.* North Sydney, New South Wales: Centre for Mental Health.

————, Lundin, T., and Weisaeth, L. (1989) A research method for the study of psychological and psychiatric aspects of disaster. *Acta Psychiatrica Scandinavica* (Suppl.) 353(80), 75.

Read, P. P. (2001). *The Templars.* London: Phoenix.

Schachner, N. (1962). *The medieval universities.* New York: Barnes.

Schuster, M. A., Stein, B. D., Jaycox, L. H., Collins, R. L., Marshall, G. N., Elliott, M. N., et al. (2001). Special report: A national survey of stress reactions after the September 11, 2001, terrorist attacks. *New England Journal of Medicine, 345*(20), 1507–1512.

Sells, M. (1996). *The bridge betrayed: Religion and genocide in Bosnia.* Berkeley: University of California Press.

Sergent, H. (2004). Intrapsychic change: Methodological problems in psychotherapy research. *Psychiatry, 67*(1), 17.

Silke, A. (Ed.). (2003). *Terrorists, victims, and society: Psychological perspectives on terrorism and its consequences.* New York: Wiley.

Sjoberg, G. (1962). Disasters and social change. In G. W. Baker & D. W. Chapman (Eds.), *Man and society in disaster* (pp.356–384). New York: Basic Books.

Sluka, J. (2002). What anthropologists should know about the concept of "terrorism." *Anthropology Today, 18*(2), 22–23.

————. (Ed.). (2000). *Death squads: The anthropology of state terror.* Philadelphia: University of Pennsylvania Press.

Smeulers, A. (2002, March 22–27). What transforms ordinary people into human rights violators? Conference paper for Workshop 9: Systematic Study of Human Rights Violations. Turin, Italy. Private circulation.

Smith, J. (2003). New Zealand's anti-terrorism campaign: Balancing civil liberties, national security, and international responsibilities. Retrieved March 2, 2004, from http://www.fulbright.org.nz voicesa/axford/smithj.html.

Stahelski, A. (2004, March). Terrorists are made, not born: Creating terrorists using social psychological conditioning. *Journal of Homeland Security,* 1–11.

Steffens, L. (1931). *The autobiography of Lincoln Steffens.* New York: Harcourt Brace.

Strenz, T. (1979). The Stockholm syndrome: Law enforcement policy and ego defenses of the hostage. *Law Enforcement Bulletin,* 1–11.

Sullivan, R. E. (2002). World Bank's Wolfensohn says that poverty and inequality are at the root of global ills. *Conference News Daily.* Retrieved January 29, 2006, from http://www.earthtimes.org/sep/sustainabledevelopment worldsep18_01.htm.

Taylor, A. J. W. (1984). Architecture and society: Disaster studies and human stress. *Journal of Ekistics: The Problems and Science of Human Settlements, 308,* 446–451.

————. (1987). Mortuary ministrations. *Bereavement Care, 6*(2), 18–20.

————. (1992). Research questions arising from the 1989 student protest in Beijing. In J. Westerink (Ed.), *Critical incident stress management across the life span* (pp. 149–173). Turamurra, New South Wales: Australasian Critical Incident Stress Association.

————. (1998). Observations from a cyclone/stress assignment in the Cook Islands. *Traumatology, 4*(1), article 3. Retrieved March 3, 2006, from http://www.greencross.org/_Research/TraumatologyJournal.asp#Back%20Issues.

————. (1999). *Value-conflict arising from a disaster.* Australasian Journal of Disaster and Trauma Studies, 2. *Retrieved March 3, 2006, from http://www.massey.ac.nz/~trauma/.*

————. (2000). Tragedy and trauma in Tuvalu. *Australasian Journal of Disaster and Trauma Studies,* 2. Retrieved March 3, 2006, from http://www.massey.ac.nz/~trauma/.

————. (2001) Spirituality and personal values: Neglected components of trauma treatment, *Traumatology, 7*(3). Retrieved March 3, 2006, from http://www.greencross.org/_Research/TraumatologyJournal.asp#Back%20Issues.

————. (2003a). Traumatic stress and the differential diagnosis of malingering. *Traumatology, 9*(4), 197–215.

————. (2003b). Cross-cultural interactions in the treatment of trauma. *Asia Pacific Viewpoint, 44*(2), 177–193.

————. (2003c). Justice as a basic human need. *New Ideas in Psychology, 21*(3), 209–219.

————. (2006a). Consolidating the role of the fourth estate in disaster work. *International Journal of Mass Emergencies & Disasters, 14*(1).

————. (Ed.). (2006b). *Justice as a basic human need.* New York: Nova Science.

Taylor, A. J. W., & Frazer, A. G. (1981). *Psychological sequelae of Operation Overdue following the DC 10 aircrash in Antarctica.* Pub. no. 27. Wellington, New Zealand: Victoria University Department of Psychology.

———. (1982). The stress of post-disaster body handling and victim identification work. *Journal of Human Stress, 8*(4), 4–12.

Taylor, A. J. W., Nailatikau, E., and Walkey, F. H. (2002) A hostage assignment in Fiji. *Australasian Journal of Disaster and Trauma Studies, 2.* Retrieved March 3, 2006, from http://www.massey.ac.nz/~trauma/.

Tedeschi, R. G., Park, C. L., & Calhoun, L. G. (Eds.). (1998). *Posttraumatic growth: Positive changes in the aftermath of crisis.* Mahwah, NJ: Erlbaum.

Turner, J. T. (1985). Factors influencing the development of hostage identification syndrome. *Political Psychology, 6*(4), 705–711.

UN Standard Minimum Rules for the Treatment of Prisoners. (1977). Retrieved May 7, 2004 from http://www.hrw.org/advocacy/prisons/un-smrs.htm.

Ursano, R. J., Tzu-Cheg, K., & Fullerton, C. S. (1992). Posttraumatic disorder and meaning: Structuring human chaos. *Journal of Nervous and Mental Disease, 180*(12), 756–759.

U.S. Department of Justice. (2000). *Responding to terrorism victims: Oklahoma City and beyond.* Washington, DC: Office for Victims of Crime.

———. (2001). *Providing services to victims of fraud: Resources for victim/witness coordinators.* Washington, DC: Office of Justice Programs.

van der Kolk, B. A. (1996). The body keeps the score: Approaches to the psychobiology of post-traumatic stress disorder. In B. A. van der Kolk, A. C. McFarlane, & L. Weisaeth (Eds.), *Traumatic stress: The effects of overwhelming experience on mind, body, and society* (pp. 214–241). New York: Guilford.

Wallace, S., & Pritchard, C. (2004). "Coalition in Iraq" countries "internal" civil violent deaths compared to the USA "external" violence of September 11, 2001. *Medical Science Monitor, 10*(5), 1–4.

Waxler-Morrison, N., Richardson, E., Anderson, J., and Chambers, N.A. (2001). *Cross-cultural caring: A handbook for health professionals.* 2d ed. Vancouver: University of British Columbia Press.

Wessely, S. & Krasnov, V. (2002, March 25–27). Nato-Russia advanced workshop on social and psychological consequences of chemical, biological, and radiological terrorism: Preliminary notes. Retrieved January 20, 2003, from http://www.nato.int/science/e/020325-arw2.htm.

Wilson, J. P., & Lindy, J. D. (Eds.). (1994). *Countertransference in the treatment of PTSD.* New York: Guilford.

Woodall, J. (2006). The hidden dangers of fundamentalism: A connection exists between disease outbreaks and extreme religious practice. *The Scientist: Magazine of the Life Sciences, 20*(2), 59.

World Health Organization. (1997). *Ottawa charter for health promotion.* WHO Regional Office for Europe. Retrieved July 26, 2000, from http://who.dk/policy/ottawa.htm.

———. (1997). *Management of mental disorders: Treatment protocol project.* 2d ed. Darlinghurst, New South Wales: WHO Collaborating Centre for Mental Health and Substance Abuse.

———. (2003). *Mental health in emergencies.* Geneva: Department of Mental Health and Substance Dependence.

World terrorism and political violence: Implications for New Zealand. (2002). Background papers for the symposium. Wellington, New Zealand: Department of Continuing Education, Victoria University of Wellington.

Young, B. H., Ford, J. D., Ruzek, J., Friedman, M. J., & Gusman, F. D. (1998). *Disaster mental health services: A guidebook for clinicians and administrators.* White River Junction, VT: Department of Veterans Affairs.

Young, M. A. (2001). *The community crisis response team training manual* (2d ed.). Washington, DC: National Organization for Victim Assistance.

Zaoui, A. (2004). Refugee status appeals authority New Zealand. Refugee Appeal no. 74540, decision of August 1, 2003. Auckland: Human Rights Foundation and Legal Search.

25

Psychological Resilience in the Face of Terrorism

Lisa D. Butler
Leslie A. Morland
Gregory A. Leskin

Psychological resilience in the context of terrorism was little studied by U.S. researchers before September 11, 2001. Prior to that, the United States had suffered a number of terrorist attacks at home and abroad, including the 1993 bombing of the World Trade Center in New York, the 1995 bombing of the Murrah Federal Building in Oklahoma City, the 1996 truck bombing of a U.S. Air Force barracks in Dhahran, Saudi Arabia, and the 1998 bombings of U.S. embassies in Kenya and Tanzania, among others, each of which would certainly qualify as "terrorist spectaculars" (dramatic, attention-riveting, deadly acts that seize the interest of the media and public; Hoffman, 1999).

However, the impact of the terrorist attacks on New York and Washington, DC, in September, 2001, seemed to be of another order. These events were incomparably and indelibly etched into the national consciousness, and they ushered in a new psychological zeitgeist in U.S. political and personal life. The unique psychological potency of these attacks may be attributable to the searing real-time and repetitive media coverage, the extent of their lethality and breadth of their physical and economic destruction, and the deeply disturbing malignancy of the attacks, which included deliberate assaults on cherished symbols of U.S. economic

and military preeminence. This convergence of effects, both tangible and symbolic, tore through any possible cultural membrane of denial, forcing citizens to contemplate existential vulnerability and threat (Becker, 1973; Pyszcznski, Solomon, & Greenberg, 2003) and to consider what might enhance resilience in the face of possible terrorist attacks in the future.

Experts in terrorism (Kaplan, 1981) have observed that such acts are intended to create a *fearful state of mind* in an audience far wider than the immediate victims. In fact, terrorism is "aimed at noncombatants" with the objective of the "deliberate creation of dread" (Stern, 2003, p. xx). Clearly, terrorism is political warfare on a psychological field of battle. And in this modern electronic era of virtually simultaneous mass communication, terrorism's reach (and thus its impact) has extended—everyone with a television or an Internet connection can be witness to a "virtual ground zero" (Butler, Garlan, & Spiegel, 2005). Indeed, in one nationally representative sample, assessed 3–5 days after the attacks (Schuster et al., 2001), each of the 560 people interviewed already knew of the attacks when contacted for the survey (B. Stein, personal communication, January 17, 2005). This development underscores the need to elucidate the effects of exposure—whether direct or indirect—to terrorism and to identify factors that may allow individuals to be more resilient to such experiences.

The specter of terrorism has another critical aspect. Present distress can stem not only from events that have occurred but also from anticipation of events that may yet occur. As Miller (2002) has observed, "Essentially, terrorism is the 'perfect' traumatic stressor, because it combines the elements of malevolent intent, actual or threatened extreme harm, and unending fear of the future" (p. 296). Acute concern about the possibility of a new attack can be heightened by feelings of unpredictability and baleful inevitability and fueled by past and current experiences of stress or trauma and the anticipated impact of a future event, all telescoped into present fearful preoccupations (Butler, Field, et al., 2005). In the months following September 11, more than half of a large national probability sample reported fears of future terrorism and harm to their families, and a substantial minority continued to report these fears 6 months after the attacks (Silver, Holman, McIntosh, Poulin, & Gil-Rivas, 2002). In fact, Zimbardo and Kluger (2003) have argued that efforts ostensibly directed at the nation's protection, such as the national color-coded warning system, have compounded rather than dispelled distress about future possible attacks, leaving Americans feeling frightened and helpless, a condition they describe as a "pre-traumatic stress syndrome." Thus the effort to understand and promote resilience must confront both adjustment to an attack that has happened and the ongoing management of anxiety in the face of an uncertain future.

Resilience

The 1990s were witness to an important expansion in emphasis on the variety of possible outcomes following traumatic experience. Perhaps not surprisingly, most previous research has focused on the clinically significant end of the distribution—those most affected by the event and the factors that put them at risk for such outcomes. However, in their seminal contributions, O'Leary and Ickovics (1995; see also Carver, 1998) urged researchers to move beyond a vulnerability and deficit model to one that encompasses successful adaptation (resilience) and thriving, and Tedeschi and Calhoun (1995) and others (e.g., Joseph, Williams, & Yule, 1993) began to enumerate the benefits and positive changes that some people report following adversity.

Origins of Resilience Research

The empirical study of resilience originated in developmental research (e.g., Garmezy & Rutter, 1983; Garmezy, Masten, & Tellegen, 1984; Werner & Smith, 1982) and was initially described as "stress resistance" among children at risk for poor outcomes due to genetic or environmental circumstances. "The observation of unexpectedly good development among high-risk children gave rise to the study of resilience, an effort to identify the processes underlying successful adaptation under adverse conditions" (Masten & Wright, 1998, p. 13).

Investigations in two other research streams paralleled these developments. Researchers in life-span development (e.g., Rowe & Kahn, 1987) sought to identify factors that fostered successful (i.e., quick and thorough) recovery from the challenges of aging. In research on intrapsychic aspects of adaptation, personality psychologists began to identify resilience potentials in the ego resources available to or mobilized by some people under a variety of challenging circumstances (e.g., ego strength, reviewed in Meyer & Handler, 1997; ego resiliency, Block & Block, 1980) and in personalities characterized by traits of hardiness (Kobasa, 1979) and a sense of coherence (Antonovsky, 1987). Both hardiness and coherence involve individual approaches to action and meaning that are associated with physical and psychological health under conditions of stress. The impetus for this research was observations of successful or superior adaptation demonstrated by some individuals who were facing difficult or stressful circumstances. The goal was to discern the intrapersonal and environmental factors associated with such adaptation.

The study of resilience related specifically to *traumatic events* (rather than generally stressful or challenging experiences) began in earnest as the study of traumatic stress got its theoretical and empirical footing, prompted in part by prospective developmental research involving child maltreatment (reviewed in Masten & Wright, 1998), but has since been applied to the range of traumatic experience. In this sense, the study of resilience and thriving is the complement to research on the negative effects of trauma that has flourished in the past several decades. To understand responses to trauma, the full spectrum of possible outcomes must be considered, along with the factors that may affect those outcomes, including those that increase vulnerability or risk and those that confer protection or enhance resilience.

Functional Outcomes Following Psychological Trauma

In calling for this "paradigm shift" to include positive adaptation among the foci of research, O'Leary and Ickovics (1995; see also Carver, 1998) noted a range of possible functional endpoints following exposure to a traumatic or other adverse life experience (see Figure 25.1, adapted from O'Leary & Ickovics, 1995). Of note, only two of these outcomes are negative; the other two involve maintenance, recovery, and/or enhancement of psychological functioning following a significant life challenge.

In the most dire instance, the individual *succumbs* to the effects of the experience. Based in a health outcome perspective, O'Leary and Ickovics (1995) employ the term *succumb* to describe reduced functioning that ultimately ceases, sometimes following additional postevent decline (Carver, 1998). In the case of a serious psychological challenge, succumbing could also refer, for example, to an event-related deteriorating depression that results in the death of the individual

through deliberate suicidal action, physical injury secondary to maladaptive behaviors (such as substance use or recklessness), or possibly direct physical decline.

The second negative outcome—*survival with impairment*—characterizes a postevent diminution in functioning coupled with a failure to return to previous levels over the long term. This is the condition to which much of the traumatic stress literature applies, such as when someone experiences chronic and disabling posttraumatic stress or depression symptoms. In the National Comorbidity Survey (Kessler, Sonnega, Bromet, Hughes, & Nelson, 1995), for example, more than one-third of those who reported an index episode of posttraumatic stress disorder (PTSD) failed to fully recover over the next decade, even among those who had sought treatment for their symptoms.

The third outcome, and the one most commonly understood as *resilience*, refers to "good adaptation under extenuating circumstances" (Masten & Reed, 2002, p. 76) and may be seen in a recovery trajectory that involves a return to baseline functioning following challenge. Resilient people are less vulnerable; they bend rather than break in the face of adversity. Findings from the traumatic stress literature suggest that, despite the fact that most people will face a serious life-threatening or loss event during their lives, the majority will bear few long-term impairments (Kessler et al., 1995; Norris et al., 2002). Indeed, resilient outcomes are

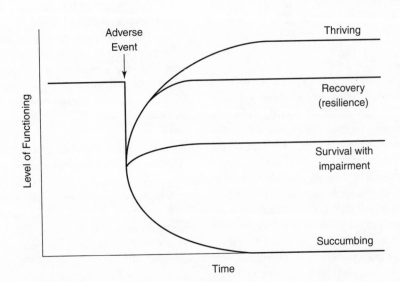

Figure 25.1. Potential outcomes following adversity.

so common that Masten (2001) has referred to the phenomenon in the developmental literature as "ordinary magic."

The final outcome, termed *thriving* (O'Leary & Ickovics, 1995; also known as posttraumatic growth [Tedeschi & Calhoun, 1995]; stress-related growth [Park, Cohen, & Murch, 1996]; or adversarial growth [Linley & Joseph, 2004]), refers to postevent adaptation that exceeds preevent levels. The readjustment experience, in other words, is transformative and represents a "value-added" end state (O'Leary & Ickovics 1995; see also Carver, 1998). Carver has suggested that the term *resilience* should be applied to cases of "homeostatic return to prior condition," while *thriving* should be reserved for cases in which an individual is judged to be "better-off-afterward" (Carver, 1988, p. 247).

In the present chapter, we examine the domain of resilience and factors that may augment or undermine adaptive functioning. While there is no singular way to describe or measure resilience, it can be defined by a set of *outcomes* that involve recovery following challenge. There are also important aspects to the *process* of that recovery that signal or instantiate elements of resilience. In other words, resilience, broadly defined, refers to the fact that an individual recovers and also the ways in which that person responds to the event over time. We believe that this process emphasis allows for a more complete investigation of the means and mechanisms of recovery.

Resilience as Outcome

In the traditional view of resilience as endpoint, Masten (2001, p. 228) has defined resilience as "a class of phenomena characterized by good outcomes in spite of serious threats to adaptation or survival." This view represents a snapshot of outcome interpreted in the context of antecedent circumstances. Consequently, resilience has been variably defined as, for example, achievement in educational and social settings, age-appropriate accomplishments or behaviors, and the presence of desirable outcomes (e.g., well-being, happiness) or the absence of undesirable ones (e.g., mental illness, distress, risky or criminal behaviors; Masten & Reed, 2002). With this emphasis on outcome, research has focused on identifying risk and protective factors that moderate or predict adjustment.

Resilience as Process

Resilience phenomena may also be identified in *trajectories of recovery.* In this way, resilience can connote features of an initial reaction to a traumatic event and characteristics of the recovery path associated with achieving a return to baseline functioning. This is a relatively uncommon research focus, however, as those who report few negative sequelae, uncomplicated recovery, or even enhanced health are generally ignored in the clinical literature because of the (understandable) clinical focus on those suffering the negative effects of a psychological challenge. As Rowe and Kahn (1987) have noted with respect to aging, few distinctions are made within the category of healthy individuals, despite substantial heterogeneity (see also O'Leary & Ickovics, 1995). In addition to the distinction between those who recover and those who thrive, we believe it is important to investigate the varied ways in which people respond and recover.

As Figure 25.2 (adapted from Carver, 1998) illustrates, resilient individuals demonstrate improvement and ultimately recovery following challenge (Lines A–C). Among those who recover, there are presumably differing degrees of resilient adaptation. Those who are most resilient may, for example, react initially with less disruption (Line A) or recover more quickly despite a significant initial setback (Line B compared to Line C). Additionally, some may show an enhanced adaptability in the face of future events (for example, if Line C were the recovery trajectory for the first event and then Lines A or B were observed for the second event)—a result that Carver (1998) conceptualizes as evidence of posttraumatic thriving.

Bonanno (2004) has recently argued that "resilience represents a distinct trajectory from the process of recovery" (p. 20), one in which the person maintains a relatively stable equilibrium, and consequently little or no *recovery* is required, something akin to the "stress resistant" category described in the early developmental literature (Garmezy, 1985). Bonanno's assertion clearly hinges on what "relatively stable" means (which he does not fully specify), and it raises questions about the requirements of the situational challenge that would make it a candidate for a potentially resilient outcome, including the nature of the event experienced, the degree of exposure endured, and the

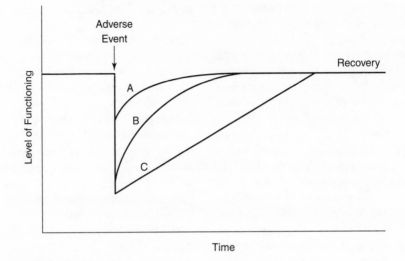

Figure 25.2. Trajectories of recovery.

extent to which the event actually challenged the individual's resources. However, stress resistance is only one among a range of possible resilient adaptations following highly stressful or traumatic experiences, and we believe that it is best understood in the context of this range.

Resilience and Risk in Trauma

In the context of exposure to terrorism or disaster, the risk of distress may be understood as a function of the interplay of a number of factors, among them the individual's personality, demographic, and historical characteristics, the degree of exposure to the event and its aftermath, the level of actual or threatened loss due to the event, initial reactions to the event, and the resources (psychological, social, and material) available to the person both during and following the event. Indeed, an emphasis on the construct of resources in conceptualizing the impact of trauma, as delineated by Hobfoll (1991), may be a useful way of understanding risk and resilience with respect to terrorism. Many of the factors that put people at risk for negative outcomes (e.g., poor premorbid functioning) or that challenge resilience (e.g., significant losses) can be viewed in the context of resource insufficiency or loss, while factors associated with higher resilience (e.g., active engagement, social support) represent resources themselves— both personal and environmental. Many of these resources can be cultivated at any time, so they may be drawn upon in times of need (i.e., when other resources are lost or at risk).

Although little empirical work has been done to examine correlates and predictors of resilience in the context of terrorism, much of the trauma literature generally (and the terrorism and disaster literatures specifically) provide applicable information. In the simplest sense, every finding regarding a poor outcome provides information about who was spared. To paraphrase Masten and Wright (1998), risk (or vulnerability) and compensatory (or protective) factors are often different names for the same continuous variables (e.g., the quality of social support). However, some assets and resources may operate only at the positive end (by their presence; e.g., benefit finding); similarly, there are factors that may harm you if they occur (e.g., a panic attack during a trauma) but do not help you if they do not occur. In this section we briefly review characteristics of the individual known to confer protection or increase psychological risk in the face of trauma.

Characteristics of the Individual

Much research has sought to characterize people who are resilient under conditions of stress (and, in some cases, traumatic stress). In general it may be said that resilience appears to be an interactive process involving beliefs, attitudes, approaches, and behaviors that determine the way the person views and engages the world.

Features of Resilient People

Pioneering developmental research initiated by Emmy Werner and colleagues in the 1950s laid the conceptual groundwork for much of the adult research that was to follow. In her longitudinal study of high-risk Hawaiian children (Werner & Smith, 1982), Werner identified four characteristics of resilient children: (1) They utilized an active problem-solving approach; (2) they employed a constructive approach to perceiving challenging or even painful experiences; (3) they relied on personal faith that maintained meaningfulness in life; and (4) they had the ability to gain positive attention from others.

Echoing the first three of these themes, Antonovsky (1987) proposed that resilient people have a *sense of coherence* characterized by the belief that the events in one's life will be comprehensible, manageable, and meaningful. Comprehensibility assumes an order and explicability to what happens in life. The belief in manageability presupposes that one will have the resources—both personal and interpersonal—to meet the demands of the event. The notion of meaningfulness applies both to finding significance in the adversity and to believing that the challenge is deserving of engagement, even when difficult.

Tedeschi and Calhoun (1995) have noted that these elements may be the keys to successful adaptation to trauma because they are precisely the domains that traumatic experiences challenge. For example, among variables found to contribute to maladaptation following a large-scale traumatic event are violations of existential assumptions about the worthiness of the self and the benevolence and meaningfulness of the world (Janoff-Bulman, 1992). Following the terrorist attacks on September 11, negative changes in existential outlook were strongly associated with higher distress and lower levels a of well-being (Butler et al., under review), while positive changes were associated with self-reported posttraumatic growth (Butler, Blasey, et al., 2005).

Indeed, finding benefits and meaning in the experience appear to be significant in successful adaptation to adversity (Janoff-Bulman, 1992; Taylor, 1983; Tennen & Affleck, 2002), including cancer (e.g., Carver & Antoni, 2004), bereavement (e.g., Davis, Nolen-Hoeksema, & Larson, 1998), and trauma (e.g. Fontana & Rosenheck, 1998). In addition, the construction of meaning may be an active ingredient in the beneficial effects of disclosing trauma through writing (Park & Blumberg, 2002). Although little research has examined personality correlates of these approaches, there is some evidence for an association with optimism (Davis et al., 1998).

Elements similar to those identified by Antonovsky (1987) are also present in Kobasa's (1979) description of *hardiness,* which involves dispositions to commitment, control, and challenge that are associated with better physical and psychological outcomes (see also, Manning, Williams, & Wolfe, 1988). Hardy people are committed to their lives and engage actively in responding to the tasks that confront them; they believe that they can influence events, and they accept change as a challenge (rather than a threat) that can result in benefits. Hardiness has been found to enhance resilience under conditions of traumatic stress (e.g., King, King, Fairbank, Keane, & Adams, 1998).

Additionally, the related constructs of self-efficacy (Bandura, 1982), a sense of mastery (Meichenbaum, 1985) with respect to challenges, and optimism about the future (Scheier, Weintraub, & Carver, 1986) can contribute to resilience. Each involves beliefs that one's skills and actions will have positive effects on circumstances, which may lead to sustained problem-focused efforts and, consequently, improve the odds of success.

More recently, research has begun to examine the role of positive emotions in coping and resilience. Fredrickson (2001) has delineated a broaden-and-build theory, proposing that positive emotions may quiet or even undo negative emotions that narrow response options, while the cognitive broadening that accompanies states of positive emotion may expand the range of thought-action repertoires. In a prospective study examining resilience and positive emotions following the terrorist attacks of September 11, Fredrickson, Tugade, Waugh, and Larkin (2003) found that positive emotions mediated the relationships between ego resiliency (measured prior to the event) and two outcomes: lower depression and greater growth in psychological resources.

The development of resilient personality features may also rely in part on the experience of stressful (but not overwhelming) life events. Rutter (1987) has asserted that successful adaptation in the past may have a "steeling" effect and therefore increase the likelihood of mastery in meeting future challenges. In other words, "protection develops not through the evasion of risk, but in the successful engagement with it" (O'Leary & Ickovics, 1995, p. 127). This is an eminently plausible prediction, stemming from the developmental literature and related to the notion of stress inoculation (Meichenbaum, 1985), that could have important implications for differentiating trajectories of adaptation to trauma. As yet, the steeling effect has been little studied in the traumatic stress or posttraumatic growth literatures.

It is worth noting that the previously mentioned personality features and approaches can be, at least in theory, learned, cultivated, and practiced. However, research indicates that there are some fixed personal characteristics that also predict outcomes following traumatic experience.

Demographic Factors Associated With Risk and Resilience

Some static individual characteristics, identified in the wider trauma and disaster literatures as risk factors for distress (Brewin, Andrews, & Valentine, 2000; Norris et al., 2002), have also been confirmed in terrorism samples. For example, females and to a lesser extent those of lower socioeconomic status or with less education and those who are middle aged are at higher risk for a variety of negative outcomes following terrorism than are males, those who are affluent and well educated, or those who are older (DeLisi et al., 2003; Galea et al., 2002; Njenga, Nicholls, Nyamai, Kigamwa, & Davidson, 2004; North et al., 1999; Schlenger et al., 2002; Verger et al., 2004). The positive relationship between age and adjustment may be due to the tendency for older individuals to have more experience with stress and coping and fewer drains on coping resources, compared to middle-aged people (Norris et al., 2002).

There are mixed findings in the disaster and trauma literature with respect to ethnicity and marital status. Norris and colleagues (2002) report that in most disaster studies those in the ethnic *majority* group fared best, a finding borne out in some recent terrorism studies (e.g., Schuster et al., 2001; Galea et al., 2002). The findings with respect to marital status sometimes indicate that being married (versus unmarried, divorced, separated, or living alone) decreases risk (Njenga et al., 2004; Verger et al., 2004); however this association may

be stronger for men (Norris et al., 2002) and may also, in part, reflect the availability of emotional support.

In addition to personality and demographic characteristics, historical features may also contribute to a person's response to trauma. Their presence may indicate compromised resources or poor learning histories with respect to dealing with trauma, resulting in less resilience when confronted with threat or possible future terrorism. Efforts to bolster resilience in such cases would be especially important.

History of Traumatic Experience

Prior trauma, including both childhood and adult experiences, may reduce one's resilience to later traumatic events. Several studies, for example, have shown that combat-exposed veterans diagnosed with PTSD have higher rates of childhood trauma, such as physical abuse, than combat-exposed veterans without PTSD (e.g., Bremner, Southwick, Johnson, Yehuda & Charney, 1993). Additionally, King and colleagues (King, King, Foy, & Gudanowski, 1996) found that other previous life traumas (e.g., motor vehicle accidents, physical assault, natural disasters) also predicted PTSD in veterans. Prior trauma (such as physical or sexual assault) may also extend risk to women exposed to later trauma (Resnick, Kilpatrick, Dansky, Saunders, & Best, 1993). Similarly, studies following September 11 reported elevations in trauma symptoms, depression symptoms, and general distress among those with histories of trauma (Silver et al., 2002) and stressful life events (Galea et al., 2002). As previously mentioned, research is needed to determine whether there is a subset of people who are actually steeled by these experiences and thus are more resilient (than they would have been otherwise) when faced with later adversity.

Psychological Functioning

Adjustment problems prior to a traumatic event may also predispose one to greater difficulties in coping or further psychopathology, including anxiety, depression, PTSD, neuroticism, and other symptom or personality states. For example, North et al. (1994) found that survivors of a shooting spree with preexisting major depression were at a significantly higher risk for PTSD 1–6 months after the event (see also Schnurr, Lunney, & Sengupta, 2004). Similarly, a number of retrospective studies of the effects of September 11 found that reports of prior maladjustment were associated with trauma and depression symptoms (e.g., Blanchard et al., 2004; DeLisi et al., 2003; Schuster et al., 2001). Prospective studies (which eliminate the possibility of a retrospective bias in reporting) have found that neuroticism and elevated MMPI clinical scale scores predicted PTSD in veterans (Lee, Vaillant, Torrey, & Elder, 1995; Schnurr, Friedman, & Rosenberg, 1993), and preexisting mental disorders predicted increased trauma symptoms and general distress after September 11 (Silver et al., 2002).

Family Characteristics

Family psychopathology and/or instability have also been found to contribute to psychosocial outcomes following traumatic stress (Ozer, Best, Lipsey, & Weiss, 2003). For example, firefighters with a family history of psychopathology were found to be at greater risk for PTSD 4 months following exposure to massive fires and death (McFarlane, 1988), and premilitary family instability (mental disorder, contact with mental health professionals, substance use) was associated with higher risk of developing PTSD among Vietnam veterans (Schnurr et al., 2004).

Overall, meta-analytic studies have found that prior trauma history, psychiatric history, and family psychopathology make a small but significant contribution to the development of trauma symptoms in both military and civilian samples following subsequent adversity (Brewin et al., 2000; Ozer et al., 2003). These analyses indicate that factors operating during or after the trauma (such as trauma severity, peritraumatic responses, coping, social support, or additional life stressors) tend to have stronger effects on outcomes than do pretrauma factors (Brewin et al., 2000; Ozer et al., 2003). As Rutter (1987) has observed, "resilience cannot be seen as a fixed attribute of the individual. . . . If circumstances change, resilience alters" (p. 317).

Characteristics of the Event

Although unique in many ways, acts of terrorism have much in common with other traumatic events, including features of criminal assaults, disasters, and acts of war (Miller, 2002). Examining the broader traumatic stress literature, the dimensions of traumatic events found to be associated with the poorest outcomes (Green, 1993) may all be present

in the experience of a terrorist attack or its aftermath (i.e., a military response): threat to life and limb; severe physical harm or injury; receipt of intentional injury or harm; exposure to the grotesque; violent or sudden loss of a loved one; witnessing or learning of violence to a loved one; learning of exposure to a noxious agent, and/or causing death or severe harm to another. Because event characteristics are significant contributors to outcomes, identifying their harmful features can improve our understanding of the challenge they pose to resilience and indicate where preventative interventions may be aimed.

Direct Event Exposure

Indisputably, those who are *directly* exposed to terrorist acts through threat or injury to themselves, the death or injury of loved ones, or witnessing the death or injury of others, along with those who tend to the injured or recover the dead, face the greatest challenges to their emotional well-being. Findings from around the world, including Ireland, Israel, France (reviewed in Gidron, 2002; Verger et al., 2004), Nairobi, Kenya (Njenga et al., 2004), and the United States (North et al., 1999; Galea et al., 2002) indicate that a sizable subgroup, ranging from 18% to 50% of directly exposed citizen survivors of terrorist attacks, develop posttraumatic stress symptoms indicative of a PTSD diagnosis (with rates typically highest among those most seriously injured). Additionally, disaster research suggests that symptom levels in the early phases of recovery are likely to determine subsequent symptom levels (Norris et al., 2002), highlighting the importance of early intervention. Training and experience in facing such events appear to promote resilience (and may also reflect the previously mentioned steeling effect): Several studies have found much lower rates of PTSD among police officers (Wilson et al., 1997, cited in Gidron, 2002) and firefighters involved in rescue operations (North et al., 2002) following terrorist attacks, although career self-selection is also likely a contributing factor.

The intensity of stressor exposure (often operationalized as proximity) is typically related to outcomes; thus, higher levels of exposure predict greater subsequent distress. Schlenger and colleagues (2002) found that levels of PTSD symptoms were significantly higher in the New York City metropolitan area than in other major cities or the rest of the country. This association was noted even among those who resided in Manhattan during the attacks: Those living south of Canal Street (the area closest to the attacks) reported significantly higher PTSD symptoms than those living north of this area (Galea et al., 2002; see also DeLisi et al., 2003). The degree of perceived threat, injury, and material losses are each also consistent predictors of traumatic stress symptoms across traumas generally (Brewin et al., 2000; Ozer et al., 2003) and with respect to terrorism (Galea et al., 2002; Njenga et al., 2004; North et al., 1999; Verger et al., 2004).

Indirect Event Exposure

Terrorism is not directed only at those who will experience the attacks firsthand or suffer personal losses due to them, however. Terrorism's magnitude is also gauged by the extent to which the acts terrorize those who are more distant from the events. *Indirect* exposure, particularly through mass media, is the type of exposure that the greatest number of people are likely to experience in the event of future terrorist attacks, as it was in the case of September 11.

Not surprisingly given the ubiquitous media coverage during and after September 11, most studies included media exposure as a variable in their assessments. As predicted, the amount of television viewed during and shortly after the attacks was associated with levels of trauma symptoms, depression, panic, and/or distress in the perievent period and in the following months (e.g., Ahern, Galea, Resnick, & Vlahov, 2004; Schlenger et al., 2002; Schuster et al., 2001), even among those without firsthand exposure or losses. However, the relationship between distress and media exposure has yet to be fully delineated. Some have proposed that TV viewing may represent an effort to cope with distress about the event, rather than a cause of it (Schlenger et al., 2002), while others have suggested that "vulnerable victims may have attempted to use information gathered via television as a coping mechanism but instead ended up retraumatizing themselves" (Kalb, 2002, cited in Miller, 2002). If the latter is the case, then limiting media viewing of such events may be a way of conserving resources and remaining more resilient during and following the event.

Because not everyone who is directly exposed—and some who are only indirectly exposed—suffer adverse consequences, exposure alone does not account for all who will have difficulties. Individual variations in psychological response, approaches to coping, and available social support may also play a role in determining a given person's outcome.

Psychological Responses During and After the Trauma

Individuals respond in very different ways during and immediately following a traumatic event (termed "peritraumatic" responses; Marmar, Weiss, & Metzler, 1997), and these differences can have significant implications for subsequent adjustment (Ozer et al., 2003). The importance of the subjective responses of fear, helplessness, and horror during a distressing event has been demonstrated across a number of traumatic experiences (reviewed in Ozer et al., 2003), including terrorism (Njenga et al., 2004), and their centrality is captured in the DSM-IV (American Psychiatric Association [APA], 1994) diagnostic criteria for acute stress disorder (ASD) or PTSD. However, other psychological reactions during and immediately after a traumatic event may be reported. In one study following the Oklahoma City bombing (Tucker, Dickson, Pfefferbaum, McDonald, & Allen, 1997), peritraumatic hyperarousal symptoms, dissociative reactions, fear for self and family, and feelings of upset about one's own actions or those of others (retrospectively reported) were each significantly correlated with posttraumatic stress symptoms 6 months later.

Peritraumatic Dissociation

One peritraumatic phenomenon is the response of dissociation, which includes altered experiences of self (depersonalization, numbing, feeling dazed) and the world (derealization, particularly time distortion) and episodic memory difficulties (amnesia; Koopman, Classen, & Spiegel, 1994; Marmar et al., 1994; APA, 1994). Although acute dissociation is common in the context of extreme distress (APA, 1994), considerable research indicates that it may herald postevent pathology, including PTSD (reviewed in Ozer et al., 2003). Following the Oklahoma City bombing, dissociative and avoidance symptoms were also strongly associated with psychiatric comorbidity, impairment, and need for treatment (North et al., 1999).

Peritraumatic Panic

Panic is another potential peritraumatic response. Panic attacks occur in 53%–90% of survivors (Nixon & Bryant, 2003; Falsetti & Resnick, 1997) and may persist among those who develop PTSD and even predict that development (Falsetti & Resnick, 1997). Some researchers have proposed that acute panic reactions during a trauma may condition cues that later trigger panic attacks (Falsetti, Resnick, Dansky, Lydiard, & Kilpatrick, 1995), which may explain findings that peritraumatic panic can persist into the postevent period (Nixon & Bryant, 2003). Research following September 11 found that peritraumatic panic was associated with both depression and PTSD (Galea et al., 2002) and with higher levels of television viewing (Ahern et al., 2004), although the direction of the relationships could not be determined.

Peritraumatic reactions may challenge resilient functioning because some (e.g., hyperarousal, panic) may exacerbate the feeling of life threat, while others (e.g., dissociation) may bar access to adaptive behavioral options and coping strategies and impede cognitive processing of the event. Although such reactions are immediate and unbidden during the event, they are important risk factors that may be open to intervention once the acute crisis is over. It is not known what distinguishes those who experience peritraumatic panic or dissociation yet remain resilient. The utilization of personal and interpersonal resources in the early posttraumatic period is likely critical.

Coping During and After the Event

Although many factors can influence the way one responds to a major stressor, a central component in determining variability in psychological outcomes is the manner in which the individual attempts to cope. Coping has been defined as "efforts, both action oriented and intrapsychic, to manage (that is, master, tolerate, minimize) environmental and internal demands, and conflicts among them, which tax or exceed a person's resources" (Cohen & Lazarus, 1979, p. 219). Coping is frequently conceptualized in terms of broad coping styles, often dichotomous, such as approach versus avoidance (Roth & Cohen, 1986), and research has consistently found approach-monitoring-vigilant coping styles to be associated with better outcomes in a variety of situations, when compared to repression-avoidant-blunting styles (Aldwin, 1999; Roth & Cohen, 1986). Dichotomizing coping styles into two broad modalities has both conceptual and psychometric appeal; however, it does not capture the fluctuating and at times alternating nature of coping. For example, Folkman and Lazarus (1980) have found that, in highly stressful situations, there is often vacillation between approach and avoidance in attempts to manage the crisis.

Considerable research has focused on examining the ways in which different coping approaches can help a person minimize or avoid adverse outcomes following a major stressor. Although there may be no one right way to cope with traumatic events initially (Norris et al., 2002), research suggests that some coping strategies are more or less adaptive over time. Substance use, for example, is one way of coping aimed at avoiding or blunting experience or managing aversive feelings associated with trauma, but it has been associated with indicators of poor functioning in this context (North et al., 2002). In contrast, spiritual faith is central to psychological recovery for many following trauma (Tedeschi & Calhoun, 1995), and religious coping was found to be associated with lower levels of distress and greater self-reported growth among survivors of the Oklahoma City bombing (Pargament, Smith, Koenig, & Pérez, 1998).

Problem-Focused Versus Emotion-Focused Coping

Research has also examined problem-focused versus emotion-focused coping (e.g., Folkman & Lazarus, 1980) and found that these coping *styles* are more stable than other ways of conceptualizing coping (Endler & Parker, 1990). Problem-focused coping includes strategies for gathering information and other resources (skills, tools) to help deal with the underlying problem, identifying objectives, planning future actions, making decisions, and resolving conflict. In contrast, emotion-focused coping typically involves managing feelings, sometimes through avoidance, distraction, withdrawal, and disengagement from coping efforts. Emotion-focused coping strategies may be relatively consistent across time, suggesting that some people may have a characteristic way of dealing with their emotions (Aldwin, 1999).

Although people often focus on trying to control their emotions in the grip of a crisis, longer-term adjustment usually requires a more problem-focused approach, during which the difficulties posed by the stressor can be actively addressed. Problem-focused coping has the potential of resolving or successfully managing the challenge, and active engagement in the situation may minimize the feelings of helplessness often associated with trauma and replace them with an increased sense of control and personal mastery—factors associated with resilience. This may be the reason active or problem-focused coping is typically associated with better psychological outcomes than avoidant coping (Holahan & Moos, 1985; reviewed in Norris et al., 2002). For example, in one study following the Oklahoma City bombing in 1993 (Sprang, 2000), those who reported task-oriented coping indicated significantly lower levels of perceived future risk and feelings of victimization than those who engaged in avoidance or emotion-oriented coping.

However, some coping requirements may be situation specific, particularly when the stressor is uncontrollable and unpredictable (Lazarus & Folkman, 1984), as in the case of dread regarding a possible terrorist attack. A study of coping and terrorism-related anxiety among Israeli bus commuters (Gidron, Gal, & Zahavi, 1999) found that problem-focused coping while commuting (i.e., checking behaviors such as observing other passengers and looking under seats for suspicious packages) was positively associated with anxiety, whereas emotion-focused behaviors (i.e., trying to calm or distract oneself or minimizing the threat) were not. Moreover, analyses indicated that the ratio of use of these different coping strategies was key: Higher levels of problem-focused relative to emotion-focused coping were associated with terrorism distress. Gidron and colleagues suggest that combining minimal problem-focused preventative acts with distraction and reduced perceived vulnerability may be the most beneficial strategy under these circumstances.

Appraisal and Coping

Coping may also be conceptualized as a process that depends on the way a person cognitively appraises a situation. According to Lazarus and Folkman (1984), cognitive appraisals associated with stress may be categorized as harm/loss, threat, and challenge, and these appraisals are influenced by environmental demands and individual beliefs, values, and commitments. Of note, one way in

which the personality feature of hardiness may enhance resilience is through its influence on stress appraisal; hardiness has been associated with the minimization of threat, less negative affect, and increased active coping (Wiebe, 1991, cited in Tedeschi & Calhoun, 1995).

Coping Following September 11

Research following the terrorist attacks of September 11 has shed further light on the relationship between coping strategies and psychosocial outcomes such as general distress, PTSD, anxiety, and well-being. In a nationwide longitudinal study examining psychological responses to September 11 (Silver et al., 2002), the use of specific coping strategies in the immediate aftermath consistently predicted psychological outcomes over time. After controlling for demographics, time, and severity of loss experienced in the attack, people who used denial, self-distraction, or self-blame; sought social support; or disengaged from coping efforts had significantly higher levels of distress and/or trauma symptoms, whereas those who engaged in active coping or acceptance reported significantly lower levels of distress and symptoms. In fact, coping strategies shortly after the attacks were the strongest predictor of PTSD and the second strongest predictor of global distress (after prior mental health), with immediate disengagement from coping efforts markedly increasing the likelihood of ongoing distress and posttraumatic symptoms. In this study, active coping was the only strategy that appeared to be protective against ongoing distress (when prior mental health was controlled for). In fact, Silver and colleagues note that the absence of greater numbers of protective coping strategies was surprising.

Interestingly, while the *receipt* of social support is almost always associated with better mental and physical health outcomes (Cohen & Wills, 1985; Ozer et al., 2003), the *seeking* of social support as a coping strategy is almost always associated with poorer outcomes (Monroe & Steiner, 1986), as it was in the study by Silver et al. (2002) mentioned earlier. In many cases, this association may simply reflect the possibility that those who are more distressed (and therefore more likely to have poor outcomes) are more likely to seek support. In the first few days after September 11, those who reported the highest stress levels were significantly more likely to have talked to someone about their feelings at least "a medium amount," as well as turned to prayer and religion, made donations, and checked on the safety of their loved ones (Schuster et al., 2001) as ways of coping. Seeking out others to talk at least "a little bit" following the trauma was a virtually universal reaction (98%).

Consistent with these overall findings, in another study examining responses after September 11, denial, behavioral disengagement, mental disengagement, and focus on and venting of emotions was predictive of anxiety 2 months after the attacks among indirectly exposed college students, with venting of emotions uniquely predictive of long-term anxiety (Liverant, Hofmann, & Litz, 2004). Similarly, a study examining resilience in an indirectly exposed Internet sample following September 11 (Butler et al., under review) found that higher levels of psychological well-being and/or lower distress in the first few months were associated with less emotional suppression, denial, self-blame, emotional venting, substance use, and seeking of social support; and more active coping and planning. Less self-blame remained a predictor of positive outcomes at 6 months, highlighting the importance of cognitive appraisal and attribution to resilience.

In sum, research suggests that active, problem-focused coping strategies are most likely to promote outcomes of resilience, whereas avoidant, emotion-focused coping strategies contribute to outcomes of distress. In addition, cognitive factors such as appraisal and attribution of blame seem to be important in determining how coping may operate as a protective factor against ongoing distress. In the next section we turn from the domain of intrapersonal resources to those that may be found in the environment, specifically social support.

Social Support During and After the Event

One of the most consistent contributors to recovery and psychological well-being during and following stress or trauma is social support (Brewin et al., 2000; Cohen & Wills, 1985; Holahan & Moos, 1985; Norris et al., 2002; Ozer et al., 2003). Social support's stress-buffering effects (Cohen & Wills, 1985) may reduce the experience or impact of stress and thereby increase the individual's ability to function adaptively in difficult times. In one study following September 11, higher levels of social support in the 6 months *before the attacks* was associated with less attack-related depression

and PTSD (Galea et al., 2002), suggesting that having a supportive environment in place enhances resilience directly or by providing assistance to draw on when needed.

One benefit of social contact is that it allows survivors to communicate their experience to others, which may normalize and modulate their emotional reactions through experiencing them in combination with social support (Spiegel, 1999). Conversely, lack of social support (reviewed in Brewin et al., 2000) and the presence of social environments that inhibit direct discussion of the event are clear risk factors for distress, including terrorism-related distress (Butler et al., under review; Wayment, 2004). Communication also requires that the experience be put into words, which may elicit emotional and instrumental social support from the listener, as well as promote cognitive processing through structuring, elaborating, and differentiating the cognitive representation of the experience (Harber & Pennebaker, 1992). Emotional support is typically provided by friends and family, as well as by support and therapy groups, while instrumental support refers to the receipt of practical help from others in accomplishing needed tasks. Ozer and colleagues' (2003) meta-analysis concludes that the beneficial effects of perceived social support (primarily emotional support) may be cumulative or function as secondary prevention following trauma, as these effects are seen more distinctly as time since the event increases.

Personality and Support

Personality factors may influence one's ability to maintain interpersonal relationships following a traumatic event or develop and accept new social supports in the days and months after the incident. Regehr and colleagues (2001) found that firefighters who indicated more *relational capacity* (basic trust in others, less sensitivity to rejection, and ease in making friends) had less severe PTSD and depression. Coupled with cognitive appraisal of social support, these factors accounted for 88% of variance in distress. Similarly, in a study of risk and resilience factors among male and female Vietnam veterans (King et al., 1998), functional social support (the quality of the support, including perceived emotional sustenance and instrumental assistance) and hardiness were directly related to the development of PTSD, while structural social support (the size of the support system) predicted functional social support. Hardiness also contributed to PTSD outcomes through its relationship to both types of support. That is, hardiness appeared to enhance individuals' abilities to build and utilize social support, and those with more intact, well-functioning support networks exhibited fewer PTSD symptoms.

Community Involvement and Prosocial Actions

Community involvement and altruism are aspects of social contact that may help both the actor and the recipient. Large social networks can provide information and tangible help in managing event-related stressors (Cohen & Wills, 1985), and reaffirming ties to social and religious institutions may provide emotional and spiritual comfort in addition to beneficial community engagement. Indeed, *providing* emotional and instrumental support to others during times of crisis can be as helpful as receiving it (Taylor, Falke, Mazel, & Hilsberg, 1988) and may account in part for the outpouring of prosocial actions (such as donating blood, money, and time) following September 11 (Schuster et al., 2001). Of note is the finding, in a sample without direct connection to September 11, that attack-specific distress (grief, survivor guilt, and intrusive thoughts) was found to be positively associated with collective helping behaviors (e.g., giving blood, goods, or money; volunteering) in the first few weeks following the attacks, and engagement in those activities was associated with greater decreases in grief and survivor guilt over time (Wayment, 2004).

Thus, drawing on social resources during times of crisis is one of the ways people can shore up emotional support and other sources of aid to meet the challenge and cope on an ongoing basis. However, resilience resources may be strained during and following trauma, and the addition of other life stressors in the aftermath of the event can exacerbate difficulties (Brewin et al., 2000; King et al., 1998) and undermine hardiness and the availability of functional support (King et al., 1998), suggesting that a large support network should be developed before the event.

Conclusions

Masten and colleagues (Masten et al., 1999) have noted that, "to study resilience, investigators must specify the threat to [adjustment], the criteria by which adaptation is judged to be successful, and the features of the individual or the environment that may help to explain resilient outcomes" (p. 144). We have discussed the danger to well-being that terrorism (in threat and deed) poses, and we have described possible trajectories of functioning after trauma, with successful recovery representing resilience. We have also identified factors in the empirical literature found to be important contributors to positive and negative outcomes following stress and traumatic stress. Some appear to be risk or vulnerability factors for poor adaptation (e.g., poor premorbid functioning, direct exposure, certain peritraumatic reactions, avoidant coping), whereas others seem to confer protection or enhance one's ability to successfully negotiate the experience without long-term psychosocial disability (e.g., positive attitude and active engagement, previous successes in adaptation, finding meaning and benefits in adversity, problem-focused coping), and still others can either support or undermine resilience depending on their quality (e.g., appraisals, functional social support) or, in some cases, quantity (e.g., structural social support). Not surprisingly, many of these factors are interactive and that must be taken into account (and modeled in analyses) for a full appreciation of the dynamics of resilience to emerge.

Resilience may be seen as an issue of resources: the quality and quantity of psychological and interpersonal assets that can be drawn upon and brought to bear in traversing life's most difficult experiences. Such resources may be circumstantial or dispositional, learned through successes or life's knocks, or provided by supports we have in place or that come to our aid in times of need. However, resources may be limited by experience or situation, and they may be drained, inaccessible, or overwhelmed by traumatic events. Moreover, identifying these resource domains is only a first step in elucidating the underpinnings of resilience.

Clearly, additional research is needed to fully delineate the protective processes and mechanisms that enable resilient functioning and to examine their interrelationships and their effects under conditions of traumatic stress. Rutter (1987) has noted that protective elements include factors that reduce the risk itself or exposure to it; decrease the likelihood of negative chain reactions during and after the event; promote self-esteem and self-efficacy through successful task accomplishment or social supports; and open up positive opportunities that may change the initial risk trajectory.

However, to date, the majority of research on resilience and risk has been descriptive. Certain personality features, cognitive approaches, coping styles, and social supports appear to contribute to resilience, but little has been done experimentally (with adults) to examine the effects of developing or augmenting these qualities on subsequent long-term adjustment, particularly under conditions of traumatic stress. Rutter has also pointed to the need to identify and specify the parameters of difficult life experiences that ultimately bolster resilient functioning. This could take research into the realm of longitudinal studies examining *trajectories* of adaptation—succumbing, surviving with impairment, recovering, and thriving—and their predictors and mechanisms, rather than simply focusing on functional endpoints.

In their comprehensive review of disaster trauma, Norris, Friedman, and Watson (2002) conclude that distress is most likely when two or more of the following features are present: human perpetrators; intentional violence; high prevalence of injuries; threat to life; loss of life; severe, extensive property damage; and significant, ongoing financial difficulties for the community. All of these conditions are likely to be present in any future large-scale terrorist assault, as they were in the attacks of September 11. Nonetheless, most traumatic events leave in their wake a range of levels of functioning due to differences in exposure to the event and the personal resources that were available and brought to bear on adaptation. We concur, therefore, with Rowe and Kahn's (1987; see also O'Leary & Ickovics, 1995) urging that research examine this range of psychosocial outcomes and undertake the task of explaining their heterogeneity. In doing so, much will be added to our understanding of resilience and to the potential for fostering it in the face of threat and possible future acts of terrorism.

Acknowledgment. The authors wish to thank Robert W. Garlan for his tremendous help with and thoughtful contributions to this chapter.

References

Ahern, J., Galea, S., Resnick, H., & Vlahov, D. (2004). Television images and probable posttraumatic stress disorder after September 11: The role of background characteristics, event exposures, and perievent panic. *Journal of Nervous and Mental Disease, 192,* 217–226.

Aldwin, C. M. (1999). *Stress, coping, and development: An integrative approach.* New York: Guilford.

American Psychiatric Association. (1994). *Diagnostic and statistical manual of mental disorders* (4th ed.). Washington, DC: Author.

Antonovsky, A. (1987). *Unraveling the mystery of health: How people manage stress and stay well.* San Francisco: Jossey-Bass.

Bandura, A. (1982). Self-efficacy mechanism in human agency. *American Psychologist, 37,* 747–755.

Becker, E. (1973). *The denial of death.* New York: Free Press.

Blanchard, E. B., Kuhn, E., Rowell, D. L., Hickling, E. J., Wittrock, D., Rogers, R. L., et al. (2004). Studies of the vicarious traumatization of college students by the September 11th attacks: Effects of proximity, exposure, and connectedness. *Behaviour Research and Therapy, 42,* 191–205.

Block, J. H., & Block, J. (1980). The role of ego-control and ego-resiliency in the origination of behavior. In W. A. Collins (Ed.), *The Minnesota Symposia on Child Psychology, Vol. 13* (pp. 39–101). Hillsdale, NJ: Erlbaum.

Bonanno, G. A. (2004). Loss, trauma, and human resilience: Have we underestimated the human capacity to thrive after extremely aversive events? *American Psychologist, 59,* 20–28.

Bremner, J. D., Southwick, S. M., Johnson, D. R., Yehuda, R., & Charney, D. S. (1993). Childhood physical abuse and combat-related posttraumatic stress disorder in Vietnam veterans. *American Journal of Psychiatry, 150,* 235–239.

Brewin, C. R., Andrews, B., & Valentine, J. D. (2000). Meta-analysis of risk factors for posttraumatic stress disorder in trauma-exposed adults. *Journal of Consulting and Clinical Psychology, 68,* 748–766.

Butler, L. D., Blasey, C. M., Garlan, R. W., McCaslin, S. E., Azarow, J., Chen, X. H., et al. (2005). Posttraumatic growth following the terrorist attacks of September 11, 2001: Cognitive, coping, and trauma symptom predictors in an Internet convenience sample. *Traumatology, 11,* 247–267.

Butler, L. D., Field, N. P., Busch, A. L., Seplaki, J. E., Hastings, T. A., & Spiegel, D. (2005). Anticipating loss and other temporal stressors predict traumatic stress symptoms among partners of metastatic/recurrent breast cancer patients. *Psycho-Oncology, 14,* 492–502.

Butler, L. D., Garlan, R. W., & Spiegel, D. (2005). Virtual 9/11: Managing terror in an electronic era. In Y. Danieli & R. L. Dingman (Eds.), *On the* ground after September 11: Mental health responses and practical knowledge gained (pp. 575–581). New York: Haworth Maltreatment and Trauma Press.

Butler, L. D., Koopman, C., Azarow, J., Blasey, C. M., Desjardins, J. C., Dimiceli, S., et al. (under review). Psychosocial predictors of resilience following the September 11, 2001, terrorist attacks. Manuscript submitted for publication.

Carver, C. S. (1998). Resilience and thriving: Issues, models, and linkages. Journal of Social Issues, 54, 245–266.

———, & Antoni, M. H. (2004). Finding benefit in breast cancer during the year after diagnosis predicts better adjustment 5 to 8 years after diagnosis. Health Psychology, 23, 595–598.

Cohen, F., & Lazarus, R. S. (1979). Coping with the stress of illness. In G. Stone, F. Cohen, & N. Adler (Eds.), Health psychology (pp. 217–225). San Francisco: Jossey-Bass.

Cohen, S., & Wills, T. A. (1985). Stress, social support, and the buffering hypothesis. Psychological Bulletin, 98, 310–357.

Davis, C. J., Nolen-Hoeksema, S., & Larson, J. (1998). Making sense of loss and benefiting from the experience: Two construals of meaning. Journal of Personality and Social Psychology, 75, 561–574.

DeLisi, L. E., Maurizio, A., Yost, M., Papparozzi, C. F., Fulchino, C., Katz, C. L., et al. (2003). A survey of New Yorkers after the Sept. 11, 2001, terrorist attacks. American Journal of Psychiatry, 160, 780–783.

Endler, N. S., & Parker, J. D. (1990). Multidimensional assessment of coping: A critical evaluation. Journal of Personality and Social Psychology, 58, 844–854.

Falsetti, S. A., & Resnick, H. S. (1997). Frequency and severity of panic attack symptoms in a treatment-seeking sample of trauma victims. Journal of Traumatic Stress, 10, 683–689.

———, Dansky, B. S., Lydiard, R. B., & Kilpatrick, D. G. (1995). The relationship of stress to panic disorder: Cause or effect? In C. M. Mazure (Ed.), Does stress cause psychiatric illness? Vol. 46 (pp. 111–147). Washington, DC: American Psychiatric Association.

Folkman, S., & Lazarus, R. (1980). An analysis of coping in a middle-aged community sample. Journal of Health and Social Behavior, 21, 219–239.

Fontana, A., & Rosenheck, R. (1998). Psychological benefits and liability of traumatic exposure in the war zone. Journal of Traumatic Stress, 11, 485–503.

Fredrickson, B. L. (2001). Positive emotions in positive psychology: The broaden-and-build theory of positive emotions. American Psychologist, 56, 218–226.

———, Tugade, M. M., Waugh, C. E., & Larkin, G. R. (2003). What good are positive emotions in crises? A prospective study of resilience and emotions following the terrorist attacks on the United States on September 11, 2001. Journal of Personality and Social Psychology, 84, 365–376.

Galea, S., Ahern, J., Resnick, H., Kilpatrick, D., Bucuvalas, M., Gold, J., et al. (2002). Psychological sequelae of the September 11 terrorist attacks in New York City. New England Journal of Medicine, 346, 982–987.

Garmezy, N. (1985). Stress-resistant children: The search for protective factors. In J. E. Stevenson (Ed.), Recent research in developmental psychopathology (pp. 213–233). New York: Pergamon Press.

———, Masten, A. S., & Tellegen, A. (1984). The study of stress and competence in children: A building block for developmental psychopathology. Child Development, 55, 97–111.

Garmezy, N., & Rutter, M. (Eds.). (1983). Stress, coping, and development in children. New York: McGraw-Hill.

Gidron, Y. (2002). Posttraumatic stress disorder after terrorist attacks: A review. Journal of Nervous and Mental Disease, 190, 118–121.

———, Gal, R., & Zahavi, S. (1999). Bus commuters' coping strategies and anxiety from terrorism: An example of the Israeli experience. Journal of Traumatic Stress, 12, 185–192.

Green, B. L. (1993). Identifying survivors at risk: Trauma and stressors across events. In J. P. Wilson & B. Raphael (Eds.), International handbook of traumatic stress syndromes (pp. 135–144). New York: Plenum Press.

Harber, K. D., & Pennebaker, J. W. (1992). Overcoming traumatic memories. In S. Christianson (Ed.), Handbook of emotion and memory: Research and theory (pp. 359–387). Hillsdale, NJ: Erlbaum.

Hobfoll, S. E. (1991). Traumatic stress: A theory based on rapid loss of resources. Anxiety Research, 4, 187–197.

Hoffman, B. (1999). Terrorism trends and prospects. In I. Lesser, B. Hoffman, J. Arquilla, D. Ronfeldt, & M. Zanini (Eds.), Countering the new terrorism (pp. 7–38). Santa Monica, CA: RAND.

Holahan, C. J., & Moos, R. H. (1985). Life stress and health: Personality, coping, and family support in stress resistance. Journal of Personality and Social Psychology, 49, 739–747.

Janoff-Bulman, R. (1992). Shattered assumptions: Toward a new psychology of trauma. New York: Free Press.

Joseph, S., Williams, R., & Yule, W. (1993). Changes in outlook following disaster: The preliminary development of a measure to assess positive and negative responses. *Journal of Traumatic Stress, 6,* 271–279.

Kaplan, A. (1981). The psychodynamics of terrorism. In Y. Alexander & J. Gleason (Eds.), *Behavioral and quantitative perspectives on terrorism* (pp. 35–50). New York: Pergamon Press.

Kessler, R. C., Sonnega, A., Bromet, E., Hughes, M., & Nelson C. B. (1995). Posttraumatic stress disorder in the National Comorbidity Survey. *Archives of General Psychiatry, 52,* 1048–1060.

King, D. W., King, L. A., Foy, D. W., & Gudanowski, D. M. (1996). Prewar factors in combat-related posttraumatic stress disorder: Structural equation modeling with a national sample of female and male Vietnam veterans. *Journal of Consulting and Clinical Psychology, 64,* 520–531.

King, L. A., King, D. W., Fairbank, J. A., Keane, T. M., & Adams, G. A. (1998). Resilience-recovery factors in post-traumatic stress disorder among female and male Vietnam veterans: Hardiness, postwar social support, and additional stressful life events. *Journal of Personality and Social Psychology, 74,* 420–434.

Kobasa, S. C. (1979). Stressful life events, personality, and health: An inquiry into hardiness. *Journal of Personality and Social Psychology, 37,* 1–11.

Koopman, C., Classen, C., & Spiegel, D. (1994). Predictors of posttraumatic stress symptoms among survivors of the Oakland/Berkeley, Calif., firestorm. *Journal of Consulting and Clinical Psychology, 64,* 1054–1059.

Lazarus, R. S., & Folkman, S. (1984). *Stress, appraisal, and coping.* New York: Springer.

Lee, K. A., Vaillant, G. E., Torrey, W. C., & Elder, G. H. (1995). A 50-year prospective study of the psychological sequelae of World War II combat. *American Journal of Psychiatry, 152,* 516–522.

Linley, P. A., & Joseph, S. (2004). Positive change following trauma and adversity: A review. *Journal of Traumatic Stress, 17,* 11–21.

Liverant, G., Hofmann, S., & Litz, B. (2004). Coping and anxiety in college students after the September 11th terrorist attack. *Anxiety, Stress, and Coping: An International Journal, 17,* 127–139.

Manning, M. R., Williams, R. F., & Wolfe, D. M. (1988). Hardiness and the relationship between stressors and outcomes. *Work and Stress, 2,* 205–216.

Marmar, C. R., Weiss, D. S., & Metzler, T. J. (1997). The Peritraumatic Dissociative Experience Questionnaire. In J. P. Wilson & T. M. Keane (Eds.), *Assessing psychological trauma and PTSD* (pp. 412–428). New York: Guilford Press.

Masten, A. S. (2001). Ordinary magic: Resilience processes in development. *American Psychologist, 56,* 227–238.

————, Hubbard, J. J., Gest, S. D., Tellegen, A., Garmezy, N., & Ramirez, M. (1999). Competence in the context of adversity: Pathways to resilience and maladaption from childhood to late adolescence. *Development and Psychopathology, 11,* 143–169.

Masten, A. S., & Reed, M. J. (2002). Resilience in development. In C. R. Snyder & S. J. Lopez (Eds.), *Handbook of positive psychology* (pp. 74–88). New York: Oxford University Press.

Masten, A. S., & Wright, M. O. (1998). Cumulative risk and protection models of child maltreatment. *Journal of Aggression, Maltreatment, and Trauma, 2,* 7–30.

McFarlane, A. C. (1988). The aetiology of post-traumatic stress disorders following a natural disaster. *British Journal of Psychiatry, 152,* 116–121.

Meichenbaum, D. (1985). *Stress inoculation training.* New York: Pergamon Press.

Meyer, G. J., & Handler, L. (1997). The ability of the Rorschach to predict subsequent outcome: A meta-analysis of the Rorschach Prognostic Rating Scale. *Journal of Personality Assessment, 69*(1), 1–38.

Miller, L. (2002). Psychological interventions for terroristic trauma: Symptoms, syndromes, and treatment strategies. *Psychotherapy: Theory/ Research/Practice/Training, 39,* 283–296.

Monroe, S. E., & Steiner, S. C. (1986). Social support and psychopathology: Interrelations with preexisting disorder, stress, and personality. *Journal of Abnormal Psychology, 95,* 29–39.

Nixon, R. D., & Bryant, R. A. (2003). Peritraumatic and persistent panic attacks in acute stress disorder. *Behaviour Research and Therapy, 41,* 1237–1242.

Njenga, F. G., Nicholls, P. J., Nyamai, C., Kigamwa, P., & Davidson, J. (2004). Post-traumatic stress after terrorist attack: Psychological reactions following the U.S. embassy bombing in Nairobi. *British Journal of Psychiatry, 185,* 328–333.

Norris, F. H., Friedman, M. J., & Watson, P. J. (2002). 60,000 disaster victims speak: Part 2. Summary and implications of the disaster mental health research. *Psychiatry, 65,* 240–260.

————, Byrne, C. M., Díaz, E., & Kaniasty, K. (2002). 60,000 disaster victims speak: Part 1. An empirical review of the empirical literature, 1981–2001. *Psychiatry, 65,* 207–239.

North, C. S., Nixon, S. J., Shariat, S., Mallonee, S., McMillen, J. C., Spitznagel, E. L., et al. (1999). Psychiatric disorders among survivors of the Oklahoma City bombing. *Journal of the American Medical Association, 282,* 755–762.

North, C. S., Smith, E. M., & Spitznagel, E. L. (1994). Posttraumatic stress disorder in survivors of a mass shooting. *American Journal of Psychiatry, 151,* 82–88.

North, C. S., Tivis, L., McMillen, J. C., Pfefferbaum, B., Spitznagel, E. L., Cox, J., et al. (2002). Psychiatric disorders in rescue workers after the Oklahoma City bombing. *American Journal of Psychiatry, 159,* 857–859.

O'Leary, V. E., & Ickovics, J. R. (1995). Resilience and thriving in response to challenge: An opportunity for a paradigm shift in women's health. *Women's Health: Research on Gender, Behavior, and Policy, 1,* 121–142.

Ozer, E. J., Best, S. R., Lipsey, T. L., & Weiss, D. S. (2003). Predictors of posttraumatic stress disorder and symptoms in adults: A meta-analysis. *Psychological Bulletin, 129,* 52–73.

Pargament, K. I., Smith, B. W., Koenig, H. G., & Pérez, L. (1998). Patterns of positive and negative religious coping with major life stressors. *Journal for the Scientific Study of Religion, 37,* 710–724.

Park, C. L., & Blumberg, C. J. (2002). Disclosing trauma through writing: Testing the meaning-making hypothesis. *Cognitive Therapy and Research, 26,* 597–616.

Park, C. L., Cohen, L. H., & Murch, R. L. (1996). Assessment and prediction of stress-related growth. *Journal of Personality, 64,* 71–105.

Pyszcznski, T., Solomon, S., & Greenberg, J. (2003). *In the wake of 9/11: The psychology of terror.* Washington, DC: American Psychological Association.

Regehr, C., Hemsworth, D., & Hill, J. (2001). Individual predictors of posttraumatic distress: A structural equation model. *Canadian Journal of Psychiatry, 46,* 156–161.

Resnick, H. S., Kilpatrick, D. G., Dansky, B. S., Saunders, B. E., & Best, C. L. (1993). Prevalence of civilian trauma and posttraumatic stress disorder in a representative national sample of women. *Journal of Consulting and Clinical Psychology, 61,* 984–991.

Roth, S., & Cohen, L. J. (1986). Approach, avoidance, and coping with stress. *American Psychologist, 41,* 813–819.

Rowe, J. W., & Kahn, R. L. (1987). Human aging: Usual and successful. *Science, 237,* 143–149.

Rutter, M. (1987). Psychosocial resilience and protective mechanisms. *American Journal of Orthopsychiatry, 57,* 316–331.

Scheier, M. F., Weintraub, J. K., & Carver, C. S. (1986). Coping with stress: Divergent strategies of optimists and pessimists. *Journal of Personality and Social Psychology, 51,* 1257–1264.

Schlenger, W. E., Caddell, J. M., Ebert, L., Jordan, K., Rourke, K. M., Wilson, D., et al. (2002). Psychological reactions to terrorist attacks: Findings from the National Study of Americans'

Reactions to September 11. *Journal of the American Medical Association, 288,* 581–588.

Schnurr, P. P., Friedman, M. J., & Rosenberg, S. D. (1993). Premilitary MMPI scores as predictors of combat-related PTSD symptoms. *American Journal of Psychiatry, 150,* 479–483.

Schnurr, P. P., Lunney, C. A., & Sengupta, A. (2004). Risk factors for the development versus maintenance of posttraumatic stress disorder. *Journal of Traumatic Stress, 17,* 85–95.

Schuster, M. A., Stein, B. D., Jaycox, L. H., Collins, R. L., Marshall, G. N., Elliott, M. N., et al. (2001). A national survey of stress reactions after the September 11, 2001, terrorist attacks. *New England Journal of Medicine, 345,* 1507–1512.

Silver, R. C., Holman, E. A., McIntosh, D. N., Poulin, M., & Gil-Rivas, V. (2002). Nationwide longitudinal study of psychological responses to September 11. *Journal of the American Medical Association, 288,* 1235–1244.

Spiegel, D. (1999). Healing words: Emotional expression and disease outcome. *Journal of the American Medical Association, 281,* 1328–1329.

Sprang, G. (2000). Coping strategies and traumatic stress symptomatology following the Oklahoma City bombing. *Social Work and Social Sciences Review, 8,* 207–218.

Stern, J. (2003). *Terror in the name of God: Why religious militants kill.* New York: HarperCollins.

Taylor, S. E. (1983). Adjustment to threatening events: A theory of cognitive adaptation. *American Psychologist, 38,* 1161–1173.

———, Falke, R. L., Mazel, R. M., & Hilsberg, B. L. (1988). Sources of satisfaction and dissatisfaction among members of cancer support groups. In B. H. Gottlieb (Ed.), *Marshaling social support* (pp. 187–208). Newbury Park, CA: Sage.

Tedeschi, R. G., & Calhoun, L. G. (1995). *Trauma and transformation: Growing in the aftermath of suffering.* Thousand Oaks, CA: Sage.

Tennen, H., & Affleck, G. (2002). Benefit-finding and benefit-reminding. In C. R. Snyder & S. J. López (Eds.), *Handbook of positive psychology* (pp. 584–597). New York: Oxford University Press.

Tucker, P., Dickson, W., Pfefferbaum, B., McDonald, N. B., & Allen, G. (1997). Traumatic reactions as predictors of posttraumatic stress six months after the Oklahoma city bombing. *Psychiatric Services, 48,* 1191–1194.

Verger, P., Dab, W., Lamping, D. L., Loze, J., Deschaseaux-Voinet, C., Abenhaim, L., et al. (2004). The psychological impact of terrorism: An epidemiological study of posttraumatic stress disorder and associated factors in victims of the 1995–1996 bombings in France. *American Journal of Psychiatry, 161,* 1384–1389.

Wayment, H. A. (2004). It could have been me: Vicarious victims and disaster-focused distress. *Personality and Social Psychology Bulletin, 30,* 515–528.

Werner, E. E., & Smith, R. S. (1982). *Vulnerable but invincible: A longitudinal study of resilient children and youth.* New York: McGraw-Hill.

Zimbardo, P. G., & Kluger, B. (2003). Overcoming terror. *Psychology Today.* Retrieved January 31, 2006, from http://www.psychologytoday.com/ articles/pto-20030724–000001.html.

26

Promoting Resilience and Recovery in First Responders

Richard Gist

It has become almost axiomatic in the field of trauma response to assert that first responders—law enforcement officers and agents, firefighters, rescue specialists, emergency medical technicians, and paramedics—are at severely heightened risk for posttraumatic stress disorder (PTSD) and related psychiatric maladies because of the nature and emotional impact of their work. While a number of reports have appeared indicating higher rates of endorsed reactivity and probable caseness (see, for example, Clohessy & Ehlers, 1999), several reports have also concluded that first responders are, in fact, uncommonly resilient (cf. Gist & Woodall, 2000). Moreover, while programs such as critical incident stress debriefing, which are designed to mitigate traumatic impacts and prevent PTSD, have permeated these fields and even extended into an ever-broadening range of other workplaces (see Mitchell [2004] with regard to claims of penetration and range for the intervention set in question), the key intervention has become increasingly controversial as empirical reports have accumulated, showing it to be inert at best and possibly even detrimental to some (cf. Rose, Bisson, Churchill, & Wessely, 2004 or Van Emmerik, Kamphuis, Hulsbosch, & Emmelkamp, 2002; see also McNally, Bryant, & Ehlers, 2003, for a comprehensive overview).

Inherent in these seeming contradictions is an array of issues that must be teased out and carefully considered if we are to understand the interaction between the nature of these occupations, the people who perform within them, the structure of their work and encounters, and the impact of those encounters on their career growth and personal functioning. Some of those issues include matters related to the construction of the PTSD diagnosis and its application to a population wherein exposure to situations often deemed traumatic is expected and sometimes daily fare. When does such exposure fall outside the range of ordinary experience for those who are so situated?

Other issues involve identifying, operationalizing, and effectively impacting the most salient sources of occupational stress and especially plumbing the interaction of persistent *strain* with episodic *stress*. Still others involve the nature of stress mitigators in these particular occupations. Secondary interventions imposed after the fact are generally less likely to provide meaningful preventive impact than are primary interventions deployed to mitigate the impact of the nearly inevitable exposure inherent in the social roles and primary functions these occupations represent. It is also necessary to consider a range of contextual issues because the impacts of these events on individual providers reflect the interactions of workplace experience with personal, interpersonal, social, and community features of each provider's life and circumstances, as well as the roles such experiences play in personal and professional development across the life cycle of individual and career growth. It is by no means a simple portrait to paint.

The prospect of terrorist events, especially those that might involve weapons of mass destruction or actions intended to instigate fear and disequilibrium, complicates the matter further. These events, by nature and design, are likely to fall outside the ordinary experience of even veteran first responders. However, it is the practiced capacity to deal with the ordinary and usual challenges of the occupations that must provide the skill base that enables these professionals to respond effectively and provides the capability for their resilience in the aftermath.

The Nature of the Work

Law enforcement and firefighting are more than occupations or professions. These enterprises represent essential social functions that must be exercised for any community to prosper. Law enforcement represents the formalized embodiment of a community's need for social regulation to ensure that balance is maintained between the prerogatives of the individual and the priorities of the commonwealth; firefighting evolves as the extension of the needs of the collective to come together with precision and effectiveness to facilitate the protection of its members from threats too large for any one to master by oneself. Each finds its roots in the voluntarism that de Tocqueville ([1835–1840] 2001) celebrated in his early commentaries on American life, but each has evolved into formal governmental structures and entities that hold increasingly proscribed roles in a complex, technologically based society.

The complexity of their modern roles is reflected in the size and responsibilities of contemporary law enforcement and fire service organizations, as well as in the wide range of events in which their response is expected. Law enforcement includes duties that range from daily patrol and traffic management to counterterrorism, forensic science, and tactical operations. Fire service organizations are their communities' first resource for most issues related to hazards and safety, but now they must also provide expertise for hazardous material identification and mitigation, mass casualty triage, decontamination, and technical rescue in the event of structural collapse or environmental contamination. Because the occupations have extended on both ends of their spectra, the practitioner's contact with the ordinary citizen has become more frequent and more personal at the same time that issues and impacts of a more global and technical nature have become increasingly critical elements of social role and expectations.

What draws people to these jobs and shapes their careers within them continues to hold features of idealism and service—these are constantly challenged, however, by confrontation with the very elements of life from which their social roles daily insulate their fellow citizens. Law enforcement officers are consistently confronted with those who prey upon the social order. Firefighters and medics quickly learn that death is an omnipresent and ultimately inescapable part of daily life. Nested within that constant strain are periodic episodes that stand out as particularly challenging.

Such circumstances result almost unavoidably in cognitive disequilibrium. The manifestations of such disequilibrium are not generally inconsonant with those of other forms of distress, making it facile to describe them as symptoms of any number of conditions in which generalized distress plays a presumed etiologic and diagnostic role. Since this disequilibrium tends to manifest itself most visibly following exposure to emotionally laden occupational events, it is equally simplistic to attribute the distress to the essential nature of the seemingly precipitating event. It may, however, prove counterproductive to couch such disequilibrium as a symptom of psychic injury resultant of some particular exposure. Superior utility and understanding may appertain from couching it instead as a sign of processes that hold at least an equal propensity to stimulate personal and professional adaptation and growth (Gist & Woodall, 1999).

Such growth does not necessarily come gently, nor can it always be expected to come without distress. How that distress is characterized, however, is a central attributional feature that likely holds a strong capacity to influence its perceived nature and its ultimate impact. While the distress of such disequilibration is typically cast as pathognomonic in the literature of traumatic stress, cognitive disequilibrium is well recognized in educational development as a salutatory if sometimes discomfiting factor that motivates people to reexamine their understanding of a situation or circumstance, embrace broader and alternative views, and emerge with a fuller understanding and appreciation of the matter at issue (cf. Mills & Keil, 2004). When viewed in this light, it can emerge as the essence of the enterprise's rewards even more than the reservoir of its liabilities.

Woodall (1997), as a career firefighter completing a doctorate in human and organizational development, garnered the Student Paper of the Year award from the Sociological Practice Association for his ethnographic treatment of the role of these "critical incidents" in the career development of successful professional firefighters. He collated data from interviews with a wide range of students and alumnae of the National Fire Academy's Executive Fire Officer program to investigate how such incidents were remembered, accommodated, and incorporated into the occupational understanding of those who had objectively advanced in their organizations and profession. He summarized the conundrum in the following fashion:

> It is the very nature of a firefighter's journey, the seemingly endless exposure to human pain and suffering, that has afforded them the opportunity to appreciate the joys of life by knowing and understanding human tragedy. By experiencing, although most times vicariously, the emotional and physical pain of the sick, injured, and dying, they become capable of experiencing the true meaning of life. These resilient emotional skills serve them both at home and on the job. Their experiences afford them the emotional skills required to function in dangerous and tragic environments. By the same token, these skills also afford them the opportunity to take that little extra moment to appreciate the joys of life, understanding all the while just how fleeting those joys can be. (p. 155)

Such resolution might be better conceptualized as a dynamic equilibrium between the cognitive and emotional challenges inherent in the occupations and the cognitive resolution one can achieve by asking progressively better questions about the nature of things each time one's understanding encounters significant conceptual challenge (cf.

Graesser & Olde, 2003). While successful for most people over time, such resolution may indeed prove to be difficult for everyone at various points and too challenging for some at particular junctures. How to anticipate, mitigate, mediate, and accommodate those challenges becomes pivotal to effective management of human capital in these enterprises.

Dealing With Occupational Stress

Recognition of stress as a significant factor affecting the health and safety of public safety providers no longer meets macho resistance within the industry; no longer do stress management or behavioral wellness programs encounter denial so intense as to demand or justify missionary zeal to secure their endorsement or adoption. Behavioral wellness, including personal and occupational stress management, was accorded direct recognition and standing in the Joint Wellness Initiative of the International Association of Fire Fighters, AFL-CIO, and the International Association of Fire Chiefs (IAFF/IAFC, 1997, Chapter 5); these are also recognized components within the National Fire Protection Association standards regarding occupational health and safety for firefighters (NFPA, 1997, Standard 1500).

Most of the attention initially afforded these topics centered around a relatively singular and narrow construction of occupational stress and occupational stressors (dubbed "critical incident stress") and a specific popularized model of peer intervention (critical incident stress debriefing [CISD]). Much like the suicide prevention and crisis intervention movement of a quarter century ago (cf. Echterling & Wylie, 1981), the CISD phenomenon arose primarily as a grassroots amalgam spurred by a few charismatic leaders without standing or recognition in mainstream medicine or psychology.

The core contentions on which the enterprise was erected derived from an essential assumption that occupational events function on an individual level as psychic traumata, "wounding" the psyche of people confronting them in such a way as to disrupt their capacity to function normally in the aftermath (cf. Mitchell, 1983, 1988; Mitchell & Bray, 1990; Mitchell & Everly, 1995). The premise that these exposures, if not contravened through direct and focused rapid interventions, would lead to posttraumatic stress disorder and related psychiatric maladies (cf. Mitchell, 1992) quickly became an unquestioned axiom.

Critical Incident Stress Debriefing

When distilled to its essence, CISD is a simple application of an objectively rather loose amalgam of rudimentary notions regarding structured re-exposure, proximal early catharsis, anticipatory guidance, and peer modeling folded into an otherwise unremarkable group-process approach (cf. Mitchell & Everly, 1995). This blending of widely venerated but generally untested axioms regarding crisis intervention (e.g., temporal and physical proximity of intervention to stressor exposure; cathartic utility of early narrative reconstruction and emotional expression) with popularized self-help standbys such as peer-mediated disclosure and psychoeducational information lent the procedure both an attractive familiarity and a strong dose of presumptive face validity. Since its first formal articulation in a proprietary trade magazine of the emergency medical services (Mitchell, 1983), the technique has been aggressively marketed on the following express premises:

- Even singular exposure to certain critical incidents could reliably give direct rise to post-traumatic stress disorder and other psychiatric morbidity.
- Nearly immediate (within 24–72 hours) application of this specific intervention procedure would reliably prevent such transition.
- Failure to provide such specific intervention (or even the provision of other intervention approaches) would potentiate or exacerbate traumatic reactions and their sequelae (cf. Mitchell, 1992).

These assertions were repeatedly published and proclaimed in the trade venues of fire service and public safety occupations, and a wide following grew around debriefing as an almost evangelical self-help program. Debriefing seemed, on its face, to be benign at its very worst and to represent a reasonably caring organizational response to the impact of difficult duty. Despite the claims of its principals and their disciples that it enjoyed a detailed and specific grounding in empirical research, these contentions—especially those regarding its purported preventive efficacy—had not been established in the usual venues of objective academic research. Proclamations made in that regard, when investigated to any depth, proved not to have been derived from the sorts of systematic testing and study normally associated with evidence-based practice (Gist et al., 1997; Gist & Woodall, 1995, 1999; Gist, Woodall, & Magenheimer, 1999).

The intensive marketing of the rubric and the broadening range of its application, especially as contrasted with observations from serious practitioners regarding limitations or misadventures in actual application, eventually led these claims to be subjected to direct scientific scrutiny. Initial studies in several parts of the globe clearly suggested that the claims of preventive impact had been seriously overstated—indeed, systematic studies repeatedly found no evidence of preventive impact compared to nonintervention controls (see, for example, Deahl, Gillham, Thomas, Dearle, & Srinivasan, 1994; Lee, Slade, & Lygo, 1996; McFarlane, 1988) or compared against informal vehicles of social support (cf. Hytten & Hasle, 1989). Even more disturbing, though, were findings—ultimately repeated across a range of studies—that specific applications of debriefing interventions resulted in paradoxically inhibited courses of recovery for significant numbers of recipients (Griffith & Watts, 1992; Kenardy et al., 1996; Mayou, Ehlers, & Hobbs, 2000).

These reports have increasingly appeared in mainstream journals of the psychological and psychiatric disciplines and have now coalesced into a strengthening body of scientific information. The overall direction of the empirical data has now become decidedly clear:

- The *Cochrane Reviews*—Oxford-based systematic, critical reviews of research reports covering a range of medical treatments—again updated their report regarding debriefing after traumatic exposure in May 2001; that iteration evaluated 11 randomized, controlled trials (RCTs) of the intervention genre (Rose, Bisson, Churchill, & Wessely, 2006). Conclusions have been very strong that debriefing has proven ineffective at best with respect to preventing PTSD and may actually inhibit the normal course of recovery. The closing recommendation from that update specifically states, "There is no evidence that psychological debriefing is a useful treatment for the prevention of post-traumatic stress disorder after traumatic incidents. Compulsory debriefing of victims of trauma should cease."

- Several well-partitioned field studies (quasi experiments, rather than RCTs) of debriefing following occupational incidents in law enforcement, fire and rescue services, and emergency medical workers have also been reported in refereed research venues. These studies, too, found debriefing inert at best with respect to preventing PTSD (Carlier, Lamberts, van Uchlen, & Gersons, 1998; Macnab, Russell, Lowe, & Gagnon, 1998), and at least two studies echoed findings of the RCTs regarding paradoxical outcomes for some debriefed participants (Carlier, Voerman, & Gersons, 2000; Gist, Lubin, & Redburn, 1998).

- A more recent and thorough meta-analysis, including both RCTs and partitioned-field studies (Van Emmerick et al., 2002) has established that effect sizes for debriefing showed no significant preventive efficacy, held the possibility of paradoxical impacts, were generally smaller than those found for nonintervention controls, and were notably smaller than those of other interventions against which it had been contrasted. Though these confidence intervals overlapped and hence could not be conclusively stated as statistically significant differences, the authors noted that the mean effect size for natural resilience with respect to PTSD was at least moderate, while that of the contrasted interventions was moderate to strong; only the confidence interval for debriefing effect sizes included zero and negative values (indicating an inert or even a paradoxical intervention).

- The rejoinder that these conclusions relied principally on data from individual applications rather than intact occupational groups has been severely weakened with preliminary reporting of the largest and most tightly controlled study to date, involving military personnel studied in intact units before and after deployment (Litz, Adler, Castro, Suvek, & Williams, 2004). More than a thousand personnel attached to multiple military units received either group CISD from fully trained debriefers using precisely managed protocols, a traditional "stress education" handout and talk, or an "assessment only" control condition. Postdeployment measures were compared against predeployment baselines utilizing contemporary growth curve modeling techniques to measure the impact of interventions on trajectory of change over time. CISD yielded no preventive impact in any of the dimensions measured.

The Empirical Imperative

These data have compelled an increasing range of scientific bodies and professional organizations—including many originally quite supportive of the notion—to reexamine the assumptions and recommendations related to the application of interventions styled on the principles of debriefing and have led, in their turn, to a number of published statements prescribing limitation or contraindication (e.g., Bisson, McFarlane, & Rose, 1998); Parry, 1999; Raphael, 1999; Wessely & Krasnov, 2002). Current guidance from the United Kingdom's National Institute for Clinical Excellence (2005) specifically contraindicates offering debriefing to trauma victims, and an advisory bulletin from the World Health Organization (2005) echoes that contraindication. The findings of the largest consensus panel convened to date (Ritchie, 2002) specifies that the term "debriefing" should be restricted to operational review of responder activities for purposes of incident management (specifically nonpsychological in nature) and does not recommend any use of approaches based on narrative reconstruction or cathartic ventilation in the immediate aftermath period (Watson, 2004).

Emerging studies reported in a variety of first-tier journals and symposia have indicated additional concerns that prove particularly troublesome. Those experiencing increases in hyperarousal symptoms, for example—those who are generally those most likely to perceive themselves and be perceived by others as distressed and needing intervention—have been particularly prone to paradoxical impacts from these interventions, no matter how constructed (Sijbrandij, Olff, Gersons, & Carlier, 2002). Those who favor repressive coping styles—again, among those most often prodded to participate—may do quite well absent intervention but deteriorate with supportive and educational approaches that most others would find helpful and reassuring, a repeated finding with cardiac patients across several studies and locations (Frasure-Smith et al., 2002; Ginzburg et al., 2002; Shaw, Cohen, Doyle, & Palesky, 1985). Still other studies have suggested that those who most endorse these encounters may also be among those most likely to experience paradoxical inhibition of resolution relative to similarly situated persons to whom no intervention was provided (Mayou, Ehlers, & Hobbs, 2000).

Deconstructing Debriefing

Why should something with such seeming face validity and close congruence to dominant notions of traumatic reactivity and intervention prove almost universally to have been nonefficacious? Why would such a procedure be counterproductive for some, potentially yielding paradoxical inhibition of resolution trajectories for those most particularly disturbed by their experiences? To understand this calamity, we must first deconstruct the process. The dominant model (Mitchell and Everly, 1999) prescribes seven phases:

Introduction Phase

The standard CISD protocol begins by having the practitioner outline the process and prescribe certain ground rules for the session. Included in these instructions are statements of purpose and presumption intended to encourage participants to engage themselves in the process and participate in the phases to follow. Rather than the statements of limitation and potential risk that fully informed consent would ordinarily demand before proceeding with an intervention widely reported to be inert at best and paradoxical for some, these instructions have tended instead to promote claims of exaggerated preventive efficacy. Rather than the proviso that one should carefully consider one's decision to participate in light of these concerns, participants in group encounters are instead told that their participation may be helpful not only to them but also to others. Participants are typically promised confidentiality, despite being told that the intervention is not a therapeutic one (hence negating the precise relationship required to invoke any such protection). They are also generally told that no records will be kept, contravening strict ethical and legal prescriptions regarding documentation of services.

"Facts" Phase

The CISD protocol calls next for the specific reporting of what participants saw and heard during the traumatic episode. The goal of this exercise is generally described in terms of creating a calibrated perspective of the event. Such reconstruction may serve to intensify already disturbing reactions by reconnecting the individual with sources of profound discomfort and disequilibrium well before sufficient distancing has had an opportunity to develop. This revivification is unlikely to serve its intended purpose and may, especially for parties disposed toward repressive coping styles, be more likely to arrest than to accelerate the processes inherent in normal resolution.

Group applications of debriefing, rather than creating a shared picture of circumstances and events, may further compound these issues by exposing those who are struggling to keep their own arousal in check to additional, potentially even more vivid and arousing constructions of the event and its images. Especially when the process is invoked within the frequently recommended postimpact envelope of 24–72 hours, the potential for these paradoxical impacts may be heightened as one progresses from this element through the "thoughts" and "reactions" phases to follow. Given that Charlton and Thompson (1996) found only positive reappraisal and distancing to be coping strategies predictive of successful adaptation, this early insistence on reconstruction may well run counter to the very processes most likely to promote eventual resolution, problems that may be systematically compounded in the following two phases of the classic CISD rubric.

"Thoughts" Phase

This phase asks participants to articulate their initial thoughts as the impact and magnitude of the traumatic event first came to their awareness. This is apparently intended to establish a sort of cognitive baseline from which subsequent reappraisals might emerge. It may instead present, at least for some, the potential to paradoxically solidify negative elements of events resurrected through the narrative reconstruction of the "facts" phase. This can again be compounded in group applications, where some participants may not have been fully cognizant of the level of danger to which they were exposed or may not have construed their experience in as threatening or unnerving a fashion as that which may be heard from others. The impact of this paradox may be further exacerbated by immediate implementation of the intervention attempt, leading readily to situations in which the encounter serves to encourage dissemination of idiosyncratic, unsubstantiated, and/or disconcerting information among those immersed in distressing and disequilibrating circumstances.

Such postevent processes can lead to reappraisal of one's memory of the event in ways that may increase one's subjective estimation of the threat. Such reappraisals have been posited as central in the derivation of fear responses (Davey, 1993), and others have shown that such increased subjective appraisal of danger correlates with pathologic outcomes (Solomon, Mikulincer, & Benbenishty, 1989; Stallard, Velleman, & Baldwin, 2000). This may be exacerbated in vulnerable individuals, as these cognitions are again paired with arousal sensations when the process moves into the "reactions" or "feelings" phase.

"Reactions" (or "Feelings") Phase

This phase invites participants to articulate their emotional responses to the event, often through queries such as "What was the worst part of the experience for you?" This serial progression from narrative reconstruction of events ("facts" phase) through cognitive retrieval of proximal perceptions ("thoughts" phase) to reconnection of these with the immediate emotional impact of the experience in the "reactions" phase completes a process of revivification. Those who fully submit themselves to the procedure, especially the most vulnerable, can find themselves intolerably close to those states of terror, helplessness, and confusion from which distancing is most vital. When instituted before reliable pictures of fact have been established and early arousal has had an opportunity to abate, this process of revivification—especially when delivered to people who might normally have gone on to process the information successfully if left unassisted—runs the risk of sensitizing such persons to intrusive internal stimuli at a time when desensitization is vital to immediate stabilization.

The processes of desensitization necessary to address pathological elements inherent in diagnosable PTSD require systematically graded exposure to defined stimuli and progressive habituation to them. This serves to extinguish the fear response and provide corrective information to challenge aberrantly held beliefs (Foa & Kozac, 1986). This is unlikely to be accomplished in a one-shot, ostensibly prophylactic group encounter and cannot reasonably be attempted until initial reactions have had sufficient time to stabilize and abate. Indeed, such short-term and short-lived exposure to memories of threat in people who may not currently have a pathological condition but who present with pronounced subjective distress conceivably introduces a risk of generalizing these memories and priming certain stimuli that are, or could become, triggers for consolidating the fear response (McNally et al., 1987). Regardless of any intention to subsequently normalize this subjective arousal, those already struggling to regulate arousal, intrusion, and reexperiencing may find that these elements of the debriefing rubric reinforce, entrench, and exacerbate their subjective discomfort rather than mitigate or diminish it.

"Symptoms" Phase

Narrative reconstruction of the traumatic episode and the various reactions it may have engendered is followed by a descriptive exercise in which participants are queried regarding "symptoms" they may be experiencing. While the rhetorical justification for this phase is to normalize whatever reactions may be felt, there is a subtle but possibly profound difference to be drawn between discussing common manifestations of postimpact distress and priming people to consider these discomfitures as if they were pathologic indicators associated with psychological dysfunction. Moreover, repeatedly labeling the event "traumatic" superimposes a set of attributions and expectations that might not otherwise apply. Such attributions may dispose vulnerable people to interpret the inescapable disequilibrium of disruptive life events as pathological anxiety—becoming, in effect, a self-fulfilling prophecy of despair. Once again, this is particularly pertinent when the topic is introduced before the normal processes of identification and attribution of subjective discomfort have begun, much less stabilized. The greatest risk may reside with those who are already experiencing heightened distress.

The very labeling of subjective experiences that are, in most cases, *signs* of inescapable disequilibrium as if they are *symptoms* of pathology may contribute to a "medicalization" of the experience—to wit, "I didn't think of myself as sick until you sent for a remedy" (Gist, 2002). Here again, the combined impact of one phase (in this case, the "symptoms" phase) with that of its succeeding phase (the "teaching" phase) holds even further potential to compound complications for vulnerable participants, especially when implemented at a juncture where the strongest susceptibility to suggestion is likely to be present.

"Teaching" Phase

Debriefing protocols provide for a psychoeducation element intended to provide modeling of and information about adaptive approaches to addressing the trauma and its sequelae. This discussion generally centers around colloquialized discussions of PTSD and its symptomatology. Debriefers have frequently been known to distribute lists of problems that participants are told they may expect to experience (e.g., increased irritability, avoidance of reminders of the trauma, disturbed sleep, intrusive memories of the event) and then to provide suggestions, often simplistic at best, regarding coping strategies and approaches. Such a narrow focus on the core constructs of PTSD may lead one somewhat astray from dealing with disaster as a social experience (see Staab, Fullerton, & Ursano, 1999, for an alternative construction). Social comparison under threat, however, may prove a more salient construction for understanding both successful adaptation and the paradoxical impacts sometimes associated with debriefing.

Perceived threat lends a unique urgency to the search for affiliation and social comparison (Kulik, Mahler, & Moore, 1996). These contacts tend to follow particular patterns that underscore the need for specifically appropriate models (see also Taylor, 1983). Given that Gump and Kulik (1997) found that settings composed of those who share traumatic exposure contain demonstrable elements of social contagion, blanket application of an indiscriminate group process may stand particularly prone to stimulation of negative outcomes, especially when invoked before constructive coping strategies have had time to fully evolve in the affected individual or population. Add to this the hypothesis that overestimation of threat and fear expectation play a causal role in the origins and maintenance of anxiety (Wiedemann, Pauli, & Dengler, 2001) and that for people with panic disorder, the expectation of panic is associated with actual panic occurrence (Kenardy & Taylor, 1999), and the potential for selective misadventure again increases.

"Reentry" Phase

This is intended as a time to reinforce consolidation of material learned from the group experience, a typical element of any group-process model. Where the information communicated in a group setting is valid and useful, such consolidation is likely to be productive. Consolidation of counterproductive ideas and information, however, is no less likely an outcome than consolidation of productive learning. Where there is likely at best to have been a liberal mixture of both, the resulting outcome would seem destined to be nonproductive at best.

Reconsidering Occupational Stress

Particularly with respect to occupational and organizational events, context and circumstance may prove much more determinant of impact than the nature or magnitude of a given incident (Alexander & Wells, 1991; Gist et al., 1998), while individual circumstances and proclivities preextant to the event have proven decidedly more predictive of lasting sequelae than have features such as proximity and exposure alone (Cook & Bickman, 1990; McFarlane, 1988, 1989). More than two decades ago Taylor (1983) posited that cognitive adaptation to stressful events might be more effectively characterized from a salutogenic, developmental perspective rather than being presumed pathognomonic of psychopathologic risk.

A rigorous and very productive line of empirical research emerging since that time (see, for example, Taylor & Brown, 1988; Taylor & Lobel, 1989) provided affirmation and considerable refinement to these propositions and melded them into an alternative, more discernable and testable construction for the operation of such stressors in both individual and collective adjustment to negative events (Taylor, 1991). Those constructions recognize the unique salience and impact of extraordinary threat as a stressor while still embracing the long-standing conventional wisdom that adversity can, and in fact most commonly will, provide challenges from which character and resilience are built.

Exposure to critical incidents is not only unavoidable in fire and rescue work; it is in fact the essence of the enterprise. For most providers in most situations, these encounters are not sources of *threat* or *loss* but are rather episodes of *challenge*, in which skills and effort central to one's personal and professional role identity are focused on the legitimate demands of the occupation (see McCrae, 1984, for an overview of situational determinants of coping strategy). The organization may be argued to hold a range of responsibilities to ensure that personnel are adequately prepared, equipped, deployed, and configured for effective response and for ensuring that the impact of equivocal events is effectively addressed in organizational and operational review (Gist & Taylor, 1996), but individual decisions, actions, coping patterns, and responses are also highly determinant of adjustment. These interact with organizational determinants in complex and sometimes unpredictable ways that render uniform approaches to remediation suspect, if not overtly dangerous (Moran, 1998). Accordingly, appropriate strategies for intervention and assistance must separately and distinctly address organizational, situational, and individual factors and determinants and must be capable of effectively addressing both the unique contributions of each and the interactions among them.

Distinction must also be drawn between approaches focused on issues and assumptions related to presumed vulnerability factors versus those focused on building and enhancing resilience. Despite the presumptions of the debriefing movement and its conceptual cousins in disaster response regarding exposure, risk, and causation, an increasing body of empirical research has focused on consistent finding of remarkable resilience in a sizable, often strongly dominant, portion of those exposed to ostensibly traumatizing events. The distinctions between these competing views reach much further than simple twists of title or subtle shifts of attention and became a principal focus of the National Institute of Mental Health's proposed plan for basic behavioral science research (Basic Behavioral Science Task Force, 1996).

Effective strategies for intervention and assistance, then, must begin with strategies to enhance resilience and integrate these strategies with approaches that supplement and reinforce resilient responses of individuals and organizations. When specific interventions are undertaken, they must occur without supplanting natural contacts and supports that promote autonomy and resilience with artificial structures that may instead reinforce vulnerability or encourage reliance on inappropriate, ineffective, or ill-timed strategies of coping and resolution.

A Systems View of Occupational Stress

It is not some specific and conceptually isolated set of critical incidents that can be posited to determine the most salient links in the processes of reaction and resolution. It is, in fact, the backdrop of daily hassles in the form of personal and organizational *strain* that can ultimately be said to define the relative impact of a given stressor. This was highlighted in a thorough study of more than 200 firefighter/paramedics and firefighter EMTs in the State of Washington (Beaton & Murphy, 1993), in which past critical incidents ranked well below obvious concerns such as sleep disruption, wages and benefits, labor/management issues, personal safety, equipment, job skill concerns, and family/financial strains as elements of perceived job stress. Past critical incidents failed to significantly enter regression equations that predict job satisfaction and morale for paramedic firefighters and barely achieved significance for firefighter/EMTs. Moreover, Wright (1993) reported in a preliminary study of successful career paramedics that the principal factors influencing perceptions of stress in a series of hypothetical calls hinged not on the manifest content of the encounter or even on patient outcome but rather were driven by perceptions of personal and organizational success in the address of component evolutions.

The most promising strategy for primary prevention of problems related to occupational stress interventions in these professions must deal with enhancing those features of organizational performance, personal conditioning and development, and social support that provide effective response and promote personal and organizational resilience. Similarly, strategies for incident-specific interventions must look to support the operation and, if necessary, the regeneration of these same factors through the least intrusive vehicles consistent with the given circumstance. Moreover, they must at the same time carefully consider and evaluate the interactions between individual circumstances of the affected people and broader organizational impacts and needs. Inherent conflicts between personal and organizational interests cannot be avoided, and separate routes of intervention with clearly specified client relationships will generally be required for the system to operate ethically and effectively.

Organizational Factors

Gist and Taylor (1996) outlined a series of organizationally based strategies that, they argued, should be considered before, during, and after particularly stressful operations to promote maximum resilience within both the formal and the informal organizations of the workplace, which, in turn, would help to support maximum resilience in those exposed to stressful occupational events. These focused on the incorporation of enhanced information and more effective practices into existing organizational relationships affecting management, command, supervision, and human resource support and on the addition of skills and resources to supplement existing patterns where deficits might exist or develop. The recommended approaches advocated empowerment in daily activities and responses over remedial interventions, which they described metaphorically as opting to promote flood control engineering rather than sandbagging as a better strategy for advancing risk management.

Adoption and consistent utilization of practiced incident management systems represent major factors favoring organizational resilience (Alexander & Wells, 1991; Gist, Lubin, & Redburn, 1998). These systems have achieved increasing sophistication over the past two decades, culminating in a synthesized approach that has emerged as a national standard (Federal Emergency Management Agency, 2004). The protective benefit lies in providing a well-rehearsed, systematic vehicle by which the command systems used each day in routine operations expand to anticipate and address the needs of complex and escalating situations. When coupled to a consistent program of operational review such as the military's After Action Review protocols (see Gist & Woodall, in press, for discussion of its application to fire and rescue service), this provides a strong foundation both to mitigate and contain the stress of the operation and to reframe its personal impacts in the context of coordinated occupational activity (providing, in essence, distancing and reframing; see Charlton & Thompson, 1996).

However, events occur that require coordinated strategies of response. The range of possibilities for reasoned intervention is broad indeed, and a number of suggestions have emerged. The most detailed recommendation set to date has emerged from the consensus panel convened by the National Institute of Mental Health, the U.S. Department of Defense, and a number of other agencies charged to examine early interventions following mass violence and terrorist events (Ritchie, 2002). While *psychological* debriefing was not recommended for first responders, *operational* debriefing was recognized both for its critical role in the management of events and for the widely recognized palliative effects that accrue to participants in the process.

Ørner (2003) has described an evidence base for early intervention in emergency services populations constructed on determining and supporting natural adjustment and coping patterns of these personnel. Macnab, Sun, and Lowe (2003) note that, while debriefing and related interventions had shown little preventive impact on personnel following a fatal air ambulance crash, preexisting stress management and coping strategies showed a noteworthy mediating effect. Systems of intervention and assistance that reflect help-seeking and attribution patterns of affected persons are more likely to be utilized by those in need and to support resilient responses (Yates, Axsom, & Tiedeman, 1999). Avery and King (2003) describe an effort in a program initially modeled around debriefing and related interventions to reshape its initiatives along these lines.

This program focused on the inherent resilience of emergency responders. Hands-on, practical ways of preparing responders to adjust to the stressors encountered in their work were coupled to the realization that frequent exposure to intense and varied stressors can create service needs that are often more determined by the nature of the individual's world at the time of a critical exposure than by the nature of the exposure itself. Service possibilities with potential to address those situations and needs are also a strong part of the initiative.

Psychological First Aid

Ruzek (2002) proposes a strategy for postevent intervention with response personnel based on pragmatic elements of education and practical support. These approaches are consistent with the general tone of *psychological first aid* (PFA) notions currently gaining favor as supportive responses in the immediate aftermath of stressful events. There has been little clarity of specific objectives or systematic definition of technique regarding PFA, hence little can be adduced in the way of empirical data regarding efficacy. But the intent of PFA centers on practical and palliative impacts rather than the prevention of later PTSD, and appreciation for these less specific impacts has been suggested as the principal source of positive endorsements given most visible early interventions, including debriefing (Gist, 2002).

Such impacts should not be slighted. Data now suggest that fewer persons may be likely to develop diagnosable PTSD than has often been suggested and that many who do may resolve to subclinical levels without overt intervention (cf. Galea et al., 2002; Galea et al., 2003). The dominant resolution trajectory of early resilience was posited by Bonanno (2004) as parallel to the trajectory of recovery, differing principally in the extent of early arousal and distress and in the length of the refractory period. It is reasonable to suggest, then, that early efforts to mitigate initial distress may hold potential to at least moderate the subjective experience of impact.

Traditional approaches to first aid in the physical domain concentrated on similarly basic ideas. The intent was not to prevent some single, specific consequence through some single, specific technique. First aid represented instead the capacity to apply any or several in a range of techniques to provide basic practical and palliative care where injury was not sufficient to warrant definitive care, and the capability to provide critical life support where needed until definitive care could be rendered. The former case entailed a kit filled with band aids, light antiseptics, gauze pads, and other simple remedies; the latter centered on the most basic interventions to preserve life organized along a simple mnemonic of "ABC":

- airway
- breathing
- circulation

With respect to PFA, Gist, Jackson, and Song (2004) have suggested a loose set of concepts clearly modeled on a metaphor, and a similar construction may be apt:

- attenuation of initial distress
- basic needs
- compassion

This does not necessarily require orchestrated attempts at visible psychological intervention, especially in occupational settings. The objective in occupational encounters is generally to ensure that the organization acknowledges the difficulty of the encounter, that adequate information is provided to evaluate its context and learn from its implications, and that avenues for future assistance, should they be needed, are noted and made available. This can be accomplished in many ways, tailored to the organization, the personnel, and the circumstances. More importantly, it can be crafted from routine interactions in understated fashions, helping to ensure the most unintrusive form of support congruent with the situation at hand.

Early Assessment

Identification of those for whom resilience proves insufficient demands a simple but effective early screening device. Brewin et al. (2002) reported a simple 10-item screen to be given 3–4 weeks post-impact. Centered on intrusion and arousal symptoms consistent with active PTSD, the screen simply asks whether the respondent has experienced any of the noted reactions at least twice within the past week. Six or more positive endorsements is determined to represent a positive screen.

Despite its simplicity, the instrument has achieved very promising utility in early trials. Sensitivity and specificity have been above 0.9, with screening efficiency at 0.92. The most direct advantage, however, is that the instrument can be administered quickly and easily in a variety of settings (e.g., general practice), and scoring requires only simple counting of affirmative responses. Since the outcome is referral for more intensive screening, it could feasibly be used as self-screening tool and might even be delivered through online and similar mass distribution venues.

Efficacious Early Intervention Following a Positive Screen

The most widely endorsed treatment for those developing diagnosable PTSD is trauma-focused cognitive behavioral therapy (CBT) (see, for example, National Institute for Clinical Excellence, 2005; Litz, Gray, Bryant, & Adler, 2002; Ritchie, 2001; Watson, 2004; World Health Organization, 2005). Current protocols recommend a short cycle (approximately five sessions) commencing somewhere near the 4-week diagnostic point regarding symptom duration.

Despite widespread recognition of superior efficacy, providers who are suitably trained and prepared to administer trauma-focused CBT are not easily found among the resources most often available to rescue personnel. Available providers are most likely to be employee assistance counselors, agency-based counselors, or similar providers who are more likely to be trained in supportive techniques requiring much less intensive training and supervision to acquire or apply. These techniques, however, have been shown repeatedly to be inert relative to trauma-focused CBT (Bisson, 2001). Programs to provide "just in time" training and preparation in these approaches are being explored in several settings.

Stepped Care

An effective program of services requires that objectives be mapped for development of resilience, enhancement of adjustment skills before exposure, management of exposure factors, metered support congruent with coping styles and preferences following exposure, early assessment to identify those for whom additional services may be required, and accessible services with strongly demonstrated efficacy for those who require such intervention. Such a system needs to be based in a thorough understanding of the organizational systems .involved, the culture and traditions within which the systems operate, the groups and individuals who compose the organization, and the tasks and encounters they engage.

A more subtle but in many ways more critical limitation of traditional programs of support for emergency workers has been a tacit assumption of homogeneity within emergency responders. This may be driven by an implicit focus on a perceived strong commonality in the situations and stressors they seemingly face *as seen from the perspective of those outside the experience.* While law enforcement officers, fire suppression personnel, emergency medical responders, and other providers of emergency response may indeed confront similar situations and often do so together, the impacts of those exposures may well be determined at least as much by the organizational contexts surrounding that exposure than by any individual factors of the experience. Where specific factors rise to strong salience, these may often be better understood, defined, and ameliorated when viewed in the broader contexts of interpersonal and organizational systems. While personal reactivity may indeed reach clinical levels for some, it is equally important to realize that resilience is strong, especially in this population, and

that "watchful waiting" with instrumental and palliative support frequently proves to be the best practice.

Summary Observations

There is no question that emergency response work is demanding. There is also no question, however, that those challenges bring their own rewards. Undoubtedly emergency workers are strongly impacted by the situations they encounter, and certainly those impacts yield meaning and strength more often than they engender pathology and disturbance. Helping prepare emergency responders and their organizations to build resilience, enhance systems, create responsiveness, anticipate resource needs, and design accessible mechanisms to facilitate the balanced operation of these options requires a much more proactive, consultative, and organizationally driven approach than traditional intervention-driven, reactive approaches have provided.

Even more important than the differences in orientation and technique may be the underlying difference in humility. The roles prescribed for the interventionists in traditional models are central, visible, self-affirming, and even aggrandizing. The roles prescribed for the consultant in the emerging approaches are much more circumspect and require that one seek and maintain a much less central and visible presence. The intent is not to rescue but to facilitate strength among those for whom rescue is their daily fare.

Resilience is not simply recovery in shorter time (Bonanno, 2004; Rutter, 1987). Resilience is a complex set of interactions that allows people not to avoid the discomforts of adversity and challenge but to manage their ways through them, often to discover enhanced strength as a consequence. The efforts to build pathways to resilience, design systems to support them, and provide graded support to promote their operation must complement cautious, evidence-based approaches to assessment of perturbation in exposed people and the provision of timely, efficacious intervention when and to whom indicated. The challenge to first responder organizations is to shift from simple ideas and simplistic approaches toward deeper understanding and multilayered approaches that can help these vital organizations and their personnel meet the demands of their increasingly difficult work.

References

Alexander, D. A., & Wells, A. (1991). Reactions of police officers to body handling after a major disaster: A before and after comparison. *British Journal of Psychiatry, 159,* 547–555.

Avery, A., & King, S. (2003). The Lincolnshire Joint Emergency Services Initiative: An early intervention protocol for emergency services staff. In R. Ørner & U. Schnyder (Eds.), *Reconstructing early intervention after trauma: Innovations in the care of survivors* (pp. 212–219). New York: Oxford University Press.

Basic Behavioral Science Task Force. (1996). Basic behavioral science research for mental health: Vulnerability and resistance. *American Psychologist, 51,* 22–28.

Beaton, R. D., & Murphy, S. A. (1993). Sources of occupational stress among firefighter/EMTs and firefighter/paramedics and correlations with job-related outcomes. *Prehospital and Disaster Medicine, 8,* 140–150.

Bisson, J. I. (2001, December 6–9). Providing an evidence-based early psychological response following physical injury. In P. J. Watson, Early intervention to prevent the development of PTSD. Symposium presented at 17th Annual Meeting of the International Society for Traumatic Stress Studies, New Orleans, LA.

———, McFarlane, A. C., & Rose, S. (1998). (Paper Position). Psychological Debriefing. International Society for Traumatic Stress Studies. PTSD Treatment Guidelines Committee.

Bonanno, G. A. (2004). Loss, trauma, and human resilience: Have we underestimated the human capacity to thrive after extremely aversive events? *American Psychologist, 59,* 20–28.

Brewin, C. R., Rose, S., Andrews, B., Green, J., Tata, P., McEvedy, C., et al. (2002). A brief screening instrument for post-traumatic stress disorder. *British Journal of Psychiatry, 181,* 158–162.

Carlier, I. V. E., Lamberts, R. G., van Uchlen, A. J., & Gersons, B. P. R. (1998). Disaster-related post-traumatic stress in police officers: A field study of the impact of debriefing. *Stress Medicine, 14,* 143–148.

Carlier, I. V. E., Voerman, A. E., & Gersons, B. P. E. (2000). The influence of occupational debriefing on post-traumatic stress symptomology in traumatized police officers. *British Journal of Medical Psychology, 73,* 87–98.

Charlton, P. F. C., & Thompson, J. A. (1996). Ways of coping with psychological distress after trauma. *British Journal of Clinical Psychology, 35,* 517–530.

Clohessy, S., & Ehlers, A. (1999). PTSD symptoms, responses to intrusive memories, and coping in ambulance service workers. *British Journal of Clinical Psychology, 38,* 251–265.

Cook, J. D., & Bickman, L. (1990). Social support and psychological symptomatology following a natural disaster. *Journal of Traumatic Stress, 3,* 541–556.

Davey, G. C. L. (1993). Trauma revaluation, conditioning, and anxiety disorders. *Behavior Change, 10,* 131–140.

Deahl, M. P., Gillham, A. B., Thomas, J., Dearle, M. M., & Srinivasan, M. (1994). Psychological sequelae following the Gulf War: Factors associated with subsequent morbidity and the effectiveness of psychological debriefing. *British Journal of Psychiatry, 165,* 60–65.

de Tocqueville, A. ([1835–1840] 2001). *Democracy in America.* New York: Penguin Putnam.

Echterling, L., & Wylie, M. L. (1981). Crisis centers: A social movement perspective. *Journal of Community Psychology, 9,* 342–346.

Federal Emergency Management Agency. (2004). *National Incident Management System.* Washington, DC: Author.

Foa, E. B., and Kozac, M. J. (1986). Emotional processing of fear: Exposure to corrective information. *Psychological Bulletin, 99,* 20–35.

Frasure-Smith, N., Lespérance, F., Gravel, G., Masson, A., Juneau, M., & Bourassa, M. G. (2002). Long-term survival differences among low-anxious, high-anxious, and repressive copers enrolled in the Montreal heart attack readjustment trial. *Psychosomatic Medicine, 64,* 571–579.

Galea, S., Ahern, J., Resnick, H., Kilpatrick, D., Bucuvalas, M., Gold, J., et al. (2002). Psychological sequelae of the September 11 terrorist attacks in New York City. *New England Journal of Medicine, 346,* 982–987.

Galea, S., Vlahov, D., Resnick, H., Ahern, J., Susser, E., Gold, J., et al. (2003). Trends of probable post-traumatic stress disorder in New York City after the September 11 terrorist attacks. *American Journal of Epidemiology, 158,* 514–524.

Ginzburg, K., Solomon, Z., & Bleich, A. (2002). Repressive coping style and adjustment following myocardial infarction (MI). *Psychosomatic Medicine, 64,* 748–757.

Gist, R. (2002). What have they done to my song? Social science, social movements, and the debriefing debates. *Cognitive and Behavioral Practice, 9,* 272–279.

————, Jackson, C. M., & Song, J. K. (2004, November 14). Integrating research and practice to foster community resilience. In R. Gist, Response to disaster: New research, ageless wisdom, and efficacy. Symposium presented at 20th Annual Meeting of the International Society for Traumatic Stress Studies, New Orleans, LA.

Gist, R., Lohr, J. M., Kenardy, J. A., Bergmann, L., Meldrum, L., Redburn, B. G., et al. (1997). Researchers speak on CISM. Journal of Emergency Medical Services, 22(5), 27–28.

Gist, R., Lubin, B., & Redburn, B. G. (1998). Psychosocial, ecological, and community perspectives on disaster response. Journal of Personal and Interpersonal Loss, 3, 25–51.

Gist, R., & Taylor, V. H. (1996). Line of duty deaths and their effects on coworkers and their families. Police Chief, 63(5), 34–37.

Gist, R., & Woodall, S. J. (1995). Occupational stress in contemporary fire service. Occupational Medicine: State of the Art Reviews, 10, 763–787.

————. (1999). There are no simple solutions to complex problems: The rise and fall of critical incident stress debriefing as a response to occupational stress in the fire service. In R. Gist & B. Lubin (Eds.), Response to disaster: Psychosocial, community, and ecological approaches (pp. 211–235). Philadelphia: Brunner/Mazel.

————. (2000). There are no simple solutions to complex problems. In J. M. Violanti & P. Douglas (Eds.), Posttraumatic stress intervention: Challenges, issues, and perspectives (pp. 81–95). Springfield, IL: Charles C. Thomas.

————. (In press). Occupational stress in the fire and rescue professions: Evidence informed approaches for individual, operational, and organizations initiatives. Clifton Park, NY: Thomson Delmar Learning.

————, & Magenheimer, L. K. (1999). And then you do the hokey-pokey and you turn yourself about. In R. Gist & B. Lubin (Eds.), Response to disaster: Psychosocial, community, and ecological approaches (pp. 269–290). Philadelphia: Brunner/Mazel.

Graesser, A. C., & Olde, B. A. (2003). How does one know whether a person understands a device? The quality of the questions the person asks when the device breaks down. Journal of Educational Psychology, 95, 524–536.

Griffith, J., & Watts, R. (1992). The Kempsey and Grafton bus crashes: The aftermath. East Lismore, Australia: Instructional Design Solutions.

Gump, B. B., & Kulik, J. A. (1997). Stress, affiliation, and emotional contagion. Journal of Personality and Social Psychology, 72, 305–319.

Hytten, K., & Hasle, A. (1989). Firefighters: A study of stress and coping. Acta Psychiatrica Scandinavia, 355(Suppl.), 50–55.

International Association of Fire Fighters and International Association of Fire Chiefs. (1997). Joint Labor Management Health, Wellness, and Fitness Initiative. Washington, DC: Author.

Kenardy, J. A., & Taylor, C. B. (1999). Expected versus unexpected panic attacks: A naturalistic prospective study. Journal of Anxiety Disorders, 13, 435–445.

Kenardy, J. A., Webster, R. A., Lewin, T. J., Carr, V. J., Hazell, P. L., & Carter, G. L. (1996). Stress debriefing and patterns of recovery following a natural disaster. Journal of Traumatic Stress, 9, 37–49.

Kulik, J. A., Mahler, H. I. M., & Moore, P. J. (1996). Social comparison and affiliation under threat: Effects on recovery from major surgery. Journal of Personality and Social Psychology, 71, 967–979.

Lee, C., Slade, P., & Lygo, V. (1996). The influence of psychological debriefing on emotional adaptation in women following early miscarriage: A preliminary study. British Journal of Medical Psychology, 69, 47–58.

Litz, B. T., Adler, A. B., Castro. C. A., Suvek, M., & Williams, L. (2004, November). A randomized controlled trial of critical incident stress debriefing. In M. Friedman, Military psychiatry, then and now. Plenary session presented at the 20th annual meeting of the International Society for Traumatic Stress Studies, New Orleans, LA.

————, Gray, M. J., Bryant, R., & Adler, A. B. (2002). Early intervention for trauma: Current status and future directions. Clinical Psychology: Science and Practice, 9, 112–134.

Macnab, A. J., Russell, J. A., Lowe, J. P., & Gagnon, F. (1998). Critical incident stress intervention after loss of an air ambulance: Two-year follow-up. Prehospital and Disaster Medicine, 14, 8–12.

Macnab, A. J., Sun, C., & Lowe, J. (2003). Randomized controlled trial of three levels of critical incident stress intervention. Prehospital and Disaster Medicine, 18, 365–369.

Mayou, R. A., Ehlers, A., & Hobbs, M. (2000). Psychological debriefing for road traffic accident victims: Three-year follow-up of a randomized controlled trial. British Journal of Psychiatry, 176, 589–593.

McCrae, R. R. (1984). Situational determinants of coping responses: Loss, threat, and challenge. Journal of Personality and Social Psychology, 46, 919–928.

McFarlane, A. C. (1988). The longitudinal course of posttraumatic morbidity: The range of outcomes and their predictors. *Journal of Nervous and Mental Disease, 176,* 30–39.

McFarlane, A. C. (1989). The aetiology of post-traumatic morbidity: Predisposing, precipitating, and perpetuating factors. *British Journal of Psychiatry, 154,* 221–228.

McNally, R. J., Bryant, R. A., & Ehlers, A. (2003). Does early psychological intervention promote recovery from posttraumatic stress? *Psychological Science in the Public Interest, 4*(2).

McNally, R. J., Luedke, D. L., Besyner, J. K., Peterson, R. A., Bohm, K., & Lips, O. J. (1987). Sensitivity to stress-relevant stimuli in post-traumatic stress disorder. *Journal of Anxiety Disorders, 1,* 105–116.

Mills, C. M., & Keil, F. C. (2004). Knowing the limits of one's understanding: The development of an awareness of an illusion of explanatory depth. *Journal of Experimental Child Psychology, 87,* 1–32.

Mitchell, J. T. (1983). When disaster strikes . . . the critical incident stress debriefing process. *Journal of Emergency Medical Services, 8*(1), 36–39.

———. (1988). The history, status, and future of critical incident stress debriefing. *Journal of Emergency Medical Services, 13*(11), 49–52.

———. (1992). Protecting your people from critical incident stress. *Fire Chief, 36*(5), 61–67.

———. (2004). Crisis intervention: A defense of the field. Retrieved February 1, 2006, from http://www.icisf.org/articles/Acrobat%20Documents/CISM_Defense_of_Field.pdf

———, & Bray, G. (1990). *Emergency services stress.* Englewood Cliffs, NJ: Brady.

Mitchell, J. T., & Everly, G. S. (1993, 1999). *Critical incident stress debriefing: An operations manual for the prevention of traumatic stress among emergency services and disaster workers.* Ellicott City, MD: Chevron.

Moran, C. C. (1998). Individual differences and debriefing effectiveness. *Australasian Journal of Disaster and Trauma Studies,* 1998–1. Retrieved February 1, 2006, from http://www.massey.ac.nz/~trauma/issues/1998–1/moran1.htm.

National Fire Protection Association. (1997). *Standard on Fire Department Occupational Safety and Health Program* (NFPA Standard 1500). Quincy, MA: Author.

National Institute for Clinical Excellence. (2005). *Management of post-traumatic stress disorder in adults in primary, secondary, and community care.* London: Author.

Ørner, R. (2003). A new evidence base for making early intervention in emergency services complementary to officers' preferred adjustment and coping strategies. In R. Ørner & U. Schnyder, Eds., *Reconstructing early intervention after trauma: In-* *novations in the care of survivors* (pp. 143–153). New York: Oxford University Press.

Parry, G. (Chair).(2001). Evidence-based clinical practice guidelines for treatment choice in psychological therapies and counselling. London, UK: Department of Health, National Health Service.

Raphael, B. (Chair). (1999). Mental health disaster training manual. Sydney, Australia: New-South Wales Department of Health.

Ritchie, E. C. (Chair). (2001). *Mental health and mass violence: Evidence-based intervention for victims/survivors of mass violence* (NIH Publication no. 02–5138). Washington, DC: U.S. Government Printing Office.

Rose, S., Bisson, J., Churchill, R., & Wessely, S. (2006). Psychological debriefing for preventing posttraumatic stress disorder. Cochrane Database of Systematic Reviews (2006:1). New York: John Wiley & Sons.

Rutter, M. (1987). Psychosocial resilience and protective mechanisms. *American Journal of Orthopsychiatry, 57,* 316–331.

Ruzek, J. I. (2002). Providing "brief education and support" for emergency response workers: An alternative to debriefing. *Military Medicine, 167*(9, Suppl.), 73–75.

Shaw, R. E., Cohen, F., Doyle, B., & Palesky, J. (1985). The impact of denial and repressive style on information gain and rehabilitation outcomes in myocardial infarction patients. *Psychosomatic Medicine, 47,* 262–273.

Sijbrandij, M., Olff, M., Gersons, B., & Carlier, I. V. E. (2002, November 10). A closer look at debriefing: Emotional ventilation vs. psychoeducation. In M. Olff, Early interventions: New contributions to outcome research. Symposium presented at 18th Annual Meeting of the International Society for Traumatic Stress Studies, Baltimore, MD.

Solomon, Z., Mikulincer, M., & Benbenishty, R. (1989). Locus of control and combat-related post-traumatic stress disorder: The intervening role of battle intensity, threat appraisal, and coping. *British Journal of Clinical Psychology, 28,* 131–144.

Staab, J. P., Fullerton, C. S., & Ursano, R. (1999). A critical look at PTSD: Constructs, concepts, epidemiology, and implications. In R. Gist & B. Lubin (Eds.), *Response to disaster: Psychosocial, community, and ecological approaches* (pp. 101–128). Philadelphia: Brunner/Mazel.

Stallard, P., Velleman, R., & Baldwin, S. (2000). Prospective study of post-traumatic stress disorder in children involved in road traffic accidents. *British Medical Journal, 7173,* 1619–1623.

Taylor, S. E. (1983). Adjustment to threatening events: A theory of cognitive adaptation. *American Psychologist, 38,* 1161–1174.

———. (1991). Asymmetrical effects of positive and negative events: The mobilization-minimization hypothesis. *Psychological Bulletin, 110,* 67–85.

———, & Brown, J. D. (1988). Illusion and well-being: A social psychological perspective on mental health. *Psychological Bulletin, 103,* 193–211.

Taylor, S. E., & Lobel, M. (1989). Social comparison activity under threat: Downward evaluation and upward contacts. *Psychological Review, 96,* 569–575.

Van Emmerik, A. A. P., Kamphuis, J. H., Hulsbosch, A. M., & Emmelkamp, P. M. G. (2002). Single-session debriefing following psychotrauma, help or harm: A meta-analysis. *Lancet, 360,* 766–771.

Watson, P. J. (2004). Behavioral health interventions following mass violence. *Traumatic Stress Points, 18,* 8–9.

Wessely, S., & Krasnov, V. (2002, March 25–27). NATO-Russia advanced workshop on social and psychological consequences of chemical, biological, and radiological terrorism. Retrieved February 1, 2006, from http://www.nato.int/science-old/e/020325-arw2.htm.

Wiedemann, G., Pauli, P., & Dengler, W. (2001). A priori expectancy bias in patients with panic disorder. *Journal of Anxiety Disorders, 15,* 401–412.

Woodall, S. J. (1997). Hearts on fire: An exploration of the emotional world of firefighters. *Clinical Sociology Review, 15,* 153–162.

World Health Organization. (2005). Single-session psychological debriefing: Not recommended. Retrieved February 1, 2006, from http://www.who.int/mental_health/media/en/note_on_debriefing.pdf.

Wright, R. M. (1993, May). Any fool can face a crisis: A look at the daily issues that make an incident critical. In R. Gist, *New information, new approaches, new ideas.* Overland Park, KS: Center for Continuing Professional Education, Johnson County Community College.

Yates, S., Axsom, D., & Tiedeman, K. (1999). The help-seeking process for distress after disasters. In R. Gist & B. Lubin (Eds.), *Response to disaster: Psychosocial, community, and ecological approaches* (pp. 133–165). Philadelphia: Brunner/Mazel.

27

Integrating Medical, Public Health, and Mental Health Assets into a National Response Strategy

Dori B. Reissman
Stephan G. Reissman
Brian W. Flynn

Because terrorism is a federal crime and grabs national attention, management of a terrorist attack is complicated. In a terrorist event, the Federal Bureau of Investigation (FBI) is in charge of managing the criminal investigation (U.S. Department of Homeland Security, 2004b). The jurisdictional Emergency Management Agency coordinates various groups (i.e., response and recovery operations) to manage the consequences of such events. State and federal resources can be called upon to support local response efforts if the scope or severity of the impact overextends the capabilities of local agencies. In 2003, Homeland Security Presidential Directive number 5 (Office of the President of the United States, 2003a) called for a single, comprehensive national approach for use by all levels of government by integrating emergency management principles in response to a terrorist attack or other disaster:

- The Secretary of the U.S. Department Homeland Security (DHS), or designee, is the principal federal official for domestic incident management.
- A standardized incident management system will be used for all levels of government and

private service sectors involved in disaster response (including terrorism).
- A national strategy for disaster and terrorism preparedness planning will address the core health, safety, and infrastructure needs of those affected

Local Emergency Management

The local emergency management agency (EMA) supports the on-scene efforts of the first-response agencies by obtaining and coordinating the resources and personnel needed to do their jobs. They coordinate the available resources (e.g., public works) to deal with emergencies effectively, "thereby saving lives, avoiding injury, and minimizing economic loss" (Haddow & Bullock, 2003, p. 55). The first responder's role in an event is coordinated in proximity to the event. For example, if an attack is a localized explosion, the first responders' activities are handled at the "incident command post," which is set up near the affected area. If there are multiple sites, responders will be coordinated through an "area command" (Emergency Management Institute, 2005). The local EMA hosts and collocates key decision makers from multiple response agencies (e.g., police, fire, EMS, environmental protection, Red Cross, hospital associations, public health and medical agencies, public works) at an emergency operations center (EOC) to jointly manage the overall response.

An important part of the EMA's efforts revolves around preparedness planning for all types of emergencies (see Table 27.1). Rather than developing separate plans for terrorist attacks and other disasters (e.g., hurricanes, hazardous industrial explosions, major transportation crashes), emergency managers use an "all-hazards" response-planning strategy for disaster preparedness. The all-hazards approach addresses the commonly anticipated essential needs of an impacted community and standardizes operations. Issues that are unique to a particular hazard (e.g., chemical, radiological, biological, nuclear, explosive) are addressed as part of an "annex" (or appendix) to the jurisdiction's response plan. These plans should be written in collaboration with the community's response partners and need to be exercised, reviewed, and updated regularly (Federal Emergency Management Agency [FEMA], 1996a).

Incident Management

An incident command system (ICS) or incident management system (IMS) is used by the EMA, public safety officers, and emergency response partners to integrate strategic analysis and planning, daily tactical operations, logistical support, and financial accountability into the response and recovery efforts (FEMA, 1996; Emergency Management Institute, 2005). Disasters and other large-scale events may require shared leadership or unified command among multiple agencies. Unified command brings together entities with different jurisdictional and/or functional responsibilities "to work together to develop a common set of incident objectives and strategies, share information, maximize the utilization of available resources, and enhance the efficiency of the individual response organizations" (National Response Team, 2004). All of the various groups involved in the response are obligated to support the leading agencies, and different ones may be in charge or share leadership (or support) of the incident at different times during the same event or for different types of events.

Table 27.1. Example of a local EMA's responsibilities, as delineated by statutory authority (City of Des Moines [Iowa] Emergency Management Agency, 2004)

---

1. *Hazard identification and planning:* Conduct hazard identification and vulnerability analyses that identify the hazards presenting the greatest danger to the jurisdiction and the consequences and impact of the occurrences.

2. *Maintenance of the emergency partnership:* Develop and maintain effective relationships with emergency response agencies, as well as government, private, and voluntary sectors of the community. The objectives of the relationships are to facilitate mutual consultation, exchange information, and provide agreements for cooperative action.

3. *Emergency response systems:* Develop and maintain such systems as communications, warning, emergency public information, damage assessment, shelter, resource management, radiological defense, and the emergency operations center.

4. *Coordination:* Coordinate the response and recovery activities of the departments and organizations involved in emergencies. One role for the emergency management coordinator is to serve as chief of staff to the responsible executive, be it a city manager, mayor, or county executive, during a disaster or emergency situation.

5. *Hazard mitigation:* Provide oversight and motivation to departments and agencies to carry out their duties in ways that avoid or minimize potential emergency conditions.

   Regulatory: Participate in and contribute to the legislative and regulatory process as it relates to emergency management.

6. *Information:* Develop and implement public information and public relations activities.

7. *Administration:* Oversee budget and finance, personnel, programs, supplies, and reporting systems.

8. *Training:* Identify training needs and develop, participate in, and provide training programs.

9. *Planning:* Review and revise operations, recovery, mitigation, and other supporting plans on a regular basis.

10. *Drills:* Coordinate drills that test the written plans and procedures of emergency management and supporting agencies that are involved in emergency response and recovery.

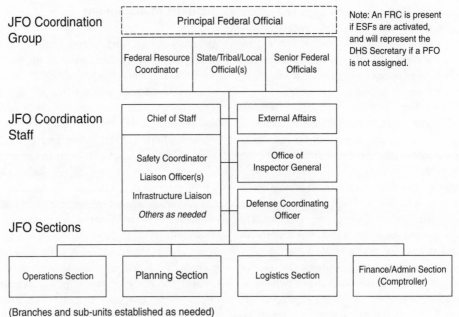

Figure 27.1. Joint Field Office (JFO) for federal-to-federal support (U.S. Department of Homeland Security, 2004b, p. 39, figure 9).

Traditionally, the ICS is composed of five organizational management sections: the incident manager (called the "principle federal official" for federal-to-federal coordination), and the operations, planning, logistics, and finance/administration sections (Figure 27.1; Emergency Management Institute, 2005). The incident manager sets the objectives and priorities of the event and has the overall responsibility for coordination. The operations section carries out the day-to-day tactical operations of the response. The planning section develops daily action plans during the event, is kept informed of investigative and operational details, and anticipates needs as the event evolves. The logistics section provides the resources and other services needed to support the incident response. The finance/administration section monitors and documents all of the costs related to the incident.

Such a command or management structure needs to be scalable and flexible to account for the unique characteristics of an unfolding situation. Although a variety of incident management or command systems are used all over the country, there has not been a standard approach for managing emergencies or disasters. The absence of standardized terminology, concepts, and strategic approaches to managing incidents can lead to

confusion and delays in providing services during large-scale events (e.g., acts of terrorism, natural disasters). This deficiency may compromise public health, safety, and security. Therefore, all first responder agencies and federal agencies were officially advised to use a nationally standardized model for incident management based on the principles of ICS (Office of the President of the United States, 2003a; U.S. Department of Homeland Security, 2003a).

The National Incident Management System

In 2004, the U.S. Department of Homeland Security introduced the official version of the National Incident Management System (U.S. Department of Homeland Security, 2004a). Future federal funding for state and local response agencies may rest on their adoption and implementation of NIMS. NIMS provides standard terminology, protocols, and procedures for all responders at the scene of an event. The system is designed to address all types of hazards, including those involved in terrorism (see Figure 27.2). The scope of NIMS includes responder training and certification, compatible

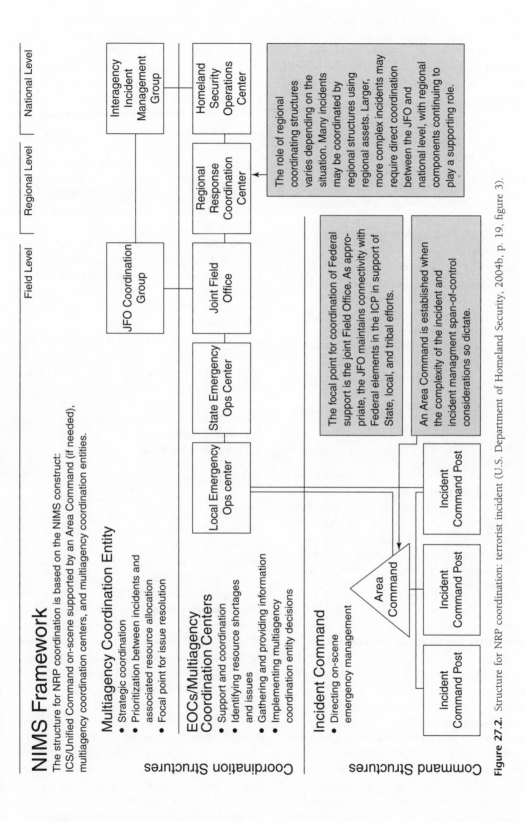

NIMS Framework

The structure for NRP coordination is based on the NIMS construct: ICS/Unified Command on-scene supported by an Area Command (if needed), multiagency coordination centers, and multiagency coordination entities.

| | Field Level | Regional Level | National Level |

Multiagency Coordination Entity

- Strategic coordination
- Prioritization between incidents and associated resource allocation
- Focal point for issue resolution

Interagency Incident Management Group

JFO Coordination Group

Homeland Security Operations Center

Regional Response Coordination Center

Joint Field Office

The role of regional coordinating structures varies depending on the situation. Many incidents may be coordinated by regional structures using regional assets. Larger, more complex incidents may require direct coordination between the JFO and national level, with regional components continuing to play a supporting role.

EOCs/Multiagency Coordination Centers

- Support and coordination
- Identifying resource shortages and issues
- Gathering and providing information
- Implementing multiagency coordination entity decisions

State Emergency Ops Center

Local Emergency Ops center

The focal point for coordination of Federal support is the Joint Field Office. As appropriate, the JFO maintains connectivity with Federal elements in the ICP in support of State, local, and tribal efforts.

Incident Command

- Directing on-scene emergency management

Area Command

An Area Command is established when the complexity of the incident and incident managment span-of-control considerations so dictate.

Incident Command Post

Incident Command Post

Incident Command Post

Incident Command Post

Coordination Structures

Command Structures

Figure 27.2. Structure for NRP coordination: terrorist incident (U.S. Department of Homeland Security, 2004b, p. 19, figure 3).

437

communication systems for use by response agencies (i.e., interoperability), and ongoing evaluation and quality improvement of the NIMS products. Some of the key features of the system include the following (U.S. Department of Homeland Security, 2004a):

- Command and management: to delineate the chain and sharing of command and leadership in managing the event to coordinate multiple agencies (and jurisdictions), according to a standard platform of ICS
- Preparedness: to demand that specific measures, actions, and processes be included in emergency management plans by designated agencies
- Resource management: to identify, track, and deploy resources (using standardized terminology and terms of reference)
- Communications and information management: to ensure and expedite information sharing among the various agencies involved in a response. This aids in establishing a common view of the incident by all of the involved agencies and also encourages the crafting of accurate, consistent, and unified messages for public dissemination.
- Supporting technologies: to ensure that equipment and technology selected by the various response agencies function in a compatible (interoperable) fashion
- Ongoing management and maintenance: to support the refinement of NIMS through best practices research and lessons learned from exercises and actual responses. This component also includes setting national standards for responder training and credentialing.

Requests for Federal Assistance

Every state now has an Office of Homeland Security (or a similarly titled entity) to link with the federal counterpart, DHS, and to address issues surrounding terrorism. These offices are often connected to the state's EMA and/or to a state law enforcement agency. The DHS is charged with leading federal preparedness for, response to, and recovery from terrorist attacks, major disasters, and other emergencies (U.S. Department of Homeland Security, 2004b). The Robert T. Stafford Disaster Relief and Emergency Assistance Act ("Stafford Act"; 2000) specifies procedures for requesting federal assistance (see Figure 27.3).

Each state has an emergency management agency that represents the governor in coordinating state-level disaster response. In addition to providing training and developing statewide response plans, the state EMA can request personnel and equipment through the National Guard, mutual aid resources from both inside and outside the state, and petition for federal assets to be deployed to the state. The Federal Emergency Management Agency (FEMA), now part of DHS, assesses the extent of the damage and the appropriate types of federal assistance needed by a petitioning state. Then FEMA forwards the state's request and FEMA's assessment to both the President of the United States and the Secretary of DHS. In some cases, the Stafford Act can authorize deployment of federal assets to a state without a governor's request. Once the assistance is deployed, a demobilization strategy is formulated to guide the release and return of federal response personnel and other deployed federal assets.

Federal Response to a Terrorism Incident

The U.S. government has the primary authority to prevent and respond to acts or potential acts of terrorism against the people or possessions of the United States. This responsibility is assigned to the U.S. Attorney General and carried out through the Federal Bureau of Investigation. "Crisis management" refers to law enforcement "measures to identify, acquire, and plan the use of resources needed to anticipate, prevent, and/or resolve a threat or act of terrorism" (U.S. Department of Homeland Security, 2004b, p. 82). This can include intelligence, criminal surveillance, forensic investigations, and tactical operations. "Consequence management" refers to "measures to protect public health and safety, restore essential government services, and provide emergency relief to governments, businesses, and individuals affected by the consequences of terrorism" (U.S. Department of Homeland Security, 2004b, p. 82). Crisis management and consequence management often take place concurrently.

In an actual or potential terrorist incident, local jurisdictions, followed by state authorities, have

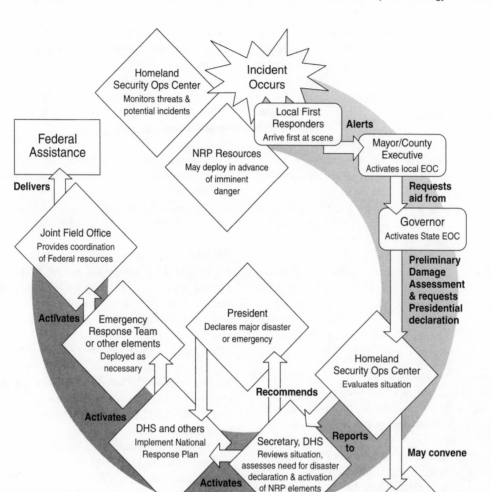

Figure 27.3. Overview of initial federal involvement under the Stafford Act (U.S. Department of Homeland Security, 2004b, p. 93, figure 11).

the primary authority to respond to the consequences. In the past, the federal response to terrorism and other disasters was governed by four principal federal response plans and other supporting strategies:

- The Federal Response Plan (FRP) was used to provide federal assistance for major disasters or emergencies (FEMA, 1999).

  The FRP outlines the ways in which the federal government assists state and local

governments when a major disaster or emergency overwhelms their capacity to respond. The FRP describes the activities and responsibilities of the federal government and the American Red Cross following a presidential declaration of a major disaster or emergency under the Stafford Act. Initially issued in 1992, the FRP was updated in 1999, then again in 2002 to reflect changes due to the passage of the Homeland Security Act of that year.

- The National Oil and Hazardous Substances Pollution Contingency Plan (NCP) addresses the federal response to oil spills and hazardous substance releases (U.S. Environmental Protection Agency, 1994).

   The first NCP was introduced in 1968 in order for the United States to have a coordinated approach to oil spills in U.S. waters. The scope of the plan was later expanded to include spills and releases of hazardous substances or wastes.
- The Federal Radiological Emergency Response Plan (FRERP) addresses the federal response to peacetime radiological emergencies (FEMA, 1996b).
- The U.S. Government Interagency Domestic Terrorism Concept of Operations Plan (CONPLAN) coordinates crisis management (law enforcement investigation) and consequence management (life safety response) during a federal response to terrorism (FEMA, 2001).

Enacted by separate legislation, each of these plans has over time resulted in overlapping authorities and confusion of role by the assigned federal agencies. Therefore, a single comprehensive strategy was developed to unify domestic national response, thus becoming the National Response Plan (NRP) utilizing NIMS (Office of the President of the United States, 2003a; U.S. Department of Homeland Security, 2004a, 2004b). Enacted by the U.S. Congress, the NRP supercedes the previous federal response plans.

National Response Plan

In 2003, DHS introduced the Initial National Response Plan (INRP) as a general and conceptual document to address broad issues of consolidation and structure (U.S. Department of Homeland Security, 2003a, 2003b), followed by a draft NRP in May 2004. The NRP is designed to establish a "single, comprehensive approach required to enhance the ability of the United States to manage domestic incidents" (ibid., 2004b). The NRP describes the manner of coordination and the available federal resources that can be used to assist state and local government responses during terrorist attacks or other disasters. The primary goals of the NRP are as follows:

- to save lives and protect the health and safety of the public, responders, and recovery workers
- to protect and restore critical infrastructure
- to conduct law enforcement investigation to resolve the incident, apprehend the subjects, and collect and preserve evidence for prosecution
- to protect property and mitigate damages and impacts to individuals, communities, and the environment
- to facilitate the recovery of individuals, families, businesses, and governments

The NRP begins with an initial description of the role of the federal government and the DHS in an incident response. It addresses the issues of organization, leadership, and coordination of incident resources. This includes the designation of the secretary of the DHS as the "principal federal official" (PFO) charged with coordinating the overall federal response to a terrorist attack. A critical section of the NRP identifies 15 functional response components called "emergency support function" annexes (ESFs), which address specific categories of assistance that are common to all disasters (see Table 27.2). Each ESF is headed by a lead federal agency that is responsible for coordinating the delivery of goods, personnel, and services to the affected area and is supported by numerous other federal agencies. Public health, mental health, and medical issues are coordinated by the U.S. Department of Health and Human Services (DHHS). Depending upon the size and scope of the event, some or all of the ESFs may be activated during a response (U.S. Department of Homeland Security, 2004b; see Table 27.2).

Special incident annexes are adjunct management protocols to the NRP that account for unique aspects of specific hazards or their exposure pathways and include the following (DHS/NRP annexes, 2004):

- biological incident annex
- catastrophic incident annex
- cyber incident annex
- food security and agriculture incident annex
- oil and hazardous materials incident annex
- nuclear and radiological incident annex
- terrorism incident annex

Table 27.2. Essential support functions of the National Response Plan
(U.S. Department of Homeland Security, 2004b)

ESF Responsible Federal Department	Scope
ESF 1. Transportation Department of Transportation	Federal and civil transportation support Transportation safety Restoration/recovery of transportation infrastructure Movement restrictions
ESF 2. Telecommunications and Information Technology Department of Homeland Security	Coordination with telecommunication industry Restoration/repair of telecommunications network Cyber and information technology
ESF 3. Public Works and Engineering Department of Defense: U.S. Army Corps of Engineers	Infrastructure protection and emergency repair Infrastructure restoration Engineering services, construction management Critical infrastructure liaison Natural resources restoration
ESF 4. Fire Fighting U.S. Department of Agriculture: Forest Service	Fire-fighting activities on federal lands Resource support for rural and urban fire-fighting operations
ESF 5. Emergency Management Department of Homeland Security: FEMA	Information collection, analysis, and dissemination Reports, bulletins, advisories, and assessments Action planning and tracking Resource tracking Science and technology support (modeling, information provision, and interpretation)
ESF 6. Mass Care, Housing, and Human Services Department of HomelandSecurity: FEMA	Shelter Feeding Emergency first aid Disaster welfare information Bulk distribution of emergency relief items
ESF 7. Resource Support and Logistics Management General Services Administration	Resource support Logistics
ESF 8. Public Health and Medical Services Department of Health and Human Services	Public health Medical Behavioral health care services Assays, disease models
ESF 9. Urban Search and Rescue Department of Homeland Security: FEMA	Lifesaving assistance Urban search and rescue
ESF 10. Oil and Hazardous Materials Response Environmental Protection Agency	Hazardous materials (hazardous substances, oil, etc.) response Environmental safety; short- and long-term cleanup
ESF 11. Agriculture U.S. Department of Agriculture	Nutritional services Agricultural production Animal health
ESF 12. Energy Department of Energy	Energy system assessment Repair/restoration Energy industry utilities coordination Energy forecast
ESF 13. Public Safety and Security	Operational and personnel security Liaison between criminal investigation and response/recovery ops Inspector general activities
ESF 14. Economic Stabilization, Community Recovery, and Mitigation Department of Homeland Security: FEMA	Assess economic impacts and/or assist states and local governments and the private sector in addressing impacts Long-term community recovery Mitigation response and program implementation
ESF 15. Emergency Public Information and External Communications Annex Department of Homeland Security	Emergency public information and protective action guidance Media and community relations Congressional affairs International affairs Tribal and insular affairs

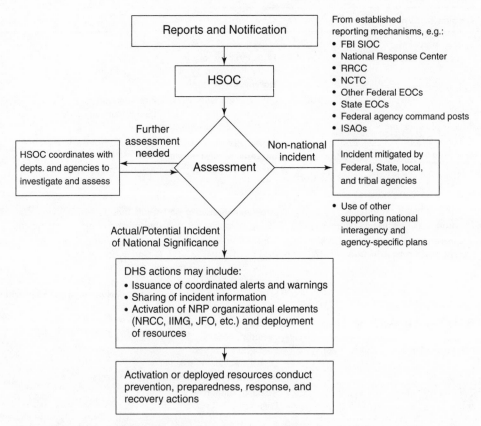

Figure 27.4. Flow of initial national-level incident management actions (U.S. Department of Homeland Security, 2004b, p.47, figure 10).

National Level Coordination

The secretary of the DHS is charged with coordinating and integrating federal assets with state, local, tribal, and nongovernmental efforts during a response (see Figure 27.4; DHS/NRP, 2004). The interagency incident management group (IIMG) coordinates and manages federal operational resources during incidents of national significance. The IIMG is composed of senior representatives from the DHS, other federal departments and agencies, and nongovernmental organizations and national experts as required, including appropriate subject matter expertise. The group serves as the focal point for federal strategic and operational coordination and decision making.

The Homeland Security Operations Center (HSOC) is the "primary national-level hub for operational communications, information, and resource coordination pertaining to domestic incident management" (DHS/NRP, 2004). The HSOC maintains daily situational awareness and shares

intelligence and operational information with federal, state, local, and tribal intelligence and law enforcement agencies as appropriate. It also monitors nonterrorist hazards and receives reports regarding natural hazards (e.g., severe storms, floods), oil spills, and other hazardous materials releases. When notified of an incident with possible national-level implications, the HSOC assesses the situation and briefs the secretary of the DHS, who determines the need for NRP activation (see Figure 27.4). The HSOC also houses the National Resource Coordination Center (NRCC), which coordinates and tracks federal resources.

The Stafford Act also authorizes the president to use the military to assist civilian authorities in responding to disasters (see Figure 27.3). The Department of Defense (DOD) supplies what the NRP refers to as defense support to civil authorities (DSCA), which offers support during domestic incidents, including terrorist attacks. DOD support is dependent upon the request not interfering with the department's military readiness or operations (ibid.). The military, through its various assets, routinely provides support to civilian disaster operations, including Hurricane Katrina in 2005; air patrols after 9/11, and supporting security activities for the 2002 Olympics and at Super Bowl games.

The Joint Field Office

The Joint Field Office (JFO) collocates all of the federal agencies that are essential to enhance coordination and communication in a temporary facility close to state and local emergency operations centers (see Figure 27.2; DHS/NRP, 2004). The organization of the JFO is scaled to match the magnitude of the incident and incorporates NIMS principles regarding the span of control and the functions of ICS (see Figure 27.1). The JFO coordination group is led by the principal federal official and consists of the federal coordinating officer; the senior federal law enforcement official; state, local, and tribal officials; and senior federal officials. This group "provides strategic guidance and resolution of any conflicts in priorities for allocation of critical Federal resources" (U.S. Department of Homeland Security, 2004b, p. 33).

The federal coordinating officer manages federal resource support activities related to disasters and emergencies as authorized by the Stafford Act, assists the unified command and/or the area command, and coordinates with state operations. The senior federal law enforcement official is a member of the agency with primary jurisdictional responsibility and is typically the "FBI special agent in charge" during a terrorist event. A public information function is coordinated through a joint information center (JIC), which acts as a central point for coordination and the issuing of public information. In a terrorist incident, there may be two operations sections: one focusing on law enforcement and criminal investigation and the other focusing on response and recovery operations.

Response Actions

Initial response activities are focused on rescue and the preservation of life, property, the environment, and the critical community infrastructure. Federal, state, and local governments will implement their agencies' response plan based on NIMS principles (see Figures 27.2, 27.3, and 27.4). Activity levels

at the HSOC will be elevated. National and regional coordination centers will activate the necessary ESFs to mobilize and deploy personnel and resources to support the incident manager (see Table 27.2). These centers also assess the need for and facilitate the deployment of medical and specialty teams composing the National Disaster Medical System. They also support teams that assist with incident management or the setting up of emergency facilities. Other response actions include the establishment of the JFO and other field facilities.

At the regional level, the required resources will depend upon the size and scope of the event. The regional resources coordination center (RRCC) will begin the local federal response coordination, while the JFO is established in the affected area. During a terrorist response, law enforcement activities occur concurrently with life safety operations and must be coordinated to ensure the primacy of these activities. Once the immediate response missions and lifesaving activities conclude, the emphasis shifts from response to recovery operations and hazard mitigation. The JFO planning section develops a demobilization plan for the release of appropriate components. Additionally, the JFO initiates a disaster recovery center to provide information about assistance and recovery programs to the victims. These efforts are coordinated with local jurisdictional authorities through state and local government emergency operations centers.

Federal Health and Medical Assets

There are numerous federal public health, mental health, and medical assets that can be deployed to the scene of a terrorist attack through the emergency support functions of the National Response Plan. Of these, ESF 8, 10, and 6 are the most closely associated with public health, mental health, and medical response (see Table 27.2).

ESF 8: Health and Medical Services

ESF 8, the most comprehensive of the ESFs, provides coordinated federal assistance to supplement state and local resources in response to public health and medical care needs following a terrorist attack or other disaster or emergency. These assets can also be activated and predeployed in anticipation of an emergency event. The U.S. Department of Health and Human Services coordinates this ESF, which provides support from numerous federal agencies including the Veterans Administration (VA), the Department of Defense, the Department of Transportation (DOT), and the Department of Homeland Security. Included in ESF 8 are the overall public health response; triage, treatment, and transportation of victims; and evacuation of patients out of the disaster area. The ESF 8 functions in the NRP include the following:

1. Public health and medical needs are assessed, and any impact to the public health care system and health care facility infrastructure is determined.
2. The general population and special high-risk groups are monitored for injury and disease patterns, as well as potential disease outbreaks.
3. Medical care personnel, including federal personnel and volunteers from unaffected areas, provide care for ill or injured victims on site.
4. Health and medical equipment and supplies may be requested from DHS and includes materiel from the Strategic National Stockpile, as well as other medical supplies.
5. Patient evacuation and movement of seriously ill and injured patients to other areas are arranged through ESF 1.
6. For situations requiring ongoing patient care, additional medical personnel can be brought in to support the existing medical infrastructure and provide definitive medical care to victims in the affected community.
7. The safety and security of human drugs, biologics (including blood and vaccines), medical devices (including radiation-emitting and screening devices), veterinary drugs, and other federally regulated products following a major disaster or emergency are addressed.
8. Food safety and security personnel assess the safety and security of federally regulated foods following a major disaster or emergency.
9. Agricultural safety and security refers to ensuring the safety and security of animal feed and therapeutics following a major disaster or emergency.
10. Worker health and safety refer to assistance in monitoring the health and well-being of emergency workers; they also entail addressing precautions to ensure the health and safety of other workers.

11. All-hazard public health and medical consultation, technical assistance, and support refer to assistance in assessing public health and medical effects of all hazards on both the general population and high-risk groups. This can include field investigations, collection and analysis of samples, and advice on medical treatments and protective actions with regard to health, medical, and sanitation issues.
12. Behavioral health care involves assessments of mental health and substance abuse treatment needs; the provision of disaster mental health training materials for disaster workers; and liaison with assessment, training, and program development activities undertaken by federal, state, and local mental health officials.
13. Public health and medical information refers to assistance provided to state and local communities for developing and issuing public health, disease, and injury prevention information that can be transmitted to members of the general public who are located in or near the affected area.
14. Vector control assistance is provided for threat assessment, as well as for the collection and analysis of samples and recommendations for protective actions and medical treatment.
15. Potable water and wastewater, solid waste disposal, and other environmental health issues include field investigations, sample collection, and analysis. This includes the provision of supplies and technical assistance.
16. Victim identification and mortuary services come from DHS and DOD and include disaster mortuary teams (DMORTs) from the National Disaster Medical System (NDMS); temporary morgue facilities; victim identification by fingerprint, forensic dental, and/or forensic pathology methods; and the processing, preparation, and disposition of remains.
17. Protection of animal health by delivering health care to injured or abandoned animals and performing preventive veterinary medicine following a major disaster or emergency. This includes the examination and care of animals used for search-and-rescue efforts.
18. The blood and blood products function includes assessing the availability of blood products and the taking of emergency measures to augment or replenish existing supplies.

ESF 10: Hazardous Materials

This function is designed to provide federal support to state and local governments in response to an actual or potential discharge and/or release of hazardous materials following a major disaster or emergency. ESF 10 is closely connected to the National Contingency Plan. The health and medical issues in ESF 10 are statutorily addressed by the DHHS through its Agency for Toxic Substances and Disease Registry (ATSDR) and through the U.S. Environmental Protection Agency (EPA) with a specific focus on the following:

- providing assistance in the assessment of health hazards
- determining whether illnesses, diseases, or complaints may be attributable to exposure to a hazardous substance
- establishing disease and exposure registries and conducting appropriate tests
- developing, maintaining, and providing information on the health effects of toxic substances

ESF 6: Mass Care

This function is coordinated by the DHS, and the primary functional leadership is through the American Red Cross, a nongovernmental entity. ESF 6 is designed to coordinate federal assistance in support of state and local efforts to meet the mass care needs of disaster victims such as shelter, food, and emergency first aid. It also provides for the establishment of systems to distribute bulk emergency relief supplies. Moreover, it provides for the collection of information to operate a disaster welfare information (DWI) system for the purpose of reporting victims' status and assisting in family reunification. Recovery issues may be handled by the American Red Cross but under different congressional authorities. As recovery operations are introduced, close coordination is required between those federal agencies responsible for recovery operations and the voluntary organizations, including the American Red Cross, that are providing recovery assistance.

FEMA's National Disaster Medical System (NDMS) is a nationwide medical mutual aid network of both federal and nonfederal health care personnel who can be deployed from anywhere in the country to provide on-site medical care in an area affected by a terrorist attack or other disaster (National Disaster Medical System website, http://www.ndms.fema.gov/). Federal partners in the NDMS include the DHS, DHHS, DOD, and the VA; nonfederal sources include major pharmaceutical suppliers, hospital supply vendors, the National Foundation for Mortuary Care, international disaster response organizations, and international health organizations.

The NDMS was developed to assist state and local agencies, address medical and public health effects of major disasters, and provide support to the military medical system in caring for casualties resulting from overseas armed conflicts. The NDMS consists of specialty medical teams that deploy personnel, supplies, and equipment anywhere in the country. These teams typically arrive with enough personnel, supplies, equipment, and shelters to be self-supporting for up to 72 hours. The personnel are a mix of clinicians and support staff. These responders are employed in other jobs, both in the government and in other areas of health care. They have volunteered to be part of their teams and are paid by the federal government for their time when they are activated.

Of the more than 70 teams that have been formed, more than half are disaster medical assistance teams (DMATs) that provide primary care in the affected area. Additionally, the NDMS has specialty teams that can be deployed to handle the following:

- burns
- pediatrics
- trauma care
- mental health
- veterinary medical assistance
- disaster mortuary operations
- pharmaceutical distribution
- search-and-rescue operations

In addition to sending personnel to the affected area, another component of the NDMS is a system to evacuate patients from a disaster site to a voluntary network of government, public, and private hospitals. The NDMS is designed to be activated when states have been overwhelmed by a disaster and a request has been made for federal assistance, although its members can be predeployed in anticipation of an impending disaster or to support medical needs at a large event (e.g., the Olympics).

Mental Health Functions

The need to consider the mental health sequelae of major disasters was first institutionalized by FEMA many years ago. As that agency began to encounter disaster victims and to provide basic disaster recovery services, it became clear that many of these victims were under extreme stress. Their psychological reactions were so severe that they were unable even to properly complete the paperwork necessary to obtain relief. Their behavior was disorganized, and they were generally having difficulty with their own recovery and that of their family and other community members.

Although the vast majority of people who survive these extraordinary events sometimes experience very significant fear and distress, they do not necessarily develop a mental disorder that requires ongoing formal treatment by a licensed mental health professional. While there is some disagreement in this arena, there is little evidence that professional services significantly change the trajectory of their recovery. In most cases, trained and well-supervised nonprofessionals and paraprofessionals, as well as professionals from other disciplines (e.g., clergy, guidance counselors), can play significant roles.

As the field of disaster mental health and the sophistication of the federal disaster response have developed over the years, new roles, relationships, and programs have emerged. The primary locus of responsibility for responding to the mental health needs of disaster victims rests within ESF 8 of the FRP and NRP. The Substance Abuse and Mental Health Services Administration (SAMHSA) within the DHHS is the lead federal agency for the federal mental health response. Under ESF 8 the primary mental health missions are to "assist in assessing mental health needs; provide disaster mental health training materials for disaster workers; and provide liaison with assessment, training, and program development activities undertaken by Federal, State, and local mental health officials" (FEMA, 1999; Gerrity & Flynn, 1997).

Needs Assessment

SAMHSA has designed a methodology that is used to assess needs in impacted areas to inform the design of crisis counseling programs. Upon critical review of the needs assessment methodology,

modifications have been recommended and are likely to be implemented in future disaster response (Norris, Donohue, & Felton, et. al., in press). A wide variety of training and educational materials and tools have been developed by SAMHSA (http://www.samhsa.gov/Matrix/matrix_disaster.aspx), the SAMHSA Disaster Mental Health Technical Assistance Center (http://www.mentalhealth.samhsa.gov/dtac), the SAMHSA-funded National Child Traumatic Stress Network (http://www.nctsn.org), the National Institute of Mental Health (NIMH; http://www.nimh.nih.gov/healthinformation/index.cfm), the VA's National Center for PTSD (http://www.ncptsd.va.gov), and the Centers for Disease Control and Prevention (CDC; http://www.bt.cdc.gov/mentalhealth). In the future, more attention is needed to ensure the appropriate integration of psychosocial issues into the assessment of public health and medical needs as part of the overall response efforts among affected populations (Reissman, Spencer, Tanielian, & Stein, 2005).

Crisis Counseling and Support

The United States was certainly the first (and is perhaps the only) country to establish a federally authorized and funded program to meet the mental health needs of disaster victims (Gerrity & Flynn, 1997). First implemented in the mid-1970s, the Crisis Counseling Assistance and Training Program (CCP), which FEMA administers, is included in its enabling legislation (Stafford Act, 2000). A presidential disaster declaration is required for states to be eligible for activation of the crisis counseling provisions. The CCP provides short-term, informal crisis counseling services, general and targeted information and education outreach to individuals and communities, and referral for those who may need formal treatment for a mental disorder. A more complete description of this program can be found at http://www.mentalhealth.samhsa.gov/cmhs/EmergencyServices/progguide.asp.

Funding is provided through the states to local service providers. The program is based upon the belief that fear and distress are widespread after disasters, that relatively few people will develop a full-blown mental disorder from their exposure to disaster, and that those who do can be treated within the capacity of existing mental health resources. As a result, the program makes extensive use of trained nonprofessionals (who are supervised by mental health specialists) for many services and provides informal counseling for a relatively short time. The program also relies heavily on assertive outreach to the general public and special needs populations using psychoeducational approaches.

However, the program does *not* include formal, ongoing professional psychological or psychiatric (i.e., clinical) treatment. Those who need formal care for diagnosed disorders are referred to existing mental health services. However, the scope and scale of the terrorist attacks in September 2001 led to the provision of enhanced services through the crisis counseling mechanism. These were provided contingent upon assessments that were conducted using a 12-item "SPRINT-E" tool (Norris Donohue, & Felton et. al., in press). A manual has now been prepared to standardize the implementation of SPRINT-E to identify persons in need of further evaluation and treatment by assessing demographics, risk categories, and psychological reactions surrounding a disaster or terrorist action (VA/National Center for PTSD, White River Junction, VT).

Other Federal Disaster Mental Health Programs

While no program is as large and frequently activated to meet the needs of disaster victims and survivors as the Crisis Counseling Program, in recent years a few other federal programs have become available to help address mental health needs. The most significant ones are listed here:

- SAMHSA established a limited grant program to meet both mental health and substance abuse needs following events that do not activate eligibility for the Crisis Counseling Program (e.g., an event that results in significant psychosocial distress yet does not receive a presidential disaster declaration). As an example, this program was used to fund services for survivors, families of deceased victims, and other impacted community members following the nightclub fire in Warwick, Rhode Island, in February 2003. Additional information is available at http://www.samhsa.gov/Matrix/matrix_disaster.aspx.
- Manualized "psychological first aid" for children and adults, funded by SAMHSA (National Center for Child Traumatic Stress and National Center for PTSD, 2005). Additional information can be obtained at http://www.ncptsd.va.gov/pfa/PFA.html and http://www.nctsn.org.
- The Office for Victims of Crime (OVC) in the Justice Department supports services (including mental health services) for victims of crimes. While these programs are not activated in natural disasters, they have been a critical part of the service array following acts of terrorism.
- Project School Emergency Response to Violence (SERV) within the Safe and Drug-free Schools Program in the Department of Education provides support for services (including mental health) to local education agencies following acts of violence in schools. Project SERV provides assistance to help children recover from a violent or traumatic event in which the learning environment has been disrupted. Immediate assistance lasts for up to 60 days from the date of the incident. Extended services last for up to a year from the incident. Additional information is available at http://www.ed.gov/programs/dvppserv/index.html.
- Disaster research, education, mentoring, and training grants in disaster mental health are sponsored by the National Institute of Mental Health (NIMH). Additional information is available at http://www.redmh.org.

Promoting Behavioral Health Preparedness

The federal role in the delivery of mental health services in large-scale emergency situations is complex. As this chapter documents, the federal response environment is increasingly formal and ever changing. Integration of effort and resources is essential but complicated given the size, compartmentalization, territoriality, and diverse funding streams inherent in the federal structure. In addition, significant planning and preparation are needed to effectively coordinate the multiple disciplines that may be involved in offering disaster mental health services at the local and state level (Compton, Gard, Kaslow, Kotwicki, & Reissman, et al., 2005).

Among the most important roles in integrating medical, public health, and mental health in disaster and emergency response are the following:

- Direct service delivery (e.g., through general and specialized NDMS teams) that facilitates the integration of effort
- Consultation to leadership in the preparedness and response phases to ensure that mental health issues are appropriately recognized and integrated
- Training that cuts across specialty and disciplinary lines
- An integrated federal approach that facilitates the development of a comprehensive strategy and integrates state and local preparedness and response efforts

One of the most overlooked, yet critical, opportunities for mental health providers is the provision of technical assistance, consultation, and training (Reissman, 2004; Reissman, Spencer, Tanielian & Stein, 2005; Ursano, Norwood, & Fullerton, 2004). When one thinks of the roles mental health professionals can play, too often the direct service intervention role is what comes to mind. However, major contributions can be made in other areas as well. In addition to the resources already identified in this section, several publications may be especially helpful to those wishing to focus more on the theory, challenges, opportunities, and status of the field of disaster mental health.

The first publication is *Mental Health and Mass Violence* (National Institute of Mental Health, 2002), which is the result of a consensus workshop held in the fall of 2001 that brought together 58 disaster mental health experts from six countries to attempt to reach consensus on what works and what does not and to identify the knowledge gaps. Aside from reflecting a very intensive and credible process, one of the primary contributions of the document is its articulation of the important roles mental health can play in addition to those roles most commonly known.

The second is *Preparing for the Psychological Consequences of Terrorism: A Public Health Strategy* (Butler, Panzer, & Goldfrank, 2003), which was developed by the Institute of Medicine (IOM) with the involvement of experts. This publication is especially helpful in both describing the reasons mental health should be fully integrated into health care and public health systems and outlining a public health model for disaster mental health.

The consensus workshop suggested that technical assistance can be provided to help improve the capacity of organizations and caregivers to offer what is needed to reestablish community structures, foster family recovery and resilience, and safeguard the community (NIMH, 2002). It also proposed giving assistance, consultation, and training to relevant organizations, caregivers, responders, and leaders. The training content might include the following topics:

- identification of normal psychological responses
- suggestions on when to refer someone to a mental health professional
- stress identification and management
- communication in a crisis
- needs of special populations
- changes in psychological issues over time
- integration of systems of care
- management of survivors in the workplace

Basic to the establishment of psychological health is the perception that one is safe and secure. By definition, when one experiences extraordinary events such as natural disasters or acts of terrorism, these feelings of safety and security are compromised (Ursano, Norwood, & Fullerton, 2004). In the case of terrorism, this erosion of the perception of safety and security is the very intent, and they create a loss of confidence in the collective well-being. It is important and legitimate work for mental health providers to ensure the provision of and monitor the perception of these needs. In doing so, the NIMH (2002) publication suggests the following priorities:

- Ensure food and shelter. While this may seem obvious, survivors must have housing and nutritional support as soon as possible. Proper rest and sustenance are essential to maintaining health psychological function.
- Provide orientation. In large-scale and/or ongoing events, obtaining a comprehensive picture of what is occurring and how people are impacted is difficult. Mental health providers should help fill in the gaps for victims and survivors so that their understanding of the event is based, as much as possible, on

credible information rather than impression and rumor.

- Facilitate communication with family members, friends, and the community. Reliable communication with and about family and friends is an important part of stress reduction in extraordinary events. It is also typically difficult to obtain, especially in the early hours and days. One of the first and most stressful questions for disaster survivors is, "are my loved ones dead, alive, injured, or safe?" Helping to answer those questions and ensuring ongoing communication is an important role in enhancing psychological health.
- Assess the environment for ongoing threats or toxins. Often when events appear to be over, they are not. If mental health providers are able to have regular and accurate information about ongoing situations, they can help ensure that this information is communicated and received by survivors in a way that helps reduce stress and leads to compliance with desired behavior.

Disaster mental health issues extend beyond the treatment needs of those with preexisting or newly emerging (because of current exposures) psychiatric illness and management of those concerned about their health. Contrary to stereotype, it is not dealing with "how people feel" about what they have experienced. In the early stages, although feelings are important to the extent that they influence behavior, they are not the primary focus of mental health's role and efforts. Our primary concern is influencing individual and collective behavior in ways that enhance compliance with direction from credible health and safety authorities (Reissman, Spencer, Tanielian, & Stein, 2005).

In addition, we want to decrease the potential for people to act in ways that are detrimental to their own health and safety and/or that adversely affect the function of public safety, medical, and public health authorities. Serious health consequences can result from actions taken by individuals and groups in reaction to disasters and terrorism, many of which completely disregard the advice and instruction of health and safety authorities. Some of the issues that have a dramatic impact on community-based strategies to contain and control health and medical emergencies (e.g.,

outbreaks of disease, hazardous exposures) are addressed by the following questions:

- Do we want people to seek immediate medical care or wait to be evaluated?
- Do we want people who are at high risk of exposure to biological pathogens to obtain medications or vaccinations to prevent illness through an emergency mass distribution and delivery system?
- Do we want people to take shelter in the affected area or to evacuate?
- Are their particular instructions appropriate to subgroups in the population such as children, those whose systems are immunosuppressed, and elderly people?

Our sense of safety and security involves processing information by means of a complex set of beliefs and perceptions. Is the event over? Am I out of harm's way? Am I confident in the ability of the government and other leaders to eliminate or reduce the threat and keep me safe? Everly and Flynn (2005) have offered a solid framework for the principles and practice of psychological first aid as one aspect of a psychological continuum of care. Further exploration of individual and community psychological resilience in the face of disasters and terrorist acts may be extremely useful for the design and evaluation of effective public health programming and services (Reissman, Klomp, Kent, & Pfefferbaum, 2004). Mental health providers can play important roles in assessing the environment, communicating that status, and helping individuals and groups to understand, believe, and be reassured by what they see and hear.

References

Butler, A. S., Panzer, A. M., & Goldfrank, L. R. (Eds.). (2003) *Preparing for the psychological consequences of terrorism: A public health strategy.* Washington, DC: Institute of Medicine, National Academies Press. Retrieved March 13, 2006, from http://www.iom.edu/CMS/3775/3895/11573.aspx.

City of Des Moines Emergency Management Agency. (2004). Duties and responsibilities. City of Des Moines, Iowa. Retrieved February 2, 2006, from http://www.co.des-moines.ia.us/EMA/EMAHome.asp#Duties.

Compton, M. T., Gard, B., Kaslow, N. J., Kotwicki, R. J., Reissman, D. B., Schor, L., & Wetterhall, S. (2005,

July–August). Incorporating mental health into bioterrorism response planning. *Public Health Reports, 120*(Suppl. 1), 16–19.

Emergency Management Institute. (2005). Introduction to Incident Command System, IS-100. Self-study course. Emmitsburg, MD: Federal Emergency Management Agency, U.S. Department of Homeland Security. Retrieved March 9, 2006, from http://www.training.fema.gov/EMIWeb/IS/is100.asp.

Everly, G. S., Jr., & Flynn, B. W. (2005). Ch 6: Principles and practice of psychological first aid. In G. S. Everly Jr. & C. I. Parker (Eds.), *Mental health and mass disasters: Public health preparedness and response* (pp. 105–112.). Baltimore: Johns Hopkins Center for Public Health Preparedness.

Federal Emergency Management Agency. (1996a). *Guide for all-hazard emergency operations planning.* Emmitsburg, MD: Author.

———. (1996b, May). Federal Radiological Emergency Response Plan (FRERP). Retrieved February 2, 2006, from http://www.fas.org/nuke/guide/usa/doctrine/national/frerp.htm

———. (1999, April). Federal Response Plan. Retrieved March 13, 2006, from http://www.disasters.org/emgold/frp.htm.

———. (2001, January). U.S. Government Interagency Domestic Terrorism Concept of Operations Plan (CONPLAN). Retrieved February 2, 2006, from http://www.fema.gov/pdf/rrr/conplan/cplncvr.pdf.

Gerrity, E. T., & Flynn, B. W. (1997). Mental health consequences of disaster. In E. K. Noji (Ed.), *The public health consequences of disasters* (pp. 101–121). New York: Oxford University Press.

Haddow, G. D., & Bullock, J. A. (2003). *Introduction to emergency management.* Burlington, MA: Elsevier Science.

National Center for Child Traumatic Stress and National Center for PTSD. (2005, September). *Psychological first aid: Field operations guide.* Retrieved February 2, 2006, from http://www.ncptsd.va.gov/pfa/PFA_9_6_05_Final.pdf.

National Disaster Medical System. (n.d.). The National Disaster Medical System. Retrieved February 2, 2006, from http://ndms.dhhs.gov/.

National Institute of Mental Health. (2002). Mental health and mass violence: Evidence-based early psychological intervention for victims/survivors of mass violence. A workshop to reach consensus on best practices. NIH Publication no. 02–5138. Washington, DC: U.S. Government Printing Office. Retrieved February 2, 2006, from http://www.nimh.nih.gov/publicat/massviolence.pdf.

National Response Team. (2000). Incident command system/Unified command technical assistance

document. Washington, DC: U.S. Environmental Protection Agency. National Response Team Consortium. Retrieved March 9, 2006, from http://www.nrt.org/Production/NRT/NRTWeb.nsf/AllAttachmentsByTitle/SA-52ICSUCTA/$File/ICSUCTA.pdf?OpenElement.

Norris F., Donahue S. A., Felton C. J., Watson P. J., Hamblen J. L., & Marshall R. D. (in press). Making and monitoring referrals to clinical treatment: A psychometric analysis of Project Liberty's Adult Enhanced Services Referral Tool. White River Junction, VT: National Center for Posttraumatic Stress Disorder, U.S. Department of Veterans Affairs and Dartmouth University.

Office of the President of the United States. (2003a). Homeland Security Presidential Directive/HSPD-5, Subject: Management of domestic incidents. Washington, DC. Retrieved July 12, 2004, from http://www.whitehouse.gov/news/releases/2003/02/print/20030228-9.html.

———. (2003b). Homeland Security Presidential Directive/HSPD-8, Subject: National preparedness. Washington, DC. Retrieved July 12, 2004, from http://www.whitehouse.gov/news/releases/2003/12/print/20031217-6.html.

Reissman, D. B. (2004). New roles for mental and behavioral health experts to enhance emergency preparedness and response readiness. *Psychiatry, 67*(2), 118–122.

———, Klomp, R. K., Kent, A. T., and Pfefferbaum, B. (2004). Exploring psychological resilience in the face of terrorism. *Psychiatric Annals, 34*(8), 626–632.

Reissman, D. B., Spencer, S., Tanielian, T., & Stein, B. D. (2005). Integrating behavioral aspects into community preparedness and response systems. Co-published simultaneously in *Journal of Aggression, Maltreatment, and Trauma, 10*(3/4), 707–720, and in Y. Danieli, D. Brom, & J. Sills. (Eds.), *The trauma of terrorism: Sharing knowledge and shared care, an international handbook.* New York: Haworth Maltreatment and Trauma Press.

Robert T. Stafford Disaster Relief and Emergency Assistance Act, 42 U.S.C. 68. (2000, October 30). (As amended by Pub. L. 103–181, Pub. L. 103–337, and Pub. L. 106–390, October 30, 2000, 114 Stat. 1552–1575). Retrieved February 2, 2006, from http://www.fema.gov/library/stafact.shtm.

Substance Abuse and Mental Health Services Administration (SAMHSA). (2003). Mental health all-hazards disaster planning guidance. DHHS Publication no. SMA 3829. Washington, DC: U.S. Government Printing Office.

————. Emergency mental health and traumatic stress crisis counseling training and assistance program guidance. Retrieved February 2, 2006, from http://www.mentalhealth.samhsa.gov/cmhs/Emergency Services/progguide.asp.

Ursano, R., Norwood, A., & Fullerton, C. (Eds.) (2004). *Bioterrorism: Psychological and public health interventions.* New York: Cambridge University Press.

U.S. Department of Homeland Security. (2003a, September 30). The initial national response plan (INRP). Retrieved February 2, 2006, from http://www.dhs.gov/interweb/assetlibrary/Initial_NRP_100903.pdf.

————. (2003b, October 10). Homeland Security Secretary Ridge approves initial national response plan. Press release. Retrieved February 2, 2006, from http://www.dhs.gov/dhspublic/display?content=1935.

————. (2004a, March 1). The National Incident Management System (NIMS). Retrieved February 2, 2006, from http://www.dhs.gov/interweb/assetlibrary/NIMS-90-web.pdf.

————. (2004b, December). National Response Plan (NRP). Retrieved February 2, 2006, from http://www.dhs.gov/interweb/assetlibrary/NRP_FullText.pdf.

U.S. Environmental Protection Agency. (1994). The national oil and hazardous substances pollution contingency plan. Retrieved February 2, 2006, from http://www.epa.gov/oilspill/ncpover.htm.

28

Reflections on the Psychology of Terrorism

Laura Pratchett
Lisa M. Brown
Bruce Bongar

One ought never to turn one's back on a threatened danger and try to run away from it. If you do that, you will double the danger. But if you meet it promptly and without flinching, you will reduce the danger by half. Never run away from anything. Never!

Ralph Waldo Emerson, 1803–1882

Terrorism is about one thing: Psychology. It is the psychology of fear.

Philip G. Zimbardo, 2004

The chapters in this book attest to the emergence of the psychology of terrorism as a comprehensive discipline with an interdisciplinary perspective. Although this is a relatively new discipline, it is a quickly evolving field that strives to apply psychological theory and concepts to foster scientific advancement. Ideally, scientific research progresses at a steady pace, building on new methodologies, technologies, and theoretical insights and benefiting from multiple perspectives and converging evidence. However, since the events of September 11, 2001, U.S. government agencies, policy makers, and academic research centers have been seeking empirical evidence to identify service priorities, guide decisions regarding resource allocation, and develop, administer, and evaluate antiterrorism programs with new urgency. To encompass the entire realm of psychological factors associated with terrorist acts, the field of terrorism psychology now contends with problems of a historic nature and others that come from growing pains.

Although other professions can provide research expertise, psychologists offer the best explanations of and theoretical insights into behaviors that can be translated into testable propositions and useful predictions. Psychological theories should be used to guide the development and refinement of models of human behavior that promote our knowledge of generalizable principles of human behavior across a wide array of settings and situations. For example, to derive the psychological underpinnings of terrorist acts, an understanding of how political and belief systems have evolved over time, and the consequences of these changes, is imperative. This insight provides clues that can be used to prevent the recurrence of some types of terrorism and offers cautionary signs about the potential for new forms of terrorist activity. A historical and psychological analysis of change helps us begin to comprehend the problems we encounter today. An integrated, multidisciplinary approach benefits stakeholders because it provides a faster understanding of emerging trends and provides an interface between academic research and applied settings. The goal of this book is to provide a comprehensive overview of systems, responders, and personal reactions to terrorism and to demonstrate the collaborative role that psychology plays across various settings and situations.

Bongar (Chapter 1) discusses some of the tasks that psychologists face with respect to contemporary terrorism. These roles include defining and studying anticipated psychological reactions to mass trauma that might occur in the population following a terrorist attack; preparing society for acts of terror by sharing an understanding of collective responses such as panic and mass psychogenic illness; studying and disseminating information about the motivations, dynamics, and strategies of terrorists; and assessing and treating those who are exposed to terrorist attacks.

Taylor (Chapter 24) describes the way in which political and moral questions interfere with conducting research in this area, particularly field research. He argues that terrorism can be categorized as a type of disaster, allowing for a conceptualization of casualties, reaction phases, and cross-cultural issues. He states that individuals, groups, and nations have different needs and priorities at any of four phases—preparedness, response, recovery, and mitigation. He cogently argues that further attention needs to be paid to the subject of terrorism to adequately address the needs of various affected populations.

The Psychology of the Terrorist

Terrorism as a decision and an action are also evaluated and discussed in a number of chapters. McCauley (Chapter 2) discusses three theories commonly postulated to account for an individual's motivation to conduct acts of terrorism. He dismisses the notion of individual psychopathology of terrorists based on the lack of supporting literature and points out that the idea of terrorists as psychopaths is contradicted by the lack of impulsivity and the existence of cooperation with others and a willingness to die for a cause. He argues that the letters found in the luggage of the September 11, 2001, attackers provides evidence that undermines the theory that terrorism is an emotional response of anger to perceived group or individual frustrations. Rather, he contends that the motivations of terrorists in undertaking their actions are often reflective of those normal responses exhibited by combat veterans—attachment to each other and to a "greater cause"—and draws parallels between the training of armed forces and the path an individual may take on the route to employing terrorist violence. McCauley asserts that the dual strategies of terrorism are to recruit sympathy from the constituent population and to undermine civilian confidence in the enemy authority.

A second theory is offered by Moghaddam (Chapter 5). He conceptualizes the trajectory of

civilian to terrorist as a developmental process in which the person proceeds through a number of stages that offer progressively fewer solutions. In the first stage, the individual perceives a lack of fairness or relative deprivation of society toward the group with which the person identifies. For those who have a tendency to displace their frustration as anger directed at others, a lack of procedural means or personal ability to address an injustice can create a sense of moral justification in the means used to advance their cause. Moghaddam highlights the social influence of the group members who are becoming increasingly disaffiliated with and disengaged from mainstream society through isolation, their new attachment, and fear. They then develop a dichotomous moral position that is unintentionally reinforced by authorities who espouse the same rhetoric but from an opposing perspective. The final, intensive step in the developmental process is the removal of personal reservations to undertaking acts of terror.

In Chapter 8, Merari emphasizes the importance of social dynamics and group processes in promoting suicide terrorism. He discusses and rejects theories that propose religion as a prerequisite for suicide terrorism and for poverty, revenge, or suicide-related pathologies as etiologies for suicide terrorism. Merari describes the demographic variables associated with suicide terrorism, such as age, gender, and marital status, but cautions that these factors may be a function of the terrorist groups' policies rather than a trait profile of an individual who is most likely to commit an act of suicide terrorism. Echoing the messages of earlier chapters, Merari emphasizes the role of social influence both in motivating people to join terrorist organizations and in the indoctrination process leading to a commitment to perpetrate an act of suicide terrorism.

The Strategy of Terrorism

The importance of fear as a weapon utilized in the tactics of terrorism is discussed in a number of chapters. Breckenridge and Zimbardo (Chapter 9) illustrate the way that fear is used when a group has insufficient material power to wage a conventional war. This tactical disadvantage is overcome by their ability to evoke a disproportionate level of fear in the enemy community. This in turn serves to weaken the authority of the enemy leaders by undermining the public's confidence in their ability to ensure people's safety. The mechanisms by which this fear operates—availability heuristics, affect heuristics, bias for negatively valenced information and social amplification—are discussed in detail.

Embry (Chapter 12) explains how the principles of classical conditioning were used to great effect on September 11, 2001, to create an association between fear and anxiety and the symbols of everyday life in the United States. The chapter maintains that targeting strong iconic symbols, such as the Twin Towers, whose name echoes their visual appearance, and the use of airlines that are verbally associated with the country's name increased the impact of the connection. The association of fear was magnified by the timing of the events and the subsequent media coverage, which was inevitable. The impact of this fear is designed to undermine government authorities, reduce productive capacity, increase healthcare costs, and diminish society's capacity to accurately detect future threats.

Terrorism is interpreted within the paradigm of a social influence campaign in Chapter 7. Gerwehr and Hubbard argue that even the most heinous of terrorist acts have little military value and are actually messages communicated through acts of violence to multiple target audiences. These message are intended to manipulate the emotions, motives, reasoning, perceptions, and ultimately the behavior of the audience. They posit that the success or failure of a terrorist campaign depends on the ability to achieve each of the six stages outlined in the Yale model of social influence: exposure, attention, comprehension, acceptance, retention, and translation.

The main vehicle for disseminating the message of contemporary terrorism is the media, and in Chapter 6, Shurkin deals with the conflicting roles the media faces—both as an instrument for the delivery of the terrorists' message and as a channel to be utilized in combating terrorism. Shurkin discusses the challenge that the media face in balancing these roles and its influence on public response. Using the example of the nuclear incident at Three Mile Island in 1979, he illustrates the difficulties inherent in reporting evolving, novel incidents that threaten public safety and notes that the authorities

need to be honest and provide timely information that in turn is disseminated by the media in an accurate and nonsensational fashion.

Institutional Responses to Terrorism

In Chapter 4 McCauley compares the implications of two opposing frames of reference used by authorities in response to acts of terrorism: that of a criminal justice response, such as the response that occurred after the World Trade Center bombing of 1993, versus that of a war against terrorism. He contends that framing makes a difference in determining whether people are more likely to endorse a risk-averse response (such as one involving the criminal justice system) or a more risk-taking response (such as war). He compares the strengths and weakness of these two approaches and concludes that, despite the positive aspects of resorting to a war on terrorism, (i.e., increased patriotism, resource allocation, public perception of action), war is not the best solution for fighting a chronic problem involving an enemy that is difficult to find and identify.

Banks and James (Chapter 16) describe the role that psychology plays in warfare and terrorism. They discuss and define the issues of military threat, psychological threat, terrorism, and psychological resilience and highlight the relationships among these concepts. Using examples from history, they argue that war is usually an action designed to impose the will of one group on another as opposed to the direct annihilation of the group. In this context, the group that attains psychological control over its opponent is the victor. Terrorism can be viewed within the same framework. Because most terrorists do not have the resources to conduct a full-scale war, the psychological threat they pose to society must be large in order to compensate for the small likelihood of direct military action.

McDermott and Zimbardo (Chapter 23) critique and voice concern about the terror alarm system used by the authorities to communicate the level of threat to the public. They argue that a successful alarm system should be moderately arousing, incorporate reliable evidence, and be communicated by a single credible source that provides specific information about the level of threat and recommendations for action. In situations of an ongoing threat, misinformation should be corrected, recommendations modified, citizens' responses to alarms reinforced, and efforts for continuing collaborative to ensure security reiterated.

Individual Responses to Terrorism

As terrorism psychology moves beyond its initial dependence on research conducted with victims of natural disasters, it has become increasingly clear that it is important to determine how individuals will respond psychologically to acts of terrorism. Beutler and colleagues (Chapter 3) maintain that natural disasters differ from terrorism in key ways that can impact psychological sequelae because of causal attributions, heuristics, and risk assessments used by individuals. While the majority of people are unlikely to develop symptoms that reach pathological levels, some may go on to develop trauma-spectrum disorders such as acute stress disorder, posttraumatic stress disorder (PTSD), major depressive disorder, or substance abuse disorders. The authors propose a model for understanding the development of psychopathologies in terms of three stages of individual risk assessment. They also discuss intervention approaches such as psychological first aid and critical incident stress debriefing (CISD). In the absence of more empirically supported treatments, guidelines are given for recommended interventions and those that are to be avoided immediately following a mass-trauma incident.

In Chapter 19, Yehuda and colleagues describe the existing knowledge and some of the unique problems associated with differentiating normal, adaptive responses to terrorist attacks from serious psychopathology. They discuss the literature on the neurobiological, affective, and behavioral symptoms suggestive of PTSD and describe pre- and peritraumatic risk factors identified in the literature.

Sullivan and Bongar (Chapter 11) describe how the general public is likely to experience the psychological impact of an actual or threatened use of chemical, biological, radiological, nuclear, or high-yield explosion weapons by terrorists. The psychological consequences of such an attack are likely to be magnified not only because of the novelty of these weapons but also because of the

difficulty of determining immediately whether an exposure has occurred due to the lack of instantaneous physical trauma or symptoms. In addition to the expected psychopathologies in response to all terrorist attacks, widespread mass psychogenic illness is likely. The authors discuss the risk factors and impacts of occurrence. They also provide examples from recent history and guidelines for preventing and managing such responses.

Brandon and Silke (Chapter 13) discuss the three possible positive outcomes of a terrorist attack: survival, recovery, and resilience. They define the processes of dissipation, adaptation, habituation, and sensitization within the context of people's responses to the threat of and exposure to terrorism. They argue that resilience due to adaptation and habituation is the most likely outcome for the majority of individuals and suggest that the likelihood of this outcome will be increased by preparing society to expect future terrorist attacks and focusing on society's strengths and capacity for recovery.

Chapter 25 defines and describes four possible responses to an act of terrorism: the individual succumbs, survives with impairment, exhibits resilience, or thrives. Butler, Morland, and Leskin discuss a recent shift in the literature to examine the concept of resilience—by far the most common outcome associated with mass trauma. The chapter discusses the factors that contribute to resilience, including individual characteristics, event characteristics, peritraumatic responses, and the coping and social support resources that people make use of during and after an event.

An important mediating factor in the development of psychopathology or resilience following an act of terror may be the role that spirituality plays in the life of the exposed person. Kelly (Chapter 10) addresses the role of faith and involvement in a faith-based community in the aftermath of terrorism. Despite the irony that religion is often used as a justification for acts of violence, including terrorism, Kelly identifies three positive aspects to using religion in the process of coping—an openness to religious flexibility and growth rather than rigid, punitive religious beliefs; active engagement in spiritual reflection to find meaning in the event; and involvement with a faith-based community to receive social support.

Assessment and Treatment Issues

Given that some percentage of the population will develop psychopathology from exposure to an act of terrorism, several chapters in the book address issues that pertain to assessment and treatment. Ruzek, Maguen, and Litz (Chapter 18) emphasize the importance of identifying those who are at high risk for adverse psychological consequences so that intervention can occur before symptoms become chronic. A multistep protocol is recommended that includes treating with psychological first aid, following up with high-risk individuals, providing survivor education and training in coping skills, and using evidence-based treatment in an integrated plan involving group and individual therapy. Evidence-based treatments such as cognitive behavioral therapy are described, the challenges of providing such treatments in the aftermath of a terrorist attack are noted, and suggestions for improvement of existing interventions are made.

Brown et al. (Chapter 20) focus on the unique challenges faced by community-dwelling and institutionalized older adults after a terrorist attack. Using existing theoretical frameworks and models, they provide an overview of the risks and protective factors associated with age. While the literature suggests that older adults develop fewer psychological problems than younger adults, vulnerabilities that place older people at increased risk for adverse psychological consequences in the aftermath of a disaster are described. The chapter recommends steps that formal and informal caregivers can take to assist homebound, disabled, and institutionalized older people in preparing for, responding to, and recovering from disaster.

Chapter 21 describes a psychoeducational intervention that was designed to address issues faced by children and families who lost a father or husband in the attacks of September 11, 2001. Underwood, Kalafat, and Spinazzola describe the planning and implementation of the program, which focused on crisis intervention, community-based education, and personal empowerment to build resilience. A group modality was selected to make use of the supportive, sharing experience of the community and to emphasize the treatment of participants within their environment. The sessions were designed for different developmental levels and focused on resilience rather than pathology. Cognitive behavioral techniques were combined with fun activities that allowed the families to join together to commemorate their loss. The program's outcome measures indicated significant increases in hope in both children and adults.

Chapter 22 deals with issues to be considered in planning and implementing interventions with culturally diverse populations after a terrorist attack. Chiriboga discusses barriers to treatment, such as people's perception of ongoing discrimination with respect to mental health interventions provided to minority populations after a terrorist attack. The victims' culture, background, immigration status, and trauma history influence their recovery from a terrorist attack. The chapter describes guidelines produced by the U.S. Department of Health and Human Services' Office of Minority Health for providing culturally and linguistically appropriate services (CLAS). The author maintains that the guidelines may be relevant for clinicians to consider when planning for and responding to acts of terror.

First Responders to Acts of Terrorism

In Chapter 14, Clizbe and Hamilton illustrate the needs, responses, and challenges faced by government agencies and relief organizations in their efforts to collaborate in response to the attacks of September 11, 2001. The chapter highlights the preexisting relationships among some agencies and the ways in which these relationships mediated the efforts of both local and national-level organizations to work together in a cohesive fashion, despite the unique challenges the situation posed as a result of its novelty. The difficulties they faced in identifying and balancing the victims' needs with the organizations' resources is addressed, and the authors describe the utility of the Family Assistance Centers.

Pfeiffer (Chapter 15) describes the way in which organizational bias influenced communication between the police and fire departments responding to the events of September 11, 2001. Using theories of social group behaviors, he contends that positive in-group and negative out-group biases exist between the separate organizations and that these leanings contributed to the resulting diffusion of individual responsibility during this crisis situation. To help ensure that this scenario is not repeated, he makes recommendations for a unified operating procedure.

In the process of simply performing their duties, first responders cannot avoid exposure to terrorist attacks when they occur. In Chapter 17, Paton and Violanti discuss a risk management paradigm for first responders that encompasses both positive and negative outcomes. Since the specific characteristics of a situation are difficult to determine in advance, the authors describe a risk management system that focuses on both personal and organizational elements that mediate the effects of exposure to acts of terrorism and emphasize the importance of primary prevention.

Chapter 26 discusses the risk and protective factors that operate among those who are first responders to acts of terrorism. Gist explains how factors such as individual personalities, organizational structures, event characteristics, and the effect of the event on career and personal growth interact to determine the way a person will respond. He maintains that chronic exposure to stress can create a cognitive disequilibrium, which results in either psychological problems or growth. Until recently, CISD was routinely used following traumatic events. The chapter describes CISD and explains that this intervention has become controversial because some research has found that it may actually hinder the normal recovery process.

Reissman, Reissman, and Flynn (Chapter 27) also focus on recent changes in the area of first responders—organizational changes that occurred in response to the events of September 11, 2001. The chapter reviews the response situation involving the federal health infrastructure following natural disasters and terrorist acts. The authors explain the role of organizations such as the local emergency management agencies in planning and supporting first responders and the changes implemented by the Department of Homeland Security in standardizing a National Incident Management System to ensure better interagency interaction in dealing with future terrorist situations. Finally, the authors explain the system of employing all federal public health, mental health, and medical services through Emergency Support Functions 6, 8, and 10.

In each chapter of this book, the complex interaction between terrorism and psychology has been revealed to further the state of knowledge in this new and evolving discipline. Yet we must close on a cautionary note about the enormous need for sound scientific psychological data to drive our clinical and other applied endeavors in this specialty realm for psychology. It has certainly not escaped the reader's attention that the most crucial dilemma for intervention facing psychology, psychiatry, social work, public health, nursing, family therapy, and other core mental health disciplines is the critical lack of solid, replicable scientific evidence to guide our primary, secondary, and tertiary care along with scientifically grounded preventive activities. Common sense would dictate that good science be central in the development of this discipline. Thus, as the psychology of terror emerges as a crucial and vital field of study and application for psychological science and clinical care, scientists and clinicians must constantly be on guard to ensure that we recall Hippocrates' dictum, "Primum non nocere" (first do no harm), as well as Benjamin Franklin's observation that an "investment in knowledge always pays the best interest."

Appendix

Resources in Psychology of Terrorism

Matteo Bertoni
Brynne Johannsen

American Biological Safety Association (ABSA)
1202 Allanson Road
Mundelein, IL 60060
Telephone: 847–949–1517
Fax: 847–566–4580
Website: http://www.absa.org/index.shtml
Email: absa@absa.org
ABSA promotes continuing advancements in the field of biosafety and disseminates pertinent information to biosafety professionals in a timely manner. Biosafety courses are offered at the beginner and advanced levels, and an annual conference is held to apprise biosafety professionals of the most current information. A primary goal of the association is to reduce the potential effects of biologically derived materials and infectious agents.

American Psychological Association (APA), Public Policy Office
750 First Street NE
Washington, DC 20002–4242
Telephone: 202–336–6062
Fax: 202–336–6063
Website: http://www.apa.org/ppo/issues/terrorhome.html
Email: ppo@apa.org
The Public Policy Office of the APA, the largest U.S. association of psychologists, has at its website a section

specifically dedicated to combating terrorism. It provides news, reports advocacy activities on counter-terrorism, and gives visitors an opportunity to sign letters directed to important political figures who deal with terrorism-related issues.

American Radio Relay League (ARRL)
225 Main Street
Newington, CT 06111–1494
Telephone: 860–594–0200
Fax: 860–594–0529
Website: http://www.arrl.org/
Email: hq@arrl.org
The ARRL is an organization composed of amateur radio operators who provide critical communications in the event of a disaster or other emergency. Amateur radio personnel are trained to be proficient in emergency communication skills.

American Red Cross (ARC)
National Headquarters
2025 E Street NW
Washington, DC 20006
Telephone: 202–303–4498
Disaster assistance information: 866–438–4636
Website: http://www.redcross.org/services/disaster/
ARC is the major organization in charge of providing disaster relief by focusing on meeting people's immediate needs. Its website has a Homeland Security

Advisory System that provides information about the current status of the U.S. government's terrorist alert level and the implications these have for individuals, families, neighborhoods, schools, and businesses. The ARC Homeland Security Advisory System also provides publications on topics such as emergency preparedness and disaster planning.

American Safety and Health Institute (ASHI)
4148 Louis Avenue
Holiday, FL 34691
Telephone: 800–682–5067
Website: http://www.ashinstitute.org/
Email: info@ashintitute.org
ASHI is a nonprofit organization of professional educators who provide safety and health training, such as first responder and disaster preparedness training. Instruction centers include hospitals, fire departments, colleges, and schools. Current personnel who are trained through ASHI include the U.S. Border Patrol, U.S. Coast Guard, U.S. Customs Service, and federal air marshals.

Association of Traumatic Stress Specialists (ATSS)
Jo Halligan
Telephone: 512–868–3677
Fax: 512–868–3678
Website: www.atss-hq.com
Email: johalligan@atss-hq.com
ATSS is a nonprofit organization that offers professional certification and training to those who provide treatment to people suffering from traumatic stress. Training is tailored to victims of crime, natural disasters, terrorist attacks, injuries and deaths sustained in the line of duty, school and workplace violence, and political persecution; veterans; refugees; holocaust survivors; and others who have experienced traumatic stress injuries.

Citizen Corps
Website: http://www.citizencorps.gov/
Email: citizencorps@dhs.gov
Citizen Corps is a government organization associated with the USA Freedom Corps, founded by President Bush after the events of September 11 and coordinated through the Department of Homeland Security. Local, state, and tribal citizen councils make up the organization. Citizen Corps helps coordinate citizen volunteer activities to assist in homeland security issues. Citizens may volunteer to assist in activities related to crime, disaster, and terrorism prevention. Publications provide information on citizen preparedness. The main website allows one to search for local councils. Currently there are 55 state/territory Citizen Corps Coun-

cils and 1,599 county/local/tribal Citizen Corps Councils that serve 188,767,873 people, or 66% of the total U.S. population.

Civil Air Patrol
National Headquarters
105 South Hansell Street, Building 714
Maxwell AFB, AL 36112–6332
Website: http://www.cap.gov/
The Civil Air Patrol is a congressionally chartered nonprofit organization composed of civilian air patrol personnel and formed as an auxiliary to the U.S. Air Force. Services performed by the Civil Air Patrol are available to any branch in any agency of the federal government. Aerospace education, cadet training, and emergency response services are provided in order to prepare civilian volunteers to lend assistance in case of local or national emergencies. Volunteers may assist with coastal patrol, air/ground observation, search and rescue, radio communications and relay, aerial reconnaissance for homeland security, air-to-ground photography, radiological monitoring, disaster relief, and damage assessment.

Community Emergency Response Team (CERT)
U.S. Fire Administration
16825 S. Seton Ave.
Emmetsburg, MD 21727
Telephone: 301–447–1000
Website: http://training.fema.gov/emiweb/CERT/index.asp
CERT is a component of the U.S. Department of Homeland Security (DHS) and the Federal Emergency Management Agency (FEMA). CERT is composed of people who have completed its train-the-trainer course through its state training office for emergency management or FEMA's Emergency Management Institute (EMI). Team members provide support to first responders and immediate assistance to victims, organize volunteers at disaster sites, and participate in the improvement of community safety. Training includes disaster preparedness, disaster fire suppression, basic disaster medical operations, and light search-and-rescue operations.

Conflict 21 and Center for Terrorism Studies
ANG Conflict 21
Building 1451
Maxwell AFB, AL 36112
Website: http://c21.maxwell.af.mil/cts-home.htm
Part of the National Guard, the center identifies and develops innovative ideas for research and matches them up with issues and problems of the ANG, USAF, and the Department of Defense. Teaching, collaboration, and coordination through the maximum use

of technology are particularly emphasized. The website has a section dedicated to the psychology of terrorism, as well as links to reports and related articles.

Corporation for National and Community Service (CNCS)

1201 New York Avenue NW
Washington, DC 20525
Telephone: 202–606–5000
TTY: 202–565–2799
Website: http://www.nationalservice.org/
Email: webmaster@cns.gov

CNCS is part of the U.S. Freedom Corps, a presidential initiative designed to foster a sense of responsibility in its members and a commitment to service to U.S. citizens. CNCS coordinates programs such as Senior Corps, AmeriCorps, and Learn and Serve America. Volunteer members participate in programs on education, the environment, public safety, and homeland security.

Dart Center for Journalism and Trauma

Department of Communication
102 Communications Building
Box 353740
University of Washington
Seattle, WA 98195–3740
Telephone: 800–332–0565
Email: info@dartcenter.org
Website: http://www.dartcenter.org/

The Dart Center is a global network of journalists, educators, and health professionals dedicated to improving media coverage of trauma, conflict, and tragedy. The center also addresses the psychological impact and consequences of such coverage for those working in journalism.

Department of Homeland Security (DHS)

Washington, DC 20528
Operator number: 202–282–8000
Comment line: 202–282–8495
Website: http://www.dhs.gov/

DHS is ultimately responsible for ensuring that emergency response professionals are prepared for any situation. It deals with citizen preparedness, recovery, and assistance with regard to a terrorist event. The DHS established the National Response Plan (available at the website), a comprehensive all-hazard approach to enhance the ability of the United States to manage domestic incidents. The department offers grants for studies on terrorism and releases important information on weapon of mass destruction. Its website contains interesting links to articles and other government-related agencies.

E9-1-1 Institute

Gregory Rohde, Executive Director
Email: glr@e911institute.org
Telephone: 202–292–4603
Jamie Radice, Administrative Assistant
Email: jamie.radice@e911institute.org
Telephone: 202–292–4603

The E9-1-1 Institute was formed to support the congressional E9-1-1 caucus, as well as to promote public education on emergency communication issues. The congressional E9-1-1 caucus was created to increase awareness among lawmakers, constituents, and community members with regard to citizen-activated emergency response systems. The goals of the caucus include the following: (1) providing 911 emergency responders with a callback number and the location of the caller; (2) promoting the 911 system as the preferred public emergency resource; (3) promoting citizen-activated emergency response systems; (4) securing funding for 911 systems, operators, and networks; and (5) increasing awareness of emergency response issues among all levels of government. The E9-1-1 Institute provides a forum for discussion of policies related to emergency communications.

Emergency Medical Services (EMS) Magazine

Summer Communications, Inc.
7626 Densmore Ave.
Van Nuys, CA 91406–2042
Telephone: 800–224–4367; 818–786–4367
Fax: 818–786–9246
Website: http://www.emsresponder.com/publication/pub.jsp?pubId=1
Email: emsmag@earthlink.net; rtmag@earthlink.net

EMS magazine has compiled an online collection of its articles related to bioterrorism preparedness. Articles provide information on improving the delivery of prehospital emergency medical care and are directed toward paramedics, EMTs, administrators, and instructors working in private and public services.

Federal Emergency Management Agency (FEMA)

500 C Street SW
Washington, DC 20472
Telephone: 202–566–1600
Website: www.fema.gov
Email: FEMAOPA@dhs.gov

FEMA is a formerly independent agency that was incorporated into the U.S. Department of Homeland Security in 2003. It is responsible for preventing, planning for, responding to, and mitigating the consequences of disasters. FEMA teaches people how to respond to disasters, helps equip and prepare state and local emergency agencies, trains emergency personnel, and coordinates federal response to emergencies.

Fire Corps

1050 17th Street NW, Suite 490
Washington, DC 20036
Telephone: 202–887–4809
Fax: 202–887–5291
Website: http://www.firecorps.org/
The Fire Corps is managed through the National Volunteer Fire Council, the International Association of Fire Fighters, and the International Association of Fire Chiefs. It is funded through the U.S. Department of Homeland Security. Its functions include fire safety outreach, youth programs, administrative support, the provision of support to fire and rescue departments, and the promotion of citizen participation. The Fire Corps was created to assist fire and rescue departments that are constrained by limited resources.

Harvard Program in Refugee Trauma (HPRT)

Department of Psychiatry
Massachusetts General Hospital
22 Putnam Avenue
Cambridge, MA 02139
Telephone: 617–876–7879
Fax: 617–876–2360
Website: http://www.hprt-cambridge.org/Layer3
.asp?page_id=36
Email: rmollica@partners.org
The HPRT has focused on empirical research to improve the treatment of psychopathology in refugee populations and victims/survivors of disasters and terrorism. The site describes projects and research conducted by the HRPT and provides clinical guidelines, useful screening instruments, educational and training curricula for different constituency groups, policy descriptions, and humanistic survivor narrative material.

International Association of Emergency Managers (IAEM)

Beth Armstrong, Executive Director
201 Park Washington Court
Falls Church, VA 22046–4527
Telephone: 703–538–1795
Fax: 703–241–5603
Website: http://www.iaem.com/index.htm
Email: info@iaem.com
The IAEM is a nonprofit educational organization that seeks to save lives and protect property during emergencies and disasters. The association addresses issues such as terrorism preparedness, emergency preparation, and disaster assistance delivery and educates decision makers at the federal, state,

and local levels on the importance of emergency management services. Membership provides access to the top emergency management experts, as well as to a certification program in emergency management.

International Center on Responses to Catastrophes (ICORC)

1601 West Taylor Street, 5th floor
Chicago, IL 60612
Telephone: 312–355–5407
Fax: 312–996–7958
Website: www.ichrsc.org
Email: mpandey@psych.uic.edu
Established in 2002 at the University of Illinois–Chicago, ICORC promotes research and scholarships to study and improve services to people who have been affected by social catastrophes. Its primary activities focus on documentaries, ethnographic studies, and intervention.

Policy Institute for International Counter-Terrorism (ICT)

3811 N. Fairfax Drive, Suite 720
Arlington, VA 22203
Telephone: 703–797–4592
Fax: 703–797–4591
Website: http://www.ict.org.il/
Email: services@ict.org.il
The ICT is an Israeli research institute established in 1996 at the academic Interdisciplinary Center in Herzliya (IDC), which is committed to developing innovative public policy solutions to international terrorism. It also has an office in Washington, DC. The ICT takes an unconventional approach to policy research by combining academic knowledge and theory with practical field experience. News and articles, some of them related to the psychology of terrorism, are available at its website.

International Society for Traumatic Stress Studies (ISTSS)

60 Revere Drive, Suite 500
Northbrook, IL 60062
Telephone: 847–480–9028
Fax: 847–480–9282
Website: http://www.istss.org/
Email: istss@istss.org
The ISTSS, founded in 1985, is an organization that enables professionals to share information about the effects of trauma. It is involved in various activities, including publishing scientific research, consumer-oriented pamphlets, and treatment guidelines; developing worldwide networking and support systems; and promoting excellence in the field through training

and annual awards. The terrorism and trauma section of the website contains interesting and useful information and links.

International Trauma Studies Program (ITSP)

155 Avenue of the Americas, 4th Floor
New York, NY 10013
Telephone: 212–691–6499
Fax: 212–807–1809
Website: http://itspnyc.org
Email: trauma.studies@nyu.edu
The ITSP uses a multidisciplinary approach to the study, treatment, and prevention of trauma-related suffering. It was founded in 1998 as a collaboration of various departments of New York University (NYU), including the Department of Psychiatry, the Department of Applied Psychology, and the Center for War, Peace, and the News Media.

Johns Hopkins Center for Public Health Preparedness (CPHP)

615 N. Wolfe Street, Room WB030
Baltimore, MD 21205
Telephone: 443–287–6735
Fax: 443–287–6736
http://www.jhsph.edu/CPHP/index.html
Email: jsims@jhsph.edu
As part of the School of Public Health of Johns Hopkins University, the CPHP is charged with training public health providers and improving their ability to respond to terrorist-related incidents. It currently provides instruction and resources to public health professionals in Maryland, the District of Columbia, and Delaware.

Medical Reserve Corps (MRC)

Office of the Surgeon General
U.S. Department of Health and Human Services
5600 Fishers Lane, Room 18C-14
Rockville, MD 20857
Telephone: 301–443–4951
Fax: 301–480–1163
Website: http://www.medicalreservecorps.gov/
Email: MRCcontact@osophs.dhhs.gov
The MRC is composed of medical, public health, and other volunteers who work in coordination with existing local emergency response programs and community public health initiatives. Volunteers address public health needs and help their community during large-scale emergencies. Activities include outreach and prevention, provision of public health services during a crisis, assistance to emergency response teams, provision of health care to those with less serious injuries, immunization programs, blood drives, case management, and care planning.

Mercy Medical Airlift (MMA)

Box 1940
Manassas, VA 20108–0804
Telephone: 800–296–1191, ext. 2
703–296–1191, ext. 23
Fax: 703–257–1642
Patient Assistance Center:
4620 Haygood Road, Suite 1
Virginia Beach, VA 23455
Telephone: 888–675–1405
757–318–9175
Fax: 757–318–9107
Website:http://www.mercymedical.org/
Email: mercymedicalops@erols.com
The MMA is a nonprofit organization composed of volunteer pilots and office assistants who provide air transportation to those in need. Volunteer pilots work together with the Homeland Security Air Transportation System (HSATS) in times of emergency to transport priority cargo and emergency management personnel.

National Center for Injury Prevention and Control/Bioterrorism Preparedness and Response Planning

Mailstop K65
4770 Buford Highway NE
Atlanta, GA 30341–3724
Telephone: 770–488–1506
Clinician information line: 877–554–4625
Fax: 770–488–1667
Website: http://www.bt.cdc.gov/
Email: OHCINFO@cdc.gov
Mass trauma and bioterrorism preparedness and response are two of the emergency areas covered by the National Center for Disease Control and Prevention. It provides clinicians with real-time information and training opportunities to help prepare for and respond to terrorism and other emergency events.

National Center for Post-Traumatic Stress Disorder (PTSD)

Executive Division
VA Medical Center 116D
215 North Main St.
White River Junction, VT 05009
Telephone: 802–296–6300
Fax: 802–296–5135
Website: http://www.ncptsd.va.gov
Email: ptsd@dartmouth.edu
Created in 1989 within the Department of Veterans Affairs, the center addresses the needs of veterans with military-related posttraumatic stress disorder. Each of its six divisions (behavioral science, women's health science, clinical neuroscience, program evaluation,

clinic laboratory and evaluation, and Pacific Islander) deals with a different aspect of PTSD. The branches are located in different cities, but all are part of the VA Health Care System. The webpage (http://www.ncptsd .va.gov/about/divisions/index.html) provides a complete description of each division's specialty and relevant contact information. The website also offers information on how to deal with the aftereffects of terrorism.

National Center on the Psychology of Terrorism (NCPT)

795 Willow Road, Building 348
VA Palo Alto Health Care System
Menlo Park, CA 94025
Telephone/Fax: 650–618–0448
Website: http://www.terrorismpsychology.org/
Email: info@terrorismpsychology.org
The NCPT is dedicated to research, education and training, public policy, and community service to improve the ability to respond effectively to terrorism. A cornerstone initiative has been the establishment of a volunteer rapid-response medical reserve corps in Palo Alto, which has become a model for other communities in the United States.

National Memorial Institute for the Prevention of Terrorism (MIPT)

Box 889
621 North Robinson, 4th Floor
Oklahoma City, OK 73101
Telephone: 405-232-5121
Fax: 405-232-5132
Website: http://www.mipt.org/
The MIPT was established to help survivors and family members of the victims of the 1995 Murrah Federal Building bombing. The institute has several ongoing research projects that deal mainly with first responders. Even if psychological matters are addressed only tangentially, the website remains a good resource of information.

National Mental Health Information Center and Center for Mental Health Services

Box 42557
Washington, DC 20015
Telephone: 800–789–2647
Fax: 240-747-5470
Website: http://www.mentalhealth.samhsa.gov/
Through its various programs, this center, which is part of the Substance Abuse and Mental Health Administration of the U.S. Department of Health and Human Services, provides guidelines and tips to help adults, adolescents, children, families, teachers, and professionals to cope with traumatic events and manage the anxiety caused by disasters and terrorism. Of particular interest is the Disaster Technical Assistance Center (DTAC), which assists the states and territories with disaster response planning and supports collaboration between mental health and substance abuse authorities, federal agencies, and nongovernmental organizations. The website has a section in Spanish.

National Voluntary Organizations Active in Disaster (NVOAD)

Ande Miller, Executive Director
Box 151973
Alexandria, VA 22315
Telephone: 703–339–5596
Fax: 703–339–3316
Website: http://www.nvoad.org/
Email: amiller@nvoad.org
The NVOAD is a league of the major national voluntary organizations that concentrate on disaster-related activities. It provides year-round communication and coordination among these various agencies so that disaster response is provided efficiently and performed without duplication. Matters addressed by the various organizations include disaster prevention, response, recovery and mitigation, facilitation of volunteer response, and enhancement of response capabilities. Through these functions, numerous large agencies are able to work together in a collaborative and coordinated manner to ensure smooth disaster response.

Neighborhood Watch Program (NWP)

National Sheriff's Association
1450 Duke Street
Alexandria, VA 22314–3490
Telephone: 703–836–7827
Fax: 703–683–6541
Website: http://www.usaonwatch.org/
Email: info@usaonwatch.org
The NWP is administrated by the National Sheriffs' Association and is funded by the U.S. Department of Justice. In addition to crime prevention, disaster and emergency preparedness, and emergency response training, the NWP provides terrorism alertness training to citizen volunteers. Local officials, law enforcement, and citizens work together to ensure the safety and protection of their communities.

Operation HOPE, Inc. (OHI)

707 Wilshire Blvd., Suite 3030
Los Angeles, CA 90017
Telephone: 213-891-2900
Fax: 213-489-7511
Website: http://www.operationhope.org/
Email: corporate@operationHOPE.org

OHI is a nonprofit organization that was formed in the aftermath of September 11, 2001. It provides economic education to inner-city communities. HOPE Coalition America (HCA) is an initiative put forth by OHI to provide economic counseling to assist businesses, individuals, and families to prepare for and recover from disasters and emergencies.

Provincial Emergency Program (PEP) of British Columbia

Terrorism Consequence Management and Preparedness
Headquarters
455 Boleskine Road
Victoria, BC V8Z 1E7
Canada
Telephone: 250–952–4913
Mailing Address:
Box 9201 Stn. Prov. Govt.
Victoria, BC V8W 9J1
Canada
Website: http://www.pep.bc.ca/hazard_preparedness/terrorism_consequences.html
The PEP of British Columbia is a branch of the Ministry of Public Safety and Solicitor General of the Government of British Columbia. Its website provides information on the nature of terrorism, publications that describe different types of terrorism and disaster situations, emergency preparedness tips, instructions on creating a personal emergency plan, directions on steps to take in an emergency situation, and information on what to do following an emergency situation, including acts of terrorism. The agency provides brochures containing specific information about the different types of potential terrorist activities, including radiological, chemical, or biological attacks. The website also gives the current status of terrorism

alert levels, as well as links to other disaster resources in Canada.

ReadyAmerica

Department of Homeland Security
http://www.ready.gov/index.html
The ReadyAmerica website provides step-by-step instructions, as well as definitions and descriptions of the different types of homeland security threats. Citizens are instructed on how to prepare for biological, chemical, nuclear, radiological, explosive, and natural disasters.

Save a Life Foundation (SALF)

O'Hare Aerospace Center
9950 W. Lawrence Ave., Suite 300
Schiller Park, IL 60176–1216
Telephone: 847–928–9683
Fax: 847–928–9684
Website: http://www.salf.org/index.html
Email: estare@salf.org
Save a Life Foundation is a nonprofit organization that trains volunteers in the use of life-saving techniques such as cardiopulmonary resuscitation (CPR), the Heimlich maneuver, and automated external defibrillators (AEDs) in disaster and emergency situations.

Website for Weapons of Mass Destruction First Responders (WMDFR)

Website: www.WMDFR.com
Email: admin@wmdfr.com
WMDFR.com provides information, exercises, networking capabilities, planning information, and research aimed at assisting WMDFR in planning for and implementing an efficient response in the case of a biological, nuclear, chemical, radiological, or explosive terrorist attack, as well as decontamination procedures should an attack occur.

Glossary

Acculturate: to adopt the social and behavioral patterns of the surrounding culture

Acute stress disorder: a variation of posttraumatic stress disorder that includes symptoms of anxiety and significant impairment in at least one essential area of functioning

Adaptation: a general term for any process whereby behavior or subjective experience alters to fit in with a changed environment or circumstances or in response to social pressure

Agency: a business or service authorized to act for others

Alcohol abuse: excessive use of alcohol and alcoholic drinks

American Red Cross: (also known as Red Cross or the International Red Cross) a comprehensive designation used for all or one of the components of the International Red Cross and Red Crescent Movement, a worldwide organization active in humanitarian work. This organization has three components: the International Committee of the Red Cross (ICRC), which acts primarily as a neutral intermediary during armed conflict and includes the Guardian of the Geneva Conventions, an advocate for the protection of war vic-

tims; the League of the Red Cross and Red Crescent Societies (LRCS), an international federation of the national societies that is active in nonconflict disasters and natural calamities; and the National Red Cross or Red Crescent Society, a worldwide relief organization.

Amygdala: an almond-shaped neural structure involved in producing and responding to nonverbal signs of anger, avoidance, defensiveness, and fear

Analgesic: any drug or substance that induces the absence of a pain sensation

Anterior cingulate: the anterior cingulated cortex plays a role in a wide variety of autonomic functions, such as regulating heart rate and blood pressure. It is vital to cognitive functions such as reward anticipation, decision making, empathy, and emotion.

Anthrax: a serious disease caused by *Bacillus anthracis*, a bacterium that forms spores. There are three types of anthrax (skin, lungs, digestive) that can be used as a weapon. This happened in the United States in 2001, when anthrax was deliberately spread through the postal system by sending letters with powder containing anthrax.

Apollonian: in Nietzschean philosophy, of or embodying the power of critical reason as opposed to the creative-intuitive

Appraisal: a classification of someone or something with respect to the worth of the person or thing

Assimilate: to absorb (immigrants or a culturally distinct group) into the prevailing culture

Asymmetric war: a state of open, armed, often prolonged conflict carried on between nations, states, or parties utilizing asymmetric approaches that generally seek a major psychological impact, such as shock or confusion, which affects an opponent's initiative, freedom of action, or will

Atherosclerosis: a disease affecting arterial blood vessels and veins that have been surgically moved to function as arteries

Atropine reactions: allergic reactions (e.g., dry mouth, tachycardia, blurred vision, palpitations, difficulty swallowing, and death due to respiratory failure) following the injection of atropine, a premedication for anesthesia that decreases bronchial and salivary secretions

Autonomic reactivity: any behavior executed without one's conscious awareness or control

Aversive conditioning: a learning process designed to modify undesirable or antisocial habits or addictions by creating a strong association with a disagreeable or painful stimulus

Barriers to care/treatment: obstacles that a person may encounter when seeking care (e.g., cultural differences, language difficulties, rural areas without specialists, lack of insurance)

Biological pathogen: an infectious agent that can create disease in its host

Botulinum bacillus: bacteria that cause three types of botulism or a severe, sometimes fatal, food poisoning brought on by ingestion of food containing botulin and characterized by nausea, vomiting, disturbed vision, muscular weakness, and fatigue

Casus belli: an event used to justify starting a war

Catecholamine: a chemical compound derived from the amino acid tyrosine; acts as a hormone or neurotransmitter

Cause: a basis for an action or response

CBR device: a chemical, biological, or radiological instrument or apparatus used for a specific act of violence or terrorism

CBRN attack: a chemical, biological, radiological, or nuclear overt, aggressive action

Cognitive behavioral theory: an approach to psychotherapy that involves the extension of the modification and relearning procedures to cognitive processes such as imagery, fantasy, thought, and self-image

Cognitive restructuring: a therapy whose emphasis is on learning to recognize and then change or restructure thought processes, reframing thoughts in less stressful terms

Cohesion: a tendency to stick together or be united either physically or logically. The term may be used in reference to social groups, educational concepts, items in learning tasks, and so on.

Compassion fatigue: a state of tension and preoccupation with individual or cumulative trauma as manifested in one or more ways including reexperiencing a traumatic event, avoidance or numbing of reminders of the event, and persistent arousal. This often occurs among doctors, nurses, EMS personnel, police, firefighters, victim advocates, and many others.

Comrade: one who shares another person's interests or activities; a friend or companion

Constituency: the body of citizens who elect a representative for their area

Coordination: a systematic exchange of information among principal participants in order to carry out a unified response in the event of an emergency

Coping skills training: conscious, rational strategies designed to deal with the anxieties of life

Critical incident stress debriefing (CISD): a term that refers to the "Mitchell model," a seven-phase, structured group discussion, usually held 1 to 10 days after a crisis. It is designed to mitigate acute symptoms, assess the need for follow-up, and, if possible, provide a sense of postcrisis psychological closure.

Critical incident stress management (CISM): a comprehensive, integrative, multicomponent crisis intervention system

Cross-cultural issues: matters that may arise as a result of evaluating cultures according to different cultural dimensions; comparison of various practices in different cultural settings

Cult: a religion or religious sect generally considered to be extremist or false. Its followers often live in an unconventional manner under the guidance of an authoritarian, charismatic leader.

Depersonalization: a sense of disconnection from one's body and feelings (e.g., observing oneself act but feeling as if one is not actually taking part) (see **derealization**)

Derealization: the feeling that things in one's surroundings are strange, unreal, or somehow altered

Dionysian: in Nietzschean philosophy, of or displaying creative-intuitive power as opposed to critical-rational power

Disaster categories: accidents such as plane crashes, criminal acts such as terrorist bombings, and natural catastrophes such as earthquakes

Dissipation: breaking up and scattering; dispersion

Distributive justice: perceptions of the fairness of a particular outcome

Education: knowledge or skill obtained or developed by a learning process

Epidemiology: the study of the distribution and determinants of disease in human populations and the application of this study to the control of health problems

Eschatological: regarding the ultimate destiny of humankind and the world

Ethnicity: a quality or affiliation resulting from racial or cultural ties

Etiology: the branch of medicine that deals with the causes or origins of disease

Evidence-based treatment: specific clinical practices that help bridge the gaps between what researchers find to be effective treatment and what is implemented at the practice level

Exposure: condition of being subjected to an action or an influence

Extinction: reduction of or loss in the strength or rate of a conditioned response when an unconditioned stimulus or reinforcement is withheld

Fatwa: in Islam, a legal pronouncement on a specific matter issued by a religious law specialist

GABA: short for gamma-aminobutyric acid, the most important and abundant inhibitory neurotransmitter in the brain. GABA helps induce relaxation and sleep and balances excitation in the brain with inhibition.

General systems theory: an interdisciplinary field that studies relationships of systems as a whole

Glucocorticoids/cortisol: a class of steroid hormones characterized by an ability to bind with the corticol receptor and supportive of a variety of important cardiovascular, metabolic, immunologic, and homeostatic functions

Glutamatergic functioning: the support of a variety of important cardiovascular, metabolic, immunologic, and homeostatic functions

Grief: deep mental anguish, such as that arising from bereavement

Group dynamics: the driving forces that result from the interaction of individual behaviors. These may differ depending on individuals' current or prospective connections to a sociological group. Urges to belong to or identify with a particular group may make for distinctly different attitudes (recognized or unrecognized), and a group's influence may quickly increase, influencing or overwhelming individual proclivities and actions.

Group intervention: an orchestrated attempt by family and friends to persuade a family member to seek help for an addiction or other similar problem

Habituation: the process of becoming accustomed to something

Hegemony: the predominant influence (as of a state, region, or group) over others

Help seeking: acquiring support or assistance

Heuristics: a trial-and-error procedure or rule of thumb for making a decision, forming a judgment, or solving a problem

Hippocampus: a part of the brain's limbic system; plays a part in memory and navigation

HPA (hypothalamic-pituitary-adrenal) axis: the classical neuroendocrine system that responds to stress and whose final product, corticosteroids, targets components of the limbic system, particularly the hippocampus

Hypervigilance: watchfulness that is over and above what is normal or reasonable

Iatrogenic: of or pertaining to a disorder or symptom inadvertently caused by a physician's treatment or management of a patient

Identity: one's sense of self

Immunosuppression: the medical suppression of the immune system. This is usually done to prevent the body from rejecting a transplanted organ.

In vivo exposure: subjection to a harmful action or condition as a result of biological processes or experiments that occur in living organisms

Individual intervention: a conscious attempt by a person to get help for an addiction or similar problem

Indoctrination: instruction that seeks to persuade someone to accept a body of principles presented for unconditional acceptance or uncritical belief

Inhibitory mechanisms: characteristics of habitual adaptive responses of neurons that restrain other responses from firing

Insurgency: an instance of rebellion

Interactional justice: the nondiscriminatory implementation, by organizational agents, of procedures for treating people respectfully and explaining decisions adequately

Interobjectivity: mutual judgment based on observable phenomena and uninfluenced by emotions or personal prejudices

Intifada: an Arabic term for "uprising" that came into common usage in English as the popularized name for two Palestinian campaigns, the First Intifada (1987) and the Al-Aqsa Intifada (2000)

Isomorphic: having similar appearance but genetically different

Justice as a basic need: a powerful human motive that may be a necessity for human survival

Learned helplessness: a human condition in which apathy and submission prevail, causing an individual to rely fully on others for help. People in a state of learned helplessness view problems as personal (they view themselves as the problem), pervasive (they see the problem as affecting all aspects of life), or permanent (they see the problem as unchangeable).

Lessons learned: knowledge derived from the implementation and evaluation of a program that can be used to identify strengths and weaknesses of program design and implementation

Lexicon: an alphabetic listing of the words of a language; vocabulary

Mass psychogenic illness (MPI): a feeling of sickness within a group of people (such as a class in a school or workers in an office) who start feeling unwell at the same time even though no physical or environmental reason exists for ill health

Mass violence: an intentional violent criminal act that results in physical, emotional, or psychological injury to a large number of people

Myocardial infarction: sudden interruption of or insufficiency in the supply of blood to the heart, typically resulting from obstruction of a coronary artery and often characterized by severe chest pain (also known as a heart attack)

National Voluntary Organizations Active in Disaster: an organization that coordinates the relief efforts of many voluntary organizations engaged in disaster response

Nietzschean: a philosophy developed by German philosopher Friedrich Wilhelm Nietzsche that argues that the ideal human would be able to channel passions creatively instead of suppressing them

Not-for-profit: an incorporated organization that exists for educational or charitable reasons and whose shareholders and trustees do not benefit financially

Ongoing threat: a constant danger

Opiate receptors: a specialized neural cell that is responsive to or activated by a group of chemical substances that contain opium and tends to have a narcotic effect

Pathogenic: capable of causing disease

Peritraumatic: characteristic of serious injury or shock to the body around the time of an act of violence or an accident

Peritraumatic dissociation: immediate dissociation at the time of a traumatic event; occasionally develops into posttraumatic stress disorder

Pneumonic plague: a frequently fatal form of bubonic plague in which the lungs are infected and the disease is transmissible by coughing

Polemics: the branch of Christian theology devoted to the refutation of errors

Post hoc: after the fact

Posttraumatic: following or resulting from injury or trauma

Posttraumatic growth: improvement and development of people after experiencing traumatic circumstances (e.g., more intimate, emotionally open relationships with others; the recognition of new possibilities for one's life path; a more profound appreciation for what life has to offer; an enhanced sense of personal strength; religious or spiritual development)

Posttraumatic stress disorder (PTSD): a psychiatric disorder that can occur following the direct experiencing or witnessing of life-threatening events such as military combat, natural disasters, terrorist incidents, serious accidents, or violent personal assaults such as rape. People who suffer from PTSD often relive the experience through nightmares and flashbacks, have difficulty sleeping, and feel detached or estranged. These symptoms can be severe enough and last long enough to significantly impair the person's daily life.

Premorbid: the state of mind prior to the onset of physical disease or emotional illness

Prevalence rates: the number of cases of a disease or disorder within a specified population at a point in time

Procedural justice: a process by which fair and equitable decisions are made

Prophylaxis: prevention of or protective treatment for disease

Protective factors: characteristics, variables, and/ or conditions present in individuals or groups that enhance resilience, increase resistance to risk, and fortify against the development of a disorder or an adverse outcome. Examples are constitutional factors such as attractiveness or an engaging personality and bonding to family, school, and some other social institution.

Psychoeducation: education in a subject area that fosters treatment and rehabilitation. It involves teaching people about their problem, how to treat it, and how to recognize signs of relapse so that they can get necessary treatment before the difficulty worsens or reoccurs.

Psychogenic: originating in the mind or in mental or emotional processes; having a psychological rather than a physiological origin

Psychological adaptive capacity: the emotional and mental ability to function, adjust, and cope with issues that may be distressing

Psychological attenuation: the mental and emotional ability to reduce the force, effect, or value of something

Psychological debriefing: a single-session, semistructured crisis intervention designed to reduce and prevent unwanted psychological aftereffects of traumatic events by promoting emotional processing through the ventilation and normalization of reactions and preparation for possible future experiences

Psychological first aid: pragmatically oriented interventions with survivors or emergency responders targeting acute stress reactions and immediate needs. The goals of psychological first aid include the establishment of safety (objective and subjective), stress-related symptom reduction, restoration of rest and sleep, linkage to critical resources, and connection to social support

Psychological hardiness: resistance to stress, anxiety, and depression

Psychological trauma: a traumatic event that overwhelms an individual's perceived ability to cope and leaves that person fearing death, annihilation, mutilation, or psychosis. The individual feels emotionally, cognitively, and physically overcome. The triggering event commonly includes abuse of power, betrayal of trust, entrapment, helplessness, pain, confusion, and/or loss.

Psychometrics or psychometry: the branch of psychology that deals with the design, administration, and interpretation of quantitative tests for the measurement of psychological variables such as intelligence, aptitude, and personality traits

Psychopathology: (a) the study of mental illness or mental distress; (b) the manifestation of behaviors and experiences that may be indicative of mental illness or psychological impairment; (c) the name of an academic journal that specializes in the understanding and classification of mental illness in clinical psychiatry

Psychosomatic: relating to certain organic disorders such as hypertension that are believed to be caused by psychological factors such as stress

Qualitative: relating to or involving comparisons based on qualities

Quantitative: relating to or involving the measurement of quantity or amount

Race: a population of humans distinguished from other populations. The most widely used racial categories are based on visible traits (especially skin color and facial features)

Randomized control trials (RCTs): a research protocol for testing the effectiveness of a drug or other type of treatment, in which research participants are assigned randomly to either treatment and control or placebo

Reaction phases: stages in a particular pattern or course of response following an initiating event

Region-beta paradox: a general phenomenon in which intense hedonic states trigger psychological processes that are designed to attenuate them; thus, intense states may abate more quickly than mild states. Because people are unaware of these psychological processes, they may mistakenly expect intense states to last longer than mild ones. In Study 1, participants predicted that the more they initially disliked a transgressor, the longer their dislike would last. In Study 2, participants predicted that their dislike for a transgressor who hurt them a lot would last longer than their dislike for a transgressor who hurt them a little, but precisely the opposite was the case. In Study 3, participants predicted that their dislike for a transgressor who hurt them a lot would last longer than their dislike for a transgressor who hurt someone else a lot, but precisely the opposite was the case. These errors of prediction are instances of the region-beta paradox.

Relational Frame Theory: an approach designed to provide a pragmatic analysis of complex human language and cognitions that can be traced back to a single psychological process

Relief organization: an association that exists solely to give aid to a cause (e.g., disaster areas, homelessness, hunger)

Resilience: the ability to cope with stress and catastrophe

Retributive violence: physical force exerted for the purpose of violating, damaging, or abusing and given as repayment; an act of retaliation

Risk factor: a variable associated with an increased risk of disease, infection, or other illness

Role stereotypy: characteristic and expected social behavior illustrated by a high degree of stereotyped behavior and movement

Schema: a mental set or representation

Screening: examination of a great number of something (e.g., people) for the purpose of identifying those with a particular problem or feature

Secondary prevention: action aimed at mitigating the health consequences of disasters (e.g., the use of carbon monoxide detectors when operating gasoline-powered generators after the loss of electric power, employing appropriate occupant behavior in multistory structures during earthquakes, and building "safe rooms" in dwellings located in tornado-prone areas); may be instituted when disasters are imminent

Sensitization: the process of becoming highly sensitive, usually with the implication that one is not uniformly sensitive to all stimuli but only to specific events or situations

Sequela (plural sequelae): a secondary consequence or result; aftereffect

Serotonergic receptor: a specialized neural cell that is responsive to or activated by serotonin and that reliably undergoes a particular pattern of change

Sicarii: dagger bearers; members of a band of violent nationalists prepared to carry out assassination and murder in a campaign to set Palestine free

Skin conductance test: an assessment that measures changes in the skin's conductivity of a weak electrical current

Slippery slope: an argument for the likelihood of one event, given another. Invoking the "slippery slope" means arguing that one action will initiate a chain of events that will lead to a (generally undesirable) event later.

Social support: a network of family, friends, colleagues, and other acquaintances that one can turn to, whether in times of crisis or simply for fun and entertainment

Somatic cues: bodily sensations a person experiences in response to a stimulus

Steeling effect: the dialectic between over- and underprotection in development

Stepped care: a process in which people are assigned to different levels of treatment based on personal characteristics

Stress inoculation: a term for the development of anxiety-reducing techniques that can be accessed whenever needed. The goal of stress inoculation is to develop a procedure that will allow one to remain calm.

Subsyndromal: characterized by or exhibiting symptoms that are not severe enough for diagnosis as a clinically recognized syndrome

Syllogism: deductive reasoning in which a conclusion is derived from two premises

Symmetric war: a state of open, armed, often prolonged conflict carried on between nations, states, or parties utilizing similar tactics that then imply predictability

Symptom threshold: the lowest intensity at which a stimulus evokes a response; an initial subjective indication of a disorder reported by an afflicted person

Tachycardia: abnormally rapid beating of the heart, defined as a resting heart rate of more than 100 beats per minute

Technology: aspects of a culture involving the application of the findings, procedures, and principles of the systematic identification and solution of problems

Terrorism: the unlawful use of force and violence against people or property to intimidate or coerce some entity (e.g., a government or population) in the furtherance of political or social objectives

Theodicy: the branch of theology that defends God's goodness and justice in the face of the existence of evil

Thriving: making steady progress; prospering; flourishing

Thyombolytic therapy: use of a drug that breaks up or dissolves blood clots, which are the main cause of both heart attacks and stroke

Toxic exposure: subjection to chemicals or substances that are capable of causing injury or death

Trajectory of recovery: the course of returning to a normal state

Trauma: an emotional or psychological injury, usually resulting from an extremely stressful and life-threatening situation

Traumatic grief: distress and intense sorrow in response to the loss (caused by some direct external force) of someone or something to which one is strongly attached

Triage: a system used by medical or emergency personnel to ration limited medical resources when the number of injured needing care exceeds the resources available; permits the treatment of the greatest possible number of patients

Vector control: any method to limit or eradicate the mechanisms that transmit genes or diseases to one's offspring

Vicarious traumatization: see compassion fatigue

Worried well: a term applied to people who exhibit psychogenic symptoms of a disease when they are at low or no risk

Index

Boldface numbers indicate tables and figures.